Recent Advances
in Retinal Degeneration

Advances in Experimental Medicine and Biology

Recent Volumes in this Series

VOLUME 606   BIOACTIVE COMPONENTS OF MILK
              Edited by Zsuzsanna Bősze

VOLUME 607   EUKARYOTIC MEMBRANES AND CYTOSKELETON: ORIGINS AND
              EVOLUTION
              Edited by Gáspár Jékely

VOLUME 608   BREAST CANCER CHEMOSENSITIVITY
              Edited by Dihua Yu and Mien-Chie Hung

VOLUME 609   HOT TOPICS IN INFECTION AND IMMUNITY IN CHILDREN IV
              Edited by Adam Finn and Andrew J. Pollard

VOLUME 610   TARGET THERAPIES IN CANCER
              Edited by Francesco Colotta and Alberto Mantovani

VOLUME 611   PETIDES FOR YOUTH
              Edited by Susan Del Valle, Emanuel Escher, and William D. Lubell

VOLUME 612   RELAXIN AND RELATED PETIDES
              Edited by Alexander I. Agoulnik

VOLUME 613   RECENT ADVANCES IN RETINAL DEGENERATION
              Edited by Robert E. Anderson, Matthew M. LaVail, and Joe G. Hollyfield

A Continuation Order Plan is available for this series. A continuation order will bring delivery of each new volume immediately upon publication. Volumes are billed only upon actual shipment. For further information please contact the publisher.

Robert E. Anderson · Matthew M. LaVail
Joe G. Hollyfield
Editors

Recent Advances in Retinal Degeneration

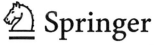 Springer

Editors

Robert E. Anderson
Dean A. McGee Eye Institute
University of Oklahoma Health Science Ctr.
608 Stanton L. Young Blvd., DMEI 409
Oklahoma City, OK 73104 USA
robert-anderson@ouhsc.edu

Matthew M. LaVail
Beckman Vision Center
UCSF School of Medicine
10 Kirkham Street
San Francisco, CA 94143 USA
matthew.lavail@ucsf.edu

Joe G. Hollyfield
Cole Eye Institute
The Cleveland Clinic Foundation
9500 Euclid Ave. (i31)
Cleveland, OH 44195
hollyfj@ccf.org

ISBN: 978-0-387-74902-0   e-ISBN: 978-0-387-74904-4

Library of Congress Control Number: 2007936186

Printed on acid-free paper

9 8 7 6 5 4 3 2 1

springer.com

Dedication

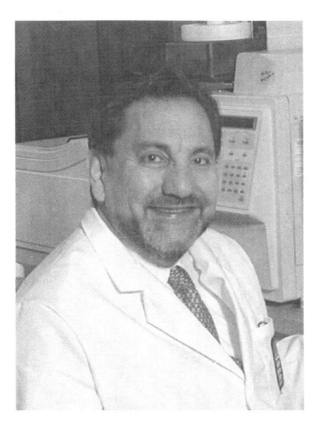

Nicolas G. Bazan, M.D., Ph.D.

Nicolas Bazan is a man of great talent and energy who has overcome many obstacles to achieve the tremendous success he now enjoys in retinal research. We are honored to dedicate this proceedings volume to him.

Preface

A Symposium on Retinal Degenerations has been held in conjunction with the biennial International Congress of Eye Research (ICER) since 1984. These Retinal Degeneration Symposia have allowed scientists and clinicians from around the world to convene and present their new research findings. The Symposia have been organized to allow sufficient time for discussions and one-on-one interactions in a relaxed atmosphere, where international friendships and collaborations would be fostered.

The XII International Symposium on Retinal Degeneration (also known as RD2006) was held from October 23–28, 2006 in San Carlos de Bariloche, Argentina. The meeting brought together 130 scientists, retinal specialists in ophthalmology and trainees in the field from all parts of the world. In the course of the meeting, 49 platform and 54 poster presentations were given, and a majority of these are presented in this proceedings volume. New discoveries and state of the art findings from most research areas in the field of retinal degenerations were presented. The RD2006 meeting was highlighted by three special lectures. The first was given by Dr. Ruben Adler, Johns Hopkins University Medical School, Baltimore, Maryland, USA. Dr. Adler discussed the hope, reality, and challenges of using stem cells to treat blinding diseases. The second was given by Prof. Pierluige Nicotera. Prof. Nicotera is a leading authority on apoptosis and presented an outstanding lecture on his latest exciting research. The last special lecture was given by Prof. Eliot Berson, Harvard Medical School, Cambridge, MA, who gave an illuminating and informative overview of his work on vitamin A and omega-3 fatty acids in treatment of retinitis pigmentosa.

The Symposium received international financial support from a number of organizations. We are particularly pleased to thank The Foundation Fighting Blindness, Owings Mills, Maryland, for its continuing support of this and the previous biennial Symposia, without which we could not have held these important meetings. In addition, for the third time, the National Eye Institute of the National Institutes of Health contributed to the meeting. We are also grateful to Dr. Konstantin Petrukhin for a travel award from Merck & Co., Inc. – USA. Funds from these organizations allowed us to provide 26 Travel Awards to young investigators and trainees working in the field of retinal degenerations. The response to the Travel Awards program was extraordinary, with 58 applicants competing for the 26 Awards.

We also acknowledge the diligent and outstanding efforts of Ms. Holly White-side, who carried out most of the administrative aspects of the RD2006 Symposium, designed and maintained the meeting website, and organized and edited the production of this volume. Holly is the Administrative Manager of Dr. Anderson's laboratory at the University of Oklahoma Health Sciences Center, and she has become the permanent Coordinator for the Retinal Degeneration Symposia. Her dedicated efforts with the Symposia since RD2000 have provided continuity heretofore not available, and we are deeply indebted to her.

We thank Ms. Maria Rosa Adamo of Zafiro Viajes, who provided extraordinary effort in arranging the travel and local program. Thanks also go to Kluwer Academic/Plenum Publishers for its publication.

Finally, we give our heart-felt thanks to our dear friend and colleague, Nicolas Bazan, for his help in every step of the organization and execution of this endeavor. He provided extraordinary input, from the selection of the meeting venue to the procurement of the wine that all of us enjoyed. He also gave an outstanding lecture. We are delighted to dedicate this volume to him.

Robert E. Anderson
Matthew M. LaVail
Joe G. Hollyfield

Travel Awards

We gratefully acknowledge the Foundation Fighting Blindness, National Eye Institute, and Merck Pharmaceuticals, Inc. for their generous support of 26 travel fellowships to attend this meeting. The travel awardees are listed below. Each awardee submitted a chapter to this proceedings volume and is identified by an asterisk in the Table of Contents.

John Alexander
William Beltran
D. Joshua Cameron
Dibyendu Chakraborty
Junping Chen
Tanja Diemer
Michael Elliott
Marina Gorbatyuk
Abigail Hackam
Takao Hashimoto
Yogita Kanan
Sukanya Karan
Linda Köhn
Adam Kundzewicz
Yun Le
Ann Morris
Gerardo Paez
Brian Raisler
Alison Reynolds
Tonia Rex
Mehrnoosh Saghizadeh
Ruifang Sui
Markus Thiersch
Ana Vanesa Torbidoni
Yumiko Umino
Vidyullatha Vasireddy

Contents

Contributors xvii

Part I   Keynote Lectures

Curing Blindness with Stem Cells: Hope, Reality, and Challenges   3
Ruben Adler

Retinal Degenerations: Planning for the Future 21
Eliot L. Berson

Part II   Neuroprotection

Neurotrophins Induce Neuroprotective Signaling in the Retinal Pigment
Epithelial Cell by Activating the Synthesis of the Anti-inflammatory and
Anti-apoptotic Neuroprotectin D1 39
Nicolas G. Bazan

On the Role of CNTF as a Potential Therapy for Retinal Degeneration:
Dr. Jekyll or Mr. Hyde? 45
William A. Beltran*

Nanoceria Particles Prevent ROI-Induced Blindness 53
Junping Chen*, Swanand Patil, Sudipta Seal, and James F. McGinnis

An in-vivo Assay to Identify Compounds Protective Against Light
Induced Apoptosis 61
Yogita Kanan*, Anne Kasus-Jacobi, Kjell Sawyer, David S. Mannel, Joyce
Tombran Tink, and Muayyad R. Al-Ubaidi

Role of BCL-XL in Photoreceptor Survival 69
Yun-Zheng Le*, Lixin Zheng, Yuwei Le, Edmund B. Rucker III,
and Robert E. Anderson

**The Hypoxic Transcriptome of the Retina: Identification of Factors with
Potential Neuroprotective Activity** 75
Markus Thiersch*, Wolfgang Raffelsberger, Enrico Frigg, Marijana
Samardzija, Patricia Blank, Olivier Poch, and Christian Grimm

Part III   Gene Therapy and Neuroprotection

**Lentiviral Gene Transfer-Mediated Cone Vision Restoration in RPE65
Knockout Mice** 89
Alexis-Pierre Bemelmans, Corinne Kostic, Maité Cachafeiro, Sylvain
V. Crippa, Dana Wanner, Meriem Tekaya, Andreas Wenzel, and
Yvan Arsenijevic

**In vitro Analysis of Ribozyme-mediated Knockdown of an ADRP
Associated Rhodopsin Mutation** 97
Dibyendu Chakraborty*, Patrick Whalen, Alfred S. Lewin, and
Muna I. Naash

Gene Therapy for Mouse Models of ADRP 107
Marina S. Gorbatyuk*, William W. Hauswirth, and Alfred S. Lewin

**Development of Viral Vectors with Optimal Transgene Expression for
Ocular Gene Therapies** 113
Takao Hashimoto*

Adeno-Associated Viral Vectors and the Retina 121
John J. Alexander* and William W. Hauswirth

**Genetic Supplementation of RDS Alleviates a Loss-of-function
Phenotype in C214S Model of Retinitis Pigmentosa** 129
May Nour, Steven J. Fliesler, and Muna I. Naash

**Morphological Aspects Related to Long-term Functional Improvement
of the Retina in the 4 Years Following rAAV-mediated Gene
Transfer in the RPE65 Null Mutation Dog** 139
Kristina Narfström, Mathias Seeliger, Chooi-May Lai, Vaegan, Martin Katz,
Elizabeth P. Rakoczy, and Charlotte Remé

Virus-mediated Gene Delivery to Neuronal Progenitors 147
Tonia S. Rex*

Part IV   Animal Models of Retinal Degeneration

Loss of Visual and Retinal Function in Light-stressed Mice 157
Drew Everhart, Ana Stachowiak, Yumiko Umino*, and Robert Barlow

ERG Responses and Microarray Analysis of Gene Expression in a Multifactorial Murine Model of Age-Related Retinal Degeneration 165
Goldis Malek, Jeffery A. Jamison, Brian Mace, Patrick Sullivan, and Catherine Bowes Rickman

Oxygen Supply and Retinal Function: Insights from a Transgenic Animal Model 171
Edda Fahl, Max Gassmann, Christian Grimm, and Mathias W. Seeliger

Characterization of Gene Expression Profiles of Normal Canine Retina and Brain Using a Retinal cDNA Microarray 179
Gerardo L. Paez*, Barbara Zangerl, Kimberly Sellers, Gregory M. Acland, and Gustavo D. Aguirre

Toward a Higher Fidelity Model of AMD 185
Brian J. Raisler*, Miho Nozaki, Judit Baffi, William W. Hauswirth, and Jayakrishna Ambati

The Potential of Ambient Light Restriction to Restore Function to the Degenerating P23H-3 Rat Retina 193
Krisztina Valter, Diana K. Kirk, and Jonathan Stone

Part V Molecular Genetics and Candidate Genes

Mutations in Known Genes Account for 58% of Autosomal Dominant Retinitis Pigmentosa (adRP) 203
Stephen P. Daiger, Lori S. Sullivan, Anisa I. Gire, David G. Birch, John R. Heckenlively, and Sara J. Bowne

Genetics of Age-related Macular Degeneration 211
Albert O. Edwards

Retinal Phenotype of an X-Linked Pseudo-usher Syndrome in Association with the G173R Mutation in the RPGR Gene 221
Alessandro Iannaccone, Mohammad I. Othman, April D. Cantrell, Barbara J. Jennings, Kari Branham, and Anand Swaroop

Mutation in the PYK2-Binding Domain of PITPNM3 Causes Autosomal Dominant Cone Dystrophy (CORD5) in Two Swedish Families 229
Linda Köhn*, Konstantin Kadzhaev, Marie S. I. Burstedt, Susann Haraldsson, Ola Sandgren, and Irina Golovleva

Identification and Characterization of Genes Expressed in Cone Photoreceptors 235
Mehrnoosh Saghizadeh*, Novrouz B. Akhmedov, and Debora B. Farber

Clinical and Genetic Characterization of a Chinese Family with CSNB1 .. 245
Ruifang Sui*, Fengrong Li, Jialiang Zhao, and Ruxin Jiang

**10q26 Is Associated with Increased Risk of Age-Related Macular
Degeneration in the Utah Population** 253
D. Joshua Cameron*, Zhenglin Yang, Zhongzhong Tong, Yu Zhao, Alissa
Praggastis, Eric Brinton, Jennifer Harmon, Yali Chen, Erik Pearson, Paul S.
Bernstein, Gregory Brinton, Xi Li, Adam Jorgensen, Sara Schneider, Daniel
Gibbs, Haoyu Chen, Changguan Wang, Kimberly Howes, Nicola J. Camp,
and Kang Zhang

**Part VI   Diagnostic, Clinical, Cytopathological and Physiologic Aspects of
Retinal Degeneration**

**Carboxyethylpyrrole Adducts, Age-related Macular Degeneration and
Neovascularization** 261
Kutralanathan Renganathan, Quteba Ebrahem, Amit Vasanji, Xiaorong Gu,
Liang Lu, Jonathan Sears, Robert G. Salomon, Bela Anand-Apte, and John
W. Crabb

**A Possible Impaired Signaling Mechanism in Human Retinal Pigment
Epithelial Cells from Patients with Macular Degeneration** 269
Piyush C. Kothary and Monte A. Del Monte

**Expression and Cell Compartmentalization of EFEMP1, a Protein
Associated with *Malattia Leventinese*** 277
Adam Kundzewicz*, Francis Munier, and Jean-Marc Matter

Role of ELOVL4 in Fatty Acid Metabolism 283
Vidyullatha Vasireddy*, Majchrzak Sharon, Norman Salem, Jr, and Radha
Ayyagari

**Organization and Molecular Interactions of Retinoschisin in
Photoreceptors** 291
Camasamudram Vijayasarathy, Yuichiro Takada, Yong Zeng,
Ronald A. Bush, and Paul A. Sieving

Part VII   Basic Science Underlying Retinal Degeneration

Proteomics Profiling of the Cone Photoreceptor Cell Line, 661W 301
Muayyad R. Al-Ubaidi, Hiroyuki Matsumoto, Sadamu Kurono,
and Anil Singh

γ-Secretase Regulates VEGFR-1 Signalling in Vascular Endothelium
and RPE 313
Michael E. Boulton, Jun Cai, Maria B. Grant, and Yadan Zhang

Analysis of the Rate of Disk Membrane Digestion by Cultured
RPE Cells 321
Tanja Diemer*, Daniel Gibbs, and David S. Williams

Functional Expression of Cone Cyclic Nucleotide-Gated Channel in
Cone Photoreceptor-Derived 661W Cells 327
J. Browning Fitzgerald, Anna P. Malykhina, Muayyad R. Al-Ubaidi,
and Xi-Qin Ding

Phosphorylation of Caveolin-1 in Bovine Rod Outer Segments in vitro
by an Endogenous Tyrosine Kinase 335
Michael H. Elliott* and Abboud J. Ghalayini

Regulation of Neurotrophin Expression and Activity in the Retina 343
Abigail S. Hackam*

Involvement of Guanylate Cyclases in Transport of Photoreceptor
Peripheral Membrane Proteins 351
Sukanya Karan*, Jeanne M. Frederick and Wolfgang Baehr

Rod Progenitor Cells in the Mature Zebrafish Retina 361
Ann C. Morris*, Tamera Scholz, and James M. Fadool

αvβ5 Integrin Receptors at the Apical Surface of the RPE: One
Receptor, Two Functions 369
Emeline F. Nandrot, Yongen Chang, and Silvia C. Finnemann

Implantation of Mouse Eyes with a Subretinal Microphotodiode Array ... 377
Machelle T. Pardue, Tiffany A. Walker, Amanda E. Faulkner, Moon K. Kim,
Christopher M. Bonner, and George Y. McLean

Variation in the Electroretinogram of C57BL/6 Substrains of Mouse 383
Alison L. Reynolds*, G. Jane Farrar, Pete Humphries, and Paul F. Kenna

A2E, A Pigment of RPE Lipofuscin, is Generated from the Precursor,
A2PE by a Lysosomal Enzyme Activity 393
Janet R. Sparrow, So Ra Kim, Ana M. Cuervo and Urmi Bandhyopadhyayand

Endothelin Receptors: Do They Have a Role in Retinal Degeneration? ... 399
Vanesa Torbidoni*, María Iribarne, and Angela M. Suburo

**CNTF Negatively Regulates the Phototransduction Machinery
in Rod Photoreceptors: Implication for Light-Induced Photostasis
Plasticity** 407
Rong Wen, Ying Song, Yun Liu, Yiwen Li, Lian Zhao, and Alan M. Laties

About the Editors 415

Index 419

Contributors

Gregory M. Acland

Baker Institute, Cornell University, Hungerford Hill Road, Ithaca, NY 14853

Ruben Adler

The Johns Hopkins University School of Medicine, Baltimore, Maryland, 410-955-7589, 410-955-0749
radler@jhmi.edu

Gustavo D. Aguirre

Department of Clinical Studies Philadelphia, School of Veterinary Medicine, University of Pennsylvania Philadelphia, PA 19104

Novrouz B. Akhmedov

Jules Stein Eye Institute, David Geffen School of Medicine and Molecular Biology Institute, UCLA, Los Angeles, California 90095

John J. Alexander

Department of Molecular Genetics & Microbiology, University of Florida College of Medicine, Gainesville, FL 32610-0266, USA

Muayyad R. Al-Ubaidi

Department of Cell Biology, University of Oklahoma Health Sciences Center, 940 Stanton L. Young Blvd. (BMSB781), Oklahoma City, OK 73104, USA, 405-271-2382, 405-271-3548
muayyad-al-ubaidi@ouhsc.edu

Jayakrishna Ambati

Department of Ophthalmology, University of Kentucky, Lexington, Kentucky, 40356

Bela Anand-Apte

Cole Eye Institute, Lerner Research Institute, Cleveland Clinic Foundation, Cleveland, Ohio

Robert E. Anderson

Cell Biology; Dean A. McGee Eye Institute, Oklahoma City, OK; Ophthalmology, University of Oklahoma Health Sciences Center, Oklahoma City, OK

Yvan Arsenijevic

Unit of Gene Therapy and Stem Cells Biology, Hôpital Ophtalmique Jules-Gonin, Lausanne, Switzerland, 41 21 626 82 60, 41 21 626 88 88
yvan.arsenijevic@ophtal.vd.ch

Radha Ayyagari

Ophthalmology and Visual Sciences, W. K. Kellogg Eye Center, University of Michigan, Ann Arbor

Wolfgang Baehr

John A. Moran Eye Center, University of Utah, Salt Lake City, UT 84132, USA

Judit Baffi

Department of Ophthalmology, University of Kentucky, Lexington, Kentucky, 40356

Urmi Bandhyopadhyayand

Department of Anatomy and Structural Biology, Albert Einstein College of Medicine, Bronx, New York, 10461

Robert Barlow

Center for Vision Research, Department of Ophthalmology, Upstate Medical University, 750 East Adams Street, Syracuse, NY 13210, USA

Nicolas G. Bazan

Louisiana State University Health Sciences Center, Neuroscience Center of Excellence and Department of Ophthalmology, 2020 Gravier Street, Suite D, New Orleans, LA 70112, USA, 504 599 0832, 504 568 5801
nbazan@lsuhsc.edu

William A. Beltran

Section of Ophthalmology, Department of Clinical Studies, School of Veterinary Medicine, University of Pennsylvania, Philadelphia, PA, 19104, USA, 1 215 898 4913, 1 215 573 2162
wbeltran@vet.upenn.edu

Alexis-Pierre Bemelmans

Unit of Gene Therapy and Stem Cells Biology, Hôpital Ophtalmique Jules-Gonin, Lausanne, Switzerland

Paul S. Bernstein
Department of Ophthalmology and Visual Sciences, Moran Eye Center and Program in Human Molecular Biology and Genetics, University of Utah School of Medicine, Salt Lake City, UT 84132, USA

Eliot L. Berson
Berman-Gund Laboratory for the Study of Retinal Degenerations, Harvard Medical School, Massachusetts Eye and Ear Infirmary, 243 Charles Street, Boston, MA 02114, USA, 617-573-3600, 617-573-3216
linda_berard@meei.harvard.edu

David G. Birch
Anderson Research Center, Retina Foundation of the Southwest, Dallas, TX, USA

Patricia Blank
Lab for Retinal Cell Biology, Dept Ophthalmology, CIHP, University of Zurich, Switzerland

Christopher M. Bonner
Optobionics, Corp, Naperville, IL 60563

Michael E. Boulton
Ophthalmology and Visual Sciences, University of Texas Medical Branch, Galveston, Texas 77550, 409-747-5410, 409-747-5402
boultonm@utmb.edu

Sara J. Bowne
Human Genetics Center, School of Public Health, The University of Texas, Houston, TX, USA

Kari Branham
Kellogg Eye Center, Department of Ophthalmology and Visual Sciences, University of Michigan, 1000 Wall Street, Ann Arbor, MI 48105, USA

Eric Brinton
Department of Ophthalmology and Visual Sciences, Moran Eye Center and Program in Human Molecular Biology and Genetics, Department of Oncological Sciences, Huntsman Cancer Institute and Department of Pediatrics, Division of Hematology/Oncology, University of Utah School of Medicine, Salt Lake City, UT 84132, USA

Marie S. I. Burstedt
Department of Clinical Sciences, Ophthalmology, Umeå University, S-901 85, Umeå, Sweden

Ronald A. Bush
Section for Translational Research in Retinal and Macular Degeneration, National Institute on Deafness and other Communication Disorders, National Institutes of Health, Bethesda, MD 20892, USA

Maité Cachafeiro
Unit of Gene Therapy and Stem Cells Biology, Hôpital Ophtalmique Jules-Gonin, Lausanne, Switzerland

Jun Cai
Ophthalmology and Visual Sciences, University of Texas Medical Branch, Galveston, Texas 77550

D. Joshua Cameron
Department of Ophthalmology and Visual Sciences, Moran Eye Center and Program in Human Molecular Biology and Genetics, University of Utah School of Medicine, Salt Lake City, UT 84132, USA, 801-363-2433
joshua.cameron@utah.edu

Nicola J. Camp
Department of Ophthalmology and Visual Sciences, Moran Eye Center and Program in Human Molecular Biology and Genetics, University of Utah School of Medicine, Salt Lake City, UT 84132, USA

April D. Cantrell
Hamilton Eye Institute, Department of Ophthalmology, University of Tennessee Health Science Center, 930 Madison Avenue, Suite 731, Memphis, TN 38163, USA

Dibyendu Chakraborty
Department of Cell Biology, University of Oklahoma Health Sciences Center, 940 Stanton L. Young Blvd. (BMSB781), Oklahoma City, OK 73104, USA, 405-271-2402, 405-271-3548
dchakrab@ouhsc.edu

Yongen Chang
Margaret M. Dyson Vision Research Institute, Department of Ophthalmology, Weill Medical College of Cornell University, Box 233, 1300 York Avenue, New York, NY10021, USA

Haoyu Chen
Department of Ophthalmology and Visual Sciences, Moran Eye Center and Program in Human Molecular Biology and Genetics, University of Utah School of Medicine, Salt Lake City, UT 84132, USA

Junping Chen
Oklahoma Center for Neuroscience; Dean A. McGee Eye Institute, University of Oklahoma Health Sciences Center, Oklahoma City, OK 73104, USA

Yali Chen
Department of Ophthalmology and Visual Sciences, Moran Eye Center and Program in Human Molecular Biology and Genetics, University of Utah School of Medicine, Salt Lake City, UT 84132, USA

John W. Crabb
Cole Eye Institute; Lerner Research Institute, Cleveland Clinic Foundation;
Department of Chemistry, Case Western Reserve University, Cleveland, Ohio,
216-445-0425, 216-445-3670
crabbj@ccf.org

Sylvain V. Crippa
Unit of Gene Therapy and Stem Cells Biology, Hôpital Ophtalmique Jules-Gonin,
Lausanne, Switzerland

Ana M. Cuervo
Department of Anatomy and Structural Biology, Albert Einstein College of
Medicine, Bronx, New York, 10461

Stephen P. Daiger
Human Genetics Center, School of Public Health; Department of Ophthalmology,
The Univ. of Texas, Houston, TX, USA, 713-500-9829, 713-500-0900
stephen.p.daiger@uth.tmc.edu

Tanja Diemer
Departments of Pharmacology and Neurosciences, UCSD School of Medicine, La
Jolla, California, 92093-0983, USA, 858-534-9550, 858-822-6950
tdiemer@ucsd.edu

Xi-Qin Ding
Departments of Cell Biology, University of Oklahoma Health Sciences Center, 940
Stanton L. Young Blvd., Oklahoma City, OK 73104, USA, 405-271-8001 x47959,
405-271-3548
xi-qin-ding@ouhsc.edu

Quteba Ebrahem
Cole Eye Institute, Case Western Reserve University, Cleveland, Ohio

Albert O. Edwards
Mayo Clinic, Department of Ophthalmology, 200 First Street, SW, Rochester, MN
55905. Supported by the NEI, FFB, and RPB, (507) 284-2787, (507) 284-4612
edwards.albert@mayo.edu

Michael H. Elliott
Department of Ophthalmology, University of Oklahoma Health Sciences Center;
Dean A. McGee Eye Institute, Oklahoma City, OK 73104, USA, 405-271-8316,
405-271-8128
michael-elliott@ouhsc.edu

Drew Everhart
Center for Vision Research, Department of Ophthalmology, Upstate Medical
University, 750 East Adams Street, Syracuse, NY 13210, USA, 315-464-7773,
315-464-8750
everhard@upstate.edu

James M. Fadool
Department of Biological Science, Florida State University, Tallahassee, FL 32306

Edda Fahl
Ocular Neurodegeneration Research Group, Centre for Ophthalmology, Institute
for Ophthalmic Research, Tuebingen, Germany D-72076, 49-7071-298-7784,
49-7071-29-4503
edda.fahl@med.uni-tuebingen.de

Debora B. Farber
Jules Stein Eye Institute, David Geffen School of Medicine and Molecular Biology
Institute, UCLA, Los Angeles, California 90095

G. Jane Farrar
Ocular Genetics Unit, Smurfit Institute of Genetics, Trinity College Dublin, Ireland

Amanda E. Faulkner
Rehab R&D, Atlanta VA Medical Center, Decatur, GA 30033, USA

Silvia C. Finnemann
Margaret M. Dyson Vision Research Institute, Department of Ophthalmology;
Department of Cell and Developmental Biology, and Department of Physiology
and Biophysics, Weill Medical College of Cornell University, Box 233, 1300 York
Avenue, New York, NY 10021, USA

J. Browning Fitzgerald
Departments of Cell Biology, University of Oklahoma Health Sciences Center, 940
Stanton L. Young Blvd., Oklahoma City, OK 73104, USA

Steven J. Fliesler
Ophthalmology and Pharmacological & Physiological Science, Saint Louis
University School of Medicine, St. Louis, MO, 63104, USA

Jeanne M. Frederick
John A. Moran Eye Center, University of Utah, Salt Lake City, UT 84132, USA

Enrico Frigg
Lab for Retinal Cell Biology, Dept Ophthalmology, CIHP, University of Zurich,
Switzerland

Max Gassmann
Institute of Veterinary Physiology, University Eye Hospital, Zurich, Switzerland,
CH-8057

Abboud J. Ghalayini
Medical University of the Americas, Nevis, West Indies

Daniel Gibbs
Department of Ophthalmology and Visual Sciences, Moran Eye Center and Program
in Human Molecular Biology and Genetics, Departments of Pharmacology and
Neurosciences, UCSD School of Medicine, La Jolla, California, 92093-0983, USA;
University of Utah School of Medicine, Salt Lake City, UT 84132, USA

Anisa I. Gire
Human Genetics Center, School of Public Health, The University of Texas, Houston, TX, USA

Irina Golovleva
Medical and Clinical Genetics, Department of Medical Biosciences, Umeå University, S-901 85 Umeå, Sweden, 46 907856820, 46 90 128163
Irina.Golovleva@vll.se

Marina S. Gorbatyuk
Department of Molecular Genetics and Microbiology, University of Florida College of Medicine, Gainesville, FL 32610-0266, USA, 1 352-392-0673, 1 352-392-3233
mari653@mgm.ufl.edu

Maria B. Grant
Pharmacology and Therapeutics, University of Florida, Gainesville, FL 32618

Christian Grimm
Lab for Retinal Cell Biology, Department of Ophthalmology, CIHP, University of Zurich, Switzerland; Lab for Retinal Cell Biology, University Eye Hospital, Zurich, CH-8091

Xiaorong Gu
Cole Eye Institute, Case Western Reserve University, Cleveland, Ohio

Abigail S. Hackam
Bascom Palmer Eye Institute, University of Miami Miller School of Medicine, 1638 NW 10th Ave., Miami, FL 33136, 305-547-3723, 305-547-3658
ahackam@med.miami.edu

Susann Haraldsson
Medical and Clinical Genetics, Department of Medical Biosciences, Umeå University, S-901 85 Umeå, Sweden

Jennifer Harmon
Department of Ophthalmology and Visual Sciences, Moran Eye Center and Program in Human Molecular Biology and Genetics, University of Utah School of Medicine, Salt Lake City, UT 84132, USA

Takao Hashimoto
Jules Stein Eye Institute, University of California Los Angeles, CA 90095, USA, 310-825-6992, 425-660-6923
takao17.hashimoto@nifty.com; gbf00573@nifty.com

William W. Hauswirth
Departments of Ophthalmology and Molecular Genetics & Microbiology, University of Florida College of Medicine, Gainesville, FL 32610-0284, USA
hauswrth@eye1.eye.ufl.edu

John R. Heckenlively
Kellogg Eye Center, University of Michigan, Ann Arbor, MI, USA

Kimberly Howes
Department of Ophthalmology and Visual Sciences, Moran Eye Center and
Program in Human Molecular Biology and Genetics, University of Utah School of
Medicine, Salt Lake City, UT 84132, USA

Pete Humphries
Ocular Genetics Unit, Smurfit Institute of Genetics, Trinity College Dublin,
Ireland

Alessandro Iannaccone
Hamilton Eye Institute, Department of Ophthalmology, University of Tennessee
Health Science Center, 930 Madison Avenue, Suite 731, Memphis, TN 38163,
USA, 901-448-7831, 901-448-5028
aiannacc@utmem.edu

María Iribarne
Facultad de Ciencias Biomédicas, Universidad Austral, Pilar B1629AHJ, Buenos
Aires, Argentina
atorbidoni@cas.austral.edu.ar

Anne Kasus-Jacobi
Department of Ophthalmology, Dean McGee Eye Institute, 608 Stanton l. Young
Blvd., Oklahoma City, OK 73104, USA

Jeffery A. Jamison
Retina Discovery Unit, Alcon Research, Ft. Worth, Texas

Barbara J. Jennings
Hamilton Eye Institute, Department of Ophthalmology, University of Tennessee
Health Science Center, 930 Madison Avenue, Suite 731, Memphis, TN 38163,
USA

Ruxin Jiang
Department of Ophthalmology, Peking Union Medical College Hospital, Beijing
100730, China

Konstantin Kadzhaev
Medical and Clinical Genetics, Department of Medical Biosciences, Umeå
University, S-901 85 Umeå, Sweden

Yogita Kanan
Department of Cell Biology, University of Oklahoma Health Sciences Center, 940
Stanton L. Young Blvd. (BMSB781), Oklahoma City, OK 73104, USA
ykanan@ouhsc.edu

Sukanya Karan
John A. Moran Eye Center, University of Utah, Salt Lake City, UT 84132,
801-585-7621, 801-585-7686
sukanyat15@yahoo.com

Martin Katz

Mason Eye Institute, University of Missouri-Columbia, Columbia, MO, USA

Paul F. Kenna

Ocular Genetics Unit, Smurfit Institute of Genetics, Trinity College Dublin, Ireland

Moon K. Kim

Rehab R&D, Atlanta VA Medical Center, Decatur, GA 30033, USA

Diana K. Kirk

CNS Stability and Degeneration Group and ARC Centre of Excellence in Vision Science, Research School of Biological Sciences, The Australian National University

Linda Köhn

Medical and Clinical Genetics, Department of Medical Biosciences, Umeå University, S-901 85 Umeå, Sweden

Corinne Kostic

Unit of Gene Therapy and Stem Cells Biology, Hôpital Ophtalmique Jules-Gonin, Lausanne, Switzerland

Piyush C. Kothary

Kellogg Eye Center, University of Michigan, Ann Arbor, MI 48105-0714, 734-936-9254, 734-647-0228
kotha@umich.edu

Adam Kundzewicz

Department of Ophthalmology, School of Medicine, University of Geneva, 22 Rue Alcide Jentzer, 1211 Geneva 14, Switzerland, 41763472742, 41216268888
Adam.Kundzewicz@unil.ch

Sadamu Kurono

Department of Biochemistry and Molecular Biology, University of Oklahoma Health Sciences Center, 940 Stanton L. Young Blvd. (BMSB781), Oklahoma City, OK 73104

Current address: IBERICA Holdings Co., Ltd, Kurume University Translational Research Center, Kurume, Fukuoka 830-0011, Japan

Chooi-May Lai

Lions Eye Institute, Centre for Ophthalmology and Visual Science, University of Western Australia, Perth, Australia

Alan M. Laties
Department of Ophthalmology, University of Pennsylvania, School of Medicine;
Philadelphia, PA 19104

Yun-Zheng Le
Departments of Medicine; Cell Biology; Dean A. McGee Eye Institute, Oklahoma
City, OK, USA, 405-271-1087, 405-271-8128
yun-le@ouhsc.edu

Yuwei Le
Dean A. McGee Eye Institute, Oklahoma City, OK; Ophthalmology, University of
Oklahoma Health Sciences Center

Alfred S. Lewin
Departments of Molecular Genetics and the Center for Vision Science, University
of Florida, Gainesville, FL 32610, USA; Department of Molecular Genetics
and Microbiology, University of Florida College of Medicine, Gainesville, FL
32610-0266, USA

Fengrong Li
Department of Ophthalmology, Peking Union Medical College Hospital, Beijing
100730, China

Xi Li
Department of Ophthalmology and Visual Sciences, Moran Eye Center and
Program in Human Molecular Biology and Genetics, University of Utah School of
Medicine, Salt Lake City, UT 84132, USA

Yiwen Li
Department of Ophthalmology, University of Pennsylvania, School of Medicine;
Philadelphia, PA 19104

Yun Liu
Department of Ophthalmology, University of Pennsylvania, School of Medicine;
Philadelphia, PA 19104

Liang Lu
Department of Chemistry, Case Western Reserve University, Cleveland, Ohio

Brian Mace
Department of Neurology, Duke University, Durham, North Carolina

Goldis Malek
Department of Ophthalmology, Duke University, Durham NC, USA
gmalek@duke.edu

Anna P. Malykhina
Physiology, University of Oklahoma Health Sciences Center, 940 Stanton L. Young
Blvd., Oklahoma City, OK 73104, USA

David S. Mannel

Department of Ophthalmology, Dean McGee Eye Institute, 608 Stanton l. Young Blvd., Oklahoma City, OK 73104, USA

Jean-Marc Matter

Department of Ophthalmology, School of Medicine, University of Geneva, 22 Rue Alcide Jentzer, 1211 Geneva 14, Switzerland

Hiroyuki Matsumoto

Department of Biochemistry and Molecular Biology, University of Oklahoma Health Sciences Center, 940 Stanton L. Young Blvd. (BMSB781), Oklahoma City, OK 73104

Current address: IBERICA Holdings Co., Ltd, Kurume University Translational Research Center, Kurume, Fukuoka 830-0011, Japan

James F. McGinnis

Oklahoma Center for Neuroscience, Dean A. McGee Eye Institute, Department of Cell Biology, Department of Ophthalmology, University of Oklahoma Health Sciences Center, Oklahoma City, OK 73104, USA, 405-271-3695, 405-271-3721 james-mcginnis@ouhsc.edu

George Y. McLean

Optobionics, Corp, Naperville, IL 60563

Monte A. Del Monte

Kellogg Eye Center, University of Michigan, Ann Arbor, MI 48105-0714

Ann C. Morris

Department of Biological Science, Florida State University, Tallahassee, FL, 32306, 850-644-5420, 850-644-0989 amorris@bio.fsu.edu

Francis Munier

Eye Hospital Jules Gonin, 15 Avenue de France, 1004 Lausanne, Switzerland

Muna I. Naash

Department of Cell Biology, University of Oklahoma Health Sciences Center, 940 Stanton L. Young Blvd. (BMSB781), Oklahoma City, OK 73104, USA muna-naash@ouhsc.edu

Emeline F. Nandrot

Margaret M. Dyson Vision Research Institute, Department of Ophthalmology, Weill Medical College of Cornell University, Box 233, 1300 York Avenue, New York, NY 10021, USA, 212-746-2327, 212-746-8101 efn2001@med.cornell.edu

Kristina Narfström

Department of Veterinary Medicine and Surgery, College of Veterinary
Medicine and Department of Ophthalmology, Mason Eye Institute, University of
Missouri-Columbia, Columbia, MO, USA, 573-882-2095, 573-884-5444
narfstromk@missouri.edu

May Nour

Cell Biology, University of Oklahoma Health Sciences Center, 940 Stanton L.
Young Blvd., Oklahoma City, OK 73104, USA

Miho Nozaki

Department of Ophthalmology, University of Kentucky, Lexington, Kentucky,
40356

Mohammad I. Othman

Kellogg Eye Center, Department of Ophthalmology and Visual Sciences, University
of Michigan, 1000 Wall Street, Ann Arbor, MI 48105, USA

Gerardo L. Paez

Department of Clinical Studies Philadelphia, School of Veterinary Medicine,
University of Pennsylvania Philadelphia. PA 19104, 215-898-7479, 215-573-2162
gpaez@vet.upenn.edu

Machelle T. Pardue

Rehab R&D, Atlanta VA Medical Center, Decatur, GA 30033, USA; Department
of Ophthalmology, Emory University, Atlanta GA 30322, USA, 404-321-6111 x
7342, 404-728-4847
mpardue@emory.edu

Swanand Patil

Surface Engineering and Nanotechnology Facility, Advanced Materials Processing
Analysis Center, Nanoscience and Technology Center, University of Central
Florida, 4000 Central Florida Blvd. Orlando, Fl 32816, USA

Erik Pearson

Department of Ophthalmology and Visual Sciences, Moran Eye Center and
Program in Human Molecular Biology and Genetics, University of Utah School of
Medicine, Salt Lake City, UT 84132, USA

Olivier Poch

Laboratoire de BioInformatique et Génomique Intégrative (IGBMC), Strasbourg,
France

Alissa Praggastis

Department of Ophthalmology and Visual Sciences, Moran Eye Center and
Program in Human Molecular Biology and Genetics, University of Utah School of
Medicine, Salt Lake City, UT 84132, USA

Wolfgang Raffelsberger
Laboratoire de BioInformatique et Génomique Intégrative (IGBMC), Strasbourg, France

Brian J. Raisler
Department of Ophthalmology, University of Kentucky, Lexington, Kentucky, 40356
raisler@uky.edu

Elizabeth P. Rakoczy
Lions Eye Institute, Centre for Ophthalmology and Visual Science, University of Western Australia, Perth, Australia

Charlotte Remé
Department of Ophthalmology, University of Zürich, Switzerland

Kutralanathan Renganathan
Cole Eye Institute, Department of Chemistry, Case Western Reserve University, Cleveland, Ohio

Tonia S. Rex
University of Pennsylvania, 422 Curie Blvd., 3e10 Stellar-Chance Labs, Philadelphia, PA 19104, USA, 215-898-0163, 215-573-8083
trex@mail.med.upenn.edu

Alison L. Reynolds
Ocular Genetics Unit, Smurfit Institute of Genetics, Trinity College Dublin, Ireland, 353 1 608 2482, 353 1 608 3848
alison.reynolds@tcd.ie

Catherine Bowes Rickman
Department of Ophthalmology, Department of Cell Biology, Duke University, Durham, North Carolina, 919-668-0648, 919-684-3687
bowes007@duke.edu

Edmund B. Rucker III
Department of Veterinary Physiology and Pharmacology, Texas A&M University, College Station, TX

Mehrnoosh Saghizadeh
Jules Stein Eye Institute, David Geffen School of Medicine and Molecular Biology Institute, UCLA, Los Angeles, California 90095, 310-206-6935, 818-986-7400
nooshs@ucla.edu

Norman Salem, Jr
Laboratory of Membrane Biochemistry and Biophysics, NIAAA, National Institutes of Health, Bethesda, MD

Robert G. Salomon
Department of Chemistry, Case Western Reserve University, Cleveland, Ohio

Marijana Samardzija
Lab for Retinal Cell Biology, Department of Ophthalmology, CIHP, University of
Zurich, Switzerland

Ola Sandgren
Department of Clinical Sciences, Ophthalmology, Umeå University, S-901 85,
Umeå, Sweden

Sara Schneider
Department of Ophthalmology and Visual Sciences, Moran Eye Center and
Program in Human Molecular Biology and Genetics, University of Utah School of
Medicine, Salt Lake City, UT 84132, USA

Tamera Scholz
Department of Biological Science, Florida State University, Tallahassee, FL, 32306

Sudipta Seal
Surface Engineering and Nanotechnology Facility, Advanced Materials Processing
Analysis Center, Nanoscience and Technology Center, University of Central
Florida, 4000 Central Florida Blvd. Orlando, Fl 32816, USA

Jonathan Sears
Cole Eye Institute, Case Western Reserve University, Cleveland, Ohio

Mathias W. Seeliger
Retinal Diagnostics Research Group, Department of Ophthalmology II, University
of Tübingen, Germany

Kimberly Sellers
Department of Mathematics, Georgetown University, Washington, DC

Majchrzak Sharon
Laboratory of Membrane Biochemistry and Biophysics, NIAAA, National
Institutes of Health, Bethesda, MD

Paul A. Sieving
National Eye Institute; National Institutes of Health, Bethesda, MD 20892, USA

Anil Singh
Department of Biochemistry and Molecular Biology, University of Oklahoma
Health Sciences Center, 940 Stanton L. Young Blvd. (BMSB781), Oklahoma City,
OK 73104.

Ying Song
Department of Ophthalmology, University of Pennsylvania, School of Medicine;
Philadelphia, PA 19104

Janet R. Sparrow
Departments of Ophthalmology; Pathology and Cell Biology, Columbia University,
New York, NY 10032, 212-305-9944, 212-305-9638
jrs88@columbia.edu

Ana Stachowiak
Institute for Sensory Research, Syracuse University, Syracuse, New York 13210, USA

Jonathan Stone
CNS Stability and Degeneration Group and ARC Centre of Excellence in Vision Science, Research School of Biological Sciences, The Australian National University

Angela M. Suburo
Facultad de Ciencias Biomédicas, Universidad Austral, Pilar B1629AHJ, Buenos Aires, Argentina
atorbidoni@cas.austral.edu.ar

Ruifang Sui
Department of Ophthalmology, Peking Union Medical College Hospital, Beijing 100730, China, 86-1065296358, 86-1065296565
hrfsui@yahoo.com

Lori S. Sullivan
Human Genetics Center, School of Public Health, The University of Texas, Houston, TX, USA

Patrick Sullivan
Department of Neurology, Duke University, Durham, North Carolina

Anand Swaroop
Kellogg Eye Center, Department of Ophthalmology and Visual Sciences, University of Michigan, 1000 Wall Street, Ann Arbor, MI 48105, USA

Yuichiro Takada
Section for Translational Research in Retinal and Macular Degeneration, National Institute on Deafness and other Communication Disorders; National Institutes of Health, Bethesda, MD 20892, USA

Meriem Tekaya
Unit of Gene Therapy and Stem Cells Biology, Hôpital Ophtalmique Jules-Gonin, Lausanne, Switzerland

Markus Thiersch
Lab for Retinal Cell Biology, Dept Ophthalmology, CIHP, University of Zurich, Switzerland, 0041 44 2553719, 0041 44 255 4385
markus.thiersch@usz.ch

Joyce Tombran Tink
Department of Ophthalmology and Visual Science, Yale University School of Medicine, New Haven, CT 06520

Zhongzhong Tong
Department of Ophthalmology and Visual Sciences, Moran Eye Center and
Program in Human Molecular Biology and Genetics, University of Utah School of
Medicine, Salt Lake City, UT 84132, USA

Vanesa Torbidoni
Facultad de Ciencias Biomédicas, Universidad Austral, Pilar B1629AHJ, Buenos
Aires, Argentina, 54-2322-482959, 54-2322-482205
atorbidoni@cas.austral.edu.ar

Yumiko Umino
Center for Vision Research, Department of Ophthalmology, Upstate Medical
University, 750 East Adams Street, Syracuse, NY 13210, USA

Vaegan
School of Optometry, University of New South Wales, Australia

Krisztina Valter
CNS Stability and Degeneration Group and ARC Centre of Excellence in Vision
Science, Research School of Biological Sciences, The Australian National
University, 02 6125 1095, 02 6125 0758
valter@rsbs.anu.edu.au

Amit Vasanji
Lerner Research Institute, Cleveland Clinic Foundation, Case Western Reserve
University, Cleveland, Ohio

Vidyullatha Vasireddy
Ophthalmology and Visual Sciences, W. K. Kellogg Eye Center, University of
Michigan, Ann Arbor, 734-647-6330, 734-936-7231
vasired@umich.edu

Camasamudram Vijayasarathy
Section for Translational Research in Retinal and Macular Degeneration, National
Institute on Deafness and other Communication Disorders, National Institutes of
Health, Bethesda, MD 20892, USA
camasamudramv@nidcd.nih.gov

Tiffany A. Walker
Rehab R&D, Atlanta VA Medical Center, Decatur, GA 30033, USA

Changguan Wang
Department of Ophthalmology and Visual Sciences, Moran Eye Center and
Program in Human Molecular Biology and Genetics, University of Utah School of
Medicine, Salt Lake City, UT 84132, USA

Dana Wanner
Unit of Gene Therapy and Stem Cells Biology, Hôpital Ophtalmique Jules-Gonin,
Lausanne, Switzerland

Rong Wen

Department of Ophthalmology, University of Pennsylvania, School of Medicine; Philadelphia, PA 19104, 215-746-0207, 215-746-0209
rwen@mail.med.upenn.edu

Andreas Wenzel

Laboratory for Retinal Cell Biology, Dept. of Ophthalmology, University of Zürich, Zürich, Switzerland

Patrick Whalen

Departments of Molecular Genetics and the Center for Vision Science, University of Florida, Gainesville, FL 32610, USA

David S. Williams

Departments of Pharmacology and Neurosciences, UCSD School of Medicine, La Jolla, California, 92093-0983, USA

Zhenglin Yang

Department of Ophthalmology and Visual Sciences, Moran Eye Center and Program in Human Molecular Biology and Genetics, University of Utah School of Medicine, Salt Lake City, UT 84132, USA

Barbara Zangerl

Department of Clinical Studies Philadelphia, School of Veterinary Medicine, University of Pennsylvania Philadelphia. PA 19104

Yong Zeng

Section for Translational Research in Retinal and Macular Degeneration, National Institute on Deafness and other Communication Disorders; National Institutes of Health, Bethesda, MD 20892, USA

Kang Zhang

Department of Ophthalmology and Visual Sciences, Moran Eye Center and Program in Human Molecular Biology and Genetics, University of Utah School of Medicine, Salt Lake City, UT 84132, USA

Yadan Zhang

Optometry and Vision Sciences, Cardiff University, Cardiff, Wales, UK

Jialiang Zhao
Department of Ophthalmology, Peking Union Medical College Hospital, Beijing 100730, China

Lian Zhao
Department of Ophthalmology, University of Pennsylvania, School of Medicine, Philadelphia, PA 19104

Yu Zhao
Department of Ophthalmology and Visual Sciences, Moran Eye Center and Program in Human Molecular Biology and Genetics, University of Utah School of Medicine, Salt Lake City, UT 84132, USA

Lixin Zheng
Dean A. McGee Eye Institute, Ophthalmology, University of Oklahoma Health Sciences Center, 608 Stanton L. Young Blvd., DMEI 409, Oklahoma City, OK 73104

Part I
Keynote Lectures

Curing Blindness with Stem Cells: Hope, Reality, and Challenges

Ruben Adler

This article is a summary of a presentation at the XII International Symposium on Retinal Degeneration in Bariloche, Argentina, in October of 2006, in which the author presented his personal views of the contributions that the study of retinal cell differentiation during normal embryonic development can make towards overcoming the limitations that have so far prevented curing blindness through stem cell transplantation. The talk was illustrated mainly with examples derived from research on retinal cell differentiation in the author's laboratory, and the same approach will be kept in this article; for a broader coverage of the field, the reader is referred to several comprehensive reviews, e.g., (Adler, 2000; Boulton and Albon, 2004; Galli-Resta, 2001; Hatakeyama and Kageyama, 2004; Jean et al., 1998; Livesey and Cepko, 2001; Lupo et al., 2000; Malicki, 2004; Marquardt and Gruss, 2002; Rapaport et al., 2004; Vetter and Brown, 2001; Zhang et al., 2002).

1 Introduction

The death of photoreceptor cells causes visual loss, and eventually blindness, in diseases such as age-related macular degeneration and retinitis pigmentosa, for which currently there is no cure. Stem cell transplantation has emerged as a potential strategy to restore vision in patients affected by these diseases; for this treatment to be effective, the transplanted stem cells would have to differentiate into rod and cone photoreceptors, which would then become synaptically connected with the appropriate cells of the host retina. Despite some promising observations in experimental animals, anatomical and functional stem cell-based restoration of the retina has not been accomplished (e.g., (Ahmad et al., 2004; Banin et al., 2006; Boulton and Albon, 2004; Canola et al., 2007; Chacko et al., 2000; Das et al., 2005; Haruta, 2005; Haynes and Del Rio-Tsonis, 2004; Klassen et al., 2004;

R. Adler
The Johns Hopkins University School of Medicine, Baltimore, Maryland, Tel: 410-955-7589, Fax: 410-955-1749
e-mail: radler@jhmi.edu

R.E. Anderson et al. (eds.), *Recent Advances in Retinal Degeneration,*
© Springer 2008

3

Limb et al., 2006; Meyer et al., 2005; Meyer et al., 2006; Qiu et al., 2005; Suzuki et al., 2006; Takahashi et al., 1998; Warfvinge et al., 2006; Young, 2005), among others). The challenge, then, is to find treatments that would "make stem cells do what we want them to do"; this would require substantial progress in three separate, but closely interrelated areas: (1) how to get "perfect" stem cells; (2) how to induce stem cells to differentiate into rod and cone photoreceptors; and (3) how to induce transplanted stem cells to form synapses with cells in the host retina.

2 How to Get "Perfect" Stem Cells

2.1 What are "Stem Cells"?

Stem cells are cells that (i) can self-renew (i.e., replicate and give rise to new stem cells), and (ii) under appropriate conditions will stop dividing and give rise to two or more (or all) of the specialized cell types of the body. As discussed in some detail below, the *developmental potential* of stem cells is an issue of great practical relevance, since it becomes progressively restricted during embryonic development and will influence what the cells do when transplanted into a patient. The fertilized egg is *totipotent*, since it can give rise to all the cell types in the body as well as to the fetal components of the placenta. The cells in the inner mass of the blastocyst (from which the so called "embryonic stem cells" are derived) are *pluripotent,* that is to say, they can give rise to all the cell types of the body, but not to those of the placenta. The stem cells found in developing organs at later embryonic stages and in the adult are *multipotent* because they can give rise to two or more, but not to all the cell types of the body (these cells are sometimes referred to as "progenitors", rather than as "stem cells"). Considerable excitement was triggered by experiments suggesting that, despite their restricted developmental potential, adult stem cells retained a considerable degree of plasticity, and could be "re-programmed" to such a degree that cells from the blood lineage, for example, could give rise to neurons. These apparent examples of "transdifferentiation" have been thrown into doubt by further studies that suggested that they could be artifactual consequences of phenomena such as cell fusion (Corti et al., 2004; Cova et al., 2004; Krabbe et al., 2005).

2.2 Stem Cells and "Cloning"

The concept of "cloning" is used in the field of stem cell biology in three different ways, which deserve separate consideration. **Clonal cultures** are populations of stem cells derived from a single cell. It is frequently assumed that *clonal* populations are homogeneous because of their origin; this assumption appears to be frequently unwarranted, however, as illustrated by the finding that among 15,000 cells in a "clonal" culture derived from a single retinal stem cell, fewer than 20 cells had retained stem cell properties (Tropepe et al., 2000). **Therapeutic cloning** refers to a strategy for generating autologous material for transplantation, with the goal of avoiding the immunological rejection that could be triggered by heterologous cells (Hall et al., 2006). In this approach, the nucleus of a cell from a patient is transplanted into an enucleated oocyte, which will thereafter develop under the genetic control of the transplanted nucleus. The cells derived from this oocyte are then grown in culture in order to establish lines of stem cells that express the patient's genetic information. *Reproductive cloning*, on the other hand, refers to a procedure that, as the one described above, begins with the transplantation of a somatic nucleus from a donor into an enucleated oocyte. In this case, however, the developing embryo is transferred to the uterus of a female, with the intention of allowing the birth of a fully developed organism. Dolly the sheep was the initial example of this approach, which has already been applied to several other animal species (Luvoni et al., 2006; Oback and Wells, 2007; Vanderwall et al., 2006). Its potential application to humans is extremely controversial (Sharma, 2004; Yoshimura, 2006) and, in the opinion of this author, it is unnecessary and undesirable.

2.3 The Need for New Stem Cell Lines

The development of methods for growing embryonic stem cells in culture (Thomson et al., 1998) brought about the possibility to generate large amounts of material for transplantation, a key step towards their possible therapeutic use. There seems to be general consensus among experts in the field that currently available stem cell culture lines are not completely devoid of features that could make their use in human patients ineffective, or even potentially risky (Amit and Itskovitz-Eldor, 2006; Findikli et al., 2005; Klimanskaya et al., 2005; Skottman et al., 2006; Stacey et al., 2006; Taupin, 2006; Trounson, 2006; Wang et al., 2005). Some of the most significant issues that remain unresolved include (but are not limited to): (i) the oncogenic potential of embryonic stem cells, (ii) the genetic and epigenetic changes that cells can undergo as they "age" upon prolonged culture, (iii) the possibility of immunological rejection, (iv) the fact that stem cells are cultured on a "feeder layer" of mouse cells, and are therefore exposed to possible infection with murine retroviruses, and (v) their heterogeneity regarding the developmental potential of the cells (see below). Given the urgent need to develop new cell lines, there has been a sense of deep disappointment and concern in the field in response to President Bush's announcement on August 9, 2001, that federal funds would be unavailable for the development of new stem cell lines, and to his decision to veto a lift of these restrictions approved by Congress with bipartisan support in 2006 (Baltimore, 2004; Holden, 2005; McCarthy, 2004; Wadman, 2007).

3 How to Induce Stem Cells to Become Photoreceptors

Cell differentiation is regulated through complex interactions between extracellular signaling molecules and intracellular genetic and epigenetic mechanisms.

A strategy for inducing stem cells to develop as photoreceptors, therefore, could involve genetic manipulation (e.g., transfection with transcription factors), and/or treatment of the cells with growth factors or similar signaling molecules. Ideally, only one or a small number of these treatments would be necessary to achieve the desired goal of inducing stem cells to develop into perfectly mature, fully differentiated, synaptically connected photoreceptors. "Magic bullets" of this type have not been identified, however, and we don't yet know how to "make stem cells do what we want them to do". A possible strategy for overcoming these limitations can be found in the words of Viktor Hamburger, a founding father of Developmental Neurobiology, who said that "Our real teacher has been and still is the embryo, who is, incidentally, the only teacher who is always right," [cited in (Purves, 1985)]. In this section I will summarize some of the lessons derived from studies of the dynamics and mechanisms of embryonic development, which are particularly relevant in the context of this article.

3.1 The Embryo does Things in a Sequence

To recapitulate the processes through which photoreceptors are normally generated, transplanted embryonic stem cells would have to go through a series of transitions similar to those that occur during normal development in the embryo, which forms ectoderm before forming a central nervous system (CNS), CNS before forming a retina, a retina before forming photoreceptors, etc. The number of such transitions would obviously be lower if the stem cells are isolated from the retina itself, but considerable complexity can be expected even in this case. The retina initially consists of a population of multipotential, dividing neuroepithelial cells; over time, increasing numbers of neuroepithelial cells become postmitotic (i.e., are "born"), and migrate to different laminar positions within the retina. The future photoreceptors don't migrate at all, and remain in the future outer nuclear layer. It has been well established in many experimental animals that *the differentiation of these cells as photoreceptors occurs in at least two distinct, independently regulated stages* (Bradford et al., 2005; Bruhn and Cepko, 1996; Johnson et al., 2001; Morrow et al., 1998; Stenkamp et al., 1997). The future photoreceptors express a small number of photoreceptor-specific molecules shortly after they are generated, but their "terminal differentiation", including the expression of most photoreceptor-specific genes, the formation of outer segments and the development of synaptic contacts between photoreceptors and post-synaptic cells, does not start until many days (or even several weeks) after the photoreceptors are generated. During the time interval between photoreceptor generation and terminal differentiation, ganglion cells send their axons to the appropriate brain centers, and the patterning of their terminals in the brain is influenced by electrical activity generated in the inner retina itself (Shatz, 1990a,b). What (if any) influences are exerted by the inner retina upon differentiating photoreceptors is not well understood, and deserves to be investigated, because it appears likely that stem cells transplanted into a degenerating retina would encounter a microenvironment completely different from that of the developing embryo. This issue will be revisited in the section on synaptogenesis.

The mechanisms that control early and late aspects of photoreceptor differentiation are incompletely understood, but two principles appear well established: (1) the initial developmental program of photoreceptor progenitors controls several important aspects of their differentiation in a cell-autonomous manner, and (2) key aspects of the terminal differentiation of photoreceptor cells are independently regulated by separate microenvironmental factors. The cell autonomous phase of photoreceptor differentiation became evident in experiments in which chick embryo retinal cells were isolated on embryonic days 5–8, before the onset of their overt differentiation, and cultured in an artificial, homogeneous microenvironment, [rev. (Adler, 2000; Adler, 2005)]. The cultured cells appeared homogeneous and undifferentiated at culture onset, but over time some of the cells developed as photoreceptors, and others as non-photoreceptor neurons (predominantly, amacrine cells). Isolated photoreceptor progenitors expressed a fairly complex set of photoreceptor-specific properties in a cell-autonomous manner. The progenitor cells initially had a circular outline, but they subsequently elongated markedly and developed structural and molecular polarity, accompanied by formation of a small outer segment-like process, the expression of several photoreceptor-specific genes, and functional activities including photomechanical responses to light.

On the other hand, a very large number of genes must be expressed in concert during the terminal differentiation of photoreceptor cells, and they are regulated through different mechanisms. These molecules include not only visual pigments, but also phototransduction cascade components, structural proteins (such as those required for outer segment and synapse assembly and maintenance), molecules related to vitamin A transport, neurotransmitters, etc. Several different experimental treatments were shown to selectively induce or repress the expression of particular visual pigment genes in cultures of chick retina photoreceptors (Adler et al., 2001; Belecky-Adams et al., 1999; Bradford et al., 2005; Xie and Adler, 2000). This made it possible to investigate whether those changes were coordinated with changes in the expression of other rod- or cone-specific genes; the results showed convincingly that they were not (Bradford et al., 2005). Rather, the data showed that visual pigments and other photoreceptor-specific genes were not co-expressed during development, were not necessarily co-induced, and were not necessarily co-repressed. Taken together, these results demonstrate that **the differentiation of photoreceptor cells is a multi-step process that appears to be regulated one step at a time, suggesting that it is unlikely that a single "magic bullet" will be found which would control the entire process of differentiation of a stem cell into a mature photoreceptor.**

3.2 Molecular Recycling During Embryonic Development

Many intracellular transcription factors and extracellular signaling molecules are used time and again in different regions of the embryo and at different stages of development, and their roles are frequently different, or even opposite, depending on the molecular context in which they act. The changing roles of the transcription factor Pax6 in photoreceptor development provide an example relevant to the topic of this article, because (i) the embryo does not form a retina without Pax6, and therefore can not generate photoreceptors, but (ii) photoreceptors will not develop if Pax6 is not down-regulated after the retina is formed.

Pax6 is expressed in both the optic vesicle and the lens ectoderm during early embryonic development, and its mutations cause complex ocular malformations such as aniridia and small eye (Glaser et al., 1994; Glaser et al., 1992; Hanson et al., 1994; Hill et al., 1991a,b; Matsuo, 1993). It has not been conclusively established whether Pax6 is normally necessary in both the optic vesicle and the lens epithelium; until recently, however, the prevailing view was that it is only needed in the ectoderm (Ashery-Padan and Gruss, 2001; Drueppel et al., 2004; Mathers and Jamrich, 2000; Ogino and Yasuda, 2000). This was re-examined in our laboratory by electroporating antisense oligonucleotide morpholinos into the chick embryo optic vesicle (Canto-Soler and Adler, 2006). Electroporation of a control morpholino did not interfere with eye development. On the other hand, a morpholino against Pax6 caused Pax6 downregulation, as expected, and this was followed by a marked increase in cell death in the optic vesicle neuroepithelium. As the embryo continued to develop, the neural retina failed to develop and, despite the fact that Pax6 expression in the lens was normal, lens development was also abortive. The experiment demonstrated that Pax6 expression in the optic vesicle was needed for retina development, and that Pax6 expression in the lens epithelium was not sufficient to support normal lens development. The experiments demonstrated, moreover, that Pax6 is critically needed in the optic vesicle during a very narrow time window: the phenotype was very severe when Pax6 morpholinos were electroporated at or before Hamburger Hamilton stage 10 (Hamburger and Hamilton, 1951), but it was quite mild when electroporation was performed at or after stage 11. It is noteworthy that only 7 hours separate stages 10 and 11. This example illustrates a general feature of experimental embryology, which is that **the consequences of a treatment depend not only on its nature, but also on the time (developmental stage) at which it is applied.**

Pax6 is initially expressed quite broadly across the undifferentiated retinal neuroepithelium; upon further development, however, Pax6 is downregulated in photoreceptor progenitors, while remaining strongly expressed in prospective amacrine and ganglion cells (Belecky-Adams et al., 1997). This led us to hypothesize that Pax6 could be both a *positive regulator* of amacrine and ganglion cell differentiation, and a *repressor* of photoreceptor development. This hypothesis was tested by experimental over-expression of Pax6 into retinal progenitor cells in culture. As predicted by this hypothesis, Pax6 decreased significantly the frequency of progenitor cells that develop as photoreceptors, while promoting their differentiation as amacrine and ganglion neurons (Toy et al., 2002). Ongoing experiments have shown similar effects of Pax6 over-expression in vivo (Canto Soler and Adler, unpublished). In addition to Pax6, other transcription factors, including Chx10 and

Six3, have also been identified as repressors of photoreceptor differentiation (Bovo-lenta et al., 1998; Livne-Bar et al., 2006). Obviously, **if repressors of this type are expressed in stem cells, it would be necessary to downregulate them in order to allow the cells to differentiate as photoreceptors.**

3.3 Transcription Factor Expression is Strongly Influenced by Microenvironmental Signals

Although experimental manipulations allow upregulating or repressing the expression of particular transcription factors in stem (or other) cells, extracellular signalling molecules present in the microenvironment into which stem cells are transplanted could have regulatory effects of their own on those genes. An example is the growth factor activin, which is present in the retinal microenvironment and appears able to influence Pax6 expression in retinal progenitors in a position-dependent manner. Activin is expressed near the vitreal surface of the developing retina, a region occupied by precursors of ganglion and amacrine neurons and located away from the layer where photoreceptors develop (Belecky-Adams et al., 1999). Activin has two complementary effects on retinal cell cultures: inhibition of photoreceptor differentiation, and increases in the frequency of Pax6 (+) amacrine neurons. In the developing retina in vivo, retrovirus-mediated overexpression of follistatin, an activin-binding protein and inhibitor, caused marked inhibition of amacrine cell differentiation, accompanied by a decrease in Pax6 expression in the inner retina (Moreira and Adler, 2006). The domains of expression of transcription factors normally restricted to horizontal and bipolar cells, such as Prox1 and Chx10, were expanded into the inner nuclear layer area where Pax6 was downregulated. These experiments suggest that, under normal circumstances, high activin concentrations near the vitreal surface of the retina induce Pax6, and repress expression of transcription factors corresponding to outer retina cells. In the case of progenitors located in the ONL, their distance from the source of activin would lead to Pax6 downregulation, thus facilitating their differentiation as photoreceptors.

3.4 The Embryo Uses Combinations of Signaling Molecules and Transcription Factors

Practically every developmental phenomenon that has been investigated in detail has been found to be regulated by an array of intracellular transcription factors and extracellular signaling molecules, acting in concert. This, of course, throws into some doubt the likelihood that there is a single "magic bullet" capable of inducing stem cells to develop as photoreceptors. Extracellular signaling molecules implicated in photoreceptor development include not only activin, but also CNTF (Ezzeddine et al., 1997; Fuhrmann et al., 1998; Fuhrmann et al., 1995; Kirsch et al., 1996; Kirsch et al., 1998; Schulz-Key et al., 2002; Xie and Adler, 2000),

BMP (Sehgal et al., 2006), retinoids (Hyatt and Dowling, 1997; Hyatt et al., 1996; Kelley et al., 1995; Roberts et al., 2005; Stenkamp et al., 1993; Wallace and Jensen, 1999), Lif (Graham et al., 2005; Neophytou et al., 1997), thyroid hormone (Ng et al., 2001; Roberts et al., 2005), docosohexanoic acid (Insua et al., 2003; Politi et al., 2001), PEDF (Jablonski et al., 2000), taurine (Altshuler et al., 1993; Wallace and Jensen, 1999; Young and Cepko, 2004), FGF (Hicks, 1996; Hicks and Courtois, 1992; Yan and Wang, 2000), and SHH (Levine et al., 1997; Stenkamp et al., 2000). These molecules have usually been tested in isolation, or at most in pairs. This probably reflects not only the technical limitations of the methods available for their study, but also the conceptual framework supporting those studies, derived from the classical neurotrophic hypothesis. This hypothesis postulated that (i) each neurotrophic factor was specific for one type, or very few types of neurons, (ii) each neuron responded to one factor, and (iii) factors derived from a restricted, unique sources (Varon et al., 1982). It is now known, however, that extracellular signaling is actually much more complicated (Davies, 1996; Henderson, 1996; Korsching, 1993): each factor can act on many cell types, each cell can respond to many factors, and the factors derive from a variety of sources. Extracellular signaling molecules, moreover, appear to be integrated in vivo into homeostatic networks, in which different factors regulate each other. Therefore, **while impressive progress has been made in elucidating the role of individual factors, we have not yet reached a clear understanding of the complex interactions between different microenvironmental signalling systems.**

3.5 Is it Possible to Predict Whether Stem Cells will Generate Photoreceptors or Some Other Types of Cells?

All the tests that are currently available for evaluating the developmental potential of cells are *retrospective*, since they ask "what did a population of cells do when it was exposed to different microenvironments?"; obviously, by the time an answer is obtained, the original population of stem cells used for the experiment no longer exist as such. In addition to being retrospective, analyses of this type only describe the behavior of cell populations, rather than that of single cells. The challenge, therefore, is to find ways to evaluate the developmental potential *of each individual cell prospectively, and at the molecular level.* High throughput molecular analysis of individual cells is now possible (Brady, 2000; Brail et al., 1999; Chiang and Melton, 2003; Iscove et al., 2002; Kamme et al., 2004; Tietjen et al., 2005), and the methods are readily applicable to differentiated photoreceptors (Wahlin et al., 2004). It is now feasible, for example, to identify morphologically different cell types (including rod and cone photoreceptors) in cell suspension of dissociated retinas; an individual cell can be captured with a micro pipet, and its RNA can be extracted and used as a template for cDNA synthesis and amplification. The identity of the cells can be corroborated by amplification of cell-specific molecules by PCR, and high throughput analysis of gene expression can be carried out by suppression subtractive hybridization or microarray technology. Similar approaches could in principle be applicable to stem cells, but they pose a special set of problems: a totipotential stem cell cannot be morphologically recognized from a more restricted stem cell, or even from a cell committed to develop as a particular cell type. Moreover, molecular markers that would allow us to identify various types of stem cell derivatives (totipotential, multipotential, lineage-restricted) are not available. The "catch-22", then, is that the cells must be identified before they can be characterized, but they should be characterized in order to be identified. Fortunately, undifferentiated progenitor cells are arranged in the future outer nuclear layer of the developing retina, and can be cleanly isolated by laser capture microdissection (LCM), without contamination with material from adjacent cells. RNA from the progenitors thus isolated can also be used for cDNA synthesis with protocols similar to those used for individual cells (see above). Therefore, it now appears possible to compare gene expression profiles not only in differentiated photoreceptor cells (for example, rods vs. cones, or green cones vs. red cones), but also to compare expression profiles of the progenitor cells for photoreceptors vs. those for other retinal cells (which are located in a different layer of embryonic retina), or even to compare changes in photoreceptor progenitors at different stages of their maturation. Together with the availability of powerful methods for gene gain-of-function and loss-of-function experiments, it can be anticipated that substantial progress will be made within the next few years in the molecular characterization of these cells.

4 How to Induce Transplanted Stem Cells to Form Synapses with the Host Retina

As mentioned in the Introduction, the lack of synapse formation between grafted and host cells is one of the fundamental roadblocks that have so far prevented the replacement of photoreceptor cells through transplantation approaches. Although frustrating and disappointing, this fact cannot be considered too surprising, considering that photoreceptor synapses are structurally and molecularly very complex (Barnes and Kelly, 2002; Brandstatter and Hack, 2001; Clegg et al., 2000; Fejtova and Gundelfinger, 2006; Harris and Lim, 2001; Heidelberger et al., 2005; Morgans, 2000a,b; Sterling and Matthews, 2005; tom Dieck and Brandstatter, 2006; von Gersdorff, 2001; Witkovsky et al., 2001). Rods and cones form specialized "ribbon" synaptic terminals, known as rod spherules and cone pedicles, which make highly stereotyped contacts with post-synaptic processes from bipolar and horizontal neurons. The "ribbons" that give these terminals their name are structures connected to the synaptic membrane by adaptor proteins, and represent specialized release sites adapted to the tonic release of glutamate in darkness. Photoreceptor synapses, like those in other regions of the central nervous system, require the synthesis and assembly of a very large number of molecules that form the pre-synaptic and the post-synaptic components; moreover, the two components must be brought together through specific adhesive interactions which are controlled by members of several families of cell adhesion molecules. Cell adhesion molecules involved in synapse formation include (but are not limited to) members of the cadherin, ephrin, β-neurexin, and neuroligin families (Akins and Biederer, 2006; Dean and Dresbach, 2006; Gerrow and El-Husseini, 2006; Grant et al., 2005; Junghans et al., 2005; Kosik et al., 2005; Lise and El-Husseini, 2006; Loers and Schachner, 2007; Martinez and Soriano, 2005; Piechotta et al., 2006; Salinas and Price, 2005; Waites et al., 2005; Washbourne et al., 2004). Although progress has been made in the study of the mechanisms of synapse formation in the hippocampus and other regions of the central nervous system(Azmitia, 2001; Cline, 2005; Garner et al., 2002; Inoue and Okabe, 2003; Kroger and Schroder, 2002; Pfrieger, 2003; Slezak and Pfrieger, 2003; Sykova, 2001; Ullian et al., 2004), **the mechanisms of photoreceptor synaptogenesis have not been similarly investigated.**.

Our laboratory has devised a strategy to search for treatments that would promote synaptogenesis between transplanted cells and a host retina. The strategy has 3 well defined stages, which need to be completed in order: (i) investigation of the molecules expressed in photoreceptors and their post-synaptic partners during synaptogenesis, (ii) gain- and loss- of – function experiments in vitro and in vivo to determine the role of those molecules in synapse formation during normal embryonic development, and (iii) extrapolation of the information derived from these embryonic studies to the promotion of synaptogenesis between transplanted stem cells and a host retina. We have chosen the chick retina for these studies because it is readily accessible and amenable to experimental manipulation, and it is rich in cones, the photoreceptors responsible for high resolution vision (Wahlin et al., 2007; Wahlin, 2006). The expression of synaptic molecules during chick embryo retinal development is being investigated using RT-PCR, laser capture microdissection, immunocytochemistry, and confocal microscopy. The studies have shown that the expression of synaptic molecules in photoreceptor cells begins at a very precise stage of development, many days after the photoreceptors are generated, and also after synaptogenesis between bipolar, amacrine, and ganglion neurons has occurred in the inner retina. Immunocytochemistry showed that most synaptic proteins first become detectable by in the inner segment (the site of protein synthesis in photoreceptors). Within 3–5 days, however, the same molecules appear in the synaptic terminal and are assembled with other synaptic components; interestingly, the proteins become undetectable in the inner segment at the same time, suggesting that their synthesis is down-regulated after synaptogenesis is completed. These very precise temporal patterns of expression provide a well-defined framework for gain- and loss-of-function experiments aimed at identifying and characterizing the signals that control synthesis, transport, and assembly of synaptic molecules. The findings, moreover, suggest that the timing of these events must be determined by endogenous photoreceptor "clocks" and/or by signals originating within the retina microenvironment. It may be relevant, in this regard, that the inner retina reaches a high degree of differentiation before photoreceptor synapses are formed, thus appearing as a likely (but hitherto unexplored) source of such hypothetical signals. Cells transplanted into a retina affected by photoreceptor degeneration are likely to encounter a microenvironment quite different from that of the embryonic retina, because the inner retina suffers extreme plastic changes and disorganization after the photoreceptors die (Marc et al., 2003). Molecular similarities and differences between the normal developing retina and the degenerating adult retina, therefore, should be investigated with high priority, and it appears likely that *both* the transplanted stem cells and the recipient retina will have to be treated in order to induce the expression of the appropriate synaptic components, and to overcome possible barriers to synaptogenesis.

5 Concluding Remarks

Three rhetorical questions can be asked about prospects for curing blindness through stem cell transplantation. First, *can retinal stem cells "make" photoreceptors?* The answer to this question is obviously *"yes"*, because this is what happens normally during embryonic development. Second, *is it conceivable that transplanted stem cells will ever make mature, synaptically connected photoreceptors?* The answer to this question cannot be as certain as the preceding one; it appears likely, however, that the answer should be *"yes, provided that we listen to the embryo in order to elucidate the mechanisms through which photoreceptors are generated during normal development"*. The final question is: *"how long will it take before we can cure blindness through stem cell transplantation?"* We don't know the answer to this question, although we certainly hope that it will be sooner, rather than later. Making this a reality is a challenge that must be answered by the vision research community, and by the governmental and private agencies that fund and promote eye research.

Acknowledgments Research in the author's laboratory was supported by NIH grants R01EY04859 and CORE Grant EY1765, by the Foundation Fighting Blindness, by an unrestricted departmental grant from Research to Prevent Blindness, Inc., by a donation from The Michael B. Panitch Macular Degeneration Laboratory at The Wilmer Eye Institute, and by a contribution from the William Weiss Endowment for Research. The author is the Arnall Patz Distinguished Professor of Ophthalmology at Johns Hopkins.

References

Adler, R., 2000. A model of retinal cell differentiation in the chick embryo. Prog Retinal Eye Res 20, 529–557.

Adler, R., 2005. Challenges in the study of neuronal differentiation: A view from the embryonic eye. Dev Dyn. 234 (3): 454–463.

Adler, R., Tamres, A., Bradford, R.L., Belecky-Adams, T.L., 2001. Microenvironmental regulation of visual pigment expression in the chick retina. Dev Biol 236, 454–464.

Ahmad, I., Das, A.V., James, J., Bhattacharya, S., Zhao, X., 2004. Neural stem cells in the mammalian eye: types and regulation. Semin Cell Dev Biol 15, 53–62.

Akins, M.R., Biederer, T., 2006. Cell-cell interactions in synaptogenesis. Curr Opin Neurobiol 16, 83–89.

Altshuler, D., Lo Turco, J.J., Rush, J., Cepko, C., 1993. Taurine promotes the differentiation of a vertebrate retinal cell type in vitro. Development 119, 1317–1328.

Amit, M., Itskovitz-Eldor, J., 2006. Sources, derivation, and culture of human embryonic stem cells. Seminars in Reproductive Medicine 24, 298–303.

Ashery-Padan, R., Gruss, P., 2001. Pax6 lights-up the way for eye development. Curr Opin Cell Biol 13, 706–714.

Azmitia, E.C., 2001. Modern views on an ancient chemical: serotonin effects on cell proliferation, maturation, and apoptosis. Brain Research Bulletin 56, 413–424.

Baltimore, D., 2004. Science and the bush administration. Science 305, 1873.

Banin, E., Obolensky, A., Idelson, M., Hemo, I., Reinhardtz, E., Pikarsky, E., Ben-Hur, T., Reubinoff, B., 2006. Retinal incorporation and differentiation of neural precursors derived from human embryonic stem cells. Stem cells (Dayton, Ohio) 24, 246–257.

Barnes, S., Kelly, M.E., 2002. Calcium channels at the photoreceptor synapse. Adv Exp Med Biol 514, 465–476.

Belecky-Adams, T., Tomarev, S., Li, H.S., Ploder, L., McInnes, R.R., Sundin, O., Adler, R., 1997. Pax-6, Prox 1, and Chx10 homeobox gene expression correlates with phenotypic fate of retinal precursor cells. Invest Ophthalmol Vis Sci 38, 1293–1303.

Belecky-Adams, T.L., Scheurer, D., Adler, R., 1999. Activin family members in the developing chick retina: expression patterns, protein distribution, and in vitro effects. Dev Biol 210, 107–123.

Boulton, M., Albon, J., 2004. Stem cells in the eye. Int J Biochem Cell Biol 36, 643–657.

Bovolenta, P., Mallamaci, A., Puelles, L., Boncinelli, E., 1998. Expression pattern of cSix3, a member of the six/sine oculis family of transcription factors. Mech Dev 70, 201–203.

Bradford, R.L., Wang, C., Zack, D.J., Adler, R., 2005. Roles of cell-intrinsic and microenvironmental factors in photoreceptor cell differentiation. Dev Biol 286, 31–45.

Brady, G., 2000. Expression profiling of single mammalian cells – small is beautiful. Yeast 17, 211–217.

Brail, L.H., Jang, A., Billia, F., Iscove, N.N., Klamut, H.J., Hill, R.P., 1999. Gene expression in individual cells: analysis using global single cell reverse transcription polymerase chain reaction (GSC RT-PCR). Mutat Res 406, 45–54.

Brandstatter, J.H., Hack, I., 2001. Localization of glutamate receptors at a complex synapse. The mammalian photoreceptor synapse. Cell Tissue Res 303, 1–14.

Bruhn, S.L., Cepko, C.L., 1996. Development of the pattern of photoreceptors in the chick retina. J Neurosci 16, 1430–1439.

Canola, K., Angenieux, B., Tekaya, M., Quiambao, A., Naash, M.I., Munier, F.L., Schorderet, D.F., Arsenijevic, Y., 2007. Retinal stem cells transplanted into models of late stages of retinitis pigmentosa preferentially adopt a glial or a retinal ganglion cell fate. Invest Ophthalmol Vis Sci 48, 446–454.

Canto-Soler, M.V., Adler, R., 2006. Optic cup and lens development requires Pax6 expression in the early optic vesicle during a narrow time window. Dev Biol 294, 119–132.

Chacko, D.M., Rogers, J.A., Turner, J.E., Ahmad, I., 2000. Survival and differentiation of cultured retinal progenitors transplanted in the subretinal space of the rat. Biochem Biophys Res Commun 268, 842–846.

Chiang, M.K., Melton, D.A., 2003. Single-cell transcript analysis of pancreas development. Dev Cell 4, 383–393.

Clegg, D.O., Mullick, L.H., Wingerd, K.L., Lin, H., Atienza, J.W., Bradshaw, A.D., Gervin, D.B., Cann, G.M., 2000. Adhesive events in retinal development and function: the role of integrin receptors. Res Probl Cell Differ 31, 141–156.

Cline, H., 2005. Synaptogenesis: a balancing act between excitation and inhibition. Curr Biol 15, R203–R205.

Corti, S., Locatelli, F., Papadimitriou, D., Strazzer, S., Comi, G.P., 2004. Somatic stem cell research for neural repair: current evidence and emerging perspectives. J Cellular Mol Med 8, 329–337.

Cova, L., Ratti, A., Volta, M., Fogh, I., Cardin, V., Corbo, M., Silani, V., 2004. Stem cell therapy for neurodegenerative diseases: the issue of transdifferentiation. Stem Cells Dev 13, 121–131.

Das, A.M., Zhao, X., Ahmad, I., 2005. Stem cell therapy for retinal degeneration: retinal neurons from heterologous sources. Semin Ophthalmol 20, 3–10.

Davies, A.M., 1996. The neurotrophic hypothesis: where does it stand? Philos Trans R Soc Lond B Biol Sci 351, 389–394.

Dean, C., Dresbach, T., 2006. Neuroligins and neurexins: linking cell adhesion, synapse formation and cognitive function. Trends Neurosci 29, 21–29.

Drueppel, L., Pfleiderer, K., Schmidt, A., Hillen, W., Berens, C., 2004. A short autonomous repression motif is located within the N-terminal domain of CTCF. FEBS letters 572, 154–158.

Ezzeddine, Z.D., Yang, X., DeChiara, T., Yancopoulos, G., Cepko, C.L., 1997. Postmitotic cells fated to become rod photoreceptors can be respecified by CNTF treatment of the retina. Development 124, 1055–1067.

Fejtova, A., Gundelfinger, E.D., 2006. Molecular organization and assembly of the presynaptic active zone of neurotransmitter release. Results Probl Cell Differ 43, 49–68.

Findikli, N., Kahraman, S., Akcin, O., Sertyel, S., Candan, Z., 2005. Establishment and characterization of new human embryonic stem cell lines. Reprod Biomed online 10, 617–627.

Fuhrmann, S., Heller, S., Rohrer, H., Hofmann, H.D., 1998. A transient role for ciliary neurotrophic factor in chick photoreceptor development. J Neurobiol 37, 672–683.

Fuhrmann, S., Kirsch, M., Hofmann, H.D., 1995. Ciliary neurotrophic factor promotes chick photoreceptor development in vitro. Development 121, 2695–2706.

Galli-Resta, L., 2001. Assembling the vertebrate retina: global patterning from short-range cellular interactions. Neuroreport 12, A103–A106.

Garner, C.C., Zhai, R.G., Gundelfinger, E.D., Ziv, N.E., 2002. Molecular mechanisms of CNS synaptogenesis. Trends Neurosci 25, 243–251.

Gerrow, K., El-Husseini, A., 2006. Cell adhesion molecules at the synapse. Front Biosci 11, 2400–2419.

Glaser, T., Jepeal, L., Edwards, J.G., Young, S.R., Favor, J., Maas, R.L., 1994. PAX6 gene dosage effect in a family with congenital cataracts, aniridia, anophthalmia and central nervous system defects. Nat Genet 7, 463–471.

Glaser, T., Walton, D.S., Maas, R.L., 1992. Genomic structure, evolutionary conservation and aniridia mutations in the human PAX6 gene. Nat Genet 2, 232–239.

Graham, D.R., Overbeek, P.A., Ash, J.D., 2005. Leukemia inhibitory factor blocks expression of Crx and Nrl transcription factors to inhibit photoreceptor differentiation. Invest Ophthalmol Vis Sci 46, 2601–2610.

Grant, S.G., Marshall, M.C., Page, K.L., Cumiskey, M.A., Armstrong, J.D., 2005. Synapse proteomics of multiprotein complexes: en route from genes to nervous system diseases. Hum Mol Genet 14 Spec No. 2, R225–R234.

Hall, V.J., Stojkovic, P., Stojkovic, M., 2006. Using therapeutic cloning to fight human disease: a conundrum or reality? Stem cells (Dayton, Ohio) 24, 1628–1637.

Hamburger, V., Hamilton, H.L., 1951. A series of normal stages in the development of the chick embryo. J Morph 88, 49–92.

Hanson, I.M., Fletcher, J.M., Jordan, T., Brown, A., Taylor, D., Adams, R.J., Punnett, H.H., van Heyningen, V., 1994. Mutations at the PAX6 locus are found in heterogeneous anterior segment malformations including Peters' anomaly. Nat Genet 6, 168–173.

Harris, B.Z., Lim, W.A., 2001. Mechanism and role of PDZ domains in signaling complex assembly. J Cell Sci 114, 3219–3231.

Haruta, M., 2005. Embryonic stem cells: potential source for ocular repair. Semin Ophthalmol 20, 17–23.

Hatakeyama, J., Kageyama, R., 2004. Retinal cell fate determination and bHLH factors. Semin Cell Dev Biol 15, 83–89.

Haynes, T., Del Rio-Tsonis, K., 2004. Retina repair, stem cells and beyond. Curr Neurovasc Res 1, 231–239.

Heidelberger, R., Thoreson, W.B., Witkovsky, P., 2005. Synaptic transmission at retinal ribbon synapses. Prog Retin Eye Res 24, 682–720.

Henderson, C.E., 1996. Role of neurotrophic factors in neuronal development. Curr Opin Neurobiol 6, 64–70.

Hicks, D., 1996. Characterization and possible roles of fibroblast growth factors in retinal photoreceptor cells. Keio J Med 45, 140–154.

Hicks, D., Courtois, Y., 1992. Fibroblast growth factor stimulates photoreceptor differentiation in vitro. J Neurosci 12, 2022–2033.

Hill, R.E., Favor, J., Hogan, B.L., Ton, C.C., Saunders, G.F., Hanson, I.M., Prosser, J., Jordan, T., Hastie, N.D., van Heyningen, V., 1991a. Mouse small eye results from mutations in a paired-like homeobox-containing gene. Nature 354, 522–525.

Hill, R.E., Favor, J., Hogan, B.L., Ton, C.C., Saunders, G.F., Hanson, I.M., Prosser, J., Jordan, T., Hastie, N.D., van Heyningen, V., 1991b. Mouse small eye results from mutations in a paired-like homeobox- containing gene [published erratum appears in Nature 1992 Feb 20;355(6362):750]. Nature 354, 522–525.

Holden, C., 2005. Stem cells. Restiveness grows at NIH over Bush research restrictions. Science 308, 334–335.

Hyatt, G.A., Dowling, J.E., 1997. Retinoic acid. A key molecule for eye and photoreceptor development. Invest Ophthalmol Vis Sci 38, 1471–1475.

Hyatt, G.A., Schmitt, E.A., Fadool, J.M., Dowling, J.E., 1996. Retinoic acid alters photoreceptor development in vivo. Proc Natl Acad Sci USA 93, 13298–13303.

Inoue, A., Okabe, S., 2003. The dynamic organization of postsynaptic proteins: translocating molecules regulate synaptic function. Curr Opin Neurobiol 13, 332–340.

Insua, M.F., Garelli, A., Rotstein, N.P., German, O.L., Arias, A., Politi, L.E., 2003. Cell cycle regulation in retinal progenitors by glia-derived neurotrophic factor and docosahexaenoic acid. Invest Ophthalmol Vis Sci 44, 2235–2244.

Iscove, N.N., Barbara, M., Gu, M., Gibson, M., Modi, C., Winegarden, N., 2002. Representation is faithfully preserved in global cDNA amplified exponentially from sub-picogram quantities of mRNA. Nat Biotechnol 20, 940–943.

Jablonski, M.M., Tombran-Tink, J., Mrazek, D.A., Iannaccone, A., 2000. Pigment epithelium-derived factor supports normal development of photoreceptor neurons and opsin expression after retinal pigment epithelium removal. J Neurosci 20, 7149–7157.

Jean, D., Ewan, K., Gruss, P., 1998. Molecular regulators involved in vertebrate eye development. Mech Dev 76, 3–18.

Johnson, P.T., Williams, R.R., Reese, B.E., 2001. Developmental patterns of protein expression in photoreceptors implicate distinct environmental versus cell-intrinsic mechanisms. Vis Neurosci 18, 157–168.

Junghans, D., Haas, I.G., Kemler, R., 2005. Mammalian cadherins and protocadherins: about cell death, synapses and processing. Curr Opin Cell Biol 17, 446–452.

Kamme, F., Zhu, J., Luo, L., Yu, J., Tran, D.T., Meurers, B., Bittner, A., Westlund, K., Carlton, S., Wan, J., 2004. Single-cell laser-capture microdissection and RNA amplification. Methods Mol Med 99, 215–223.

Kelley, M.W., Turner, J.K., Reh, T.A., 1995. Ligands of steroid/thyroid receptors induce cone photoreceptors in vertebrate retina. Development 121, 3777–3785.

Kirsch, M., Fuhrmann, S., Wiese, A., Hofmann, H.D., 1996. CNTF exerts opposite effects on in vitro development of rat and chick photoreceptors. Neuroreport 7, 697–700.

Kirsch, M., Schulz-Key, S., Wiese, A., Fuhrmann, S., Hofmann, H., 1998. Ciliary neurotrophic factor blocks rod photoreceptor differentiation from postmitotic precursor cells in vitro. Cell Tissue Res 291, 207–216.

Klassen, H., Sakaguchi, D.S., Young, M.J., 2004. Stem cells and retinal repair. Prog Retin Eye Res 23, 149–181.

Klimanskaya, I., Chung, Y., Meisner, L., Johnson, J., West, M.D., Lanza, R., 2005. Human embryonic stem cells derived without feeder cells. Lancet 365, 1636–1641.

Korsching, S., 1993. The neurotrophic factor concept: a reexamination. J Neurosci 13, 2739–2748.

Kosik, K.S., Donahue, C.P., Israely, I., Liu, X., Ochiishi, T., 2005. Delta-catenin at the synaptic-adherens junction. Trends Cell Biol 15, 172–178.

Krabbe, C., Zimmer, J., Meyer, M., 2005. Neural transdifferentiation of mesenchymal stem cells – a critical review. Apmis 113, 831-844.

Kroger, S., Schroder, J.E., 2002. Agrin in the developing CNS: new roles for a synapse organizer. News Physiol Sci 17, 207–212.

Levine, E.M., Roelink, H., Turner, J., Reh, T.A., 1997. Sonic hedgehog promotes rod photoreceptor differentiation in mammalian retinal cells in vitro. J Neurosci 17, 6277–6288.

Limb, G.A., Daniels, J.T., Cambrey, A.D., Secker, G.A., Shortt, A.J., Lawrence, J.M., Khaw, P.T., 2006. Current prospects for adult stem cell-based therapies in ocular repair and regeneration. Current Eye Res 31, 381–390.

Lise, M.F., El-Husseini, A., 2006. The neuroligin and neurexin families: from structure to function at the synapse. Cell Mol Life Sci 63, 1833–1849.

Livesey, F.J., Cepko, C.L., 2001. Vertebrate neural cell-fate determination: lessons from the retina. Nat Rev Neurosci 2, 109–118.

Livne-Bar, I., Pacal, M., Cheung, M.C., Hankin, M., Trogadis, J., Chen, D., Dorval, K.M., Bremner, R., 2006. Chx10 is required to block photoreceptor differentiation but is dispensable for progenitor proliferation in the postnatal retina. Proc Natl Acad Sci USA 103, 4988–4993.

Loers, G., Schachner, M., 2007. Recognition molecules and neural repair. J Neurochem. 101(4): 865–882.

Lupo, G., Andreazzoli, M., Gestri, G., Liu, Y., He, R.Q., Barsacchi, G., 2000. Homeobox genes in the genetic control of eye development. Int J Dev Biol 44, 627–636.

Luvoni, G.C., Chigioni, S., Beccaglia, M., 2006. Embryo production in dogs: from in vitro fertilization to cloning. Reproduction in domestic animals = Zuchthygiene 41, 286–290.

Malicki, J., 2004. Cell fate decisions and patterning in the vertebrate retina: the importance of timing, asymmetry, polarity and waves. Curr Opin Neurobiol 14, 15–21.

Marc, R.E., Jones, B.W., Watt, C.B., Strettoi, E., 2003. Neural remodeling in retinal degeneration. Prog Retin Eye Res 22, 607–655.

Marquardt, T., Gruss, P., 2002. Generating neuronal diversity in the retina: one for nearly all. Trends Neurosci 25, 32–38.

Martinez, A., Soriano, E., 2005. Functions of ephrin/Eph interactions in the development of the nervous system: emphasis on the hippocampal system. Brain Res Brain Res Rev 49, 211–226.

Mathers, P.H., Jamrich, M., 2000. Regulation of eye formation by the Rx and pax6 homeobox genes. Cell Mol Life Sci 57, 186–194.

Matsuo, T., 1993. The genes involved in the morphogenesis of the eye. Jpn J Ophthalmol 37, 215–251.

McCarthy, M., 2004. US researchers push past stem-cell restrictions. States and private sources fund research denied federal support by Bush ban. Lancet 363, 868–869.

Meyer, J.S., Katz, M.L., Kirk, M.D., 2005. Stem cells for retinal degenerative disorders. Ann N Y Acad Sci 1049, 135–145.

Meyer, J.S., Katz, M.L., Maruniak, J.A., Kirk, M.D., 2006. Embryonic stem cell-derived neural progenitors incorporate into degenerating retina and enhance survival of host photoreceptors. Stem cells (Dayton, Ohio) 24, 274–283.

Moreira, E.F., Adler, R., 2006. Effects of follistatin overexpression on cell differentiation in the chick embryo retina. Dev Biol 298, 272–284.

Morgans, C.W., 2000a. Neurotransmitter release at ribbon synapses in the retina. Immunol Cell Biol 78, 442–446.

Morgans, C.W., 2000b. Presynaptic proteins of ribbon synapses in the retina. Microsc Res Tech 50, 141–150.

Morrow, E.M., Belliveau, M.J., Cepko, C.L., 1998. Two phases of rod photoreceptor differentiation during rat retinal development. J Neurosci 18, 3738–3748.

Neophytou, C., Vernallis, A.B., Smith, A., Raff, M.C., 1997. Muller-cell-derived leukaemia inhibitory factor arrests rod photoreceptor differentiation at a postmitotic pre-rod stage of development. Development 124, 2345–2354.

Ng, L., Hurley, J.B., Dierks, B., Srinivas, M., Salto, C., Vennstrom, B., Reh, T.A., Forrest, D., 2001. A thyroid hormone receptor that is required for the development of green cone photoreceptors. Nat Genet 27, 94–98.

Oback, B., Wells, D.N., 2007. Cloning cattle: the methods in the madness. Adv Exp Med Biol 591, 30–57.

Ogino, H., Yasuda, K., 2000. Sequential activation of transcription factors in lens induction. Dev Growth Differ 42, 437–448.

Pfrieger, F.W., 2003. Role of cholesterol in synapse formation and function. Biochim Biophys Acta 1610, 271–280.

Piechotta, K., Dudanova, I., Missler, M., 2006. The resilient synapse: insights from genetic interference of synaptic cell adhesion molecules. Cell Tissue Res 326, 617–642.

Politi, L.E., Rotstein, N.P., Carri, N.G., 2001. Effect of GDNF on neuroblast proliferation and photoreceptor survival: additive protection with docosahexaenoic acid. Invest Ophthalmol Vis Sci 42, 3008–3015.

Purves, D., Lichtman, J.W., 1985. Principles of Neural Development. Sinauer, Massachussetts.

Qiu, G., Seiler, M.J., Mui, C., Arai, S., Aramant, R.B., de Juan, E., Jr., Sadda, S., 2005. Photoreceptor differentiation and integration of retinal progenitor cells transplanted into transgenic rats. Exp Eye Res 80, 515–525.

Rapaport, D.H., Wong, L.L., Wood, E.D., Yasumura, D., LaVail, M.M., 2004. Timing and topography of cell genesis in the rat retina. J Comp Neurol 474, 304–324.

Roberts, M.R., Hendrickson, A., McGuire, C.R., Reh, T.A., 2005. Retinoid X receptor (gamma) is necessary to establish the S-opsin gradient in cone photoreceptors of the developing mouse retina. Invest Ophthalmol Vis Sci 46, 2897–2904.

Salinas, P.C., Price, S.R., 2005. Cadherins and catenins in synapse development. Curr Opin Neurobiol 15, 73–80.

Schulz-Key, S., Hofmann, H.D., Beisenherz-Huss, C., Barbisch, C., Kirsch, M., 2002. Ciliary neurotrophic factor as a transient negative regulator of rod development in rat retina. Invest Ophthalmol Vis Sci 43, 3099–3108.

Sehgal, R., Andres, D.J., Adler, R., Belecky-Adams, T.L., 2006. Bone morphogenetic protein 7 increases chick photoreceptor outer segment initiation. Invest Ophthalmol Vis Sci 47, 3625–3634.

Sharma, B.R., 2004. Medicolegal and ethical issues of cloning: do we need to think again and again? Am J Forensic Med Pathol 25, 145–149.

Shatz, C.J., 1990a. Competitive interactions between retinal ganglion cells during prenatal development. J Neurobiol 21, 197–211.

Shatz, C.J., 1990b. Impulse activity and the patterning of connections during CNS development. Neuron 5, 745–756.

Skottman, H., Dilber, M.S., Hovatta, O., 2006. The derivation of clinical-grade human embryonic stem cell lines. FEBS Letters 580, 2875–2878.

Slezak, M., Pfrieger, F.W., 2003. New roles for astrocytes: regulation of CNS synaptogenesis. Trends Neurosci 26, 531–535.

Stacey, G.N., Cobo, F., Nieto, A., Talavera, P., Healy, L., Concha, A., 2006. The development of 'feeder' cells for the preparation of clinical grade hES cell lines: challenges and solutions. J Biotech 125, 583–588.

Stenkamp, D.L., Barthel, L.K., Raymond, P.A., 1997. Spatiotemporal coordination of rod and cone photoreceptor differentiation in goldfish retina. J Comp Neurol 382, 272–284.

Stenkamp, D.L., Frey, R.A., Prabhudesai, S.N., Raymond, P.A., 2000. Function for Hedgehog genes in zebrafish retinal development. Dev Biol 220, 238–252.

Stenkamp, D.L., Gregory, J.K., Adler, R., 1993. Retinoid effects in purified cultures of chick embryo retina neurons and photoreceptors. Invest Ophthalmol Vis Sci 34, 2425–2436.

Sterling, P., Matthews, G., 2005. Structure and function of ribbon synapses. Trends Neurosci 28, 20–29.

Suzuki, T., Mandai, M., Akimoto, M., Yoshimura, N., Takahashi, M., 2006. The simultaneous treatment of MMP-2 stimulants in retinal transplantation enhances grafted cell migration into the host retina. Stem cells (Dayton, Ohio) 24, 2406–2411.

Sykova, E., 2001. Glial diffusion barriers during aging and pathological states. Prog Brain Res 132, 339–363.

Takahashi, M., Palmer, T.D., Takahashi, J., Gage, F.H., 1998. Widespread integration and survival of adult-derived neural progenitor cells in the developing optic retina. Mol Cell Neurosci 12, 340–348.

Taupin, P., 2006. Derivation of embryonic stem cells for cellular therapy: challenges and new strategies. Med Sci Monit 12, RA75–RA78.

Thomson, J.A., Itskovitz-Eldor, J., Shapiro, S.S., Waknitz, M.A., Swiergiel, J.J., Marshall, V.S., Jones, J.M., 1998. Embryonic stem cell lines derived from human blastocysts. Science 282, 1145–1147.

Tietjen, I., Rihel, J., Dulac, C.G., 2005. Single-cell transcriptional profiles and spatial patterning of the mammalian olfactory epithelium. Int J Dev Biol 49, 201–207.

tom Dieck, S., Brandstatter, J.H., 2006. Ribbon synapses of the retina. Cell Tissue Res 326, 339–346.

Toy, J., Norton, J.S., Jibodh, S.R., Adler, R., 2002. Effects of homeobox genes on the differentiation of photoreceptor and nonphotoreceptor neurons. Invest Ophthalmol Vis Sci 43, 3522–3529.

Tropepe, V., Coles, B.L., Chiasson, B.J., Horsford, D.J., Elia, A.J., McInnes, R.R., van der Kooy, D., 2000. Retinal stem cells in the adult mammalian eye. Science 287, 2032–2036.

Trounson, A., 2006. The production and directed differentiation of human embryonic stem cells. Endocrine Rev 27, 208–219.

Ullian, E.M., Christopherson, K.S., Barres, B.A., 2004. Role for glia in synaptogenesis. Glia 47, 209–216.

Vanderwall, D.K., Woods, G.L., Roser, J.F., Schlafer, D.H., Sellon, D.C., Tester, D.F., White, K.L., 2006. Equine cloning: applications and outcomes. Reprod Fertil Dev 18, 91–98.

Varon, S., Manthorpe, M., Skaper, S.D., Adler, R., 1982. Neuronotrophic factors: problems and perspectives. Prog Clin Biol Res 79, 225–242.

Vetter, M.L., Brown, N.L., 2001. The role of basic helix-loop-helix genes in vertebrate retinogenesis. Semin Cell Dev Biol 12, 491–498.

von Gersdorff, H., 2001. Synaptic ribbons: versatile signal transducers. Neuron 29, 7–10.

Wadman, M., 2007. Congress and Bush set to clash on stem cells again. Nature 445, 134–135.

Wahlin, K.J., Lim, L., Grice, E.A., Campochiaro, P.A., Zack, D.J., Adler, R., 2004. A method for analysis of gene expression in isolated mouse photoreceptor and Muller cells. Mol Vis 10, 366–375.

Wahlin, K.J., Moreira, E., Huang, H. Yu, N. Adler, R., 2007. Molecular dynamics of photoreceptor synapse formation in the developing chick retina. In preparation.

Wahlin, K.J.a.A., R. 2006. Molecular dynamics of photoreceptor synapse formation in the developing chick retina. ARVO abstract # 4182.

Waites, C.L., Craig, A.M., Garner, C.C., 2005. Mechanisms of vertebrate synaptogenesis. Annu Rev Neurosci 28, 251–274.

Wallace, V.A., Jensen, A.M., 1999. IBMX, taurine and 9-cis retinoic acid all act to accelerate rhodopsin expression in postmitotic cells. Exp Eye Res 69, 617–627.

Wang, L., Li, L., Menendez, P., Cerdan, C., Bhatia, M., 2005. Human embryonic stem cells maintained in the absence of mouse embryonic fibroblasts or conditioned media are capable of hematopoietic development. Blood 105, 4598–4603.

Warfvinge, K., Kiilgaard, J.F., Klassen, H., Zamiri, P., Scherfig, E., Streilein, W., Prause, J.U., Young, M.J., 2006. Retinal progenitor cell xenografts to the pig retina: immunological reactions. Cell Transplant 15, 603–612.

Washbourne, P., Dityatev, A., Scheiffele, P., Biederer, T., Weiner, J.A., Christopherson, K.S., El-Husseini, A., 2004. Cell adhesion molecules in synapse formation. J Neurosci 24, 9244–9249.

Witkovsky, P., Thoreson, W., Tranchina, D., 2001. Transmission at the photoreceptor synapse. Prog Brain Res 131, 145–159.

Xie, H.Q., Adler, R., 2000. Green cone opsin and rhodopsin regulation by CNTF and staurosporine in cultured chick photoreceptors. Invest Ophthalmol Vis Sci 41, 4317–4323.

Yan, R.T., Wang, S.Z., 2000. Differential induction of gene expression by basic fibroblast growth factor and neuroD in cultured retinal pigment epithelial cells [In Process Citation]. Vis Neurosci 17, 157–164.

Yoshimura, Y., 2006. Bioethical aspects of regenerative and reproductive medicine. Hum Cell 19, 83–86.

Young, M.J., 2005. Stem cells in the mammalian eye: a tool for retinal repair. Apmis 113, 845–857.

Young, T.L., Cepko, C.L., 2004. A role for ligand-gated ion channels in rod photoreceptor development. Neuron 41, 867–879.

Zhang, S.S., Fu, X.Y., Barnstable, C.J., 2002. Molecular aspects of vertebrate retinal development. Mol Neurobiol 26, 137–152.

Retinal Degenerations: Planning for the Future

Eliot L. Berson

1 Introduction

Retinal degenerations are a leading cause of blindness in many parts of the world (Bunker et al., 1984; Grondahl, 1987; Berson, 1993; Klein et al., 1995; Attebo et al., 1996; Klaver et al., 1998; Novak-Laus et al., 2002). In the United States an estimated 6 million people have age-related macular degeneration with a decrease in central vision after age 60. About 100,000 people have retinitis pigmentosa or a related disease with loss of side and night vision in adolescence; they often develop tunnel vision by age 40 and lose central vision by age 60. Some 20% of patients with retinitis pigmentosa have associated hearing loss and this combination is called Usher syndrome. With increased life expectancy, the problem posed by these conditions is magnified, as affected individuals will have to endure more years of visual loss unless new treatments are found. This plenary lecture provides an overview of clinical findings and molecular genetic abnormalities in these diseases and reviews current treatments for these conditions. Selected studies of animal models of retinal degenerations will be summarized. Some proposed future therapies for human retinal degenerations will also be considered.

2 Human Retinal Degenerations: Some Clinical Findings

Fundus photographs are illustrated from patients with some forms of retinal degeneration (Fig. 1). Patients with the dry form of age-related macular degeneration have white deposits called drusen and eventual atrophy. Patients with the wet or leaky form of age-related macular degeneration show a disturbance in the appearance of the macula with hemorrhages, exudates, and scarring. Most patients with age-related macular degeneration have the dry form, but about 8% of those with the dry form

E.L. Berson
Berman-Gund Laboratory for the Study of Retinal Degenerations, Harvard Medical School, Massachusetts Eye and Ear Infirmary, 243 Charles Street, Boston, Massachusetts 02114,
Tel: 617-573-3600, Fax: 617-573-3216
e-mail: Linda_Berard@meei.harvard.edu

R.E. Anderson et al. (eds.), *Recent Advances in Retinal Degeneration,*
© Springer 2008

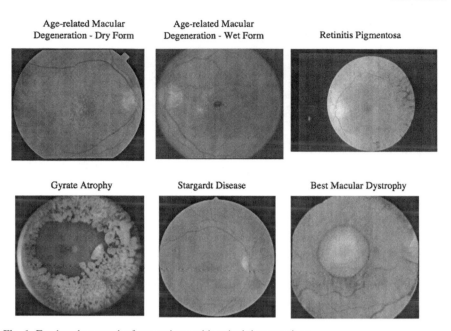

Fig. 1 Fundus photographs from patients with retinal degenerations

develop the more devastating wet form each year. Patients with retinitis pigmentosa develop pigment in a bone spicule configuration around the midperipheral retina for which the condition was named. Gyrate atrophy of the choroid and retina, a related night-blinding disorder, is characterized by areas of atrophy around the periphery that proceed toward the macula with eventual blindness often by age 50. Macular degeneration can also affect children. For example, one form called Stargardt disease results in a disturbance of macular pigmentation that can lead to visual decline by age 10. Another form called Best macular dystrophy shows a central egg-yolk like deposit that can rupture in some cases with a dramatic decline in central vision. Although these diseases appear clinically distinct on fundus examination, all affect cone and rod photoreceptors as well as the underlying retinal pigment epithelium; therefore, research on any one of them could enhance the understanding of the cellular mechanisms involved in the others.

Most retinal degenerations affect both cones and rods. To understand these conditions, it is important to know how the cones and rods are distributed across the retina and their role in vision. The cones are normally in highest concentration in the central retina or macula but cones are present across the peripheral retina as well (Fig. 2) (Osterberg, 1935). More than 90% of the cones are outside the central 10 degrees. Cones allow us sharp visual acuity and full side vision in color. Rods are also present across the retina except in the central macula and the highest concentration of rods is located 20–40 degrees eccentric to the foveola. Rods allow us to see large letters and provide us with a full visual field in shades of gray. Whereas the cones allow us to see under daylight conditions, the rods permit us to see under moonlight or starlight

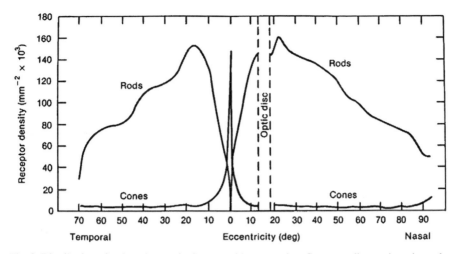

Fig. 2 Distribution of rods and cones in the normal human retina. Corresponding perimetric angles from the fovea at 0° are given. (After Osterberg from Pirenne MH: *Vision and the eye*, London. Chapman and Hall, 1967)

conditions. The normal human retina has over 100 million rods and 7 million cones. In the case of macular degeneration, both the macular cones and macular rods are compromised. In the case of retinitis pigmentosa or gyrate atrophy, both rods and cones across all or nearly all the retina are affected in the early stages as monitored by full-field electroretinograms (ERGs) (Berson, 1993).

Some hereditary retinal diseases selectively affect cone or rod function across the entire retina. For example, patients with congenital achromatopsia, who are born without color vision, have reduced cone function but retain normal rod function for their entire lives. Patients with congenital stationary night blindness are born with rod malfunction but retain normal or nearly normal cone function for their entire lives. It is important to note that these patients with stationary night blindness do not develop rod degeneration. In contrast, patients with retinitis pigmentosa develop rod degeneration and eventually cone degeneration as well. These findings lead to the conclusion that rods can live without cones but cones cannot live without rods. Why do we have a rod-dominant retina when we function most of the time with our cones? The answer has relevance to treating some retinal degenerations and we will return to this question later.

3 Molecular Genetic Abnormalities

Over 100 genes have been implicated in human hereditary retinal degenerations. For the subset of diseases called retinitis pigmentosa, over 45 causative genes have been identified that account for 50–60% of all cases. These genes can be sub-classified based on the known or presumed function of encoded proteins. Genes may affect the phototransduction cascade, vitamin A metabolism, photoreceptor structure, signaling or cell-cell interactions, RNA intron splicing factors, intracellular transport of proteins, maintenance of cilia or ciliated cells with a possible role in intracellular trafficking, regulation of the carbon dioxide-bicarbonate balance, phagocytosis, and other yet to be defined functions of the photoreceptors and pigment epithelium (Hartong et al., 2006). The most common genes causing retinitis pigmentosa are the rhodopsin (*RHO*) gene, the *USH2A* gene, and the retinitis pigmentosa GTPase regulator (*RPGR*) gene, each of which accounts for about 10% of all cases in North America (Hartong et al., 2006). In patients with gyrate atrophy, mutations have been discovered in the ornithine amino transferase (*OAT*) gene that result in a defect in the metabolism of ornithine (Ramesh et al., 1991). A current listing of mutations that cause retinitis pigmentosa and allied hereditary retinal diseases is maintained on the world wide web at *www.sph.uth.tmc.edu/RetNet/*.

With respect to age-related macular degeneration, general agreement exists that this condition is seen more frequently among individuals who have affected relatives, but a causative gene (or genes) has yet to be discovered. A DNA change in a gene encoding complement factor H increases the risk of developing age-related macular degeneration by almost four-fold (Edwards et al., 2005; Haines et al., 2005; Klein et al., 2005). In the case of juvenile macular degeneration, early detection by DNA analysis is now possible for Stargardt disease based on mutations in the *ABCA4* gene (Allikmets et al., 1997; Briggs et al., 2001) and for Best macular dystrophy based on mutations in the Bestrophin gene (Marquardt et al., 1998); although early diagnosis is possible, no treatment is yet known for these conditions.

4 Treatment of Retinal Degenerations

Progress has been made in treating some retinal degenerations. Briefly stated, the dry form of age-related macular degeneration can be slowed with a combination of beta-carotene, vitamin C, vitamin E, zinc, and copper; patients on this regimen have a 25% reduction in the risk of developing advanced macular degeneration (Age-Related Eye Disease Study Research Group, 2001). The wet form can be stabilized by laser therapy (Macular Photocoagulation Study Group, 1993). Intravitreal injections of steroids, Macugen®, Lucentis®, or more recently Avastin have been shown to interfere with blood vessel growth and can either arrest loss of vision or in some cases improve vision (Rosenfeld, 2006; Rosenfeld et al., 2006). Vitamin A palmitate can slow the common forms of retinitis pigmentosa (Berson et al., 1993). Gyrate atrophy, associated with an elevated serum ornithine level, is treatable with a low-protein, low-arginine diet or vitamin B_6 that lower the serum ornithine level toward normal with slowing of progression of the atrophy (Kaiser-Kupfer et al., 1991).

Some rare forms of retinitis pigmentosa have yielded to treatment when initiated at an early stage. Specifically, vitamins A and E have been used successfully to restore and maintain retinal function in hereditary abetalipoproteinemia (i.e. Bassen-Kornzweig disease) in the short term (Gouras et al., 1971; Bishara et al., 1982). Over the long term, some progression has been observed in these patients despite use of vitamin A and vitamin E (Chowers et al., 2001). A low phytol-low phytanic acid diet has resulted in stabilization of retinal function in patients with phytanic acid oxidase deficiency (i.e. Refsum disease) (Refsum, 1981; Hungerbuhler et al., 1985). Vitamin E supplementation has been used to stabilize retinal function in patients with isolated familial vitamin E deficiency (Yokota et al., 1997). In these conditions knowledge of the biochemical abnormalities has led to rational approaches to therapy.

5 Clinical Trials for Retinitis Pigmentosa

The typical forms of hereditary retinitis pigmentosa have been successfully treated with nutritional interventions. While studying the natural course of retinitis pigmentosa (Berson et al., 1985), those patients self-treating with a separate capsule of vitamin A and/or vitamin E showed a smaller decline in ERG amplitude than those taking a multi-vitamin or no vitamin supplement (Berson et al., 1993).The critical intake for a therapeutic effect appeared to be 16,500 IU/day of preformed vitamin A (diet plus supplements). Most patients taking a separate capsule of vitamin A were also taking a separate capsule of vitamin E so that it could not be determined whether one or the other or the combination was potentially therapeutic. No relationship was found between intake of other vitamins and ERG decline in these patients. Based on these preliminary findings, a randomized, controlled, double-masked trial was conducted for 601 patients, aged 18–49 years, from across the United States and Canada. Patients were randomized to 15,000 IU of vitamin A palmitate (Group A), 400 IU of vitamin E as *dl*-alpha-tocopherol (Group E), the two vitamins combined (Group A+E), or a control group receiving trace amounts of both (Group Trace). Patients were followed annually for 4–6 years. The main outcome variable was the full-field 30-Hz cone ERG (Fig. 3). Secondary outcome variables were visual field area with a V-4c white test light on the Goldmann perimeter and ETDRS visual

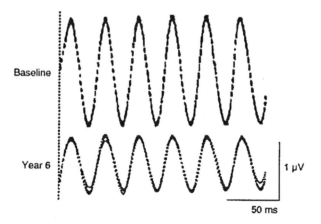

Fig. 3 Narrow bandpassed, computer-averaged full-field cone ERGs in response to 30Hz flashes (n=256 sweeps with 6 responses per sweep) from a representative patient with retinitis pigmentosa at baseline and 6 years after baseline. Three consecutive averages are superimposed. The broken vertical line indicates the onset of the train of flashes. Lower norm = 50 μV, virtual blindness ≤0.05 μV. (From Berson et al., Arch Ophthalmol 111:763, 1993)

acuity. Results were monitored by an independent Data and Safety Monitoring Committee selected by the National Eye Institute (Berson et al., 1993a).

Among all randomized patients those taking vitamin A, 15,000 IU/day, showed a slower rate of decline in remaining cone ERG amplitude than those not on this dose (p=0.01). The vitamin A treatment effect was more significant (p <0.001) in a subset of 354 patients with slightly higher initial cone amplitude (≥0.68 μV), designated as the higher amplitude cohort, who could be followed with greater precision. In this cohort a significant adverse effect (p=0.04) of vitamin E was also observed. Mean decline in 30 Hz ERG amplitude by vitamin A intake showed that the least decline occurred with an intake of about 18,000 IU/day (diet plus supplements) and that higher intake conferred no greater benefit (Fig. 4). No treatment effect could be detected with respect to visual acuity over the time interval of this study (Berson et al., 1993). In a subset of 125 patients who could perform visual fields with great precision, a significant beneficial effect of vitamin A was observed with visual field testing (Berson, 1998).

These results have led to the recommendation that most adults with retinitis pigmentosa should take vitamin A palmitate, 15,000 IU/day, and avoid high doses of vitamin E such as the 400 IU/day used in this trial (Berson et al., 1993a,b; Berson, 1998). Beta-carotene, the precursor of vitamin A, is not predictably converted to vitamin A and, therefore, is not a suitable substitute for vitamin A in the context of this treatment. No significant toxic effects have been observed with this treatment (Sibulesky et al., 1999). This treatment is not recommended for women who are pregnant or planning to become pregnant because of the increased risk of birth defects among patients on high doses of vitamin A. Since high dose vitamin A supplementation has been associated with a slight increase in the risk of hip fracture in post-menopausal women (Feskanich et al., 2002) and men over age 49

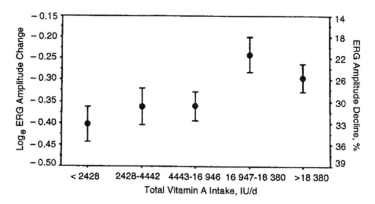

Fig. 4 Mean ± SE decline from baseline in 30Hz ERG amplitude by total vitamin A intake (diet plus capsules) irrespective of randomization assignment for all patients in the higher-amplitude cohort. The mean decline was calculated as the mean of screening and baseline minus the mean of all follow-up visits by quintile of total vitamin A intake averaged over all visits. Sample sizes were n=69, n=72, n=74, n=65, and n=74 for the lowest to highest quintiles of total vitamin A intake. Vertical bars indicate SEs. (From Berson et al. Arch Ophthalmol, 111:769, 1993a)

years (Michaelsson et al., 2003), patients who take this dose of vitamin A should be advised to monitor their bone health.

While conducting the vitamin A trial, an inverse relationship was observed in a subset of these patients between red blood cell docosahexaenoic (RBC DHA) levels and rate of progression of retinitis pigmentosa; those with higher RBC DHA levels had a significantly slower rate of decline in ERG amplitudes than those with lower levels. This led to a second randomized, controlled, double-masked trial of DHA supplementation for retinitis pigmentosa. Two hundred and twenty-one patients, aged 18–55 years, were randomly assigned to either 1200 mg/day of DHA or control fatty acid capsules; all were given 15,000 IU/day of vitamin A as retinyl palmitate. The primary outcome measure was the total point score in the Humphrey Field Analyzer monitored annually with the 30-2 program and a size V white target. Cone ERG amplitudes, ETDRS visual acuities, and combined visual fields (30-2 plus 30/60-1 programs) were assessed annually as secondary outcome measures. This study allowed at least 4 years of follow-up for each patient. Results were monitored by an independent Data and Safety Monitoring Committee selected by the National Eye Institute (Berson et al., 2004).

The primary analyses of the total study population did not reveal, on average, a beneficial effect of DHA, 1200 mg/day, for patients with retinitis pigmentosa on vitamin A over a 4-year interval as monitored by visual field sensitivities, ERG amplitudes, and visual acuities. No toxic effects attributable to DHA or vitamin A were noted (Berson et al., 2004). Subgroup analyses, however, showed that for the patients with retinitis pigmentosa beginning vitamin A therapy for the first time at the beginning of this trial (i.e. 30% of the study population), addition of DHA, 1200 mg/day, slowed the course of disease for 2 years as monitored by visual field sensitivities and cone ERG amplitudes (Table 1). Furthermore, among patients in the control group on vitamin A for at least 2 years (but not on DHA capsules), a diet rich in omega-3 fatty acids (≥ 0.20 grams per day) of which DHA is a major constituent slowed the decline in visual field sensitivity by 40–50% per year (Table 2). In the entire study population red blood cell DHA levels were inversely related to rate of decline in total field sensitivity over 4 years (Berson et al., 2004a).

The lack of a beneficial effect of DHA, 1200 mg/day, on the course of retinal degeneration among adults with typical retinitis pigmentosa on vitamin A precludes any general recommendation of DHA capsules for such patients. However, results from subgroup analyses have led to the recommendation that adults with typical retinitis pigmentosa already taking vitamin A palmitate, 15,000 IU/day, should also eat 1–2 three-ounce servings per week of omega-3 rich fish (salmon, tuna, mackerel, herring, or sardines) of which DHA is a major constituent. About three months after starting this omega-3 rich fish diet, thereby allowing sufficient time for RBC turnover, patients should have a measurement of their fasting RBC DHA through their physician to confirm that the RBC DHA level is at least 4% of total RBC fatty acids, as such patients have, on average, a slower rate of decline of visual field sensitivity than those with lower levels. With respect to adults starting vitamin A for the first time, they should also take DHA capsules 600 mg twice each day for 2 years to shorten the interval for vitamin A to achieve its benefit. After two years they should continue vitamin A palmitate, 15,000 IU/day, stop the DHA capsules

Table 1 Annual rate of decline for measures of ocular function by treatment group and vitamin A status prior to entry over a 4-year interval

	On vitamin A prior to entry		
	DHA + A	Control + A	P†
HFA 30-2 field, dB/y	39.41 ± 3.76 (74)	30.26 ± 3.93 (68)	.09
HFA total field, dB/y‡	61.01 ± 5.17 (74)	48.13 ± 5.39 (68)	.08
30-Hz ERG, log$_e$	0.11 ± 0.01 (75)	0.10 ± 0.01 (67)	.34
% Decline per year §	10.57	9.23	
ETDRS visual acuity letters per year	0.67 ± 0.13 (75)	0.68 ± 0.14 (68)	.96

	Not on vitamin A prior to entry		
	DHA + A	Control + A	P†
HFA 30-2 field, dB/y	30.70 ± 6.48 (29)	52.50 ± 5.99 (34)	.01
HFA total field, dB/y‡	47.16 ± 10.56 (28)	82.49 ± 9.58 (34)	.01
30-Hz ERG, log$_e$	0.08 ± 0.02 (26)	0.14 ± 0.02 (33)	.03
% Decline per year §	8.05	12.99	
ETDRS visual acuity letters per year	0.82 ± 0.26 (29)	0.69 ± 0.24 (34)	.70

Unless otherwise indicated, data expressed are means ± SE; numbers of patients sampled are designated in parentheses. Patients received either 1200 mg/d of docosahexaenoic acid plus 15,000 IU/d of vitamin A (DHA + A) or control capsules plus 15,000 IU/d of vitamin A (control + A). †P value calculated from PROC MIXED (SAS Institute Inc, Cary, NC) analysis comparing rates of decline in both treatment groups. ‡Total field sensitivity consists of 30-2 and 30/60-1 total point scores combined when both are available. § Derived from 100 x [1-exp(mean log change)]. Significant statistical interactions between the effect of DHA and whether or not patients were on vitamin A prior to entry were observed for HFA 30-2 field (P=.002), HFA total field (P=.001), and 30-Hz ERG (P=.02) (From Berson et al., Arch Ophthalmol 122:1308, 2004)

Table 2 Annual decline in visual field sensitivity in the control group as a function of dietary ω-3 fatty acid intake among patients on vitamin A prior to entry

Dietary ω-3 Intake	Years 0 to 4	Years 0 to 2	Years 2 to 4
30-2 Condition, dB			
<0.20 g/d	39.2 ± 5.5 (35)	32.9 ± 8.2 (35)	44.5 ± 7.5 (35)
≥ 0.20g/d	20.8 ± 5.7 (33)	14.3 ± 8.4 (33)	20.1 ± 7.7 (33)
P value ‡	.02	.12	.03
Total condition, dB §			
<0.20 g/d	57.8 ± 7.0 (35)	44.7 ± 12.4 (35)	72.9 ± 10.5 (35)
≥ 0.20g/d	37.9 ± 7.2 (33)	25.0 ± 12.7 (33)	39.3 ± 10.8 (33)
P value ‡	.05	.27	.03

Unless otherwise indicated, data expressed are means ± SE; numbers of patients sampled are designated in parentheses. Patients in the Control group received control capsules plus 15,000 IU/d of vitamin A. †Expressed as the mean of grams per day of all visits. ‡Based on PROC MIXED (SAS Institute Inc, Cary, NC) analysis comparing rates of decline in high versus low omega-3 fatty acid intake groups. § Total condition consists of the sum of 30-2 and 30/60-1 conditions when both are available. (From Berson et al., Arch Ophthalmol 122:1310, 2004b)

(because a slight tendency toward adversity over the long-term has been observed among patients concurrently on vitamin A), and also eat 1–2 three-ounce servings of omega-3 rich fish each week. They should then have a measurement of fasting RBC DHA through their physician three months later to be certain that the level is at least 4% of total RBC fatty acids. It has been estimated that the combination of vitamin A palmitate with an oily fish diet, on average, could provide almost 20 additional years of vision for the average patient who starts this regimen in their mid-thirties (Berson et al., 2004a).

It is remarkable that treatment with a single vitamin, namely vitamin A, has proven to be beneficial on average for patients with retinitis pigmentosa even though they are losing vision due to many different gene defects. To help explain this, we return to the question raised earlier, namely why do we have a rod-dominant retina when we function most of the time with our cones? Why are we using only 7% of our photoreceptors, namely our cones, to look at each other in this room; what are our rods doing under daylight conditions?

We know that both cones and rods are activated by light. The cone signal arrives first at the optic nerve and we see each other in color. The rod response to light is not wasted as the rods, in response to light, expel a twisted form of vitamin A, namely all-trans-retinol, that is reconfigured by nearby support cells called Müller cells. The reconfigured vitamin A, that is, 11-cis-retinol, is then transported to cones which contain a dehydrogenase; the cones have the capacity to further convert the vitamin A from 11-cis-retinol to 11-cis-retinal (Mata et al., 2002), the form needed for visual excitation. Therefore, one can hypothesize that under daylight conditions rods are giving cones vitamin A via Müller cells. Interphotoreceptor retinoid binding protein (IRBP) transports vitamin A between these cells and from the pigment epithelium to these cells as well. Release of vitamin A from IRBP requires DHA (Wolf, 1998), which is present in high concentration in an oily fish diet. Rod degeneration results in a retinal deficiency of vitamin A and DHA in retinitis pigmentosa, so that vitamin A plus an oily fish diet is needed to rescue remaining cones in this condition.

Taking into account this relationship between rods and cones and the fact that most forms of retinitis pigmentosa result in a final common pathway of predominant loss of rods among remaining cones, we can explain why vitamin A benefits so many patients with retinitis pigmentosa even though they are losing vision from different gene defects. Vitamin E appears to inhibit the absorption and transport of vitamin A resulting in decreased vitamin A levels in serum and presumably the retina as well; this provides an explanation for the adverse effect of vitamin E on this condition (Berson et al., 1993).

6 Studies of Animal Models of Retinal Degenerations

To understand and treat human retinal degenerations, a generally accepted plan is to find the causes of these diseases, produce these diseases in animal models, treat the animal models, and, where possible, conduct controlled clinical trials to determine whether a disease can be reversed, stabilized, or slowed in affected humans. Another therapeutic strategy is to replace the missing or abnormal photoreceptor cells or pigment epithelial cells or induce other cells in the retina to substitute for photoreceptors. Another approach is an epidemiological one; risk factor analyses of well-defined populations are performed in search of ameliorating or aggravating factors as a lead in determining possible treatments for these conditions.

Nutritional intervention with vitamin A has been evaluated in transgenic mice with rhodopsin gene defects. Specifically, mice with rhodopsin, T17M, fed a high vitamin A diet for 4 months, were found to have an outer nuclear layer that was twice as thick as that of mice fed a standard diet (Fig. 5). Furthermore, the ERG in a T17M mouse raised on a high vitamin A diet was twice as large at four months compared with the ERG from a T17M mouse on a standard diet. Stated simply, high vitamin A in the diet saved retinal structure and function in this model, and these results support the observations in humans with retinitis pigmentosa. This effect was not seen in mice with rhodopsin, P347S (Li et al., 1998). In the clinical trial of vitamins A and E, 44 patients were subsequently found to have rhodopsin mutations and vitamin A was found, on average, to have a therapeutic effect in this subgroup as monitored by the ERG, but there were insufficient patients to subdivide further this subgroup into class I (e.g. P347S) and class II (e.g. T17M) mutations. Subtracting the patients with rhodopsin mutations from the entire data set in the trial of vitamins A and E, the treatment effect of vitamin A was still significant at the p=0.01 level. Furthermore, in every subgroup analysis performed in this trial (i.e. different genetic types, older versus younger) the trend was toward benefit, so it does not appear that any one subgroup was driving the overall treatment effect of vitamin A for retinitis pigmentosa.

With respect to gene therapy, research on a canine model with an inherited RPE65 deficiency and retinal degeneration has shown that this inherited abnormality can be treated by single dose rAAV-mediated transfer of the RPE65 gene in the retina, setting a precedent for a similar attempt at therapy in humans with this gene

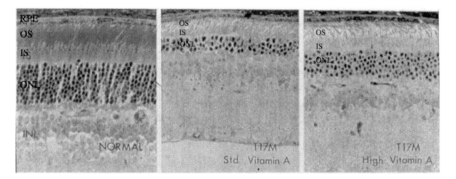

Fig. 5 Mice with a rhodopsin, T17M mutation on a high vitamin A diet for 4 months (right photo) have an outer nuclear layer (ONL) that is twice as thick as that of T17M mice on a standard vitamin A diet (middle photo). The retina from a normal mouse on a standard diet is illustrated for comparison (left photo). (Modified from Li et al., Proc Natl Acad Sci USA, 95:11936, 1998)

defect and Leber congenital amaurosis (Acland et al., 2005). Some of the genes known to cause retinitis pigmentosa have been destroyed or "knocked-out" in mice and these mice have then developed retinal degenerations. For example, knock-out of the RPGRIP gene in mice causes severe photoreceptor degeneration (Fig. 6, middle) as observed in humans with this gene defect that causes another form of Leber congenital amaurosis (Pawlyk et al., 2005). The RPGRIP knock-out or "KO" mouse has been treated by injecting a RPGRIP gene under the retina at age 1 month. At age 4 months the KO mouse that received gene therapy (Fig. 6, upper right) shows that the outer nuclear layer (ONL), containing primarily rod photoreceptors, is twice as thick as that in the KO control mouse (Fig. 6, upper middle). Comparing the lower right photograph with the lower middle photograph in Fig. 6, one can see that gene therapy has also resulted in a restoration of the organized layered structure of the photoreceptor outer segments (designated by the symbol OS) compared to the disorganization seen in the KO control mouse (Pawlyk et al., 2005). Work is in progress

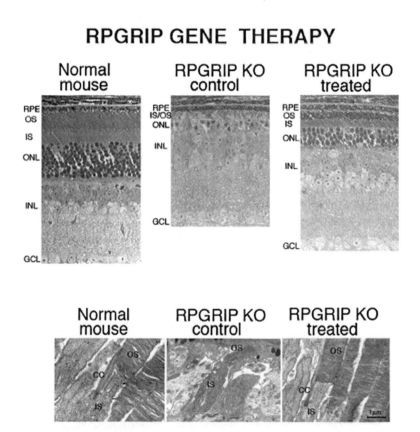

Fig. 6 Gene replacement therapy rescues photoreceptor generation in a knockout (KO) murine model of Leber congenital amaurosis lacking RPGRIP (i.e. retinitis pigmentosa GTP-ase regulator interacting protein). (Modified from Pawlyk et al., Invest Ophthalmol Vis Sci, 46:3042, 2005)

Table 3 Treatment strategies in animal models of retinal degenerations

(1)	Gene replacement therapy (for recessive gene mutations)
(2)	Ribozyme-based or RNAi based therapy (for dominant gene mutations)
(3)	Nutritional interventions
(4)	Neurotrophic or growth factors
(5)	Treatments with small molecules (e.g. aminoglycosides)
(6)	Light deprivation
(7)	Stem cell therapy
(8)	Inhibitors of apoptosis (e.g. caspase inhibitors)
(9)	Channel blockers
(10)	Retinal and or RPE transplantation
(11)	Non-viral gene therapy using nanoparticle technology

to see if cones can be rescued in this animal model in preparation for a trial of gene therapy for photoreceptors in children with this form of Leber congenital amaurosis.

Some treatment strategies for animal models of retinal degenerations are listed (Table 3) (Hartong et al., 2006). Gene replacement for recessive mutations and RNAi-based therapy, sometimes referred to as "gene silencing", for dominant mutations are of current interest. Nutritional interventions should continue to be explored. Neurotrophic factors, small molecule therapies such as aminoglycosides, and stem cell therapy have precedent of success in treating animal models or human disease. Light deprivation and inhibitors of apoptosis also deserve further study in animal models with known gene abnormalities. Channel blockers such as D-cis-diltiazem have so far not been shown to be beneficial. Retina and/or retinal pigment epithelial cell transplantation are also of theoretical interest and therefore deserve research. Nanoparticle technology has been recently described as a non-viral approach for gene transfer to ocular tissues (Farjo et al., 2006). Extending some of these studies to humans presents considerable challenges as any treatment modality proposed must not only be effective but must also be safe. In the case of gene therapy, it may be difficult to introduce genes under the retina in retinitis pigmentosa because of adhesions of the retina to the pigment epithelium in more advanced stages of this condition; moreover this approach may not prove effective in patients who no longer have rod or cone photoreceptor cells to accept gene transfection.

7 Future Treatments for Human Retinal Degenerations

With respect to the future for human retinal degenerations, some imminent new therapies hold promise for different retinal degenerations. A trial of lutein, zeaxanthine, and DHA supplementation is being considered for age-related macular degeneration. Light deprivation and pharmacologic interruption of the vitamin A cycle are possible treatments for Stargardt disease. Gene therapy is being considered for children with early stages of severe forms of retinitis pigmentosa, such as Leber congenital amaurosis and Usher syndrome, type IB, as well as for Stargardt disease. Studies in animal models and a phase I study in humans support the proposal that neuroprotective agents such as ciliary neurotrophic factor (CNTF) may stabilize retinitis pigmentosa (Sieving et al., 2006).

Other proposed therapies include optical devices to allow patients improved mobility despite constricted fields and visual prosthetic devices (such as the light-sensitive microchip) for advanced degenerations. Stem cell mediated therapy is being considered for macular degeneration or retinitis pigmentosa. It may also be possible to replace defective retinal pigment epithelium with transplanted normal pigment epithelium or stem cells and thereby benefit some patients with these conditions. For patients with advanced photoreceptor degeneration, studies are underway in an animal model of advanced disease to see if ganglion cells can be induced through gene transfection to produce melanopsin and thereby respond to light and transmit information to the brain that would allow perception of forms (Shang et al., 2007). Risk factor analyses combined with molecular genetic findings may reveal additional factors that could slow the course of these conditions with possible implications for therapy. Clearly much work remains to be done and the opportunities for rational investigations are enormous.

The scientific progress already made should encourage more investigators to enter the field of retinal degenerations. Many opportunities exist for rational laboratory studies particularly since animal models of human conditions can now be created by gene targeting manipulations. The expansion of knowledge with respect to causes and pathogenesis has created new opportunities for therapeutic interventions. Collaborations between scientists and clinicians should enhance the likelihood of developing new treatments for these diseases.

Acknowledgments This work was supported in part by National Eye Institute grant EY00169 and in part by the Foundation Fighting Blindness.

References

Acland, G.M., Aguirre, G.D., Bennett, J., Aleman, T.S., Cideciyan, A.V., Bennicelli, J., Dejneka, N.S., Pearce-Kelling, S.E., Maguire, A.M., Palczewski, K., Hauswirth, W.W., Jacobson, S.G., 2005, Long-term restoration of rod and cone vision by single dose rAAV-mediated gene transfer in the retina in a canine model of childhood blindness. *Mol. Ther.* **12**, 1072–1082.

Age-Related Eye Disease Study Research Group, 2001, A randomized, placebo-controlled, clinical trial of high-dose supplementation with vitamins C and E, beta-carotene, and zinc for age-related macular degeneration and vision loss: AREDS Report No. 8. *Arch. Ophthalmol.* **119**, 1417–1436.

Allikmets, R., Singh, N., Sun, H., Shroyer, N.F., Hutchinson, A., Chidambaram, A., Gerrard, B., Baird, L., Stauffer, D., Peiffer, A., Rattner, A., Smallwood, P., Li, Y., Anderson, K.L., Lewis, R.A., Nathans, J., Leppert, M., Dean, M., Lupski, J.R., 1997, A photoreceptor cell-specific ATP-binding transporter gene (ABCR) is mutated in recessive Stargardt macular dystrophy. *Nat. Genet.* **15**, 236–246.

Attebo, K., Mitchell, P., Smith, S., 1996, Visual acuity and the causes of visual loss in Australia: the Blue Mountains Eye Study. *Ophthalmology* **103**, 357–364.

Berson, E.L. Retinitis pigmentosa. The Friedenwald Lecture., 1993, *Invest. Ophthalmol. Vis. Sci.* **34**, 1659–1676.

Berson. E.L., 1998, Treatment of retinitis pigmentosa with vitamin A. Proceedings of the Fern-ström Symposium on Tapetoretinal Degenerations, Lund, Sweden. *Digital J. Ophthalmol.* 4(2), (http://www.djo.harvard.edu/meei/|OA/RPB/RPB.html).

Berson, E.L., Rosner, B., Sandberg, M.A., Hayes, K.C., Nicholson, B.W., Weigel-DiFranco, C., Willett, W., 1993a, A randomized trial of vitamin A and vitamin E supplementation for retinitis pigmentosa. *Arch. Ophthalmol.* **111**, 761–772.

Berson, E.L., Rosner, B., Sandberg, M.A., Hayes, K.C., Nicholson, B.W., Weigel-DiFranco, C., Willett, W., 1993b, Vitamin A supplementation for retinitis pigmentosa. *Arch. Ophthalmol.* **111**, 1456–1459.

Berson, E.L., Rosner, B., Sandberg, M.A., Weigel-DiFranco, C., Moser, A., Brockhurst, R.J., Hayes, K.C., Johnson, C.A., Anderson, E.J., Gaudio, A.R., Willett, W.C., Schaefer. E.J., 2004a, Clinical trial of docosahexaenoic acid in patients with retinitis pigmentosa receiving vitamin A treatment. *Arch. Ophthalmol.* **122**, 1297–1305.

Berson, E.L., Rosner, B., Sandberg, M.A., Weigel-DiFranco, C., Moser, A., Brockhurst, R.J., Hayes, K.C., Johnson, C.A., Anderson, E.J., Gaudio, A.R., Willett, W.C., Schaefer, E.J., 2004b, Further evaluation of docosahexaenoic acid in patients with retinitis pigmentosa receiving vita-min A treatment: Subgroup analyses. *Arch. Ophthalmol.* **122**, 1306–1314.

Berson, E.L., Sandberg, M.A., Rosner, B., Birch, D.G., Hanson, A.H., 1985, Natural course of retinitis pigmentosa over a three-year interval. *Am. J. Ophthalmol.* **99**, 240–251.

Bishara, S., Merin, S., Cooper, M., 1982, Combined vitamin A and E therapy prevents retinal electrophysiological deterioration in abetalipoproteinemia. *Br. J. Ophthalmol.* **66**, 767–770.

Briggs, C.E., Rucinski, D., Rosenfeld, P.J., Hirose, T., Berson, E.L., Dryja, T.P., 2001, Mutations in *ABCR (ABCA4)* in patients with Stargardt macular degeneration or cone-rod degeneration. *Invest. Ophthalmol. Vis. Sci.* **43**(10), 2229–2236.

Bunker, C.H., Berson, E.L., Bromley, W.C., Hayes, R.P., Roderick, T.H., 1984, Prevalence of retinitis pigmentosa in Maine. *Am. J. Ophthalmol.* **97**, 357–365.

Chowers, I., Banin, E., Merin, S., Cooper, M., Granot, E., 2001, Long-term assessment of com-bined vitamin A and E treatment for the prevention of retinal degeneration in abetalipoproteine-mia and hypobetalipoproteinaemia patients. *Eye* **15**, 525–630.

Edwards, A.O., Ritter, R., Abel, K.J., Manning, A., Panhuysen, C., Farrer, L.A., 2005, Complement factor H polymorphism and age-related macular degeneration. *Science* **308**, 421–424.

Farjo, R., Skaggs, J., Quiambao, A.B., Cooper, M.J., Naash, M.I., 2006, Efficient non-viral ocular gene transfer with compacted DNA nanoparticles. *PLoS One*, Dec 20, 1:e38.

Feskanich, D., Singh, V., Willett, W.C., Colditz, G.A., 2002, Vitamin A intake and hip fractures among postmenopausal women. *JAMA* **287**, 47–54.

Gouras, P., Carr, R.E., Gunkel, R.D., 1971, Retinitis pigmentosa in abetalipoproteinemia: Effects of vitamin A. *Invest. Ophthalmol. Vis. Sci.* **10**, 784–793.

Grondahl, J., 1987, Estimation of prognosis and prevalence of retinitis pigmentosa and Usher syn-drome in Norway. *Clin. Genet.* **31**, 255–264.

Haines, J.L., Hauser, M.A., Schmidt, S., Scott, W.K., Olson, L.M., Gallins, P., Spencer, K.L., Kwan, S.Y., Noureddine, M., Gilbert, J.R., Schnetz-Boutaud, N., Agarwal, A., Postel, E.A., Pericak-Vance, M.A., 2005, Complement factor H variant increases the risk of age-related macular degeneration. *Science* 308:419–421.

Hartong, D.T., Berson, E.L., Dryja, T.P., 2006, Retinitis pigmentosa. *Lancet*, Seminar Series **368**, 1795–1809.

Hungerbuhler, J.P., Meier, C., Rousselle, L., Quadri, P., Bogousslavsky, J., 1985, Refsum's disease: management by diet and plasmapheresis. *Eur. Neurol.* **41**, 826–832.

Kaiser-Kupfer, M.I., Caruso, R.C., Valle, D., 1991, Gyrate atrophy of the choroid and retina. Long-term reduction of ornithine slows retinal degeneration. *Arch. Ophthalmol.* **109**, 1539–1548.

Klaver, C.C., Wolfs, R.C., Vingerling, J.R., Hofman, A., deJong P.T., 1998, Age-specific preva-lence and causes of blindness and visual impairment in an older population: the Rotterdam Study. *Arch. Ophthalmol.* **116**, 653–658.

Klein, R., Wang, Q., Klein, B.E.K., Moss, S.E., Meuer, S.M., 1995, The relationship of age-related maculopathy, cataract, and glaucoma to visual acuity. *Invest. Ophthalmol. Vis. Sci.* **36**, 183–191.

Klein, R.J., Zeiss, C., Chew, E.Y., Tsai, J.-Y., Sackler, R.S., Haynes, C., Henning, A.K., SanGiovanni, J.P., Mane, S.M., Mayne, S.T., Bracken, M.B., Ferris, F.L., Ott, J., Barnstable, C., Hoh, J., 2005, Complement factor H polymorphism in age-related macular degeneration. *Science* **308**, 385–389.

Li, T., Sandberg, M.A., Pawlyk, B.S., Rosner, B., Hayes, K.C., Dryja, T.P., Berson, E.L., 1998, Effect of vitamin A supplementation on rhodopsin mutants threonine-17-methionine and proline-347-serine in transgenic mice and in cell cultures. *Proc. Natl. Acad. Sci. U.S.A.* **95**, 11933–11938.

Macular Photocoagulation Study Group, 1993, Laser photocoagulation for subfoveal lesions of age-related macular degeneration: updated findings from two clinical trials. *Arch. Ophthalmol.* **111**, 1200–1209.

Marquardt, A., Stohr, H., Passmore, L.A., Kramer, F., Rivera, A., Weber, B.H., 1998, Mutations in a novel gene, VMD2, encoding a protein of unknown properties cause juvenile-onset vitellifrom macular dystrophy (Best's disease). *Hum. Mol. Genet.* **7**(9), 1517–1525.

Mata, N.L., Radu, R.A., Clemmons, R.C., Travis, G.H., 2002, Isomerization and oxidation of vitamin a in cone-dominant retinas: a novel pathway for visual-pigment regeneration in daylight. *Neuron* **36**(1), 69–80.

Michaelsson, K., Lithell, H., Vessby, B., Melhus, H., 2003, Serum retinol levels and the risk of fracture. *N. Engl. J. Med.* **348**, 287–294.

Novak-Laus, K., Suzana-Kukulj, S., Zoric-Geber, M., Bastaic, O., 2002, Primary tapetoretinal dystrophies as the cause of blindness and impaired vision in the republic of Croatia. *Acta Clin. Croat.* **41**, 23–27.

Osterberg, G., 1935, Topography of the layer of rods and cones in the human retina. *Acta Ophthalmol.* **6**(Suppl), 1.

Pawlyk, B., Smith, A.J., Buch, P.K., Adamian, M., Hong, D., Ali, R.R., Sandberg, M.A., Li, T., 2005, Gene replacement therapy rescues photoreceptor degeneration in a murine model of Leber congenital amaurosis lacking RPGRIP. *Invest. Ophthalmol. Vis. Sci.* **46**, 3039–3045.

Ramesh, V., Gusella, J.F., Shih, V.E., 1991, Molecular pathology of gyrate atrophy of the choroid and retina due to ornithine aminotransferase deficiency. *Mol. Biol. Med.* **8**(1), 81–93.

Refsum, S., 1981, Heredopathia atactica poly neuritiformis, phytanic acid storage disease. Refsum's disease: A biochemically well-defined disease with a specific dietary treatment. *Arch. Neurol.* **38**, 605–606.

Rosenfeld, P.J., 2006, Intravitreal Avastin: the low cost alternative to Lucentis? *Am. J. Ophthalmol.* **142**(1), 141–143.

Rosenfeld, P.J., Brown, D.M., Heier, J.S., Boyer, D.S., Kaiser, P.K., Chung, C.Y., Kim, R.Y., 2006, MARINA Study Group. Ranibizumab for neovascular age-related macular degeneration. *N. Engl. J. Med.* **355**(14), 1419–1431.

Shang, Y., Meister, M., Pawlyk, B.S., Bulgakov, O.V., Li, T., Sandberg, M.A., 2007, Responses of intrinsically-photosensitive retinal ganglion cells after melanopsin-gene transfection. ARVO abstract.

Sibulesky, L., Hayes, K.C., Pronczuk, A., Weigel-DiFranco, C., Rosner, B., Berson, E.L., 1999, Safety of less than 7,500 RE/day (25,000 IU/day) of vitamin A in adults with retinitis pigmentosa. *Amer. J. Clin. Nutr.* **69**, 656–663.

Sieving, P.A., Caruso, R.C., Tao, W., Coleman, H.R., Thompson, D.J., Fullmer, K.R., Bush, R.A., 2006, Ciliary neurotrophic factor (CNTF) for human retinal degeneration: phase I trial of CNTF delivered by encapsulated cell intraocular implants. *Proc. Natl. Acad. Sci. U.S.A.* **103**, 3896–3901.

Wolf, G., 1998, Transport of retinoids by the interphotoreceptor retinoid-binding protein. *Nutr. Rev.* **56**, 156–158.

Yokota, T., Shiojiri, T., Gotoda, T., Arita, M., Arai, H., Ohga, T., Kanda, T., Suzuki, J., Imai, T., Matsumoto, S., Harino, H., Kiyosawa, M., Mizusawa, H., 1997, Friedreich-like ataxia with retinitis pigmentosa caused by the His101Gln mutation of the alpha-tocopherol transfer protein gene. *Ann. Neurol.* **41**, 826–832.

Part II
Neuroprotection

Neurotrophins Induce Neuroprotective Signaling in the Retinal Pigment Epithelial Cell by Activating the Synthesis of the Anti-inflammatory and Anti-apoptotic Neuroprotectin D1

Nicolas G. Bazan

1 Summary

The integrity of retinal pigment epithelial cells is critical for photoreceptor cell survival and vision. The essential omega-3 fatty acid, docosahexaenoic acid, attains its highest concentration in the human body in photoreceptors. Docosahexaenoic acid is the essential precursor of neuroprotectin D1 (NPD1). NPD1 acts against apoptosis mediated by A2E, a byproduct of phototransduction that becomes toxic when it accumulates in aging retinal pigment epithelial (RPE) cells and in some inherited retinal degenerations. Here we also describe that neurotrophins, mainly pigment epithelium-derived factor, induce NPD1 synthesis and its polarized apical secretion, suggesting paracrine and autocrine bioactivity of this lipid mediator. In addition, DHA elicits a concentration-dependent and selective potentiation of pigment epithelial-derived factor-stimulated NPD1 synthesis and release through the apical RPE cell surface. The bioactivity of signaling activated by PEDF and DHA demonstrates synergistic cytoprotection when cells were challenged with oxidative stress, resulting in concomitant NPD1 synthesis. Also, DHA and PEDF synergistically activate anti-apoptotic protein expression and decreased pro-apoptotic Bcl-2 protein expression and caspase 3 activation during oxidative stress. Thus, DHA-derived NPD1 protects against RPE cell damage mediated by aging/disease-induced A2E accumulation. Also, neurotrophins are regulators of NPD1 synthesis and of its polarized apical efflux from RPE cells. Therefore, NPD1 may elicit autocrine and paracrine bioactivity in cells located in the proximity of the interphotoreceptor matrix.

N.G. Bazan
Louisiana State University Health Sciences Center, Neuroscience Center of Excellence and Department of Ophthalmology, 2020 Gravier Street, Suite D, New Orleans, LA 70112, USA,
Tel: 504-599-0832, Fax: 504-568-5801
email: nbazab@Isuhsc.edu

R.E. Anderson et al. (eds.), *Recent Advances in Retinal Degeneration*,
© Springer 2008

2 Introduction

Phospholipids, enriched with docosahexaenoyl chains (22:6, n-3), and the photo-transduction molecular components are assembled at the base of the photoreceptor cell outer segment (Rodriguez de Turco et al., 1997). The oldest photoreceptor disks, at the tip of the photoreceptor, are then shed and phagocytized by the retinal pigment epithelial (RPE) cells. The RPE cells supply the photoreceptors with nutrients, including all-trans retinol, the precursor to the visual pigment chromophore for vision and docosahexaenoic acid (DHA), from the essential fatty acid family of the omega-3 series. Both are continuously recycled between the RPE and the cone and photoreceptor cells (Bazan, 2006). The RPE cell also secretes neurotrophins that are necessary for photoreceptor and RPE cell survival (Hu and Bok, 2001; LaVail et al., 1992; LaVail et al., 1998; Politi et al., 2001; Valter et al., 2005).

3 A2E-Mediated RPE Cell Apoptosis is Attenuated by NPD1

We have further investigated the A2E-mediated RPE cell damage. This bispyridinium bisretinoid is a byproduct of phototransduction that becomes toxic when it accumulates in RPE cells as a lipofuscin component. A2E accumulation in RPE cells occurs during aging (Bui et al., 2006; Cideciyan et al., 2004; Radu et al., 2004; Sparrow et al., 2003) in animal models of age-related macular degeneration as well as in the disease itself (Bui et al., 2006; Cideciyan et al., 2004; Radu et al., 2004).

As a result of A2E accumulation, RPE cells undergo apoptosis preceding photoreceptor cell dysfunction and death (Cideciyan et al., 2004). A2E (20 μM), added to ARPE-19 cells in the presence of light and O_2, was converted into oxiranes (epoxides) (Radu et al., 2004; Sparrow et al., 2003) and promoted apoptosis (Mukherjee et al., 2007). NPD1 was cytoprotective against A2E-induced ARPE-19 cell apoptosis, displaying a wide window of cytoprotection after A2E addition. NPD1 (50 nM), even 6 hrs after A2E, exerted cytoprotection. Moreover, the involvement of Bcl-2 proteins suggests that NPD1 action target the premitochondrial stage of the apoptotic cascade. The extended NPD1 window of protection indicates that the attenuation of the apoptotic cascade targets committed cell death events only relatively late upon exposure of the cells to A2E/oxiranes.

4 Neurotrophins are Activators of the Synthesis and Apical NPD1 Release from RPE Cells

Neurotrophins participate in photoreceptor survival (LaVail et al., 1992; LaVail et al., 1998; Politi et al., 2001; Valter et al., 2005). Using human RPE cells grown to confluence and a high degree of differentiation displaying apical-basolateral polarization (Hu and Bok, 2001), we have found that neurotrophins are NPD1 synthesis agonists (Mukherjee et al., 2007). Figure 1 illustrates neurotrophin (PEDF)-mediated NPD1 synthesis and bioactivity. These studies also allowed

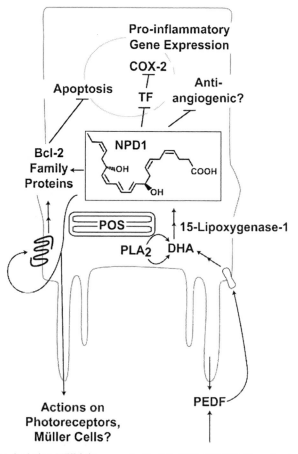

Fig. 1 Illustration depicting NPD1 (neuroprotectin D1, 10S, 17S-DHA) synthesis and bioactivity. Neurotrophins, mainly PEDF (pigment epithelium-derived factor) are NPD1 synthesis agonists in primary RPE cells in culture (Mukherjee et al., 2007). Arrows indicate that PEDF may be secreted from the RPE cell or be derived from another cell. A putative PEDF receptor is indicated. A PLA_2 (phospholipase A_2) that mediates the cleavage of docosahexaenoyl chains from phospholipids located in RPE membranes and/or phagocytized photoreceptor membranes (POS, photoreceptor outer segment) is illustrated. Likely, a very specific pool of DHA-containing phospholipids is the precursor of docosanoids. A 15-lipoxygenase-1-like enzyme mediates NPD1 synthesis. Because PEDF has antiangiogenic properties, it is likely that NPD1-evoked synthesis by this neurotrophin may participate in this process. NPD1 potently downregulates IL-1β-induced COX-2 expression (Mukherjee et al., 2004) as well as other proinflammatory genes (Lukiw et al., 2005). NPD1 action on Bcl-2 proteins may be mediated by an autocrine route or by an intracellular action. NPD1 apically released may exert bioactivity on cells in the proximity of the interphotoreceptor matrix

to show that human RPE cells in primary culture also synthesize NPD1, initially described in the ARPE-19 cell line

(Mukherjee et al., 2004). In addition, the use of human RPE cells in barrier-forming monolayers allows us to address the issue of "sidedness" of NPD1 release. Several neurotrophins (PEDF, BDNF, CNTF, FGF, GDNF, LIF, NT3, and Persephin) with bioactivities that promote neuronal and/or photoreceptor cell survival are agonists of NPD1 synthesis. These neurotrophins trigger synthesis and release of NPD1 through the apical surface of the cell. Pigment epithelium-derived factor (PEDF) was by far the most potent stimulator of NPD1 synthesis. PEDF, a member of the serine protease inhibitor (serpin) family, was initially identified in the same human retinal pigment epithelial cells (Tombran-Tink and Barnstable, 2003) used in these studies (Mukherjee et al., 2007). PEDF or ciliary neurotrophic factor (CNTF), when added to the basal medium in increasing concentrations, evoke much less NPD1 release on the apical side. Conversely, if these neurotrophins are added to the apical medium, they exert concentration-dependent increases in NPD1 release only on the apical side. These findings have relevance to retinal physiology and pathology because, when RPE cell polarization in the plane of the epithelium is disrupted, certain growth factors are believed to participate in an injury/inflammatory response, including the mediation of angiogenesis as in age-related degenerations (Bhutto et al., 2006; Kannan et al., 2006; Rattner and Nathans, 2006).

5 DHA Potentiates PEDF-Induced NPD1 Synthesis and Release

DHA exerts a remarkable potentiation by PEDF of NPD1 release to the apical media (Fig. 1). In contrast, much less NPD1 was found in the media bathing the basolateral side of the cells. Much less apical NPD1 release was observed when PEDF was applied to the media bathing the basolateral RPE surface. Regardless of the side of the cell where PEDF is added, the amount of NPD1 release through the basolateral side is similar (Mukherjee et al., 2007). Moreover, the addition of DHA to either side of the cell monolayer selectively synergized PEDF-induced NPD1 release only through the apical side. Arachidonic acid, another polyunsaturated fatty acid, did not stimulate NPD1 synthesis. The polarity of actions for the neurotrophin-mediated response suggests that NPD1 may function, at least in part, as an autocrine and paracrine signal on cells that surround the interphotoreceptor matrix, namely the photoreceptor cells and Müller cells. Moreover, the apical side of the RPE participates in the recognition and shedding of photoreceptors during outer segment phagocytosis (Bazan, 2006; Rattner and Nathans, 2006). Furthermore, interphotoreceptor matrix proteins may be acceptors of NPD1, to facilitate its diffusion and to target it to cellular site(s) of action.

6 DHA and PEDF Protects RPE Cells from Oxidative Stress with Concurrent NPD1 Synthesis

To study the consequences of the DHA/PEDF synergy in terms of bioactivity as well as to define the downstream signaling induced, we exposed ARPE-19 cells to oxidative stress. ARPE-19 cells, as human RPE cell primary cultures, up-regulated NPD1 synthesis in the presence of PEDF. Also, significant cytoprotection and increased NPD1 formation occurred synergistically when PEDF was added along with DHA under conditions of oxidative stress-induced apoptotic cell death triggered by serum starvation/H_2O_2 /TNFα (Mukherjee et al., 2007).

7 Conclusions

Because neurotrophins elicit pleiotropic bioactivity, inducing multiple pathways, it is likely that there are major signaling routes activated to promote RPE cellular integrity and preserve function. DHA-NPD1 represents a major signaling mechanism for neurotrophins in the RPE cell.

Neurotrophins, mainly PEDF, are NPD1 synthesis agonists and selective activators of the apical efflux of the lipid mediator in human RPE cells in monolayer cultures. In addition, DHA greatly potentiates PEDF-induced RPE cytoprotection against oxidative stress, with concomitant NPD1 synthesis. The synergy with PEDF and DHA indicates that the availability of the NPD1 initial precursor is critical for its synthesis.

The regulation of apoptosis is complex and comprises multiple checkpoints. The ability of DHA to potentiate PEDF bioactivity on the Bcl-2 family of proteins (Fig. 1) expression indicates that the pre-mitochondrial stage of the apoptotic cascade checkpoint is involved in cytoprotection, with concomitant NPD1 formation (Mukherjee et al., 2007). These findings are in agreement with studies in human neural progenitor cells (Lukiw et al., 2005). The regulation of pro- and anti-apoptotic proteins during a relatively prolonged window of protection (about 6 hrs in cells in culture) will help to further define NPD1 survival bioactivity in the RPE cell. These events are clinically significant because it may allow the exploration of therapeutic interventions for retinal degenerative diseases.

In retinitis pigmentosa, the expression of a mutation and the initiation of the disease is in most instances a slow process. We have an incomplete understanding of the events triggered by the expression of mutations causing retinitis pigmentosa, although impaired RPE cell function does take place. Thus, RPE cell protection may contribute to preserve photoreceptor cell integrity. Moreover, the identification of these events will allow the design of therapeutic alternatives to delay the initiation and progression of retinitis pigmentosa. The relatively wide window of NPD1-mediated cytoprotection against A2E-induced RPE cell apoptosis (Mukherjee et al., 2007) may allow the identification of potentially useful therapeutic alternatives.

Acknowledgments This work was supported by NIH, National Eye Institute grant EY005121, NIH, National Center for Research Resources grant P20 RR016816, American Health Assistance grant M2004-345, and by the Ernest C. and Ivette C. Villere Chair for Research in Retinal Degeneration.

References

Bazan, N.G., 2006, Cell survival matters: docosahexaenoic acid signaling, neuroprotection and photoreceptors, *Trends Neurosci.* **29**:263.

Bhutto, I. A., McLeod, D. S., Hasegawa, T., Kim, S. Y., Merges, C., Tong, P., and Lutty, G. A., 2006, Pigment epithelium-derived factor (PEDF) and vascular endothelial growth factor (VEGF) in aged human choroid and eyes with age-related macular degeneration, *Exp Eye Res.* **82**:99.

Bui, T. V., Han, Y., Radu, R. A., Travis, G. H., and Mata, N. L., 2006, Characterization of native retinal fluorophores involved in biosynthesis of A2E and lipofuscin-associated retinopathies, *J Biol Chem.* **281**:18112.

Cideciyan, A. V., Aleman, T. S., Swider, M., Schwartz, S. B., Steinberg, J. D., Brucker, A. J., Maguire, A. M., Bennett, J., Stone, E. M., and Jacobson, S. G., 2004, Mutations in ABCA4 result in accumulation of lipofuscin before slowing of the retinoid cycle: a reappraisal of the human disease sequence, *Hum Mol Genet.* **13**:525.

Hu, J. and Bok, D., 2001, A cell culture medium that supports the differentiation of human retinal pigment epithelium into functionally polarized monolayers, *Mol Vis.* **7**:14.

Kannan, R., Zhang, N., Sreekumar, P. G., Spee, C. K., Rodriguez, A., Barron, E., and Hinton, D. R., 2006, Stimulation of apical and basolateral VEGF-A and VEGF-C secretion by oxidative stress in polarized retinal pigment epithelial cells, *Mol Vis.* **12**:1649.

LaVail, M. M., Unoki, K., Yasumura, D., Matthes, M. T., Yancopoulos, G. D., and Steinberg R. H., 1992, Multiple growth factors, cytokines, and neurotrophins rescue photoreceptors from the damaging effects of constant light, *Proc Natl Acad Sci USA.* **89**:11249.

LaVail, M. M., Yasumura, D., Matthes, M. T., Lau-Villacorta, C., Unoki, K., Sung, C. H., and Steinberg, R. H., 1998, Protection of mouse photoreceptors by survival factors in retinal degenerations, *Invest Ophthalmol Vis Sci.* **39**:592.

Lukiw W. J., Cui, J. G., Marcheselli, V. L., Bodker, M., Botkjaer, A., Gotlinger, K., Serhan, C. N., and Bazan, N. G., 2005, A role for docosahexaenoic acid-derived neuroprotectin D1 in neural cell survival and Alzheimer disease, *J Clin Invest.* **115**:2774.

Mukherjee, P. K., Marcheselli, V. L., Serhan, C. N., and Bazan, N. G., 2004, Neuroprotectin D1: a docosahexaenoic acid-derived docosatriene protects human retinal pigment epithelial cells from oxidative stress, *Proc Natl Acad Sci USA.* **101**:8491.

Mukherjee, P. K., Marcheselli, V. L., Barreiro, S., Hu, J., Bok, D., and Bazan, N. G., 2007 Neurotrophins enhance retinal pigment epithelial cell survival through neuroprotectin D1 signaling, *Proc Natl Acad Sci USA.* **104**:13152.

Politi, L. E., Rotstein, N. P., and Carri, N. G., 2001, Effect of GDNF on neuroblast proliferation and photoreceptor survival: additive protection with docosahexaenoic acid, *Invest Ophthalmol Vis Sci.* **42**:3008.

Radu, R. A., Mata, N. L., Bagla, A., and Travis, G. H., 2004, Light exposure stimulates formation of A2E oxiranes in a mouse model of Stargardt's macular degeneration, *Proc Natl Acad Sci USA.* **101**:5928.

Rattner, A. and Nathans, J., 2006, Macular degeneration: recent advances and therapeutic opportunities, *Nat Rev Neurosci.* **7**:860.

Rodriguez de Turco, E. B., Deretic, D., Bazan, N.G., and Papermaster, D. S., 1997, Post-Golgi vesicles cotransport docosahexaenoyl-phospholipids and rhodopsin during frog photoreceptor membrane biogenesis, *J Biol Chem.* **272**:10491.

Sparrow, J. R., Vollmer-Snarr, H. R., Zhou, J., Jang, Y. P., Jockusch, S., Itagaki, Y., and Nakanishi, K., 2003, A2E-epoxides damage DNA in retinal pigment epithelial cells. Vitamin E and other antioxidants inhibit A2E-epoxide formation, *J Biol Chem.* **278**:18207.

Tombran-Tink, J. and Barnstable, C. J., 2003, PEDF: a multifaceted neurotrophic factor, *Nat Rev Neurosci* **4**:628.

Valter, K., Bisti, S., Gargini, C., Di Loreto, S., Maccarone, R., Cervetto, L., and Stone, J., 2005, Time course of neurotrophic factor upregulation and retinal protection against light-induced damage after optic nerve section, *Invest Ophthalmol Vis Sci.* **46**:1748.

On the Role of CNTF as a Potential Therapy for Retinal Degeneration: Dr. Jekyll or Mr. Hyde?

William A. Beltran

1 Introduction

Among the various neuroprotective agents, ciliary neurotrophic factor (CNTF) has been the most tested compound in animal models of retinal degeneration. CNTF was initially isolated from the chick eye as a soluble factor that promotes the survival of dissociated ciliary ganglionic neurons of 12-day chick embryos (Adler et al., 1979). Its use as a neuroprotective agent for the retina was first tested in rats 15 years ago in a light-damage model of retinal degeneration (LaVail et al., 1992). Since then, numerous studies conducted in a variety of animal models have demonstrated CNTF's pro-survival effect on photoreceptor cells. The development of a long-term intravitreal delivery device has now enabled to test this agent in humans. The results of a Phase 1 clinical trial conducted in patients with advanced stages of retinitis pigmentosa (RP) have recently been reported, and suggest that the sustained release of CNTF is well tolerated, and may improve visual acuity in some cases (Sieving et al., 2006). This has prompted the start of Phase 2 clinical trials in patients with RP and age-related macular degeneration (AMD).

Despite these encouraging results, a number of recent studies have highlighted that sustained intraocular release of CNTF in animal models of RP induces functional, cytologic, and biochemical alterations of the retina. This paper provides a brief review of our work as well as a summary of the literature on the photoreceptor rescue effect of CNTF, and on its potentially detrimental properties on retinal structure and function.

W.A. Beltran
Section of Ophthalmology, Department of Clinical Studies, School of Veterinary Medicine, University of Pennsylvania, Philadelphia, PA, 19104, USA, Tel: 1 215 898 4913, Fax: 1 215 573 2162
e-mail: wbeltran@vet.upenn.edu

2 CNTF Rescues Photoreceptors in Several Animal Models

Numerous studies conducted in transgenic, experimental (light-induced), and naturally-occurring animal models of retinal degeneration have demonstrated the neuroprotective property of CNTF on photoreceptor cells (Table 1). Although the experimental settings differed considerably between studies, CNTF rescued photoreceptors in 14 out of the 18 models in which it was tested.

Studies conducted by our group on CNTF have focused primarily on assessing its neuroprotective effect in canine models of RP as well as on its mechanism of action. Intravitreal injections of 10–15 µg of Axokine (Regeneron Inc.), a recombinant human mutein of full-length CNTF, had a positive rescue effect in the rcd1 dog model (*PDE6B* mutation). Following this unpublished pilot study, a collaboration with Neurotech Inc. was established to test the effect of prolonged intravitreal release of CNTF in this same model by means of an encapsulated cell therapy (ECT) device (Tao et al., 2002). Complete protection was achieved over the 7 week implantation period with devices that released 5–15 ng/day of CNTF. Minimal to no photoreceptor rescue was attained with lower doses (0.1–1 ng/day). This positive rescue effect led us to examine the mechanism of action of CNTF by characterizing the site of expression of its specific receptor, CNTFRα. By in situ hybridization and immunohistochemistry, we located CNTFRα to both rods and cones, as well as to cells in the INL and GCL of the adult non-mutant canine retina (Beltran et al., 2003). A similar site of expression on rods and cones was found in the human retina as well as in other mammals excluding rodents (Beltran et al., 2005), thus suggesting that a potential rescue effect may be mediated in these species through a direct mechanism of action on photoreceptor cells. This topic has been a matter of debate in rodents as studies supporting either a direct (Ju et al., 2000; Rhee and Yang, 2003) or an indirect (Peterson et al., 2000; Wahlin et al., 2000; Harada et al., 2002; Wahlin et al., 2004) mechanism of photoreceptor survival have both been reported.

As there is currently no strong evidence to support or refute the assumption that all forms of RP will be responsive to CNTF treatment, we began to address this issue by evaluating whether CNTF could rescue photoreceptors in the XLPRA2 dog. This is an early and rapidly progressive canine model for X-linked RP caused by a frameshift mutation in *RPGR* exonORF15 whose stages of disease and kinetics of photoreceptor cell death have been recently characterized (Beltran et al., 2006). Intravitreal injections of 12 µg of human recombinant CNTF failed to prevent photoreceptor cell loss in this model, while a rescue effect was observed in the rcd1 dog (Beltran et al., 2007).

3 CNTF can Cause Numerous Intraocular Side-effects

Bolus intravitreal injections of CNTF have been reported to cause corneal epitheliopathy, uveitis, cataracts, and retinal folds (Chong et al., 1999; Beltran et al., 2007). Although long-term drug delivery of CNTF by means of viral vectors or ECT

Table 1 Summary of the studies on the neuroprotective effect of CNTF in animal models of retinal degeneration [a]

Animal model	Mutation	Delivery mode	CNTF dose	Morphologic PR rescue	Function (ERG)	References
• Light-damage in Sprague-Dawley rat	None	I.-vitr. CNTF	0.5 µg	Yes		LaVail et al., 1992
		I.-vitr. CNTF	0.5–1 µg	Yes		LaVail et al., 1998
• S334ter-3 rat	Rhodopsin	I.-vitr. CNTF	1 µg	Moderate		Tao et al., 2002
		I.-vitr. NTC-201	~10 ng/day	Yes		Tao et al., 2002
• S334ter-4 rat	Rhodopsin	I.-vitr. AAV-CNTF	ND	Yes	Decreased	Liang et al., 2001a
• P23H line 1 rat	Rhodopsin	I.-vitr. AAV-CNTF	ND	Yes	Decreased	Liang et al., 2001a
• RCS rat	Mertk	Subret. CNTF	0.5 µg	Yes		Huang et al., 2004
		Subret. Adv-CNTF	ND	Yes	Increased	Huang et al., 2004
• Light-damage in BALB/c mouse	None	I.-vitr. CNTF	0.2–0.5 µg	Yes		LaVail et al., 1998
• rd/rd mouse	PDE6β	I.-vitr. CNTF	0.2–2 µg	Yes		LaVail et al., 1998
		I.-vitr. Adv-CNTF	ND	Yes		Cayouette et al., 1997
• prph2$^{Rd2/Rd2}$ mouse (= rds/rds)	Peripherin	I.-vitr. CNTF	0.2–2 µg	No	Increased	LaVail et al., 1998
		I.-vitr. Adv-CNTF	ND	Yes	Not improved	Cayouette et al., 1998
		I.-vitr. AAV-CNTF	ND	Yes	Decreased	Liang et al., 2001a
		Subret. AAV-CNTF	ND	Yes		Schlichtenbrede et al., 2003
• rds$^{+/?16L}$ mouse	Peripherin	I.-vitr. CNTF	1 µg	No	Not improved	Bok et al., 2002
		I.-vitr. AAV-CNTF	ND	moderate		Bok et al., 2002
		Subret. AAV-CNTF	ND	Yes	Decreased	Bok et al., 2002
• nr/nr mouse	ND	I.-vitr. CNTF	0.2–2 µg	Yes		LaVail et al., 1998
• Q344ter mouse	Rhodopsin	I.-vitr. CNTF	0.2–2 µg	Yes		LaVail et al., 1998
• pcd/pcd mouse	ND	I.-vitr. CNTF	0.2–2 µg	No		LaVail et al., 1998
• P23H mouse	Rhodopsin	I.-vitr. CNTF	0.2–2 µg	No		LaVail et al., 1998
• VPP mouse	Rhodopsin	I.-vitr. CNTF	0.2–2 µg	No		LaVail et al., 1998
• opsin$^{-/-}$ mouse	Rhodopsin	Subret. AAV-CNTF	ND	Yes		Liang et al., 2001b
• Rdy cat	ND	I.-vitr. CNTF	2.5–5 µg/inject.	Yes		Chong et al., 1999
• rcd1 dog	PDE6β	I.-vitr. CNTF	12 µg (2X)	Yes		Beltran et al., 2007
		I.-vitr. ECT-CNTF	5–15 ng/day	Yes		Tao et al., 2002
• XLPRA2 dog	RPGR-ORF15	I.-vitr. CNTF	12 µg	No		Beltran et al., 2007
		I.-vitr. CNTF	12 µg (2X)	No		Beltran et al., 2007

[a] The following abbreviations are used: CNTF (ciliary neurotrophic factor); PR (photoreceptor); ERG (electroretinography); ampl (amplitude); I.-vitr. (intravitreal); Subret. (subretinal); ND (not determined); AAV (adeno-associated virus); Adv (adenovirus); ECT (encapsulated cell therapy).

Table 2 Summary of the side-effects caused by intraocular delivery of CNTF in animal models of retinal degeneration[a]

Animal model	Delivery mode	CNTF dose	Clinical, morphologic, and biochemical side-effects	References
• Long Evans rat	I.-vitr. CNTF	10 μg	Reversible decrease in ERG a- and b-wave ampl. Reversible rod OS shortening and discs disorganization. Reversible decrease in rhodopsin and transducin levels. Reversible increase in arrestin levels.	Wen et al., 2006
• S334ter-4 rat	I.-vitr. AAV-CNTF	ND	Decrease in ERG b-wave ampl.	Liang et al., 2001a
• P23H line 1 rat	I.-vitr. AAV-CNTF	ND	Decrease in ERG b-wave ampl.	Liang et al., 2001a
• prph2[Rd2/Rd2] mouse (rds/rds)	Subret. AAV-CNTF	ND	Decrease in ERG b-wave ampl. ONL disorganization and increase in internuclear spacing.	Schlichtenbrede et al., 2003
• rds+/rds mouse	Subret. AAV-CNTF	ND	Decrease in ERG a- and b-wave ampl. Change in rod nuclear phenotype (increased size and euchromatin content).	Bok et al., 2002
• NZW albino rabbit	ECT-CNTF	22 ng/day	Decrease in ERG b-wave ampl. Increase in ONL thickness. Change in rod nuclear phenotype (increased size and euchromatin content).	Bush et al., 2004
• Rdy cat	I.-vitr. CNTF	2.5–5 μg/inject.	Posterior subcapsular cataracts, retinal folds.	Chong et al., 1999
• rcd1 dog	I.-vitr. CNTF I.-vitr. ECT-CNTF	12 μg (2X) >1 ng/day >2.5 ng/day	Corneal epitheliopathy, uveitis, cataract. Inner retinal thickening, ganglion cell chromatolysis. Reduced immunostaining for rhodopsin and cone arrestin. Elevation of the outer limiting membrane.	Beltran et al., 2007 Zeiss et al., 2006
• XLPRA2 dog	I.-vitr. CNTF	12 μg (1x or 2X)	Corneal epitheliopathy, uveitis, cataract. Peripheral retinal remodeling (ONL thickening, OS and IS loss; neuronal sprouting, heterotopia of retinal cells). Reversible loss of rhodopsin and cone arrestin.	Beltran et al., 2007

[a] The following abbreviations are used in this table: CNTF (ciliary neurotrophic factor); ERG (electroretinography); I.-vitr. (intravitreal); Subret. (subretinal); ND (not determined); AAV (adeno-associated virus); ECT (encapsulated cell therapy); ONL (outer nuclear layer); OS (outer segments); IS (inner segments).

technology eliminates these clinical side-effects, a number of studies have reported electroretinographic, cytological and biochemical alterations (Table 2). Rabbits implanted with ECT devices delivering a dose of 22 ng/day of CNTF showed an increase in ONL thickness and nuclear changes in rods making them appear more like cones. A similar finding was reported when delivering CNTF subretinaly by means of a rAAV vector to mice with a P216L rds/peripherin mutation (Bok et al., 2002). Changes in rod nuclear size and euchromatin content were not observed in rcd1 dogs implanted with an ECT device, although an elevation of the outer limiting membrane suggestive of intracellular swelling of photoreceptors, Müller cells, or both was recently reported (Zeiss et al., 2006). In the XLPRA2 dog, bolus intravitreal injections of CNTF did not prevent photoreceptor loss, yet prominent retinal remodeling in the peripheral retina was found (Beltran et al., 2007). There was an increase in internuclear spacing as well as in rod cell number that resulted in an abnormal increase in ONL thickness. In this same retinal area, a loss of photoreceptor outer and inner segments was also found. A panretinal, yet reversible loss of immunostaining for rod opsin and cone arrestin was also seen. Our findings suggest that at least under certain conditions (form of disease, time-window of treatment, route of administration and dose) CNTF may reveal itself as a mitogenic factor and a dedifferentiating agent.

Electroretinographic alterations mainly consisting of a decrease in b-wave amplitudes have been described by several groups following bolus intravitreal injection of CNTF, or delivery via rAAV vector or ECT (Table 2). These ERG changes are likely to be caused by a downregulation of the phototransduction machinery (Wen et al., 2006) as well as by impaired synaptic connectivity between photoreceptors and second order neurons (Beltran et al., 2007).

4 Conclusion

Despite the very encouraging results of a Phase 1 clinical trial in 10 RP patients, the retinal alterations that have been reported in animal models treated with CNTF deserve attention. Indeed, as some of these changes have been observed at doses that are within the order of magnitude of the therapeutically active doses, future clinical trials may need to monitor the occurrence of such alterations.

Acknowledgments The author thanks NIH, the FFB, and Merck for a travel award to attend RD2006.

References

Adler, R., Landa, K.B., Manthorpe, M.,Varon, S., 1979. Cholinergic neuronotrophic factors: intraocular distribution of trophic activity for ciliary neurons. Science. **204**: 1434–1436.

Beltran, W.A., Hammond, P., Acland, G.M., Aguirre, G.D., 2006. A frameshift mutation in *RPGR* exon ORF15 causes photoreceptor degeneration and inner retina remodeling in a model of X-linked retinitis pigmentosa. Invest Ophthalmol Vis Sci. **47**: 1669–1681.

Beltran, W.A., Rohrer, H., Aguirre, G.D., 2005. Immunolocalization of ciliary neurotrophic factor receptor alpha (CNTFRα) in mammalian photoreceptor cells. Mol Vis. **11**: 232–244.

Beltran, W.A., Wen, R., Acland, G.M., Aguirre, G.D., 2007. Intravitreal injection of ciliary neurotrophic factor (CNTF) causes peripheral remodeling and does not prevent photoreceptor loss in canine RPGR mutant retina. Exp Eye Res. **148**: 53–64.

Beltran, W.A., Zhang, Q., Kijas, J.W., Gu, D., et al., 2003. Cloning, mapping, and retinal expression of the canine ciliary neurotrophic factor receptor alpha (CNTFRα). Invest Ophthalmol Vis Sci. **44**: 3642–3649

Bok, D., Yasumura, D., Matthes, M.T., Ruiz, et al., 2002. Effects of AAV-vectored ciliary neurotrophic factor on retinal structure and function in mice with a P216L rds/peripherin mutation. Exp Eye Res. **74**: 719–735.

Bush, R.A., Lei, B., Tao, W., Raz, D., et al., 2004. Encapsulated cell-based intraocular delivery of CNTF in normal rabbit: dose-dependent effects on ERG and retinal histology. Invest Ophthalmol Vis Sci. **45**: 2420–2430.

Cayouette, M., Behn, D., Sendtner, M., Lachapelle, P., et al., 1998. Intraocular gene transfer of CNTF prevents death and increases responsiveness of rod photoreceptors in the retinal degeneration slow mouse. J Neurosci. **18**: 9282–9293.

Cayouette, M., Gravel, C., 1997. Adenovirus-mediated gene transfer of ciliary neurotrophic factor can prevent photoreceptor degeneration in the retinal degeneration (rd) mouse. Hum Gene Ther. **8**: 423–430.

Chong, N.H., Alexander, R.A., Waters, L., Barnett, K.C., et al., 1999. Repeated injections of a ciliary neurotrophic factor analogue leading to long-term photoreceptor survival in hereditary retinal degeneration. Invest Ophthalmol Vis Sci. **40**: 1298–1305.

Harada, T., Harada, C., Kohsaka, S., Wada, E., et al., 2002. Microglia-Muller glia cell interactions control neurotrophic factor production during light-induced retinal degeneration. J Neurosci. **22**: 9228–9236.

Huang, S.P., Lin, P.K., Liu, J.H., Khor, C.N., et al., 2004. Intraocular gene transfer of ciliary neurotrophic factor rescues photoreceptor degeneration in RCS rats. J Biomed Sci. **11**: 37–48.

Ju, W.K., Lee, M.Y., Hofmann, H.D., Kirsch, M., et al., 2000. Increased expression of ciliary neurotrophic factor receptor alpha mRNA in the ischemic rat retina. Neurosci Lett. **283**: 133–136.

LaVail, M.M., Unoki, K., Yasumura, D., Matthes, M.T., et al., 1992. Multiple growth factors, cytokines, and neurotrophins rescue photoreceptors from the damaging effects of constant light. Proc Natl Acad Sci USA. **89**: 11249–11253.

LaVail, M.M., Yasumura, D., Matthes, M.T., Lau-Villacorta, C., et al., 1998. Protection of mouse photoreceptors by survival factors in retinal degenerations. Invest Ophthalmol Vis Sci. **39**: 592–602.

Liang, F.Q., Aleman, T.S., Dejneka, N.S., Dudus, et al., 2001a. Long-term protection of retinal structure but not function using RAAV.CNTF in animal models of retinitis pigmentosa. Mol Ther. **4**: 461–472.

Liang, F.Q., Dejneka, N.S., Cohen, D.R., Krasnoperova, N.V., et al., 2001b. AAV-mediated delivery of CNTF prolongs photoreceptor survival in the rhodopsin knockout mouse. Mol Ther. **3**: 241–248.

Peterson, W.M., Wang, Q., Tzekova, R., Wiegand, S.J., 2000. Ciliary neurotrophic factor and stress stimuli activate the Jak-STAT pathway in retinal neurons and glia. J Neurosci. **20**: 4081–4090.

Rhee, K.D., Yang, X.J., 2003. Expression of cytokine signal transduction components in the postnatal mouse retina. Mol Vis. **9**: 715–722.

Schlichtenbrede, F.C., MacNeil, A., Bainbridge, J.W., Tschernutter, M., et al., 2003. Intraocular gene delivery of ciliary neurotrophic factor results in significant loss of retinal function in normal mice and in the Prph2Rd2/Rd2 model of retinal degeneration. Gene Ther. **10**: 523–527.

Sieving, P.A., Caruso, R.C., Tao, W., Coleman, H.R., et al., 2006. Ciliary neurotrophic factor (CNTF) for human retinal degeneration: Phase I trial of CNTF delivered by encapsulated cell intraocular implants. Proc Natl Acad Sci USA. **103**: 3896–3901.

Tao, W., Wen, R., Goddard, M.B., Sherman, S.D., O'Rourke, P.J., et al., 2002. Encapsulated cell based delivery of CNTF reduces photoreceptor degeneration in animal models of retinitis pigmentosa. Invest Ophthalmol Vis Sci. **43**: 3292–3298.

Wahlin, K.J., Campochiaro, P.A., Zack, D.J., Adler, R., 2000. Neurotrophic factors cause activation of intracellular signaling pathways in Muller cells and other cells of the inner retina, but not photoreceptors. Invest Ophthalmol Vis Sci. **41**: 927–936.

Wahlin, K.J., Lim, L., Grice, E.A., Campochiaro, P.A., et al., 2004. A method for analysis of gene expression in isolated mouse photoreceptor and Muller cells. Mol Vis. **10**: 366–375.

Wen, R., Song, Y., Kjellstrom, S., Tanikawa, A., et al., 2006. Regulation of rod phototransduction machinery by ciliary neurotrophic factor. J Neurosci. **26**: 13523–13530.

Zeiss, C.J., Allore, H.G., Towle, V., Tao, W., 2006. CNTF induces dose-dependent alterations in retinal morphology in normal and rcd-1 canine retina. Exp Eye Res. **82**: 395–404.

Nanoceria Particles Prevent ROI-Induced Blindness

Junping Chen, Swanand Patil, Sudipta Seal, and James F. McGinnis

1 Introduction

Retinal degeneration caused blindness, such as age-related macular degeneration (AMD), diabetic retinopathy (DR), retinitis pigmentosa (RP) and retinal detachment, is a major problem in clinical ophthalmology. Although genetic modifications are responsible for most retinal degenerative diseases, there is increasing evidence showing that reactive oxygen intermediates (ROIs), the byproducts of the oxidative metabolic reactions, are closely involved in the process of photoreceptor cell degeneration (Beatty et al., 2000; Maeda et al., 2005; Wenzel et al., 2005). These ROIs, including hydrogen peroxide, hypochlorite ions, hydroxyl radicals, hydroxyl ions and superoxide anions (Beatty et al., 2000), react with almost any nearby DNA, RNA, lipid, carbohydrate or protein. They are produced primarily by the normal oxidative metabolism that occurs in the mitochondrial respiratory chain. Photoreceptor cells are extremely sensitive to ROI-induced damage. This is not only because they are continuously exposed to the deleterious effects induced by photons of light, but also they have the highest rate of oxygen metabolism of any cells in the body (Yu and Cringle, 2005) and their outer segments contain high level of polyunsaturated fatty acids. The high consumption of oxygen results in the production of a large amount of ROIs. In consequence, ROIs result in the cytotoxic effect referred to as oxidative stress, which has been implicated as one of the initial causes of numerous eye diseases. It has been shown that, in the retinal degenerative diseases, irrespective of the initiating defect, the intracellular concentration of ROIs rises chronically or acutely and activates a cell death pathway (Lewis et al., 1991; Caldwell et al., 2003; Emerit et al., 2004).

Several therapeutic strategies have been tested to treat retinal degeneration in animal models by reducing ROIs (Wenzel et al., 2005). We are introducing a new material, vacancy engineered nanoceria particles, and testing its ability to

J.F. McGinnis
Oklahoma Center for Neuroscience, Dean A. McGee Eye Institute, Department of Department of Cell Biology, Department of Ophthalmology, University of Oklahoma Health Sciences Center, Oklahoma City, OK 73104, USA, Tel: 405-271-3695, Fax: 405-271-3721,
e-mail: james-mcginnis@ouhsc.edu

R.E. Anderson et al. (eds.), *Recent Advances in Retinal Degeneration*,
© Springer 2008

reduce ROIs (Chen, 2006). Cerium is a rare earth element in the lanthanide series. Cerium oxide (CeO_2) is the oxidized form of the element. Cerium has both +3 and +4 states and may flip-flop between the two in a redox reaction (Suzuki et al, 2001; Herman, 1999; Conesa, 1995), during which oxygen vacancies or defects are formed in the lattice structure by loss of oxygen and/or its electrons. The nanocrystalized CeO_2 molecules not only retain oxygen vacancies in the crystal structure (Patil et al., 2006), but they also are about 5nm in diameter which allows for easier passage through cell membranes. Thus we hypothesized that nanoceria particles, owing to their chemical and physical structure, can protect photoreceptor cells from light-induced ROI-mediated damage.

2 Methods

2.1 Primary Culture of Retinal Neurons

Primary dissociated cell cultures of rat retinas were established from 0- to 2-day-old rat pups as described (McGinnis et al., 1999).

2.2 Measurement of Intracellular ROI

Intracellular ROI production was measured by flow cytometry using 29,79-dichlorofluorescein diacetate (DCFH-DA), an oxidant-sensitive fluorescent probe. In the presence of intracellular peroxides, H2DCF is oxidized to a highly fluorescent compound, 2,7-dichlorofluorescein (LeBel et al., 1992). The retinal cells were exposed to nanoceria particles for 12h, and then incubated with 10mM DCFH-DA at 37°C for 30 min after washes. The cells were then incubated with 1mM H_2O_2 at 37°C for 30 min after the excess DCFH-DA was washed off with phosphate buffer saline. The cells were then harvested with trypsin. The intensity of fluorescence was detected by flow cytometry with an excitation filter of 485 nm. The ROI level was calculated as a ratio of mean intensity of experimental cells/mean intensity of control cells.

2.3 Intravitreal Injection and Light-induced Photoreceptor Degeneration

Rats were anesthetized, pupils dilated, a topical anesthetic applied to the cornea, and 2 μl of 0.1, 0.3 or 1 μM nanoceria particles in 0.9% NaCl were injected. Controls were injected with 2 μl of 0.9% NaCl. For light-induced photoreceptor degeneration, the rats were exposed to 2,700 lux (measured with a photometer) of constant light for 6 h. During light exposure, rats were maintained in transparent polycarbonate cages (one or two rats per cage) with stainless-steel wire covers. A water bottle was kept at the side of the cage and food was placed in the bottom of the cage on the bedding. They were returned to cyclic light for 7 days before the experiment was ended.

2.4 Functional Rescue of Photoreceptor Cells as Evaluated by Electroretinography

The ERG experiments were performed as described previously (Cao et al., 2001). The animals used in each set of experiments were all the same sex (males) and were taken from the same litter. They were maintained in the same room and treated identically. Animals were kept in total darkness overnight before ERGs were recorded. For quantitative analysis, the A-wave amplitude was measured as the difference between baseline and the peak of the A-wave, and the B-wave amplitude was measured as the difference between the peaks of the A- and B-waves.

2.5 Morphologic Evaluation by Quantitative Histology

After ERG recordings, the rats were killed by an overdose of carbon dioxide, the eyes enucleated, fixed in Perfix, embedded in paraffin, and 5-μm-thick sections were cut along the vertical meridian so that the superior and inferior hemispheres were separated by the optic nerve. To evaluate quantitatively the morphologic changes using H&E stained sections, we measured the ONL thickness at 220-μm intervals, starting at the optic nerve head and moving along the vertical meridian toward the superior or inferior ora serrata. The mean ONL thickness of each point was then calculated from the retinas of at least four eyes.

3 Results

3.1 Nanoceria Particles Inhibit Intracellular Accumulation of ROIs.

To study the ability of nanoceria particles scavenging intracellular ROIs, we used the intracellular ROIs maker, DCFH-DA. We found that the nanoceria particles prevent the intracellular accumulation of ROIs in cultured retinal neurons to which H_2O_2 was added. The data are shown in Fig. 1 and demonstrate that the nanoceria particles, even at 5 nM, when present for 12 h, are effective in inhibiting the H_2O_2-induced rise of intracellular ROIs.

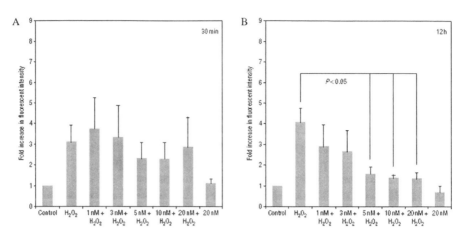

Fig. 1 Inhibition of ROIs by nanoceria particles. Pretreatment of cultured retinal neurons with nanoceria particles (1, 3, 5, 10 and 20 nM) for 12 h inhibits the intracellular accumulation of ROIs in response to exposure to 1 mM H2O2 for 30 min. The protection is dose-dependent. (Statistical analysis was done by one-way ANOVA and Newman – Keuls test for post hoc analysis. Data are shown as mean ±s.d., n=3, $P < 0.05$)

3.2 in vivo Protection of Photoreceptor Cells Morphology and Function

The cell culture data prompted us to test the efficacy of the nanoceria particles *in vivo*. We used a light-damage animal model in which albino rats are intravitreally injected with 2 μl of saline or a 0.1, 0.3 or 1.0 μM suspension of the nanoceria particles in saline and three days later were exposed to 2,700 lux of light for 6 h. The retinal function is evaluated by ERGs which were conducted 7 days after exposure. The quantification of ERG A- and B-wave amplitudes (Fig. 2A) clearly demonstrates the functional improvement of retinas following treatment with nanoceria particles from 0.1 to 1.0 μM. This is especially evident in the eyes pretreated with 1 μM nanoceria particles, which had 79% and 87% of the control A- and B-wave amplitudes, compared with 22% and 26% for the retinas with 0.9% NaCl vehicle treatment.

It is known that the superior retina is more sensitive to light damage than the inferior retina. The averages of the ONL thickness of the superior region are showed in Fig. 2B and demonstrate that the nanoceria particles are effective in protecting the photoreceptor cells in that region. Injections of 0.1 μM and 0.3 μM suspensions are partially protective, but the data obtained for a 1.0 μM suspension demonstrate almost complete protection and are essentially indistinguishable from those of the control animal, which was not exposed to light.

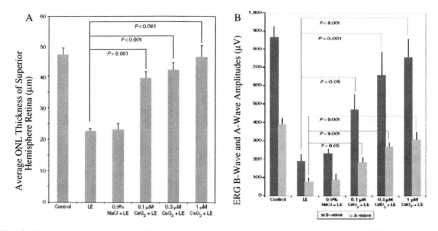

Fig. 2 Nanoceria particles provide pan-retinal protection against light damage. (A) Summation of the ONL thickness across the superior hemisphere provides a quantitative assessment of the protective effects of the nanoceria particles in the most sensitive hemisphere. (B) Mean of the ERG B-wave and A-wave amplitudes are shown for each group of animals. Statistical analysis was done by one-way ANOVA and Newman – Keuls test for post hoc analysis. The results are expressed as mean amplitude ±s.d. (n=6 for each point). Control animals had no injections and were not exposed to bright light. LE animals had no injections and were exposed to bright light

3.3 Nanoceria Particles can Rescue Retina Function After Light Damage

To determine if the nanoceria particles had any ability to rescue photoreceptor cells after they had been exposed to damaging light, rats were subjected to 6 h of 2,700 lux light and were injected intravitreally, 2 h later, with 2 µl of a 1 µM nanoceria particle suspension. The retinal function of the animals was determined seven days later using ERG. The summary of the ERG data (Fig. 3) demonstrates that a significant amount of retinal function is rescued by post-treatment with the nanoceria particles.

4 Discussion

In this report, we for the first time showed that the vacancy engineered particles have the ability to scavenge intracellular ROI, to abolish the early events in the degeneration process and to prevent photoreceptor cell degeneration induced by light. We do not know how the nanoceria particles are taken up into photoreceptor cells, nor the process by which they are eliminated. However, because ROIs are formed within the photoreceptor cells in response to light damage, and because ROIs react over very short distances, we think that the nanoceria particles enter the photoreceptor cells. Because our data demonstrate that the nanoceria particles prevent the peroxide induced increase in the intracellular concentration of ROIs in cul-

Fig. 3 Nanoceria particles
rescue photoreceptor cells
after the light exposure insult.
Each column represents the
mean of the ERG B- and
A-wave amplitudes.
Statistical analysis was done
by one-way ANOVA and
Newman – Keuls test for post
hoc analysis. The results are
expressed as mean
amplitude±s.d. (n=4;
$P < 0.01$ versus LE group).
The insets are representative
ERG waveforms from four
independent experiments

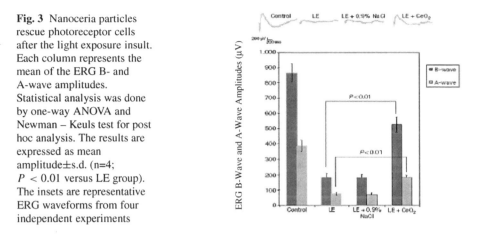

tured retinal cells, we think the nanoceria particles function by the same mechanism in vivo.

The valences of CeO_2 change spontaneously or in response to physical and environmental conditions (Conesa, 1995; Herman, 1999; Mamontov et al., 2000). It has been shown that the migration enthalpy of the oxygen vacancy in CeO_2 is smaller at the nanoscale (Conesa, 1995; Kosacki et al., 2002). Additionally, at the nanoscale, the surface area of CeO_2 particles is dramatically enlarged in relation to its volume which increases oxygen exchange and redox reactions. Thus, oxygen vacancies are likely to form more readily at the nanoscale. The nanoceria particles can act as the antioxidants similar to vitamin C, but with many more sites of spin-trap activity. In addition, the lattice defects in nanoceria particles possess the potential for regeneration and do not require repetitive dosage as seen with the use of vitamins C and E. We propose that nanoceria particles act as free-radical scavengers by switching between the +3 and +4 valence states via various surface chemical reactions. The radical-scavenging mechanism can be given by the following set of chemical reactions.

$$Ce^{3+} \Leftrightarrow Ce^{4+} + e^-$$
$$Ce^{3+} + \cdot OH \Leftrightarrow Ce^{4+} + OH^-$$
$$Ce^{4+} + \cdot O_2 \Leftrightarrow Ce^{3+} + \cdot O_2$$

This regenerative property makes utilization of the nanoceria particles a very attractive strategy for treating ROI-induced cellular damage and diseases especially because presently, other free-radical scavengers need a repetitive dosage. We know that many retinal degenerative diseases are proceeding through a mechanism that involves an increase in intracellular ROIs. We therefore think the nanoparticles have the potential to inhibit the progression of these diseases.

References

Beatty, S., Koh, H., Phil, M., Henson, D. & Boulton, M., 2000, The role of oxidative stress in the pathogenesis of age-related macular degeneration. *Surv. Ophthalmol.* 45:115–134.

Caldwell, R.B., Bartoli, M., Behzadian, M.A., El-Remessy, A.E., Al-Shabrawey, M., Platt, D.H. & Caldwell, R.W., 2003, Vascular endothelial growth factor and diabetic retinopathy: pathophysiological mechanisms and treatment perspectives. *Diabetes Metab. Res. Rev.* 19:442–455.

Cao, W., Tombran-Tink, J., Elias R., Sezate S., Mrazek, D. & McGinnis, J.F., 2001, In vivo protection of photoreceptors from light damage by pigment epithelium derived factor. *Invest Ophthalmol. Vis. Sci.* 42:1646–1652.

Chen, J., Patil, S., Seal, S. & McGinnis, J.F., 2006, Rare earth nanoparticles prevent retinal degeneration induced by intracellular peroxidase. *Nature Nanotech.* 1:142–150.

Conesa, J.C., 1995, Computer modeling of surfaces and defects on cerium dioxide. *Surf. Sci.* 339:337–352.

Deshpande, 2005, Size dependency variation in lattice parameter and valency states in nanocrystalline cerium oxide. *Appl. Phys. Lett.* 87:1–3.

Emerit, J., Edeas, M. & Bricaire, F., 2004, Neurodegenerative diseases and oxidative stress. *Biomed. Pharmacother.* 58:39–46.

Herman, G.S., 1999, Characterization of surface defects on epitaxial CeO2(001) films. *Surf. Sci.* 437:207–214.

Kosacki, I., Suzuki, T., Anderson, H.U. & Colomban, P., 2002, Raman scattering and lattice defects in nanocrystalline CeO2 thin films. *Solid State Ionics* 149:99–105.

LeBel, C.P., Ischiropoulos, H. & Bondy, S.C., 1992, Evaluation of the probe 20,70-dichlorofluorescin as an indicator of reactive oxygen species formation and oxidative stress. *Chem. Res. Toxicol.* 5:227–231.

Lewis, G.P., Erickson, P.A., Anderson, D.H. & Fisher, S.K., 1991, Opsin distribution and protein incorporation in photoreceptors after experimental retinal detachment. *Exp. Eye Res.* 53: 629–640.

Maeda, A., Crabb, J.W. & Palczewski, K., 2005, Microsomal glutathione S-transferase 1 in the retinal pigment epithelium: protection against oxidative stress and a potential role in aging. *Biochemistry.* 44(2):480–489.

Mamontov, E., Egami, T., Brezay, R., Koranne, M. & Tyagi, S., 2000, Lattice defects and oxygen storage capacity of nanocrystalline ceria and ceria-zirconia. *J. Phys. Chem.* 104:1110–1116.

McGinnis, J.F., Stepanik, P.L., Chen W., Elias R., Cao W. & Lerious V., 1999, Unique retina cell phenotypes revealed by immunological analysis of recoverin expression in rat retina cells. *J. Neurosci. Res.* 55:252–260.

Patil, S., Seal, S., Guo, Y., Schulte, A. & Norwood, J., 2006, Role of trivalent La and Nd dopants in lattice distortion and oxygen vacancy generation in cerium oxide nanoparticles. *Appl. Phys. Lett.* 88:1–3.

Suzuki, T., Kosacki, I., Anderson, H.U. & Colomban, P., 2001, Electrical conductivity and lattice defects in nanocrystalline cerium oxide thin films. *J. Am. Ceram. Soc.* 84:2007–2014.

Wenzel, A., Grimm, C., Samardzija, M. & Reme, C.E., 2005, Molecular mechanisms of light-induced photoreceptor apoptosis and neuroprotection for retinal degeneration. *Progr. Retial Eye Res.* 24:275–306.

Yu, D. & Cringle., S.J., 2005, Retinal degeneration and local oxygen metabolism. *Exp. Eye Res.* 80:745–751.

An in-vivo Assay to Identify Compounds Protective Against Light Induced Apoptosis

Yogita Kanan, Anne Kasus Jacobi, Kjell Sawyer, David S. Mannel, Joyce Tombran Tink, and Muayyad R. Al-Ubaidi

1 Introduction

Age-related macular degeneration (AMD) is the major cause of blindness in the elderly. Vision loss is caused by the death of cone photoreceptor cells in the macula. Approximately 1.65 million Americans over the age of 50 have the disease (Prevent Blindness America). Very little is known about the causes and mechanisms of photoreceptor death in this condition.

We are interested in understanding AMD and finding drugs that will alleviate this condition. In our laboratory, we have developed a cell line (661W) from a retinal tumor in mice expressing SV-40 T antigen in the photoreceptor cells (Al-Ubaidi et al., 1992). The cell line expresses cone specific antigens and therefore it is a valuable tool to study macular degeneration (Tan et al., 2004). Since light is considered to be a contributing factor in macular degeneration (Tomany et al., 2004), we designed an assay where we caused cell death in 661W by light stress in the presence of the chromophore (Kanan et al., 2007). These cells do not contain an endogenous chromophore but our previous results showed that preincubation of the cells with 10 μM 9-*cis* retinal or all-*trans* retinal potentiates the light damage, whereas all-*trans* retinol at the same concentration does not. Light causes isomerization of 9-*cis* retinal to all-*trans* retinal, making it the likely candidate that mediates light damage. Examples of the utilization of this assay to identify protective compounds against cell death are presented here. Two drugs, pigment epithelium derived factor (PEDF) and decosahexanoic acid (DHA), are tested for their protective effects against light damage.

We then tested three retinol dehydrogenases (RDH) 8, 11, and 12, upon transfection into 661W cells, for their ability to protect the cells from light induced cell death. Retinol dehydrogenases detoxify all-*trans* retinal by converting it to all-*trans* retinol.

Y. Kanan

Department of Cell Biology, University of Oklahoma Health Sciences Center, 940 Stanton L. Young Blvd. (BMSB781), Oklahoma City, OK 73104, USA Tel: 405-271-2408

e-mail: ykanan@ouhsc.edu

2 Methods

2.1 Growth of Cells for Light-Induced Apoptosis Experiments

Twenty thousand cells were added in each well of a 96-well tissue culture plate and allowed to grow overnight. The next morning, the medium was replaced with a 100-μl aliquot of fresh medium containing 10 μM 9-*cis* retinal or 9-*cis* retinal and the protective drug in the dark, and the cells were returned to the incubator for 4 hours to allow for the uptake of retinoids. After 4 hours, the media was again removed and replaced with media containing the protective drug and then exposed to light at 30,000 lux for 4 hours at room temperature. Cells kept in the dark served as dark controls. Cells replaced with media containing drug were compared to cells replaced with media alone to test the protective effects of the drug. In the case of cells transfected with retinol dehydrogenase genes, we compared these cells with cells that were not transfected to assess protection.

2.2 Expression Plasmids, Transfection and Selection of Stable Clones

RDH8-Flag, RDH11-Flag, and RDH12-Flag encoding epitope-tagged versions of these mouse RDHs were generated by PCR and cloned into the pTarget vector (Promega, Madison, WI). All expression plasmids were verified by DNA sequencing of the entire coding regions and cloning sites. 661W cells were transfected using Lipofectamine 2000 reagent (Invitrogen, Carlsbad, CA) according to the manufacturer's instructions. To select for stable transfectants, 661W cells were grown in G418-containing medium (1 mg/ml) for 3 weeks. G418-resistant colonies were collected and clonal cell lines were obtained by serial dilution in 96-well plates and assayed for Flag-tagged RDH expression by immunoblot analysis with anti-Flag antibody. Once established, stable cell lines were maintained in G418-containing medium.

2.3 Viability Assay

Viability was assessed by 3-(4,5-dimethylthiazol-2-yl)-2,5-diphenyltetrazolium bromide (MTT) according to the paper (Kanan et al., 2007). Data were graphed with commercial software (Prism; GraphPad Software). The graph was plotted by plotting the viability percent of the cells surviving compared to their dark control. The percentage of viable cells was calculated by averaging the ratios of absorbance readings of cells in the light to the dark control cells, assuming that the dark control cells were 100% viable, and the average percentage was determined.

Each experiment was performed at least three times, with 12 replicates for each treatment. Cells that underwent light treatment were compared with dark control cells. Statistical analysis was performed on the samples with Student's t-tests and one-way ANOVA followed by Bonferroni post test. All the groups were compared to each other, and statistical significance was set at $P < 0.05$.

2.4 Preparation of Membrane Fraction from 661W Cells and Assay of RDH Activity

Cells were resuspended in sucrose buffer (0.25 M sucrose, 10 mM Tris-Cl, pH 7.2, 1 mM EDTA), and a protease inhibitor mixture (2.0 µg/ml aprotinin, 5 µg/ml pepstatin A, 10 µg/ml leupeptin, and 0.5 mM phenylmethylsulfonyl fluoride) and disrupted using a Polytron. Cell homogenates were centrifuged at 800 X g for 15 min at 4°C. The resulting supernatants were then centrifuged at 100,000 X g for 30 min at 4°C, and membrane pellets were resuspended in storage buffer containing 50 mM Tris-Cl, pH 7.2, 1 mM EDTA, 20% glycerol and the protease inhibitor mixture described above. Membrane fractions were stored at –80°C after snap freezing in liquid nitrogen. Reactions with all-*trans*-retinal were carried out in 1 ml reaction buffer (100 mM Tris-HCl at pH 7.2, 200 mM NaCl, 1 mM dithiothreitol, 2 mg/ml bovine serum albumin, 1% glycerol, and 150 µM of NADPH) containing 0 or 10 µg of proteins, and 0, 1.25, 2.5, 5, 10 and 20 µM of substrate. After 4 hours incubation at room temperature, reactions were terminated by the addition of 1 volume of cold methanol. Retinoids were then extracted with 2 volumes of hexane and analyzed by HPLC. Samples were dissolved in HPLC mobile phase (11.2% ethyl acetate/2.0% dioxane/1.4% octanol in hexane) and retinoids were separated by using a Lichrosphere Sil 60A (Phenomenex) 5-µm column. The retinal peaks were identified and quantified by comparison with pure retinoid isomeric standards. All procedures were performed under dim red light. Calculation of K_m and V_{max} were done by using the direct linear plot method.

3 Results

3.1 Chromophore can Enhance Light Induced Apoptosis in 661W Cells

In the presence of 9-*cis* retinal and 30,000 lux of light, 661W cells undergo cell death. There is no change in viability at 1 and 2 hours after light exposure. At 3 hours after light stress however, 76% of the cells are viable, and at 4 and 5 hours after light stress, 50% and 27% of cells are viable, respectively, as shown in Fig. 1 Cells kept in the dark in the presence of 9-*cis* retinal for 5 hours were all viable. In the absence of chromophore, all the cells are viable at 5 hours after light stress and 68% of cells are viable after 6 hours of light stress (Kanan et al., 2007). Therefore, addition of 9-*cis* retinal, accelerates light induced damage to the cells.

Fig. 1 Viability of 661W
cells after 5 hours of light
induced apoptosis in the
presence of 9-*cis* retinal.
Statistical analysis using the
Bonferroni multiple
comparison was performed
and significant probabilities
with $P \leq 0.05$, are denoted
with asterisks

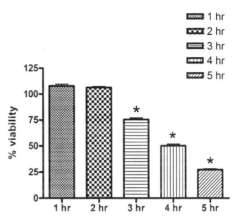

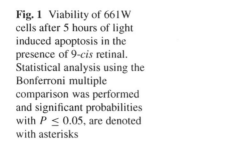

3.2 PEDF and DHA are Protective Drugs Against Light Induced Apoptosis

Using the assay outlined above, we tested 2 drugs, PEDF at 1nM and DHA at
100nM to investigate their protective effects against light induced apoptosis. We
found that both drugs offered protection against light damage. After 5 hours of light
exposure in the absence of drug, 22% of the cells are viable, however in the presence
of PEDF, 58% of cells are viable while 36% of the cells are viable in the presence of
DHA. The drug concentrations shown in Fig. 2 were the concentrations that offered
highest protection. Therefore PEDF offers more protection against light damage
compared to DHA, which offered only slight protection.

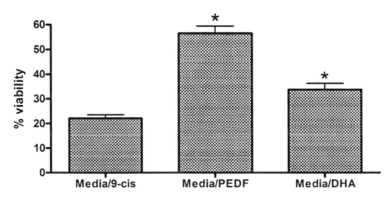

Fig. 2 Viability of 661W cells after 5 hours of light induced apoptosis in the presence of 9-*cis*
retinal. The drugs PEDF at 1 nM or DHA at 100nM was added to the media to assess protection offered by these drugs. Statistical analysis using the Bonferroni multiple comparison was
performed and significant probabilities with $P \leq 0.05$, are denoted with asterisks

3.3 Expression of RDHs in 661W Cells Provides Protection Against Light Stress

661W cells express low levels of endogenous dehydrogenases (unpublished data). We transfected these cells with RDH8, RDH11 and RDH12 and isolated pure clones of stable transfectants. We investigated the susceptibility of these clones to light stress in comparison to their untransfected counterparts. We found that only 21% of untransfected 661W cells are viable after 5 hours of light stress while 69% of cells are viable after transfection with RDH8, 34% of cells are viable after transfection with RDH11, and 42% of cells are viable after transfection with RDH12. Therefore, all three RDHs offer protection to 661W cells with RDH8 appearing to offer the highest protection as shown in Fig. 3

It is possible that RDH8 has a higher catalytic activity (V_{max}) and/or a higher affinity (K_m) towards all-*trans* retinal compared to the RDH11 and RDH12. In Table 1 we compare the apparent V_{max} and K_m of these clones, using the membrane

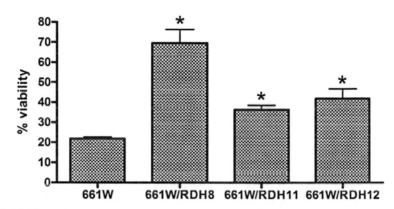

Fig. 3 Viability of 661W cells after 5 hours of light induced apoptosis in the presence of 9-*cis* retinal. 661W cells transfected with RDH8, RDH11 and RDH12 were compared to non transfected 661W cells to assess protection. Statistical analysis using the Bonferroni multiple comparison was performed and significant probabilities with $P \leq 0.05$, are denoted with asterisks

Table 1 Membrane fractions were prepared from the 4 clones used in Fig. 3. The total RDH activity was determined for each of them using 0 or 10 µg of protein in each reaction, and increasing concentrations of all-*trans* retinal. The reduction to all-*trans* retinol was quantified for each reaction, the protein-dependant production of all-*trans* retinol was calculated, and for each clone a saturation curve was plotted as well as the corresponding direct linear plot. Each clone was assayed in 3 independent experiments and the results shown are derived from one representative experiment

Transfected construct	Apparent K_m (µM)	Apparent V_{max} (pmole/min/mg protein)
None	2.1	63.9
RDH8	2.1	195.5
RDH11	3.0	105.3
RDH12	3.3	130.1

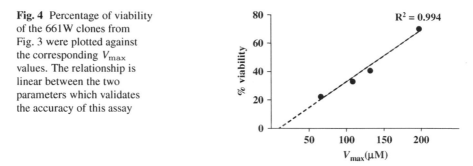

Fig. 4 Percentage of viability of the 661W clones from Fig. 3 were plotted against the corresponding V_{max} values. The relationship is linear between the two parameters which validates the accuracy of this assay

fraction of the cells as a source of enzyme, and using increasing concentrations of all-*trans* retinal to generate the saturation curves. We found that their affinities are comparable towards all-*trans* retinal. However, their catalytic activities were different. Figure 4 shows that the protection offered by these RDHs is proportional, in a linear fashion, to the amount of all-*trans* retinal that is converted to all-*trans* retinol.

4 Discussion

The assay mentioned above is a valuable way to test for the protection offered by a drug or a transfected gene against light induced stress. We found that PEDF and DHA both offer protection against light induced apoptosis. Recently it has been shown that rats that received intravitreous injection of adenoviral vector expressing PEDF offered protection to photoreceptors against light induced apoptosis and significantly reduced the number of apoptotic photoreceptor cells in the retina (Imai et al., 2005). Also, intravitreal injections of the PEDF before constant light exposure of 1500 lux, provided morphological and functional rescue to rat photoreceptors proving the efficacy of PEDF as a drug against light damage of retina (Cao et al., 2001). Though it has not been shown yet that addition of DHA can protect photoreceptor cells against light damage, it has been shown that a product of DHA metabolism, neuroprotectin D1 (NPD1), can prevent photoreceptor cells from oxidative stress (Mukherjee et al., 2004) that is resulting from light exposure (Tanito et al., 2006). Therefore DHA can reduce light induced oxidative stress by producing NPD1.

The protection offered by RDH transfection into 661W cells can be explained by the ability of RDHs to convert the photo-toxic all-*trans* retinal to the non toxic all-*trans* retinol. Loss of function mutations in the RDH12 gene were recently reported to be associated with autosomal recessive childhood-onset severe retinal dystrophy (Janecke et al., 2004). Furthermore, increased susceptibility to light-induced photoreceptor apoptosis were observed in RDH12 knockout mice (Maeda et al., 2006). Thus, visual impairments of individuals with null mutations in RDH12 may likely be caused by light damage in absence of the normal protection offered by RDH12.

Susceptibility for light damage was not tested in the RDH8 and RDH11 knockout mice. We will study these mice to assess protection offered by these RDHs under light stress condition.

Acknowledgments This publication was made possible by NIH Grant Number P20 RR 017703 from the COBRE Program of the National Center for Research Resources.

References

Al-Ubaidi, M.R., Font, R.L., Quiambao, A.B., Keener, M.J., Liou, G.I., Overbeek, P.A., and Baehr,W., 1992, Bilateral retinal and brain tumors in transgenic mice expressing simian virus 40 large T antigen under control of the human interphotoreceptor retinoid-binding protein promoter. *J. Cell Biol.* **119**:1681.

Cao, W., Tombran-Tink, J., Elias, R; Sezate, S., Mrazek, D., and McGinnis, J.F., 2001, In vivo protection of photoreceptors from light damage by pigment epithelium-derived factor. *Invest Ophthalmol. Vis. Sci.* **42**:1646.

Imai, D., Yoneya, S., Gehlbach, P.L., Wei, L.L., and Mori, K., 2005, Intraocular gene transfer of pigment epithelium-derived factor rescues photoreceptors from light-induced cell death. *J. Cell Physiol.* **202**:570.

Janecke, A.R., Thompson, D.A., Utermann, G., Becker, C., Hubner, C.A., Schmid, E., McHenry, C.L., Nair, A.R., Ruschendorf, F., Heckenlively, J., Wissinger, B., Nurnberg, P., and Gal, A., 2004, Mutations in RDH12 encoding a photoreceptor cell retinol dehydrogenase cause childhood-onset severe retinal dystrophy. *Nat. Genet.* **36**:850.

Kanan, K., Moiseyev, G., Agarwal, N., Ma., J.X., and Al-Ubaidi, M.R., 2007, Light induces programmed cell death by activating multiple independent proteases in a cone photoreceptor cell line. *Invest. Ophthalmol. Vis. Sci* **48**:40.

Maeda, A., Maeda, T., Imanishi, Y., Sun, W., Jastrzebska, B., Hatala, D.A., Winkens, H.J., Hofmann, K.P., Janssen,J.J., Baehr, W., Driessen, C.A., and Palczewski, K., 2006, Retinol dehydrogenase (RDH12) protects photoreceptors from light-induced degeneration in mice. *J.Biol.Chem.* **281**:37697.

Mukherjee, P.K., Marcheselli, V.L., Serhan, C.N., and Bazan, N.G., 2004, Neuroprotectin D1: a docosahexaenoic acid-derived docosatriene protects human retinal pigment epithelial cells from oxidative stress. *Proc. Natl. Acad. Sci. USA.* **101**:8491.

Tan, E., Ding, X.Q., Saadi, A., Agarwal, N., Naash, M.I., and Al-Ubaidi, M.R., 2004, Expression of cone-photoreceptor-specific antigens in a cell line derived from retinal tumors in transgenic mice. *Invest Ophthalmol. Vis. Sci.* **45**:764.

Tanito, M., Yoshida, Y., Kaidzu, S., Ohira, A., and Niki, E., 2006, Detection of lipid peroxidation in light-exposed mouse retina assessed by oxidative stress markers, total hydroxyoctadecadienoic acid and 8-iso-prostaglandin F2alpha. *Neurosci. Lett.* **398**:63.

Tomany, S.C., Cruickshanks, K.J., Klein, R., Klein B.E., and Knudtson, M.D., 2004, Sunlight and the 10-year incidence of age-related maculopathy: the beaver dam eye study. *Arch. Ophthalmol.* **122**:750.

Role of BCL-XL in Photoreceptor Survival

Yun-Zheng Le, Lixin Zheng, Yuwei Le, Edmund B. Rucker III,
and Robert E. Anderson

1 Introduction

Photoreceptors are post-mitotic neurons and understanding their survival mechanisms holds a key to the treatment of retinal degeneration. Many studies have demonstrated that phosphoinositide 3-kinase (PI3K) and its product phosphatidylinositol-3,4,5-trisphosphate (PIP_3) are involved in the survival of neurons through growth factor receptor-mediated activation of the serine-threonine kinase, AKT (Barber et al., 2000; D'Mello et al., 1997; Yao and Cooper, 1995). Activation of AKT further activates a number of down-stream targets, including the anti-apoptotic protein BCL-X_L, which can serve as a survival factor in a number of alternative pathways(Bui et al., 2001; Kim et al., 2005; Zha et al., 1996). For the past few years, we have investigated the roles of PI3K, insulin receptor, AKT, and BCL-X_L in photoreceptor survival. BCL-X_L was postulated as a survival factor in photoreceptors, as it was up-regulated in the bright light-stressed retina (Zheng et al., 2006). To determine the significance of BCL-X_L up-regulation in the bright light damage model, the *Bcl-x* gene was disrupted specifically in murine rod or cone photoreceptors using the Cre/*lox*-based conditional gene knockout strategy (Le and Sauer, 2000). Effects of *Bcl-x* disruption on photoreceptor function and morphology were characterized. This report reviews the results from rod-specific *Bcl-x* knockout mice and summarizes new information on cone-specific *Bcl-x* knockout mice.

2 Materials and Methods

2.1 Generation of Rod- or Cone-specific Bcl-x Knockout Mice

Albino rod- or cone-specific *Bcl-x* knockout mice were generated separately by mating floxed *Bcl-x* mice with Short Mouse Opsin Promoter-controlled *cre* (SMOPC1)

Y.-Z. Le

Departments of Medicine; Cell Biology; Dean A. McGee Eye Institute, Oklahoma City, OK, USA,
Tel: 405-271-1087, Fax: 405-271-8128
e-mail: Yun-Le@ouhsc.edu

R.E. Anderson et al. (eds.), *Recent Advances in Retinal Degeneration*,
© Springer 2008

mice or $\underline{H}$uman $\underline{R}$ed $\underline{G}$reen $\underline{P}$igment $\underline{P}$romoter-controlled $\underline{c}re$ (HRGPPC) mice, respectively,(Le et al., 2004; Le et al., 2006a; Rucker et al., 2000). The genotypes of these conditional *Bcl-x* knockout mice were verified according to the described methods (Zheng et al., 2006).

2.2 Bright Light Stress

All mice were maintained in 100-lux cyclic light after birth. Eight-week-old rod-specific *Bcl-x* knockout mice or cone-specific *Bcl-x* knockout mice were exposed to white light at an illumination of 7,000 lux for 48 h or up to 96 h, respectively. The mice were then maintained in 100-lux cyclic light. Gene expression, apoptosis, and DNA fragmentation assays were carried out 24 h after the light exposure. Morphological and functional analyses were carried out 7 days after the bright light exposure.

2.3 Analysis of the Conditional Bcl-x Knockout Mice

Immunostaining and immunoblotting for BCL-X_L, TUNEL assay, DNA fragmentation assay, retinal morphological analysis, and electroretinography (ERG) were performed as described previously (Le et al., 2006a; Zheng et al., 2006). Cone density was determined with a lectin-staining assay according to the methods described previously (Le et al., 2004; Le et al., 2006b).

3 Results

3.1 Characterization of Rod-specific Bcl-x Knockout Mice

In the rod-specific *Bcl-x* knockout mice, the loss of BCL-X_L expression was confirmed by Western blot analysis of retinal homogenates and immunohistochemistry (IHC) of retinal sections (Zheng et al., 2006). Examination of four-month-old rod-specific *Bcl-x* knockout mice demonstrated that the loss of BCL-X_L did not cause any detectable changes in retinal apoptosis, morphology, or function under normal conditions (data not shown), suggesting that BCL-X_L is not required for maintenance of the morphological and the functional integrity of the rod photoreceptors under normal conditions. Since BCL-X_L was up-regulated under the bright light stress (7,000 lux for 48 h) in the retina of the wild-type mice, we then placed the 2-month-old rod-specific *Bcl-x* knockout mice and their littermate controls under bright light stress. Apoptosis was analyzed with TUNEL, nuclear staining, and DNA fragmentation assays. Our results suggest that there were significantly more apoptotic rod photoreceptors in the bright light-stressed, rod-specific *Bcl-x* knockout mice (Zheng et al., 2006). Examination of retinal morphology and function 7 days after the bright light stress demonstrated that there was significantly greater loss of the photoreceptor outer nuclear layer (ONL) thickness and scotopic ERG amplitude in the rod-specific *Bcl-x* knockout mice (Zheng et al., 2006). In short, our results clearly demonstrated that the loss of BCL-X$_L$ caused increased susceptibility to the bright light stress in mouse rod photoreceptors.

3.2 Characterization of Cone-specific Bcl-x Knockout Mice

To address whether BCL-X$_L$ plays a protective role in the cone photoreceptors under bright light stress, we examined the effects of a genetic disruption of *Bcl-x* in mouse cone photoreceptors. Since mice have rod-dominant retinas and, since the methods to analyze both rod and cone photoreceptor-expressed genes in mouse cone photoreceptors have not been well established, it is difficult to analyze BCL-X$_L$ expression and apoptosis in the cone photoreceptors without interference from rod-expressed BCL-X$_L$. To overcome this problem, we took advantage of our cone-specific Cre mice that are capable of efficient Cre-mediated recombination in almost all S-cone and M-cone photoreceptors (Le et al., 2004). In a functional assay using double transgenic mice carrying *cre* and Cre-activatable *lacZ* reporter gene (Soriano, 1999), β-galactosidase was shown to be exclusively and efficiently expressed in the cone photoreceptors (Fig. 1). In addition, successful Cre-mediated recombination in many cell-type-specific *Bcl-x* knockout studies suggests that the chromosomal locus behaves normally and does not prevent Cre-mediated *Bcl-x* disruption in cone photoreceptors. Therefore, *Bcl-x* was disrupted genetically in cone photoreceptors in the cone-specific *Bcl-x* knockout mice.

Examination of four-month-old, albino cone-specific *Bcl-x* knockout mice demonstrated that the disruption of *Bcl-x* did not cause detectable changes in cone function or density under normal conditions (data not shown), suggesting that the BCL-X$_L$, was not required for maintenance of the structural and the functional integrity of the cone photoreceptors under normal conditions. To determine if the BCL-X$_L$ had a protective effect under light stress in cone photoreceptors, the cone-specific *Bcl-x* knockout mice were then subjected to bright light. Although bright

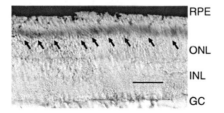

Fig. 1 Cre-mediated DNA recombination using F1 mice derived from cone-specific Cre mice and Cre-activatable *lacZ* reporter (R26R) mice. Arrows indicate a dark layer of β-galactosidase staining in a retinal section from a double transgenic mouse. ONL: outer nuclear layer; INL: inner nuclear layer; GC: ganglion cell. The scale bar represents 50 µm. Cre was efficiently expressed in the cone photoreceptors

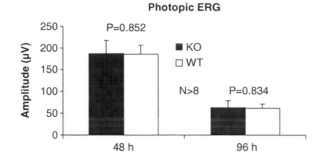

Fig. 2 Photopic ERG b-wave amplitude of age-matched cone-specific *Bcl-x* knockout (KO) mice and their wild-type (WT) littermates after exposed to bright light for 48 or 96 h, respectively. Although bright light caused significant loss of visual function, there was no significant difference in the average b-wave amplitude between the cone-specific *Bcl-x* KO mice and the WT controls

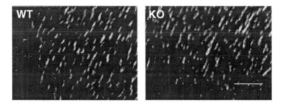

Fig. 3 Cone distribution in age-matched cone-specific *Bcl-x* knockout (KO) mice and their wild-type (WT) littermates exposed to bright light for 96 h. Similar regions of the lectin stained retinal flat-mount were used in the comparison. The scale bar equals to 50 μm. There was no significant difference in the cone distribution between the cone-specific *Bcl-x* KO mice and the WT controls

light stress caused a reduction of cone photoreceptor function in both wild-type mice and the cone-specific *Bcl-x* knockout mice, there was no detectable difference in cone photoreceptor function between the bright light-stressed, cone-specific *Bcl-x* knockout mice and their wild-type littermates (Fig. 2). Likewise, we detected no difference in the numbers of cone photoreceptors between the bright light-stressed, cone-specific *Bcl-x* knockout mice and their wild-type littermates (Fig. 3), suggesting that BCL-X$_L$ was not required for cone photoreceptor survival under bright light stress. In summary, our results demonstrates that disruption of *Bcl-x* did not affect the survivability of cone photoreceptors under normal conditions or under bright light stress. Whether BCL-X$_L$ is a survival factor for cones under other types of stress has yet to be determined and is being investigated.

4 Discussion

BCL-X$_L$ is a predominant anti-apoptotic member of BCL-2 protein family in the retina and is expressed in the mouse retina Donovan et al., 2006; Levin et al., 1997). Although the significance of BCL-X$_L$ in the adult retina under normal conditions is still not well understood, it is likely to serve as a cell death/survival checkpoint regulator of mitochondrial dysfunction. Recent evidences demonstrated that over-expression of BCL-X$_L$ protected photoreceptors from lead-induced apoptosis in mice through a blockage of the function of BAX, a pro-apoptotic protein (He et al., 2003). This is consistent with our result that loss of BCL-X$_L$ caused an increased susceptibility to bright light stress in rod photoreceptors, which is supported by the finding that loss of the pro-apoptotic proteins BAX and BAK protected photoreceptors from light damage in mice (Hahn et al., 2004). Interestingly, over-expression of BCL-X$_L$ did not appear to rescue either the inherited retinal degeneration caused by a *Rd/Rd* mutation or a dominant rhodopsin gene mutation (Joseph and Li, 1996). Therefore, the protective effect of BCL-X$_L$ is not universal and may be related to a specific stress condition. This may explain why we did not observe an increased susceptibility to bright light stress after disruption of *Bcl-x* in cone photoreceptors. In short, disruption of *Bcl-x* had no apparent effect on cone photoreceptor survival and thus BCL-X$_L$ may not play a protective role in cone photoreceptors under bright light stress.

Previous evidence demonstrates the presence of at least two independent apoptotic pathways for light-induced photoreceptor degeneration: a low light intensity caused phototransduction-related apoptosis and a high light intensity induced apoptosis via the transcription factor AP-1 (Hao et al., 2002). At present, the molecular mechanism governing bright light-induced photoreceptor protection caused by BCL-X$_L$ is not completely determined; however, BCL-X$_L$ is a down-stream target of the PI3K-AKT pathway. Genetic disruption of *Akt* also caused increased photoreceptor susceptibility to light damage (Li et al., 2007), suggesting that PI3K, AKT, and BCL-X$_L$ may act on the same pathway. BCL-X$_L$ is considered as an up-stream regulator of the caspase-dependent apoptotic pathways. Although the role of the caspase-dependent apoptotic pathways in light-induced photoreceptor degeneration is still controversial, our results suggest that BCL-X$_L$, a widely regarded up-stream regulator of the caspase-dependent apoptotic pathway, is involved in the protection of rod photoreceptors from bright light-induced stress.

Acknowledgments The authors thank W. Zheng and M. Zhu for technical assistance; Dr. Lothar Hennighausen for providing the floxed *Bcl-x* mice. This study was supported by OCAST contracts HR01-083 and HR05-133; NIH grants EY00871, EY12190, EY04149, and RR17703; ADA Grant 1-06-RA-76; the Foundation Fighting Blindness, Inc; and Unrestricted Research Awards from Hope for Vision and Research to Prevent Blindness, Inc. Y.Z. Le is supported by a Young Investigator Travel Award to attend the XIIth International Symposium on Retinal Degenerations.

References

Barber, A. J., Antonetti, D. A., and Gardner, T. W. (2000). Altered expression of retinal occludin and glial fibrillary acidic protein in experimental diabetes. The Penn State Retina Research Group. *Invest Ophthalmol Vis Sci* **41**, 3561–68.

Bui, N. T., Livolsi, A., Peyron, J. F., and Prehn, J. H. (2001). Activation of nuclear factor kappaB and Bcl-x survival gene expression by nerve growth factor requires tyrosine phosphorylation of IkappaBalpha. *J Cell Biol* **152**, 753–64.

D'Mello, S. R., Borodezt, K., and Soltoff, S. P. (1997). Insulin-like growth factor and potassium depolarization maintain neuronal survival by distinct pathways: possible involvement of PI 3-kinase in IGF-1 signaling. *J Neurosci* **17,** 1548–60.

Donovan, M., Doonan, F., and Cotter, T. G. (2006). Decreased expression of pro-apoptotic Bcl-2 family members during retinal development and differential sensitivity to cell death. *Dev Biol* **291,** 154–69.

Hahn, P., Lindsten, T., Lyubarsky, A., Ying, G. S., Pugh, E. N., Jr., Thompson, C. B., and Dunaief, J. L. (2004). Deficiency of Bax and Bak protects photoreceptors from light damage in vivo. *Cell Death Differ* **11,** 1192–97.

Hao, W., Wenzel, A., Obin, M. S., Chen, C. K., Brill, E., Krasnoperova, N. V., Eversole-Cire, P., Kleyner, Y., Taylor, A., Simon, M. I., Grimm, C., Reme, C. E., and Lem, J. (2002). Evidence for two apoptotic pathways in light-induced retinal degeneration. *Nat Genet* **32,** 254–60.

He, L., Perkins, G. A., Poblenz, A. T., Harris, J. B., Hung, M., Ellisman, M. H., and Fox, D. A. (2003). Bcl-xL overexpression blocks bax-mediated mitochondrial contact site formation and apoptosis in rod photoreceptors of lead-exposed mice. *Proc Natl Acad Sci USA* **100,** 1022–27.

Joseph, R. M., and Li, T. (1996). Overexpression of Bcl-2 or Bcl-XL transgenes and photoreceptor degeneration. *Invest Ophthalmol Vis Sci* **37,** 2434–46.

Kim, R. (2005). Unknotting the roles of Bcl-2 and Bcl-xL in cell death. *Biochem Biophys Res Commun* **333,** 336–43.

Le, Y., Ash, J. D., Al-Ubaidi, M. R., Chen, Y., Ma, J., and Anderson, R. E. (2004). Targeted expression of Cre recombinase to cone photoreceptors in transgenic mice. *Mol Vis* **10,** 1011–18.

Le, Y., and Sauer, B. (2000). Conditional gene knockout using cre recombinase. *Methods Mol Biol* **136,** 477–85.

Le, Y., Zheng, L., Zheng, W., Agbaga, M., Zhu, M., Ash, J. D., and Anderson, R. E. (2006a). Mouse opsin promoter controlled expression of Cre recombinase in transgenic mice. *Mol Vis* **12,** 389–98.

Le, Y. Z., Ash, J. D., Al-Ubaidi, M. R., Chen, Y., Ma, J. X., and Anderson, R. E. (2006b). Conditional gene knockout system in cone photoreceptors. *Adv Exp Med Biol* **572,** 173–78.

Levin, L. A., Schlamp, C. L., Spieldoch, R. L., Geszvain, K. M., and Nickells, R. W. (1997). Identification of the bcl-2 family of genes in the rat retina. *Invest Ophthalmol Vis Sci* **38,** 2545–53.

Li, G., Anderson, R. E., Tomita, H., Adler, R., Liu, X., Zack, D. J., and Rajala, R. V. (2007). Nonredundant role of Akt2 for neuroprotection of rod photoreceptor cells from light-induced cell death. *J Neurosci* **27,** 203–11.

Rucker, E. B., Dierisseau, P., Wagner, K. U., Garrett, L., Wynshaw-Boris, A., Flaws, J. A., and Hennighausen, L. (2000). Bcl-x and Bax regulate mouse primordial germ cell survival and apoptosis during embryogenesis. *Mol Endocrinol* **14,** 1038–52.

Soriano, P. (1999). Generalized lacZ expression with the ROSA26 Cre reporter strain. *Nat Genet* **21,** 70–71.

Yao, R., and Cooper, G. M. (1995). Requirement for phosphatidylinositol-3 kinase in the prevention of apoptosis by nerve growth factor. *Science* **267,** 2003–06.

Zha, J., Harada, H., Yang, E., Jockel, J., and Korsmeyer, S. J. (1996). Serine phosphorylation of death agonist BAD in response to survival factor results in binding to 14-3-3 not BCL-X(L). *Cell* **87,** 619–28.

Zheng, L., Anderson, R. E., Agbaga, M. P., Rucker, E. B., 3rd, and Le, Y. Z. (2006). Loss of BCL-XL in rod photoreceptors: increased susceptibility to bright light stress. *Invest Ophthalmol Vis Sci* **47,** 5583–89.

The Hypoxic Transcriptome of the Retina: Identification of Factors with Potential Neuroprotective Activity

Markus Thiersch, Wolfgang Raffelsberger, Enrico Frigg, Marijana Samardzija, Patricia Blank, Olivier Poch, and Christian Grimm

1 Introduction

Most blinding diseases of the retina share a common feature – the loss of photoreceptor cells by apoptosis. Although degenerative diseases like age-related macular degeneration (AMD) and Retinitis Pigmentosa (RP) are among the main causes for severe visual impairment and blindness, no effective therapeutical treatments are available to prevent loss of vision in human patients. Protection of retinal cells against cell death is a promising strategy to develop therapies aiming at the rescue of retinal function. For the successful design of neuroprotective strategies, it is essential to understand the molecular events leading to the degeneration of retinal cells. To study signaling pathways and molecular mechanisms during the degenerative processes, several mouse models of inherited retinal degeneration are used (Fauser et al., 2002). These models are complemented by models of induced photoreceptor apoptosis like the model of light-induced degeneration (Wenzel et al., 2005). The advantage of the induced models is the synchronized apoptotic response of many photoreceptor cells to the death stimulus. This might raise the activation of regulatory factors above detection threshold allowing their detailed investigation.

Recently, we showed that hypoxic preconditioning protects photoreceptor cells against light-induced cell death by preserving retinal function and morphology (Grimm et al. 2002). Similarly, hypoxic pretreatment can also protect other tissues like heart or brain against various toxic insults (Gidday et al., 1994; Emerson et al., 1999; Cai et al., 2003; Dong et al., 2003) suggesting that hypoxic preconditioning might induce a general protective response. Such a response might involve hypoxia-inducible-factor 1a (HIF-1a) which is stabilized in the retina after hypoxic exposure (Grimm et al., 2002). As a transcription factor, HIF-1a (together with HIF-2a) is a key element of the hypoxic response regulating expression of many target genes. Such genes are involved in different physiological functions like

M. Thiersch
Lab for Retinal Cell Biology, Dept Ophthalmology, CIHP, University of Zurich, Switzerland,
Tel: 0041 44 2553719, Fax: 0041 44 255 4385
e-mail: markus.thiersch@usz.ch

R.E. Anderson et al. (eds.), *Recent Advances in Retinal Degeneration*,
© Springer 2008

angiogenesis, general metabolism and apoptosis. One target gene of HIF-1a and/or HIF-2a has been identified in erythropoietin (Epo). Epo was shown to prevent death of precursor cells of erythrocytes in bone marrow and was thus recognized as a potent anti-apoptotic factor (Koury et al., 2002). Since expression of Epo is strongly induced after hypoxic preconditioning in the retina and Epo receptor expression was localized mainly to photoreceptor and ganglion cells (Bocker-Meffert et al., 2002; Grimm et al., 2002; Grimm et al., 2004), Epo was considered to be a factor protecting the retina against degeneration. Supporting this conclusion, application of recombinant Epo protected photoreceptor cells against light-induced degeneration. However, protection was not as complete as after hypoxic preconditioning suggesting that exposure to reduced oxygen levels may differentially regulate expression of additional genes involved in the protection of photoreceptor cells (Grimm et al., 2002; Grimm et al., 2004).

The goal of the present study was to analyze the retinal response to hypoxia and to identify differentially regulated genes that might be involved in retinal neuroprotection.

2 Material and Methods

2.1 Hypoxic Preconditioning and Affymetrix Microarrays

Animals were treated in accordance with the regulations of the Veterinary Authority of Zurich and with the statement of 'The Association for Research in Vision and Ophthalmology' for the use of animals in research. BALB/c mice (Harlan, The Netherlands) were exposed to 6% oxygen for 6 h. Retinas were isolated at 0 h, 2 h, 4 h or 16 h after the period of hypoxic preconditioning. Normoxic controls were treated in parallel and collected at the same time points. For each condition three retinas of three different mice were pooled. Total RNA was prepared, processed according to standard procedures and hybridized to Affymetrix GeneChip® Mouse Genome 430 2.0 microarrays. The experiment was conducted three times independently resulting in three microarray replicates per condition and a total number of 9 retinas per condition.

2.2 Quality Control and Affymetrix Chip Analyzes

To analyze the quality of the results after gene chip hybridization the online tool RACE (Remote Analysis Computation for gene Expression data) of the University of Lausanne was used.

To analyze gene expression profiles and to identify differentially regulated genes, we used Genespring 7.0 (Agilent Technologies) software based on the Mas 5.0 algorithm. In brief, hypoxic samples (H, hypoxic) were compared to their corresponding normoxic controls (N, normoxic) resulting in 4 different analyzes: N0 vs. H0, N2 vs. H2, N4 vs. H4 and N16 vs. H16. In the first step, genes were tested for their presence or absence in the samples. Genes were considered to be expressed and allowed to pass the filter only when all 3 replicates of a particular condition (normoxic, hypoxic) got a present call. Genes that passed the first filter were then analyzed and filtered according to their fold change (at least factor 2) and to their p-value (≤ 0.05). Additionally, a statistical correction according to Benjamini/Hochberg (Benjamini and Hochberg, 1995) was applied. To sort differentially regulated genes according to their biological function the online tool Onto-Express from Intelligent Systems and Bioinformatics Laboratory (Draghici et al., 2003a,b,c) was used (http://vortex.cs.wayne.edu/projects.htm).

2.3 Real-time PCR

Gene regulation was confirmed by real-time PCR on cDNA prepared from total retinal RNA, using a LightCycler 480 instrument (Roche Diagnostics AG, Rotkreuz, Switzerland) and LightCycler 480 SYBR Green I Master Mix (Roche Diagnostics AG). Primers were designed using the Universal ProbeLibrary Assay Design Centre (Roche Diagnostics AG) https://www.roche-applied-science.com. Relative expression was calculated according to the expression of b-actin using the LightCycler software package.

2.4 Light Exposure and Quantification of Cell Death

$p21^{-/-}$ mice on a mixed Bl/6;129S2 background were purchased from Jackson Laboratory (Bar Harbor, USA). Mice homozygous for the light sensitive $Rpe65_{450Leu}$ variant (Wenzel et al., 2001; Samardzija et al., 2006) were used to establish the breeding colony. After hypoxic preconditioning (see 2.1) mice were reoxygenated in darkness (dark adaptation) for 4 hours prior to illumination. 45 minutes prior to illumination, pupils were dilated in dim red light using 1% Cyclogyl (Alcon, Cham, Switzerland) and 5% Phenylephrine (Ciba Vision, Niederwangen, Switzerland). Mice were exposed to 13'000 lux of white fluorescent light for 2 hours.

36 hours after light exposure apoptotic cell death was quantified in isolated retinas using a sandwich ELISA system (Cell Death Detection ElisaPlus, Roche Diagnostics, Basel, Switzerland, used according to the manufacturer's recommendation) to determine the relative amount of free nucleosomes in the cytosolic fraction of isolated retinas.

2.5 Morphology

Eyes were removed and fixed in 2.5% glutaraldehyde in 0.1 M cacodylate buffer, pH 7.3 at 4°C overnight. For each eye, the superior central and the inferior central retina adjacent to the optic nerve were trimmed and embedded in Epon 812. Sections (0.5 μm) were prepared from the inferior central retina, stained with toluidine blue and analyzed using an Axioplan microscope (Zeiss, Oberkochen, Germany).

3 Results

3.1 Statistical Analyzes

Hypoxic preconditioning was shown to completely protect photoreceptor cells against light – induced cell death when the light stimulus was given after a reoxygenation period of 4 h (Grimm et al., 2002). In contrast, mice exposed to light at 16 h after hypoxic preconditioning were not protected suggesting that the protective effect of hypoxia is transient and short-lived. Based on these findings we decided to analyze the retinal transcriptome at 4 different time points after hypoxic preconditioning. The first three time points were within the frame of full neuroprotection (0 h, +2 h, +4 h) whereas the last time point was taken after neuroprotection has ceased (+16 h). Quality controls were used to confirm the successful performance of the experiment. Analyzes, which compare the global similarity of all gene chips indicated that hypoxic replicates were very similar within their groups and highly different to their normoxic controls (data not shown).

Genespring 7.0 software was used to detect genes that were differentially regulated by hypoxic exposure. In this first statistical analysis without mathematical correction 772 genes appeared to be differentially regulated immediately after hypoxia. This number decreased during reoxygenation to 189 genes after 2 h, 74 genes after 4 h and 24 genes 16 h after hypoxia (Table 1). After application of the highly stringent statistical method of Benjamini/Hochberg (Benjamini and Hochberg, 1995), we identified a total of 83 genes as significantly regulated immediately after hypoxic preconditioning. Already at 2 h after hypoxia, only 7 genes remained to have significantly different expression levels and at 4 h and 16 h after hypoxia the retinal transcriptome of preconditioned mice was indistinguishable from normoxic controls

Table 1 Total number of genes differentially regulated at 0 h, 2 h, 4 h and 16 h after hypoxia

Condition	Altered genes with Benjamini/ Hochberg	False positive	Altered genes without Benjamini/ Hochberg	False positive
H0 vs. N0	83	4	772	96
H2 vs. N2	7	-	189	24
H4 vs. N4	0	-	74	9
H16 vs. N16	0	-	24	3

Shown are the numbers of genes passing the stringent Benjamini/Hochberg correction in comparison to a normal t-test. The columns 'false positive' show the expected number of genes which have passed the respective test but which are nevertheless not differentially regulated. H0, H2, H4, H16: retinas at 0 h, 2 h, 4 h and 16 h, respectively, after hypoxic preconditioning. N0, N2, N4, N16: control normoxic retinas

(Table 1). Both statistical methods indicated that differential regulation of gene expression is strongest immediately after hypoxia. During reoxygenation, the retinal transcriptome quickly returned to the normoxic gene expression pattern suggesting a short-lived molecular effect of hypoxic preconditioning.

3.2 Biological Classification

It is eminent to sort differentially regulated genes according to their biological relevance. Using the statistical online tool 'Onto express' we classified the identified genes with respect to their various biological functions like apoptosis, transport, cell cycle and others (Fig. 1). The highest number of regulated genes was sorted into the group of transport-related genes followed by apoptosis-related processes. This may be of high relevance since hypoxic preconditioning induces a neuroprotective response in the retina, which most likely involves a number of genes related to the control of apoptotic events. Having in mind, that genes can be present in more than one biological group, the number of sorted genes does not reflect the real number of genes identified as differentially regulated. Individual genes of the group of 'anti-apoptotic' or the group of 'induction of apoptosis' were also found in the group 'apoptosis'. Table 2 summarizes differentially regulated genes that are considered anti-apoptotic. Note that some of these genes are repressed by the hypoxic pretreatment. Table 3 shows the most prominently regulated pro-apoptotic genes. In total, 13 genes with a known anti-apoptotic function were differentially regulated by hypoxia. Nine genes were induced whereas 4 genes were repressed (Table 2). Test of

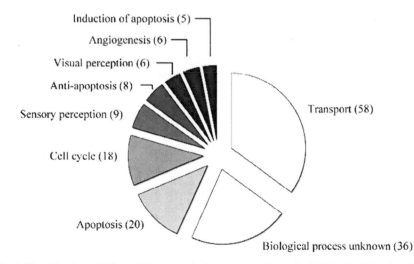

Fig. 1 Classification of differentially expressed genes according to their biological function. Genes regulated immediately after hypoxia (0 h) without statistical correction were classified using Onto-Express. Only most prominent and statistically significant ($p \leq 0.05$) groups are shown. Numbers of genes in each group are given in brackets

Table 2 Differentially regulated genes with anti-apoptotic functions

Gene	FC 0 h	FC 2 h	FC 4 h	FC 16 h
p21	34.4	–	–	–
Bcl2-like 10	6.3	–	–	–
Snai2	–	3.1	–	–
Vegfa	2.6	–	–	–
Bhlhb4	2.3	–	–	–
Bfar	2.2	–	–	–
Camk1d	–	2.2	2.0	–
Birc6	–	2.1	–	–
C/EBP	2.0	2.3	–	–
p21-activated kinase 7	0.46	–	–	–
Apoptosis inhibitor 5	0.34	–	–	–
Glutaminyl-tRNA-Synthetase	0.32	–	–	–
Birc4	0.22	–	–	–

Shown are the gene-chip deduced fold-changes (FC) at 0 h, 2 h, 4 h and 16 h after hypoxic preconditioning. p21 is the most prominently up-regulated gene within this group. -; not detected

VEGF, p21 and Bcl2l10 gene expression by real-time PCR confirmed the chip data and their up-regulation in response to the hypoxic pretreatment (Fig. 2). In addition to the anti-apoptotic genes, expression of 5 genes expected to be pro-apoptotic was induced during hypoxia (Table 3).

Having both, pro- and anti-apoptotic genes regulated by hypoxia suggests that the preconditioning protocol induces a complex response priming the tissue to resist a toxic insult but also preparing the cells to induce apoptotic cell death if needed. We hypothesize that reducing the number of cells may be required in case of prolonged hypoxic exposure to ensure that at least some cells can be supplied with sufficient oxygen to function.

3.3 The Neuroprotective Impact of p21

One of the most prominently induced genes with reported anti-apoptotic properties was p21, a cyclin-dependent kinase inhibitor. To analyze its role in neuroprotection by hypoxic preconditioning, p21 knockout mice were exposed to hypoxia,

Table 3 Differentially regulated genes with pro-apoptotic functions

Gene	FC 0 h	FC 2 h	FC 4 h	FC 16 h
Pmaip1	12.9	–	–	–
Sh3glb1 (endophilin)	5	4.7	–	–
Bnip3	2.3	–	–	–
BCL2-like 11	2.2	–	–	–
Foxo3a	2.1	–	–	–

Shown are the gene-chip deduced fold-changes (FC) at 0 h, 2 h, 4 h and 16 h after hypoxic preconditioning. -; not detected

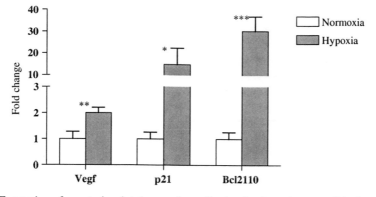

Fig. 2 Expression of apoptosis-related genes immediately after hypoxic preconditioning relative to normoxic controls as determined by real-time PCR. Expression of Vegf, p21 and Bcl2l10 (as indicated) was determined in three normoxic and three hypoxic retinas. Amplifications were done in duplicates. Normoxic samples were set to 1 and hypoxic samples represent the relative fold change due to hypoxia

reoxygenated for 4 hours and exposed to 2 hours of 13,000 lux of white light. As controls, $p21^{-/-}$ mice were kept in normoxic conditions before light exposure. Light-induced photoreceptor apoptosis was analyzed 36 hours after exposure by light microscopy (Fig. 3A) and by the semi-quantitative determination of free nucleosomes (Fig. 3B). In contrast to normoxic control mice, hypoxic preconditioned p21

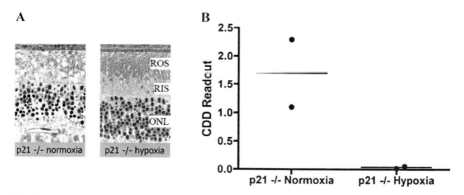

Fig. 3 Analysis of the role of p21 in retinal neuroprotection by hypoxic preconditioning. $p21^{-/-}$ mice were either kept in normoxia or were preconditioned with 6% O_2 for 6 hours before light exposure. (A) Retinal morphology was analyzed 36 hours after exposure. Normoxic mice (left panel) showed strong signs of degeneration with many pyknotic photoreceptor nuclei and severe destruction of inner and outer segments. Retinas of hypoxic preconditioned mice (right panel) were completely protected against light-induced degeneration. (B) Cell death detection (CDD) assay to analyze the amount of free nucleosomes in the cytoplasmic fraction 36 h after light exposure. Normoxic mice showed a high content of free nucleosomes whereas hypoxic preconditioned mice showed no detectable release of nucleosomes. Shown are data points of two individual mice (dots) with the respective average (line). ROS: rod outer segments; RIS: rod inner segments; ONL: outer nuclear layer

knockout animals did not produce a significant amount of free nucleosomes after light-exposure suggesting that lack of p21 did not interfere with the neuroprotection by hypoxic preconditioning. These findings were confirmed by the morphological analysis of retinal tissue after light exposure (Fig. 3A). In contrast to normoxic controls where light exposure induced the formation of pyknotic nuclei and a severe disruption of rod inner and outer segments, retinal morphology of preconditioned knockout mice was completely protected.

4 Discussion

Photoreceptor cells are among the cells with the highest need for oxygen. Highest oxygen concentrations are measured at the level of the outer segments which are closest to the choroidal blood vessels. With increasing distance from the RPE and the choroidea, oxygen concentrations drop rapidly and photoreceptor cells can experience borderline hypoxic conditions at night, the time of highest energy consumption (Yu and Cringle, 2005). To react and/or adapt to such conditions, the retina needs a system that can sense oxygen levels and induce appropriate endogenous mechanisms in response to varying conditions. In a normal physiological situation, such a response may include an adaptation of the metabolism reducing or increasing the consumption of energy. In harsher conditions, the retina may prepare the cells to survive by the induction of an endogenous neuroprotective response. If unfavorable conditions persist, the sacrifice of some individual cells may be required in order to safe the function of the retinal tissue as a whole. Understanding the retinal response to hypoxia may lead to the identification of potent endogenous neuroprotective mechanisms. Artificial and controlled stimulation of such mechanisms may be beneficial for human patients suffering from loss of vision due to retinal degeneration. Furthermore, hypoxia is one of the driving forces for neovascularization, a major complication of many retinal diseases including diabetic retinopathy and AMD (Zhang and Ma, 2007). Identification of the molecular mechanisms controlling the hypoxia-related production of angiogenic factors like VEGF may lead to the development of new and efficient treatments for these diseases.

Recently we showed that a transient period of strong hypoxia induces a molecular response in the retina which protects photoreceptors from the otherwise deleterious effect of light exposure (Grimm et al., 2002). A central regulator of this response might be the transcription factor HIF-1a which is stabilized and therefore activated in hypoxic conditions in several tissues including the retina (Grimm et al., 2002; Maxwell, 2003; Sharp and Bernaudin, 2004). However, since HIF-1a and other transcription factors modulate the expression of a large amount of genes (Ke and Costa, 2006), the molecular mechanisms involved in the tissue response to hypoxia are still poorly understood and the molecular basis for hypoxia-induced neuroprotection remains unclear. Our study was therefore designed to increase our knowledge of hypoxia-dependent gene regulation and neuroprotection by analyzing the retinal transcriptome after hypoxic preconditioning.

The highest number of differentially regulated genes was found immediately after hypoxia. At this time, HIF-1a is present at high levels suggesting that HIF-1a may indeed be one of the major factors controlling the hypoxic response in the retina. This is further supported by the rapid decline of HIF-1a levels (Grimm et al., 2002) and of differentially expressed genes during reoxygenation.

The most prominent functional group affected by hypoxia was "transport" which includes genes of general metabolic activity like Slc37a4 (glucose-6phosphate transporter) or FABP4 (fatty acid binding protein 4). This may reflect an adaptational response of the retina, which may normally occur to a rather mild change in oxygen levels. Despite the strong neuroprotective capacity of hypoxic preconditioning, we also detected a number of differentially regulated genes that are pro-apoptotic and may therefore promote cell death. As discussed above, these factors may be produced to reduce the number of oxygen-consuming cells if low levels of oxygen persist. This might secure sufficient oxygen supply and therefore energy for a smaller cell population which may thus survive and function even in unfavorable conditions. Although this may reduce the general sensitivity of the retina, it may nevertheless rescue some (reduced) function. It might be interesting to analyze whether less severe hypoxic conditions would increase the differential regulation of genes involved in general metabolism and decrease the number of pro-apoptotic genes.

Our focus, however, is the elucidation of the neuroprotective mechanisms in response to a harsh but transient hypoxic period. Therefore, we concentrated during our initial analysis on genes which might be involved in an anti-apoptotic response of the retina. Because p21 was one of the most prominently induced genes with known anti-apoptotic functions (Zaman et al., 1999; Mahyar-Roemer and Roemer, 2001), we focused on its potential role in neuroprotection after hypoxic preconditioning. We hypothesized that lack of p21 would reduce the neuroprotective effect if the gene was indeed involved in the protective response. However, mice with a functional knockout of p21 were highly protected against a toxic light insult when preconditioned with hypoxia. This suggests that this Cyclin dependent kinase inhibitor is at least not a major contributor to the neuroprotective response induced by hypoxic preconditioning.

We will continue the analysis of individual genes identified in our screen. Future studies will focus on genes like Bcl2l10 or C/EBP which were up-regulated during hypoxia and which are known to be anti-apoptotic (Song et al., 1999; Naumann et al., 2001; and Buck and Chojkier, 2003). Additionally, strongly up-regulated genes (not shown) like Paraoxonase 1, which is involved in oxidative stress response and lipid oxidation (Aviram et al., 1998) or Adrenomedullin, which was reported to be neuroprotective in ischemia models (Miyashita et al., 2006) will be studied for their relevance to retinal neuroprotection after hypoxic preconditioning.

Acknowledgments The authors thank Coni Imsand, Gaby Hoegger, Hedwig Wariwoda and Philipp Huber for excellent technical assistance. This work was supported by the Swiss National Science Foundation (SNF), the Fritz-Tobler-Foundation, the Centre of Integrative Human Physiology (CIHP) and the European Union (Evi-GenoRet).

References

Aviram, M., Rosenblat, M., Bisgaier, C.L., Newton, R.S., Primo-Parmo, S.L., and La Du, B.N. 1998. Paraoxonase inhibits high-density lipoprotein oxidation and preserves its functions. A possible peroxidative role for paraoxonase. *J Clin Invest* **101**(8): 1581–1590.

Benjamini, Y. and Hochberg, Y. 1995. Controlling the false discovery rate – a practical and powerful approach to multiple testing. *J Roy Stat Soc* **57**: 289–300.

Bocker-Meffert, S., Rosenstiel, P., Rohl, C., Warneke, N., Held-Feindt, J., Sievers, J., and Lucius, R. 2002. Erythropoietin and VEGF promote neural outgrowth from retinal explants in postnatal rats. *Invest Ophthalmol Vis Sci* **43**(6): 2021–2026.

Buck, M. and Chojkier, M. 2003. Signal transduction in the liver: C/EBPbeta modulates cell proliferation and survival. *Hepatology* **37**(4): 731–738.

Cai, Z., Manalo, D.J., Wei, G., Rodriguez, E.R., Fox-Talbot, K., Lu, H., Zweier, J.L., and Semenza, G.L. 2003. Hearts from rodents exposed to intermittent hypoxia or erythropoietin are protected against ischemia-reperfusion injury. *Circulation* **108**(1): 79–85.

Dong, J.W., Zhu, H.F., Zhu, W.Z., Ding, H.L., Ma, T.M., and Zhou, Z.N. 2003. Intermittent hypoxia attenuates ischemia/reperfusion induced apoptosis in cardiac myocytes via regulating Bcl-2/Bax expression. *Cell Res* **13**(5): 385–391.

Draghici, S., Khatri, P., Bhavsar, P., Shah, A., Krawetz, S.A., and Tainsky, M.A. 2003a. Onto-Tools, the toolkit of the modern biologist: Onto-Express, Onto-Compare, Onto-Design and Onto-Translate. *Nucleic Acids Res* **31**(13): 3775–3781.

Draghici, S., Khatri, P., Martins, R.P., Ostermeier, G.C., and Krawetz, S.A. 2003b. Global functional profiling of gene expression. *Genomics* **81**(2): 98–104.

Draghici, S., Khatri, P., Shah, A., and Tainsky, M.A. 2003c. Assessing the functional bias of commercial microarrays using the onto-compare database. *Biotechniques* **Suppl**: 55–61.

Emerson, M.R., Nelson, S.R., Samson, F.E., and Pazdernik, T.L. 1999. A global hypoxia preconditioning model: neuroprotection against seizure-induced specific gravity changes (edema) and brain damage in rats. *Brain Res Brain Res Protoc* **4**(3): 360–366.

Fauser, S., Luberichs, J., and Schuttauf, F. 2002. Genetic animal models for retinal degeneration. *Surv Ophthalmol* **47**(4): 357–367.

Gidday, J.M., Fitzgibbons, J.C., Shah, A.R., and Park, T.S. 1994. Neuroprotection from ischemic brain injury by hypoxic preconditioning in the neonatal rat. *Neurosci Lett* **168**(1–2): 221–224.

Grimm, C., Wenzel, A., Groszer, M., Mayser, H., Seeliger, M., Samardzija, M., Bauer, C., Gassmann, M., and Reme, C.E. 2002. HIF-1-induced erythropoietin in the hypoxic retina protects against light-induced retinal degeneration. *Nat Med* **8**(7): 718–724.

Grimm, C., Wenzel, A., Stanescu, D., Samardzija, M., Hotop, S., Groszer, M., Naash, M., Gassmann, M., and Reme, C. 2004. Constitutive overexpression of human erythropoietin protects the mouse retina against induced but not inherited retinal degeneration. *J Neurosci* **24**(25): 5651–5658.

Ke, Q. and Costa, M. 2006. Hypoxia-inducible factor-1 (HIF-1). *Mol Pharmacol* **70**(5): 1469–1480.

Koury, M.J., Sawyer, S.T., and Brandt, S.J. 2002. New insights into erythropoiesis. *Curr Opin Hematol* **9**(2): 93–100.

Mahyar-Roemer, M. and Roemer, K. 2001. p21 Waf1/Cip1 can protect human colon carcinoma cells against p53-dependent and p53-independent apoptosis induced by natural chemopreventive and therapeutic agents. *Oncogene* **20**(26): 3387–3398.

Maxwell, P. 2003. HIF-1: an oxygen response system with special relevance to the kidney. *J Am Soc Nephrol* **14**(11): 2712–2722.

Miyashita, K., Itoh, H., Arai, H., Suganami, T., Sawada, N., Fukunaga, Y., Sone, M., Yamahara, K., Yurugi-Kobayashi, T., Park, K., Oyamada, N., Sawada, N., Taura, D., Tsujimoto, H., Chao, T.H., Tamura, N., Mukoyama, M., and Nakao, K. 2006. The neuroprotective and vasculo-neuro-regenerative roles of adrenomedullin in ischemic brain and its therapeutic potential. *Endocrinology* **147**(4): 1642–1653.

Naumann, U., Weit, S., Wischhusen, J., and Weller, M. 2001. Diva/Boo is a negative regulator of cell death in human glioma cells. *FEBS Lett* **505**(1): 23–26.

Samardzija, M., Wenzel, A., Naash, M., Reme, C.E., and Grimm, C. 2006. Rpe65 as a modifier gene for inherited retinal degeneration. *Eur J Neurosci* **23**(4): 1028–1034.

Sharp, F.R. and Bernaudin, M. 2004. HIF1 and oxygen sensing in the brain. *Nat Rev Neurosci* **5**(6): 437–448.

Song, Q., Kuang, Y., Dixit, V.M., and Vincenz, C. 1999. Boo, a novel negative regulator of cell death, interacts with Apaf-1. *Embo J* **18**(1): 167–178.

Wenzel, A., Grimm, C., Samardzija, M., and Reme, C.E. 2005. Molecular mechanisms of light-induced photoreceptor apoptosis and neuroprotection for retinal degeneration. *Prog Retin Eye Res* **24**(2): 275–306.

Wenzel, A., Remc, C.E., Williams, T.P., Hafezi, F., and Grimm, C. 2001. The Rpe65 Leu450Met variation increases retinal resistance against light-induced degeneration by slowing rhodopsin regeneration. *J Neurosci* **21**(1): 53–58.

Yu, D.Y. and Cringle, S.J. 2005. Retinal degeneration and local oxygen metabolism. *Exp Eye Res* **80**(6): 745–751.

Zaman, K., Ryu, H., Hall, D., O'Donovan, K., Lin, K.I., Miller, M.P., Marquis, J.C., Baraban, J.M., Semenza, G.L., and Ratan, R.R. 1999. Protection from oxidative stress-induced apoptosis in cortical neuronal cultures by iron chelators is associated with enhanced DNA binding of hypoxia-inducible factor-1 and ATF-1/CREB and increased expression of glycolytic enzymes, p21(waf1/cip1), and erythropoietin. *J Neurosci* **19**(22): 9821–9830.

Zhang, S.X. and Ma, J.X. 2007. Ocular neovascularization: Implication of endogenous angiogenic inhibitors and potential therapy. *Prog Retin Eye Res* **26**(1): 1–37.

Part III
Gene Therapy and Neuroprotection

Lentiviral Gene Transfer-Mediated Cone Vision Restoration in RPE65 Knockout Mice

Alexis-Pierre Bemelmans, Corinne Kostic, Maité Cachafeiro, Sylvain V. Crippa, Dana Wanner, Meriem Tekaya, Andreas Wenzel, and Yvan Arsenijevic

1 Introduction: Cone Function in RPE65-Deficient Animal Models After AAV Gene Transfer

In photoreceptors, the photo-isomerization of 11-cis-retinal chromophore into all-trans-retinal is the first step of the photo-transduction cascade. To regain light sensitivity after light exposure, photoreceptors need to recycle their chromophore. This is done through the retinoid visual cycle, which involves a series of enzymatic reactions taking place in photoreceptors as well as in the cells of the retinal-pigmented epithelium (RPE) (reviewed by JC Saari (Saari, 2000)). *Rpe65*, a gene specifically expressed in RPE, has recently been identified as the isomerohydrolase (Jin et al., 2005; Moiseyev et al., 2005), one of the key enzymes of the retinoid visual cycle. As a consequence, when *Rpe65* is mutated, the retinoid visual cycle is disrupted, and the sensitivity to light of the photoreceptors is drastically reduced. In humans, mutations in the *RPE65* gene lead to Leber congenital amaurosis (LCA), the most severe form of retinitis pigmentosa (Gu et al., 1997; Hanein et al., 2004). Several animal models of these mutations have already been characterized, and, among them, the RPE65 deficient Briard dog (Aguirre et al., 1998), and the *Rpe65-/-* (Redmond et al., 1998) mouse have been broadly used for experimental studies. The restricted expression of RPE65 in RPE cells, the possibility to efficiently target these cells with viral vectors and the availability of animal models for RPE65 deficiency have made of *RPE65* gene therapy a widely studied field of experimental medicine (reviewed by JW Bainbridge (Bainbridge et al., 2006)).

Adeno-associated virus vectors (AAV) have been the most extensively used vectors for *Rpe65* gene transfer. Several teams have demonstrated that AAV gene transfer of *Rpe65* leads to restoration of the retinal function and vision rescue in the RPE65 deficient dog (Acland et al., 2001; Narfström et al., 2003; Le Meur et al., 2007). Furthermore, long-term studies in this canine model have shown that

A.-P. Bemelmans
Unit of Gene Therapy and Stem Cells Biology, Hôpital Ophtalmique Jules-Gonin, Lausanne, Switzerland, Tel: 41 21 626 82 60, Fax: 41 21 626 88 88
e-mail: yvan.arsenijevic@ophtal.vd.ch

this therapeutic benefit is stable (Acland et al., 2005; Narfström et al., 2005) and targeting RPE with AAV is a well-tolerated procedure (Jacobson et al., 2006). AAV gene transfer studies in the *Rpe65-/-* mouse model led to more contrasted results. Although the procedure allowed an improvement of the retinal function, the rescue observed by electroretinography (ERG) appeared limited, and the therapeutic benefit for cone survival was incomplete. Furthermore, it has been shown that cone function is abolished in *Rpe65-/-* mice (Seeliger et al., 2001), but there was no evidence that *Rpe65* gene transfer is able to restore the function of this subtype of photoreceptors in the knockout mouse model of RPE65 deficiency. This issue is however of crucial importance for any therapeutic application in humans, for whom cone photoreceptors are responsible for daylight-, color- and high-acuity vision.

In order to study the cone function after gene transfer, we have used a lentiviral vector expressing the *Rpe65* mouse cDNA under the transcriptional control of a 0.8 kbp proximal fragment of the human *RPE65* gene. Subretinal delivery of this type of vector in mammals has been shown to efficiently target the RPE over the long term, without any evidence of adverse effects (Miyoshi et al., 1997; Auricchio et al., 2001; Kostic et al., 2003; Bemelmans et al., 2005). In comparison to AAV, lentiviral vectors display a larger cloning capacity, which might be advantageous for long term gene therapy necessitating a tight regulation of the transgene expression. Classical lentiviral vectors integrate into the host genome, an interesting property for long-term transgene expression, but a disadvantage for biosafety. However it has been shown recently that lentiviral vectors can be engineered to be non-integrative, and that this type of vector is efficient for gene therapy in the knockout mouse model of RPE65 deficiency (Yanez-Munoz et al., 2006).

We have tested the feasibility of lentiviral-mediated *Rpe65* gene transfer in the *Rpe65-/-* mouse, a model in which cones degenerate quickly (Znoiko et al., 2005). We previously demonstrated (Bemelmans et al., 2006) that intra-ocular gene transfer performed at post-natal day (P) 5 led to: (1) long-lasting expression of the transgene in RPE cells, (2) long-term full protection of the cones in the treated area of the retina, (3) restoration of the functional response of rods, as well as cones. Using the optomotor response (OR), we report here that lentiviral-mediated transfer of *Rpe65* leads to vision restoration in the *Rpe65-/-* mouse model of LCA.

2 Cone- and ROD-Induced Optomotor Response

In order to quantifying vision in rodents, we evaluated the optomotor response (OR), which consists in the head movements of the subjects elicited by a moving visual stimulus. Practically, the mouse is placed at the center of a rotating drum, of which the wall is covered by a pattern of alternated vertical black and white stripes. The mouse behavior is videotaped while the drum is rotating. The experimenter then scores on the video recordings the mouse head movements, which are considered visually elicited when speed and orientation are synchronized with the drum.

To determine the sensitivity of the test, we first evaluated the OR of a group of wild type mice (C57Bl6J) in photopic as well as in scotopic conditions, and with the stripes pattern ranging from 0.025 to 0.1 cycle per degree (cpd). This allowed us to demonstrate that no significant difference occurs in the OR for a pattern ranging from 0.025 to 0.1 cpd (Fig. 1A). The visual acuity threshold (i.e. the first pattern of stripes for which it is possible to detect an OR) was above 0.1 cpd in both the scotopic and photopic conditions. Although it appeared that the OR was higher in dim light than in daylight (Fig. 1A), determination of the scotopic and photopic visual acuity thresholds will necessitate further investigation. Nonetheless, the conditions determined here will allow to assess vision restoration in *Rpe65-/-* mice after gene therapy.

To assess that OR measurement allows to discriminate cone-mediated from rod-mediated vision, we evaluated *Gnat1a-/-* mice. In this knockout strain, invalidation of the rod-specific transducin disrupts the phototransduction cascade in the rod photoreceptors. Accordingly, OR scores of *Gnat1a-/-* mice in photopic conditions were not significantly different from wild type, but were drastically reduced in scotopic conditions (Fig. 1B). This allows us to assume that the photopic conditions we have determined permit the study of cone-mediated vision independently from the rod-mediated one, as this was previously established by others (Schmucker et al., 2005).

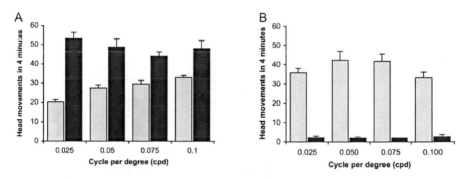

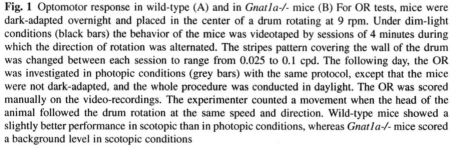

Fig. 1 Optomotor response in wild-type (A) and in *Gnat1a-/-* mice (B) For OR tests, mice were dark-adapted overnight and placed in the center of a drum rotating at 9 rpm. Under dim-light conditions (black bars) the behavior of the mice was videotaped by sessions of 4 minutes during which the direction of rotation was alternated. The stripes pattern covering the wall of the drum was changed between each session to range from 0.025 to 0.1 cpd. The following day, the OR was investigated in photopic conditions (grey bars) with the same protocol, except that the mice were not dark-adapted, and the whole procedure was conducted in daylight. The OR was scored manually on the video-recordings. The experimenter counted a movement when the head of the animal followed the drum rotation at the same speed and direction. Wild-type mice showed a slightly better performance in scotopic than in photopic conditions, whereas *Gnat1a-/-* mice scored a background level in scotopic conditions

3 Optomotor Response in RPE65-/- Mice

We previously reported that, in the *Rpe65-/-* model, early restoration of RPE65 levels is needed to rescue the function of cones and to prevent their degeneration (Bemelmans et al., 2006). We thus treated a group of 6 *Rpe65-/-* mice with a subretinal injection at postnatal day 5 (P5) of a lentiviral vector expressing the mouse *Rpe65* cDNA
    under the transcriptional control of a 800 bp fragment of the human *RPE65* gene (LV-RPE65 (Bemelmans et al., 2006)). To evaluate cone-mediated vision, we quantified the photopic OR of these mice three months after gene transfer treatment, i.e. at three months of age, when the cones have almost completely degenerated in untreated *Rpe65-/-* mice (Rohrer et al., 2005; Znoiko et al., 2005). When compared to untreated *Rpe65-/-* mice, we observed a significant improvement of the OR scores with a stripes pattern of 0.025 and 0.1 cpd, the two conditions tested (Fig. 2). This demonstrates that the lentiviral-mediated transfer of a functional *Rpe65* gene leads to restoration of a visually elicited behavior in the *Rpe65-/-* mouse model of LCA and of the entire visual pathway from the retina to the brain.
    To study the efficiency of gene transfer, we sacrificed the mice at four months of age, and studied transgene expression by immunofluorescent detection on cryostat sections. As we previously reported, intraocular injection at postnatal day 5 led to long-lasting expression of *Rpe65* in the cells of the RPE (Fig. 3A). This study also confirmed that early treatment with LV-RPE65 led to a complete protection of the cone photoreceptors in the transduced area, as demonstrated by detection of GNAT2, the cone specific transducin (Fig. 3C). In the untreated knockout, GNAT2, as well as other cone specific markers, are indeed drastically down-regulated already

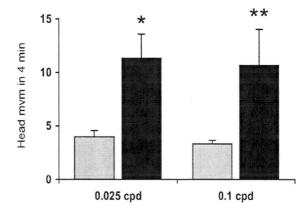

Fig. 2 *Rpe65* gene transfer improves vision in *Rpe65-/-* mice. The mice were left untreated (grey bars) or received an intraocular injection of LV-RPE65 at postnatal day 5 (black bars). The optomotor response was evaluated three months later at 0.025 and 0.1 cpd under photopic conditions. Although LV-RPE65-treated knockout animals did not reached the score of wild type animals (compare with figure 1A), they were significantly improved in comparison to untreated knockouts. *: $p < 0.05$ and **: $p < 0.01$ vs untreated knockout mice in student's *t*-test

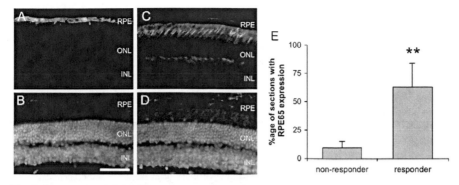

Fig. 3 Improvement of the OR scores correlates with RPE65 expression. Mice were sacrificed at 4 months for a histological study of transgene expression and rescue of cones on cryostat sections. (A) Immunofluorescent detection revealed a strong expression of RPE65 in the retinal pigment epithelium after LV-RPE65 treatment at P5. (C) GNAT2-positive outer segments in the area of transgene expression after LV-RPE65 treatment. (B, D) dapi counterstaining of the sections shown in A and C respectively. Scale bar: 50 μm. (E) the group of LV-RPE65 was arbitrary divided in two subgroups based on OR performance (see section 3), and quantification of RPE65 expression demonstrated that the animals showing the best OR scores also exhibited the strongest level of RPE65 expression. **: $p < 0.001$ in student's t-test

at one month of age due to cone degeneration (Znoiko et al., 2005; Bemelmans et al., 2006).

In order to correlate the scores of the OR study with the efficiency of gene transfer, we quantified the extent of RPE65 expression in the group of LV-RPE65-treated animals. For each eye, we examined a complete series of sections and determined that on average 27 ±11% of the sections display a positive staining for RPE65. Nevertheless, an important variability was noted: we detected no expression in certain eyes, whereas in the best case 94% of the sections exhibited RPE65 expression. A lack of reproducibility of the intraocular injections done at P5 might be at the origin of this heterogeneity. This led us to divide the group of LV-RPE65 treated animals into two subgroups, the first one being composed of the animals showing unequivocal responses in the OR test (responder group), and the second including the animals showing no or equivocal responses in the OR test (non-responder group). A significant difference was observed in the extent of transgene expression between these two groups (Fig. 3E).

Interestingly, we determined for one animal of the non-responder group that one eye displayed 42% of the sections positive for RPE65. This might indicate that, in the *Rpe65-/-* mouse model of LCA, a large portion of the eye has to be treated to lead to an improvement in the OR test, although a greater number of animals needs to be evaluated to confirm this hypothesis. Other mechanisms could explain this phenomenon. For example, exogenous factors, such as stress, can influence the results of the OR scores and may also greatly vary between animals. Another possibility is that the localization of the treated area in the retina, or a certain degree of binocular vision may also be determinant to allow a good OR.

4 Conclusion

We showed that lentiviral gene transfer of *Rpe65* cDNA at postnatal day 5 in the *Rpe65-/-* mouse leads to long-term expression of the transgene, which allows (1) to protect cones from the degeneration occurring in this model (Bemelmans et al., 2006), (2) to restore the function of these cells as assessed by electroretinography (Bemelmans et al., 2006), (3) to restore the vision of the mice in photopic conditions (Fig. 2 and 3). As demonstrated by the comparison of the OR scores between wild type and *Gnat1a-/-* mice, the vision of the mice mostly relies on cones in photopic conditions (Fig 1). Thus, the improvement in photopic vision of *Rpe65-/-* mice after LV-RPE65 treatment is probably be cone-driven. This reinforces the therapeutic value of *RPE65* gene transfer for Leber congenital amaurosis caused by mutation of the *RPE65* gene.

Acknowledgments This work was supported by the ProVisu Foundation.

References

Acland, G. M., Aguirre, G. D., Bennett, J., et al., 2005, Long-term restoration of rod and cone vision by single dose rAAV-mediated gene transfer to the retina in a canine model of childhood blindness, *Mol Ther.* **12**: 1072–1082.

Acland, G. M., Aguirre, G. D., Ray, J., et al., 2001, Gene therapy restores vision in a canine model of childhood blindness, *Nat Genet* **28**: 92–95.

Aguirre, G. D., Baldwin, V., Pearce-Kelling, S., et al., 1998, Congenital stationary night blindness in the dog: common mutation in the RPE65 gene indicates founder effect, *Mol Vis* **4**: 23.

Auricchio, A., Kobinger, G., Anand, V., et al., 2001, Exchange of surface proteins impacts on viral vector cellular specificity and transduction characteristics: the retina as a model, *Hum Mol Genet* **10**: 3075–81.

Bainbridge, J. W., Tan, M. H. and Ali, R. R., 2006, Gene therapy progress and prospects: the eye, *Gene Ther* **13**: 1191–97.

Bemelmans, A. P., Bonnel, S., Houhou, L., et al., 2005, Retinal cell type expression specificity of HIV-1-derived gene transfer vectors upon subretinal injection in the adult rat: influence of pseudotyping and promoter, *J Gene Med* **7**: 1367–74.

Bemelmans, A. P., Kostic, C., Crippa, S. V., et al., 2006, Lentiviral gene transfer of RPE65 rescues survival and function of cones in a mouse model of Leber congenital amaurosis, *PLoS Med* **3**: e347.

Gu, S. M., Thompson, D. A., Srikumari, C. R., et al., 1997, Mutations in RPE65 cause autosomal recessive childhood-onset severe retinal dystrophy, *Nat Genet* **17**: 194–97.

Hanein, S., Perrault, I., Gerber, S., et al., 2004, Leber congenital amaurosis: comprehensive survey of the genetic heterogeneity, refinement of the clinical definition, and genotype-phenotype correlations as a strategy for molecular diagnosis, *Hum Mutat* **23**: 306–17.

Jacobson, S. G., Boye, S. L., Aleman, T. S., et al., 2006, Safety in nonhuman primates of ocular AAV2-RPE65, a candidate treatment for blindness in Leber congenital amaurosis, *Hum Gene Ther* **17**: 845–58.

Jin, M., Li, S., Moghrabi, W. N., et al., 2005, Rpe65 is the retinoid isomerase in bovine retinal pigment epithelium, *Cell* **122**: 449–59.

Kostic, C., Chiodini, F., Salmon, P., et al., 2003, Activity analysis of housekeeping promoters using self-inactivating lentiviral vector delivery into the mouse retina, *Gene Ther* **10**: 818–21.

Le Meur, G., Stieger, K., Smith, A. J., et al., 2007, Restoration of vision in RPE65-deficient Briard dogs using an AAV serotype 4 vector that specifically targets the retinal pigmented epithelium, *Gene Ther* **14**: 292–303.

Miyoshi, H., Takahashi, M., Gage, F. H. and Verma, I. M., 1997, Stable and efficient gene transfer into the retina using an HIV-based lentiviral vector, *Proc Natl Acad Sci U S A* **94**: 10319–23.

Moiseyev, G., Chen, Y., Takahashi, Y., et al., 2005, RPE65 is the isomerohydrolase in the retinoid visual cycle, *Proc Natl Acad Sci U S A* **102**: 12413–8.

Narfström, K., Katz, M. L., Bragadottir, R., et al., 2003, Functional and structural recovery of the retina after gene therapy in the RPE65 null mutation dog, *Invest Ophthalmol Vis Sci* **44**: 1663–72.

Narfström, K., Vaegan, Katz, M., et al., 2005, Assessment of structure and function Over a 3-year period after gene transfer in RPE65-/- dogs, *Doc Ophthalmol* **111**: 39–48.

Redmond, T. M., Yu, S., Lee, E., et al., 1998, Rpe65 is necessary for production of 11-cis-vitamin A in the retinal visual cycle, *Nat Genet* **20**: 344–51.

Rohrer, B., Lohr, H. R., Humphries, P., et al., 2005, Cone opsin mislocalization in Rpe65-/- Mice: A defect that can be corrected by 11-cis retinal, *Invest Ophthalmol Vis Sci* **46**: 3876–82.

Saari, J. C., 2000, Biochemistry of visual pigment regeneration: the Friedenwald lecture, *Invest Ophthalmol Vis Sci* **41**: 337–48.

Schmucker, C., Seeliger, M., Humphries, P., et al., 2005, Grating acuity at different luminances in wild-type mice and in mice lacking rod or cone function, *Invest Ophthalmol Vis Sci* **46**: 398–407.

Seeliger, M. W., Grimm, C., Stahlberg, F., et al., 2001, New views on RPE65 deficiency: the rod system is the source of vision in a mouse model of Leber congenital amaurosis, *Nat Genet* **29**: 70–74.

Yanez-Munoz, R. J., Balaggan, K. S., Macneil, A., et al., 2006, Effective gene therapy with nonintegrating lentiviral vectors, *Nat Med* **12**: 348–53.

Znoiko, S. L., Rohrer, B., Lu, K., et al., 2005, Downregulation of cone-specific gene expression and degeneration of cone photoreceptors in the Rpe65-/- mouse at early ages, *Invest Ophthalmol Vis Sci* **46**: 1473–79.

In vitro Analysis of Ribozyme-mediated Knockdown of an ADRP Associated Rhodopsin Mutation

Dibyendu Chakraborty, Patrick Whalen, Alfred S. Lewin, and Muna I. Naash

1 Introduction

Retinitis Pigmentosa (RP) is a group of retinal degenerative diseases that are characterized mainly by the loss of rod photoreceptor cells. RP can be sub divided into 3 classes, autosomal dominant, autosomal recessive, and X- linked RP, where the mutant gene exists on the sex chromosome (X) (Hartong et al., 2006; Wang et al., 2005). Mutations in rhodopsin are the most common cause of the autosomal-dominant form of RP (ADRP). More than 100 mutations in rhodopsin account for approximately 30% of ADRP cases with varying severity of visual impairment (Dryja et al., 1991). Based on *in vitro* studies (Sung et al., 1993; Sung et al., 1991), rhodopsin mutations that are similar to wild-type in terms of expression levels, folding and formation of functional photopigment are considered Class 1 mutations. On the other hand Class 2 mutants are those in which the opsin protein is inefficiently transported or is retained in the endoplasmic reticulum (ER). The mutation of Proline to Histidine at the 23rd amino acid of rhodopsin (P23H) is a Class 2 mutation. The Xenopus laevis in vivo model for P23H (Tam and Moritz, 2006) shows that the protein is misfolded and that is accumulated in the inner segment (IS) causing ER overload and cellular stress thus supporting its categorization as Class 2. It has been shown that the P23H substitution reduces the binding capacity for 11-*cis* retinal and causes a defect in glycosylation (Noorwez et al., 2004). The first symptom of ADRP associated with the P23H mutation is impaired night vision that appears between 10 to 30 years of age. The majority of these individuals became blind by the age of 60.

Gene therapy is one of the most promising treatments for inherited retinal diseases. At the beginning it was a challenge to achieve successful gene therapy in the retina due to the lack of cell specific and efficient targeting as well as the lack of a delivery method that would cause minimum damage to the eye. Additionally,

D. Chakraborty
Department of Cell Biology, University of Oklahoma Health Sciences Center, 940 Stanton L. Young Blvd. (BMSB781), Oklahoma City, OK 73104, Tel: 405-271-2402, Fax: 405-271-3548
email: dchakrab@ouhsc.edu

there were no specific animal models that closely mimicked the human disease presentations. So far, two types of approaches have been considered for gene therapy in ADRP animal models. The first is delivery of genes for neurotrophic factors such as GDNF (McGee Sanftner et al., 2001) and antiapoptotic proteins such as XIAP (Petrin et al., 2003) to prevent the ongoing death of the photoreceptors. The second approach is to block the synthesis of mutant proteins and increasing the ratio of wild-type vs mutant rhodopsin to delay the onset of retinal degeneration (Drenser et al., 1998; LaVail et al., 2000). For instance, Lewin and his colleagues used AAV2 to deliver ribozymes that cleaved the P23H rhodopsin mRNA and showed an effective treatment in a rat model of ADRP (LaVail et al., 2000).

Recently various reports demonstrate the robust efficacy of RNA interference (RNAi) in animal models of human disease and support the RNAi based new therapeutic approach as one with the potential to change the treatment of human disease (Bumcrot et al., 2006). RNAi has been used to silence P23H human rhodopsin alleles by 94.9% in human embryonic retinoblasts (Cashman et al., 2005) thus providing further evidence that this approach is a viable one to treat specific human disease causing mutations.

2 Animal Model

Genetic diseases can result from both the expression of a mutant protein or the failure to express its normal form. The development of molecular biology and transgenic mouse technology has enabled researchers to generate multiple relevant animal models for the study of genetic eye diseases (including P23H) (Nour and Naash, 2003). The functional and structural defects in these models can closely mimic the human disease phenotypes. We have generated three rhodopsin transgenic disease models: one carrying the P23H mutation (Late onset ADRP) (Naash et al., 1993; Naash et al., 1996a, b; Wang et al., 1997; Wu et al., 1998) one carrying the ΔI-255/256 deletion which causes early onset ADRP (Penn et al., 2000), and one with the G90D mutation which causes congenital stationary night blindness (CSNB) (Naash et al., 2004). These animal models allow us to conduct the extensive biochemical, histological and physiological studies which necessarily underlie the development of effective therapeutic interventions.

3 Gene Therapy

Since the P23H retinal degeneration is inherited as an autosomal dominant fashion and very often caused by the product of a single mutant allele that may interferes with the function of the protein encoded by the wild-type allele, a reduction in the expression of the mutant allele may prevent or delayed the disease phenotype. While currently no therapies exist for the treatment of ADRP, gene therapy may serve the best and direct way for future therapeutic intervention. Researchers have investigated ribozyme technologies to reduce the expression of mutant gene products. It has been shown that ribozyme therapy can successfully reduce the P23H mutant protein in the rat retina (Fritz et al., 2004; Gorbatyuk et al. M., 2007; LaVail et al., 2000; Lewin et al., 1998).

3.1 Ribozymes

The discovery of naturally occurring RNA molecules which were able to regulate gene expression led to the idea that oligonucleotides could be used for gene therapy (Blake et al., 1985; Zamecnik and Stephenson, 1978). These discoveries consequently generated the hypothesis that oligonucleotides could be designed to down-regulate the expression of genes responsible for pathogenesis. At about the same time, the study of RNA processing led to the finding of naturally occurring RNA sequences that possessed catalytic properties (Inoue et al., 1985). These RNA molecules were called ribozymes, an abbreviation for ribonucleotide enzyme, stressing the ability of these RNA molecules to act as endonucleases. Ribozymes form base pair specific complexes with their RNA substrates and are able to catalyze the hydrolysis or phosphoryl exchange at a phosphodiester bond. Furthermore, the observation that ribozymes could be designed to act in *trans* led to the development of antisense technology. In addition, ribozymes do not rely on the host cellular machinery to degrade their substrate, and they can be classified into different groups based on their catalytic activities. The three main groups of ribozymes are the self-splicing introns, RNase P, and the small self-cleaving ribozymes. Each type of ribozyme is being examined for its possible use as a genetic therapy, but the hammerhead and hairpin ribozymes have received most attention for potential clinical applications. The hammerhead ribozyme recognizes the substrate sequence on either side of an NUX cleavage site by means of two flanking arms that hybridize to form helices III and I (Fig. 1). Cleavage occurs at 3' of the NUX consensus sequence, where N = any nucleotide, and X = any nucleotide except G. Cleavage sites do not all show the same efficiency. In general, GUC is the most efficient cleavage site, followed by CUC, UUC, and AUC. The rest of the cleavage sites are cleaved at least ten-fold more slowly than the GUC site (Shimayama et al., 1995).

The hairpin ribozyme binds its substrate to form a structure with four helices and two loops. The arms of the hairpin ribozyme hybridize to the substrate molecule to form a six base pair helix 1 and a four base pair helix 2 (Fig. 1). The sequence of these arms can be manipulated to allow binding to a variety of RNA substrates. Loop A contains the BNGUC target sequence required for cleavage where B = G, C, or U and N is any nucleotide (Hampel et al., 1990). There are no conserved nucleotides in any of the helices, although a G in the substrate portion of helix 2 adjacent to loop A leads to an increased rate of cleavage (Joseph and Burke, 1993). There are a number of conserved nucleotides found in loop A and loop B, which fold on top of one another to form the catalytic core (Esteban et al., 1998).

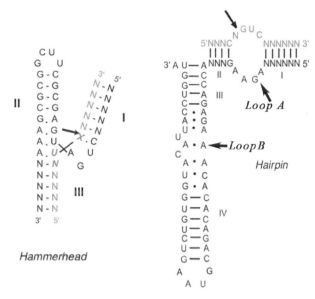

Fig. 1 The sequence and structure of the hammerhead and hairpin ribozyme

3.2 VPP Transgenic Mouse Models of ADRP

The P23H mutation in the opsin gene is one of the most prevalent mutations found in the United States, and accounts for over 12% ADRP patients (Wang et al., 2005). To examine the link between the P23H genotype and its phenotype, we have created a transgenic line named VPP that expresses mutant rhodopsin containing three substituted amino acids in the N-terminus [Val20→Gly (V20G), Pro23→His (P23H) and Pro27→Leu (P27L)] (Naash et al., 1993). These mice express equal amounts of mutant and wild-type transcripts, and develop progressive photoreceptor degeneration (Goto et al., 1996; Wang et al., 1997).

Retinal degeneration in the VPP mice appears as early as postnatal day 20 (Fig. 2) and continues to degenerate in a light-dependent manner (Wang et al., 1997). Several studies have shown that the P23H protein can traffic to the outer segments of rod photoreceptors only in the presence of the wild-type rhodopsin and can bind to the chromophore, 11-cis retinal (Qtaishat et al., 1999; Wu et al., 1998). Since it cannot transport to the outer segment on its own, it failed to support outer segment formation in the rhodopsin null background (Rho$^{-/-}$) (Fig. 2). The VPP protein in the Rho$^{-/-}$ background was found trapped in the ER and the animals showed no scotopic ERG a- wave and accelerated photoreceptor degeneration. Interestingly, this degeneration occurs more rapidly than degeneration associated with rhodopsin knockout alone (Frederick et al., 2001).

A number of factors make the VPP mouse model ideal for the evaluation of the efficiency of ribozymes in vivo. First, the retinal degeneration in these animals is slow, which gives adequate time for the ribozyme to have an effect. Second, the

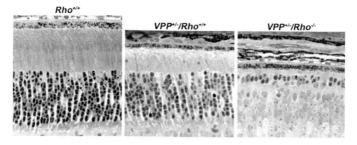

Fig. 2 Retinal structure in VPP transgenics. Histological evaluation (light microscopy) at postnatal day 20 shows retinal degeneration of the VPP$^{+/-}$/$Rho^{+/+}$ mice when compared to non-transgenic $Rho^{+/+}$ littermate. Expression of the VPP transgene on the Rho$^{-/-}$ background resulted in a faster rate of photoreceptor degeneration and an absence of outer segment structures

level of mutant message is equivalent to that of the wild-type, a situation similar to that seen in patients. Consequently, injecting the right eye of a mouse with the ribozyme construct and the left eye with a construct that acts as a control should allow an accurate determination of the activity of a ribozyme in vivo. The change in ERG can be used to measure the efficiency of a ribozyme without having to sacrifice mice that have been injected with the treatment. Thus, the effects of a ribozyme can be followed over time. This in turn will aid in the design of future ribozymes with increased therapeutic activity. This will be especially important for ribozymes designed to treat autosomal dominant genetic diseases.

3.3 Design of Ribozymes for the Treatment of P23H Associated ADRP

In ADRP, expression of the mutant protein results in retinal dystrophy (Dryja et al., 1990). The hypothesis underlying ribozyme therapy for this model is that decreasing the expression of the mutant protein will delay or prevent the disease. The success of ribozyme therapy depends on the identification of an RNA target site within the mutant allele. The hammerhead ribozyme is able to cleave an NUX target sequence, but the efficiency of the cleavage reaction can vary by as much as 100-fold depending on the precise cleavage triplet. The most efficient cleavage triplet is a GUC sequence followed by CUC, which is five-fold less efficient, and UUC, which is 10 times less efficient. The hairpin ribozyme has slightly different target site requirements than the hammerhead ribozyme. The target cleavage site of the hairpin is less flexible. Mutational analysis demonstrated that only the GUC triplet is cleaved efficiently (Hampel et al., 1990).

Two strategies were used to ensure that a ribozyme was able to specifically cleave the mRNA of the mutant but not the wild-type. The first approach was to identify a mutation that creates a cleavage triplet target in the mRNA of the mutant gene. The second strategy was to identify a mutation in close proximity to the cleavage triplet in the substrate. These mutations allow cleavage of the mutant mRNA but not the wild-type mRNA because the mismatched base pairs disrupt the formation of the catalytic core of the ribozyme (Grasby et al., 1995). Werner and Uhlenbeck (Werner and Uhlenbeck, 1995) have shown that a mismatch in any of the first four innermost nucleotides of helix III of a hammerhead ribozyme prevented cleavage. Only a mismatch in the innermost nucleotide of helix I prevented cleavage.

One hammerhead and three different hairpin ribozymes, HP1, HP2 and HP3 were designed to target the P23H message (Table 1). The specificity of the cleavage reaction catalyzed by these ribozyme was primarily due to the GUC cleavage triplet found in the transgene sequence of the VPP model but not in the wild-type rhodopsin gene (Naash et al., 1993). The hammerhead and hairpin ribozymes were both designed against the VPP transgene because ribozymes cleave different substrates with different catalytic efficiencies. For instance in the Tang et al study (Tang et al., 1994), hammerhead ribozymes cleaved the same substrates better than the hairpin ribozymes. The design of the three hairpin ribozymes was different. HP1 is the hairpin ribozyme found in the negative strand of the Tobacco Ringspot virus (Hampel et al., 1990) while the HP2 has a helix 4 with three additional base pairs and a stable loop to stabilize its secondary structure and to increases its catalytic activity. The third hairpin ribozyme, HP3, also has the modifications found in HP2 with the addition of a stem loop between helix 2 and helix 3. This stem loop was reported to increase the ability of the hairpin ribozyme to fold into its proper conformation (Esteban et al., 1998).

3.4 *Catalytic Efficiency of the Ribozyme* in vitro

All the ribozymes targeting the VPP transgene were able to specifically cleave the mutant oligonucleotide in vitro. HH1 cleaved 10% of their substrate in 24 hours

Table 1 The following deoxynucleotides were used to clone the ribozymes. Sense Strand – Oligonucleotide which has the same sequence as the ribozyme mRNA. Antisense – Oligonucleotide which has a sequence complimentary to ribozyme mRNA

Ribozyme	Sense strand	Antisense strand
HH1 Hammerhead	5'CTC CGG CCG AAG TCT G	5'GAG CAG CGT CGG AGT TTC GCG CTT TCG CGC TCA TCA GAC TTC GGC CGG AG
HP1 Hairpin	5'GCA GAA TTC AGC GGC CGC ACG AAG TAG AAC CGA ACC AGA GAA ACA CAC G	5'GCC ACG CGT ACC AGG TAA TAT ACC ACA ACG TGT GTT TCT CTG G
HP2 Hairpin	5'GCA GAA TTC AGC GGC CGC ACG AAG TAG AAC CGA ACC AGA GAA ACA CAC G	5'GCC ACG CGT TAC CAG GTA ATG TAC CAC GAC TTA CGT CGT GTG TTT CTC TGG
HP3 Hairpin	5'AGC GGC CGC ACG AAG TAG AAC CGA CCC GAC GAC GTA AGT CGT CCC CAC CAG AGA AAC ACA CG	5'GCC ACG CGT TAC CAG GTA ATG TAC CAC GAC TTA CGT CGT GTG TTT CTC TGG

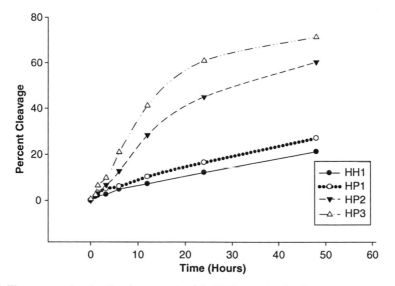

Fig. 3 Time course showing the cleavage rate of the VPP target by the ribozymes

while HP1 cleaved 10% of its substrate by 12 hours showing HP1 was twice as efficient as HH1 and 3–4 times less active than HP2 and HP3, respectively (Fig. 3). The HP2 and HP3 ribozyme cleaves 10% substrate in 5 and 3 hours respectively (Figs. 4A and 4B).

The kinetic experiments were performed with 10 mM transcribed ribozyme and increasing concentrations of substrate. For the HP2 ribozyme, the kinetic reactions were analyses 5 hours after starting the reaction. (Fig. 5A). Eadiee-Hofstee analysis was used to calculate V_{max} and K_M by performing linear regression analysis of $1/V_0$ versus $V_0/[S]$ (Fig. 5B)

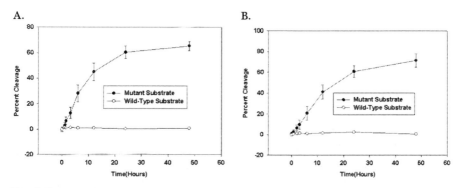

Fig. 4 Cleavage rate of the HP2 (A) and HP3 (B) hairpin ribozyme. The time courses of the cleavage reactions for the mutant and wild-type oligonucleotides are shown

(A)   (B)

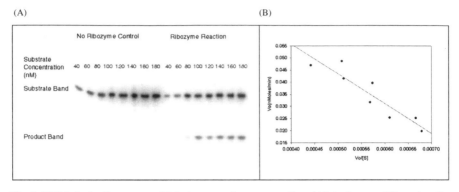

Fig. 5 HP2 hairpin ribozyme multiple turnover cleavage reaction. (A) An image of the autoradiogram of the HP2 multiple turnover cleavage reaction. (B) A graph of the Eadiee-Hofstee plot used to calculate the kinetic coefficients of the HP2 ribozyme

4 Summary of the Effectiveness of Ribozyme Therapy

Rhodopsin associated ADRP cases are mainly gain-of-function phenotypes and not a haploinsufficency disorder due to the loss of one allele. Therefore, a knockdown of mutant rhodopsin using ribozyme may be one of the best therapeutic approaches. The first test of the efficacy of ribozymes in mouse retinas was done by Lewin's group (LaVail et al., 2000). Later, they showed rhodopsin (Gorbatyuk et al., 2005) and PDE-γ (γ-subunit of rod cGMP phosphodiesterase) (Liu et al., 2005) specific ribozyme knockdown of their target genes. Very recently the use of ribozyme Rz525 in the P23H transgenic rats was able to reduce mutant transcript by 46% which resulted in a partial rescue of the retinal degeneration. The relative rescue was 50% for both a-wave and b-wave amplitudes in ribozyme treated eyes when compared to control eye. They also observed an increase in the photoreceptor outer nuclear layer (ONL) thickness (Gorbatyuk et al., 2007). This P23H transgenic animal model allowed accurate in vivo studies to evaluate the efficacy and safety of novel therapies. Such features make these models invaluable tools for the development of potential therapeutic interventions. Since there is a high level of genetic heterogeneity in rhodopsin-linked RP, mutation-independent ribozyme therapy approaches will be highly preferable strategy for future therapy.

References

Blake, K. R., Murakami, A., and Miller, P. S., 1985, Inhibition of rabbit globin mRNA translation by sequence-specific oligodeoxyribonucleotides, *Biochemistry.* **24**:6132.
Bumcrot, D., Manoharan, M., Koteliansky, V., and Sah, D. W., 2006, RNAi therapeutics: a potential new class of pharmaceutical drugs, *Nat Chem Biol.* **2**:711
Cashman, S. M., Binkley, E. A., and Kumar-Singh, R.,2005, Towards mutation-independent silencing of genes involved in retinal degeneration by RNA interference, *Gene Ther.* **12**:1223.

Drenser, K. A., Timmers, A. M., Hauswirth, W. W., and Lewin, A. S.,1998, Ribozyme-targeted destruction of RNA associated with autosomal-dominant retinitis pigmentosa, *Invest Ophthalmol Vis Sci.* **39**:681.

Dryja, T. P., Hahn, L. B., Cowley, G. S., McGee, T. L., and Berson, E. L., 1991, Mutation spectrum of the rhodopsin gene among patients with autosomal dominant retinitis pigmentosa, *Proc Natl Acad Sci U S A.* **88**:9370.

Dryja, T. P., McGee, T. L., Hahn, L. B., Cowley, G. S., Olsson, J. E., Reichel, E., Sandberg, M. A., and Berson, E. L., 1990, Mutations within the rhodopsin gene in patients with autosomal dominant retinitis pigmentosa, *N Engl J Med.* **323**:1302.

Esteban, J. A., Walter, N. G., Kotzorek, G., Heckman, J. E., and Burke, J. M., 1998, Structural basis for heterogeneous kinetics: reengineering the hairpin ribozyme, *Proc Natl Acad Sci U S A.* **95**:6091.

Frederick, J. M., Krasnoperova, N. V., Hoffmann, K., Church-Kopish, J., Ruther, K., Howes, K., Lem, J., and Baehr, W., 2001, Mutant rhodopsin transgene expression on a null background, *Invest Ophthalmolo Vis Sci.* **42**:826

Fritz, J. J., Gorbatyuk, M., Lewin, A. S., and Hauswirth, W. W., 2004, Design and validation of therapeutic hammerhead ribozymes for autosomal dominant diseases, *Methods Mol Biol.* **252**:221.

Gorbatyuk, M., Justilien, V., Liu, J., Hauswirth, W. W., and Lewin, A. S., 2007, Preservation of photoreceptor morphology and function in P23H rats using an allele independent ribozyme, *Exp Eye Res.* **84**:44.

Gorbatyuk, M. S., Pang, J. J., Thomas, J., Jr., Hauswirth, W. W., and Lewin, A. S., 2005, Knockdown of wild-type mouse rhodopsin using an AAV vectored ribozyme as part of an RNA replacement approach, *Mol Vis.* **11**:648.

Goto, Y., Peachey, N. S., Ziroli, N. E., Seiple, W. H., Gryczan, C., Pepperberg, D. R., and Naash, M. I., 1996, Rod phototransduction in transgenic mice expressing a mutant opsin gene, *J Opt Soc Am A Opt Image Sci Vis.* **13**:577.

Grasby, J. A., Mersmann, K., Singh, M., and Gait, M. J., 1995, Purine functional groups in essential residues of the hairpin ribozyme required for catalytic cleavage of RNA, *Biochemistry.* **34**:4068.

Hampel, A., Tritz, R., Hicks, M., and Cruz, P., 1990, 'Hairpin' catalytic RNA model: evidence for helices and sequence requirement for substrate RNA, *Nucleic Acids Res.* **18**:299.

Hartong, D. T., Berson, E. L., and Dryja, T. P., 2006, Retinitis pigmentosa, *Lancet.* **368**:1795.

Inoue, T., Sullivan, F. X., and Cech, T. R., 1985, Intermolecular exon ligation of the rRNA precursor of Tetrahymena: oligonucleotides can function as 5' exons, *Cell.* **43**:431

Joseph, S., and Burke, J. M., 1993, Optimization of an anti-HIV hairpin ribozyme by in vitro selection, *J Biol Chem.* **268**:24515.

LaVail, M. M., Yasumura, D., Matthes, M. T., Drenser, K. A., Flannery, J. G., Lewin, A. S., and Hauswirth, W. W., 2000, Ribozyme rescue of photoreceptor cells in P23H transgenic rats: long-term survival and late-stage therapy, *Proc Natl Acad Sci U S A.* **97**:11488.

Lewin, A. S., Drenser, K. A., Hauswirth, W. W., Nishikawa, S., Yasumura, D., Flannery, J. G., and LaVail, M. M., 1998, Ribozyme rescue of photoreceptor cells in a transgenic rat model of autosomal dominant retinitis pigmentosa, *Nat Med.* **4**:967.

Liu, J., Timmers, A. M., Lewin, A. S., and Hauswirth, W. W., 2005, Ribozyme knockdown of the gamma-subunit of rod cGMP phosphodiesterase alters the ERG and retinal morphology in wild-type mice, *Invest Ophthalmol Vis Sci.* **46**:3836.

McGee Sanftner, L. H., Abel, H., Hauswirth, W. W., and Flannery, J. G., 2001, Glial cell line derived neurotrophic factor delays photoreceptor degeneration in a transgenic rat model of retinitis pigmentosa, *Mol Ther.* **4**:622.

Naash, M. I., Hollyfield, J. G., al-Ubaidi, M. R., and Baehr, W., 1993, Simulation of human autosomal dominant retinitis pigmentosa in transgenic mice expressing a mutated murine opsin gene, *Proc Natl Acad Sci U S A.* **90**:5499.

Naash, M. L., Peachey, N. S., Li, Z. Y., Gryczan, C. C., Goto, Y., Blanks, J., Milam, A. H., and Ripps, H., 1996a, Light-induced acceleration of photoreceptor degeneration in transgenic mice expressing mutant rhodopsin, *Invest Ophthalmology Visual Sci.* **37**:775.

Naash, M. I., Ripps, H., Li, S., Goto, Y., and Peachey, N. S., 1996b, Polygenic disease and retinitis pigmentosa: albinism exacerbates photoreceptor degeneration induced by the expression of a mutant opsin in transgenic mice, *J Neurosci.* **16**:7853.

Naash, M. I., Wu, T. H., Chakraborty, D., Fliesler, S. J., Ding, X. Q., Nour, M., Peachey, N. S., Lem, J., Qtaishat, N., Al-Ubaidi, M. R., and Ripps, H., 2004, Retinal abnormalities associated with the G90D mutation in opsin, *The Journal of comparative neurology.***478**:149.

Noorwez, S. M., Malhotra, R., McDowell, J. H., Smith, K. A., Krebs, M. P., and Kaushal, S., 2004, Retinoids assist the cellular folding of the autosomal dominant retinitis pigmentosa opsin mutant P23H, *J Biol Chem.* **279**:16278.

Nour, M., and Naash, M. I., 2003, Mouse models of human retinal disease caused by expression of mutant rhodopsin. A valuable tool for the assessment of novel gene therapies, *Adv Exp Med Bio.* **533**:173.

Penn, J. S., Li, S., and Naash, M. I., 2000, Ambient hypoxia reverses retinal vascular attenuation in a transgenic mouse model of autosomal dominant retinitis pigmentosa, *Invest Ophthalmol Vis Sci.* **41**:4007.

Petrin, D., Baker, A., Coupland, S. G., Liston, P., Narang, M., Damji, K., Leonard, B., Chiodo, V. A., Timmers, A., Hauswirth, W., Korneluk, R. G., and Tsilfidis, C., 2003, Structural and functional protection of photoreceptors from MNU-induced retinal degeneration by the X-linked inhibitor of apoptosis, *Invest Ophthalmol Vis Sci.* **44**:2757.

Qtaishat, N. M., Okajima, T. I., Li, S., Naash, M. I., and Pepperberg, D. R., 1999, Retinoid kinetics in eye tissues of VPP transgenic mice and their normal littermates, *Invest Ophthalmol Vis Sci.* **40**:1040.

Shimayama, T., Nishikawa, S., and Taira, K., 1995, Generality of the NUX rule: kinetic analysis of the results of systematic mutations in the trinucleotide at the cleavage site of hammerhead ribozymes, *Biochemistry.* **34**:3649.

Sung, C. H., Davenport, C. M., and Nathans, J., 1993, Rhodopsin mutations responsible for autosomal dominant retinitis pigmentosa. Clustering of functional classes along the polypeptide chain, *J Biol Chem.* **268**:26645.

Sung, C. H., Schneider, B. G., Agarwal, N., Papermaster, D. S., and Nathans, J., 1991, Functional heterogeneity of mutant rhodopsins responsible for autosomal dominant retinitis pigmentosa, *Proc Natl Acad Sci U S A.* **88**:8840.

Tam, B. M., and Moritz, O. L., 2006, Characterization of rhodopsin P23H-induced retinal degeneration in a Xenopus laevis model of retinitis pigmentosa, *Invest Ophthalmol Vis Sci.* **47**:3234.

Tang, X. B., Hobom, G., and Luo, D., 1994, Ribozyme mediated destruction of influenza A virus in vitro and in vivo, *J Med Virol.* **42**:385.

Wang, D. Y., Chan, W. M., Tam, P. O., Baum, L., Lam, D. S., Chong, K. K., Fan, B. J., and Pang, C. P., 2005, Gene mutations in retinitis pigmentosa and their clinical implications, *Clin Chim Acta.* **351**:16.

Wang, M., Lam, T. T., Tso, M. O., and Naash, M. I., 1997, Expression of a mutant opsin gene increases the susceptibility of the retina to light damage, *Vis Neurosci.* **14**:55.

Werner, M., and Uhlenbeck, O. C., 1995, The effect of base mismatches in the substrate recognition helices of hammerhead ribozymes on binding and catalysis, *Nucleic Acids Res.* **23**:2092.

Wu, T. H., Ting, T. D., Okajima, T. I., Pepperberg, D. R., Ho, Y. K., Ripps, H., and Naash, M. I., 1998, Opsin localization and rhodopsin photochemistry in a transgenic mouse model of retinitis pigmentosa, *Neuroscience.***87**:709.

Zamecnik, P. C., and Stephenson, M. L., 1978, Inhibition of Rous sarcoma virus replication and cell transformation by a specific oligodeoxynucleotide, *Proc Natl Acad Sci U S A.* **75**:280.

Gene Therapy for Mouse Models of ADRP

Marina S. Gorbatyuk, William W. Hauswirth, and Alfred S. Lewin

1 Introduction

Autosomal Dominant Retinitis Pigmentosa (ADRP) is caused by mutations in the rhodopsin gene (*RHO*) in 30% of patients, and dominant negative mutations are often associated with toxicity of the mutated protein. Preventing or retarding ADRP progression may require the repair or silencing of the defective *RHO* gene. Two strategies for *RHO* mRNA silencing have recently been proposed (Millington-Ward et al., 1997; Lewin and Hauswirth, 2001). They are based on the application of therapeutic molecules such as ribozymes (Rz) and small interfering RNA (siRNA) that inhibit *RHO* expression.

The first approach permits the use of allele-specific regulators preferentially blocking the expression of mutated RHO mRNA. In contrast, the silencing of both alleles (mutant and wild-type) in an allele-independent strategy is more widely applicable, since the treatment takes into account the heterogeneity of RP mutations affecting the *RHO* gene. Knocking down the expression of *RHO* mRNA is the first step toward the allele-independent ADRP gene therapy. Whether ribozymes or siRNAs are used for this, gene therapy requires the delivery of the *RHO* gene resistant to the action of the therapeutic RNA in order to provide a complete supply of rhodopsin.

Mice and rats models have become extremely helpful for the study and the development of treatments for ADRP (LaVail et al., 2000; Machida et al., 2000; Kijas et al., 2002). Progress has been made in the silencing of mouse RHO mRNA in vivo (Gorbatyuk et al., 2005; Tessitore et al., 2006; Gorbatyuk et al., 2007). In this paper, we would like to highlight the results achieved in this first round using allele-independent ribozymes and siRNA, and describe the perspectives for the second step. Since the results were obtained from different experiments, they could not be used to compare the relative efficiencies of ribozymes and siRNAs in the first step of allele-independent gene therapy for ADRP.

M.S. Gorbatyuk
Department of Molecular Genetics and Microbiology, Tel: 1 352-392-0673, Fax: 1 352-392-3233,
e-mail: mari653@mgm.ufl.edu

R.E. Anderson et al. (eds.), *Recent Advances in Retinal Degeneration*,
© Springer 2008

2 Methods

The methods for ribozyme and siRNA design, vector construction for testing them in cultured cells and in vivo as well as descriptions of subretinal injections, electroretinographic (ERG) analysis, retinal RNA and protein extractions, morphological analysis were described earlier (Gorbatyuk et al., 2005; Gorbatyuk et al., 2007). As the control to ribozyme we used an irrelevant Rz. For an siRNA control we used an siRNA against the cardiac specific phospholambdan gene. Normalization of *RHO* mRNA and RHO protein was done by using internal controls: β-actin mRNA and β-actin protein.

3 Results

3.1 Testing Ribozymes and siRNA in the Cultured Cells

In HEK 293 cells, both ribozyme and an siRNA efficiently reduced accumulation of *RHO* mRNA (Fig. 1). Rz397 showed about 70% reduction, siRNA301 demonstrated 50% knock down of mouse *RHO* mRNA compared to their controls. siRNA301 was not the most effective one among tested siRNAs, but since it targets also the dog *RHO* mRNA we decided to proceed with it in mice as a prelude to large animal testing.

3.2 Attenuation of a- and b-wave Amplitudes of ERG in Response to Ribozyme and siRNA Treatment

The results of the scotopic full filed ERG analysis of animals injected with Rz397 and siRNA301 are shown the Fig. 2 A,B. We measured the ERG response at 1 and 2 months after injection and observed consistent degradation of a- and b-waves ampli-

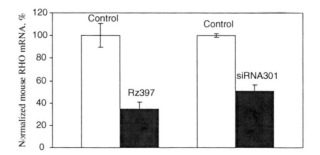

Fig. 1 Expression of Rz397 and siRNA301 in cultured HEK 293 cells led to reduction of mouse *RHO* mRNA 48 hours after co-transfection of plasmids expressing *RHO* and the knockdown of RNA. The molar ratio of plasmids expressing Rz or irrelevant Rz and target was 1:10. Concentration of siRNA301 and control siRNA was 75nM

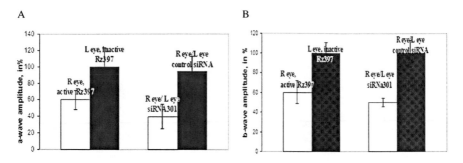

Fig. 2 Delivery of Rz397 and siRNA301 to animals retinas led to significant changes in a- and b- waves amplitudes of ERG at 2 months after injection. (A) The reduction of a-wave amplitude in RHO+/− mice injected with AAV2Rz397 and AAV5siRNA301. (B) The reduction in b-wave amplitudes of the RHO+/− retinas injected with the same vectors. Right eyes were injected with Rz397 or with siRNA301

tudes in right eyes injected with Rz397 and siRNA301. In case of Rz397, we discovered a small but statistically insignificant difference in a-wave amplitudes ($P < 0.19$) (Fig. 2A). However, we did detect a significant drop in the b-wave amplitude in treated eyes by 60% ($P < 0.037$) (Fig. 2B). With siRNA301 we found a reduction of a-and b-waves amplitude as well. At 2 months the reductions of a- and b-wave amplitudes were about 50% ($P < 0.027$, $P < 0.005$ respectively).

3.3 Ribozymes and siRNA Reduce the Mouse RHO mRNA and RHO Protein in vivo

Representative results of *RHO* mRNA and RHO protein reduction in response to AAV5siRNA301 expression in the retina are shown. Analysis of data revealed reduction by 40% of mouse RHO mRNA in RHO+/− mice at 2 months after injection the retina with AAV5siRNA301 ($P < 0.042$). Figure 3B demonstrates the results of protein analysis in the treated retinas and shows that the content of RHO protein was diminished in the RHO+/− retinas by 60% ($P < 0.013$).

3.4 The Thinning of the Outer Nuclear Layer in the Retinas of Animals Treated with Rz397 and siRNA301

The superior and the inferior regions of the retinas were analyzed. Figure 4 presents the result of measurements in the corresponded sectors of the superior retinas treated with AAV2Rz397 and AAV5siRN301. In the right eye treated with AAV2Rz397 and AAV5siRNA301 we observed reduction in the Outer Nuclear Layer (ONL) length compare to their controls by 33% and 32% correspondingly (p value < 0.04 and 0.002).

A   B

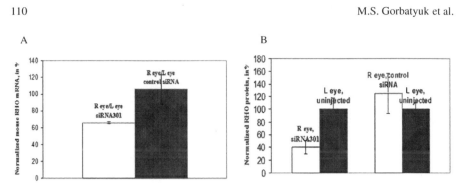

Fig. 3 Expression of siRNA301 causes the degradation of mouse normalized *RHO* mRNA (panel A). Results are expressed as ratios of normalized mouse *RHO* mRNA of right eye versus left eye measurement. Panel B shows the results of protein analysis. A significant difference in RHO protein between experimental and control eyes was observed in RHO+/–mice treated with Rz397 and siRNA301

3.5 Creation of the RHO301 Gene for the Replacement Step in ADRP Gene Therapy

To start the replacement step for ADRP gene therapy we attempted to find a suitable expression cassette to deliver the wild-type *RHO* gene to the retina. The *RHO* cDNA was placed under control of the mouse opsin proximal promoter in a plasmid with AAV2 terminal repeats and packaged in AAV capsids. We injected P23H *RHO* transgenic mice at postnatal day 16 into right eye, left eyes were intact. Animals were monitored during 2 months. At 1 month after injection, we observed the partial rescue of ERG amplitudes (Fig. 5). The b-wave amplitudes of the injected right eyes were consistently higher compared to the left eyes measurements at one month and two months post-injection.

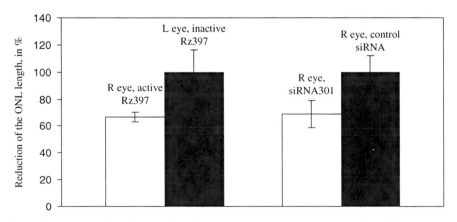

Fig. 4 Expression of Rz397 and siRNA301 digesting endogenous mouse *RHO* mRNA leads to reduction of the ONL thickness in injected eyes

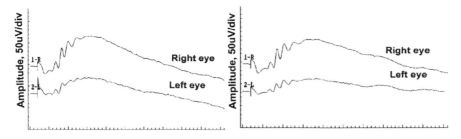

Fig. 5 Typical wave forms of scotopic ERG recordings in P23H transgenic mice after subretinal injection with AAV5RHO in the right eyes

We designed and created the *RHO*301 resistant gene by placing 5 mismatches in the coding region. The production of the RHO protein was confirmed by the immunoassay of 293 cells co-transfected with plasmid expressing the *RHO* gene under control of CMV promoter and an AAV plasmid expressing siRNA301. The *RHO*301 gene expression was resistant to siRNA301 under these conditions (data not shown).

4 Discussion

The variety of the *RHO* gene mutations leading to ADRP presents an obstacle to nucleotide sequence specific treatments based on RNA inhibitors: It is probably impossible to design of effective allele specific ribozymes or siRNAs for each disease-causing *RHO* mutation. Therefore, we and other groups are trying to design RNA inhibitors that do not discriminate between mutant and wild-type transcripts, but reduce the expression of both. In this paper, we summarize some of our results demonstrating that mouse *RHO* gene expression can be inhibited in vivo using ribozymes and siRNAs. The sustained expression of such inhibitors was provided by AAV, a virus that has been widely used for stable gene transfer to the retina, However, an allele-independent RNA replacement strategy also requires the expression of an siRNA- or ribozyme-resistant *RHO* gene later that can be delivered by a separate virus injection or can be delivered as part of a combination vector expressing both the inhibitor and the replacement gene.

We choose the RHO+/− mice carrying one allele of the RHO gene as working models. Our preferences were based on the fact that the RHO+/− mice already contain a 40% reduction in the level of RHO protein. It was therefore easier to detect an ERG phenotype in these animals, even though RNA and protein knockdown could also be detected in wild-type mice (data not shown). Expression of Rz397 and siRNA301 in wild type mice did not cause significant reduction in ERG amplitudes. In RHO+/− mice, using Rz397, the ERG b-wave amplitude was more affected than was the a-wave. In case of siRNA301 we observed decline of a-wave amplitudes whose onset was more rapidly than the decline in b-wave amplitude. The

ERG data correlated with the reduction in the ONL thickness (Figs. 2 and 4). The extent in the reduction of the ONL thickness in retinas injected with AAV2Rz397 and AAV5siRNA301 was similar.

Since we have been able to achieve allele-independent knockdown of rhodopsin in vivo, we are now working on the second step of the RNA-replacement strategy – providing an inhibitor-resistant wild-type *RHO* gene. Constructing siRNA-resistant or ribozyme *RHO* genes using a series of silent mutations has not been a major obstacle. Indeed, two other groups have also constructed RNAi resistant *RHO* cDNAs (Cashman et al., 2005 ; Kiang et al., 2005). A more important issue is balancing the expression of the RNA inhibitor and the replacement *RHO* gene so that rhodopsin synthesis is sufficiently high but not harmful due to over-expression. The appropriate timing may vary and be crucial with the animal model, since the damage caused by the endogenous mutated *RHO* may have been initiated before substantial evidence of retinal degeneration has begun.

References

Cashman, S.M., Binkley, E.A., and Kumar-Singh, R., 2005, Towards mutation-independent silencing of genes involved in retinal degeneration by RNA interference, *Gene Ther.*, **12**: 1223.

Gorbatyuk, M.S., Pang, J.J., Thomas, J., Jr., Hauswirth, W.W., and Lewin, A.S., 2005, Knockdown of wild-type mouse rhodopsin using an AAV vectored ribozyme as part of an RNA replacement approach, *Mol. Vis.*, **11**: 648.

Gorbatyuk, M., Justilien, V., Liu, J., Hauswirth, W.W., and Lewin, A.S., 2007, Preservation of photoreceptor morphology and function in P23H rats using an allele independent ribozyme, *Exp. Eye Res.*, **84**: 44.

Kiang, A.S., Palfi, A., Ader, M., Kenna, P.F., Millington-Ward, S., Clark, G., Kennan, A., O'Reilly, M., Tam, L.C., Aherne, A., McNally, N., Humphries, P., and Farrar, G.J., 2005, Toward a gene therapy for dominant disease: validation of an RNA interference-based mutation-independent approach, *Mol. Ther.*, **12**: 555.

Kijas, J.W., Cideciyan, A.V., Aleman, T.S., Pianta, M.J., Pearce-Kelling, S.E., Miller, B.J., Jacobson, S.G., Aguirre, G.D., and Acland, G.M., 2002, Naturally occurring rhodopsin mutation in the dog causes retinal dysfunction and degeneration mimicking human dominant retinitis pigmentosa, *Proc. Natl. Acad. Sci. U.S.A.*, **99**: 6328.

LaVail, M.M., Yasumura, D., Matthes, M.T., Drenser, K.A., Flannery, J.G., Lewin, A.S., and Hauswirth, W.W., 2000, Ribozyme rescue of photoreceptor cells in P23H transgenic rats: long-term survival and late-stage therapy, *Proc. Natl. Acad. Sci. U.S.A.*, **97**: 11488.

Lewin, A.S. and Hauswirth, W.W., 2001, Ribozyme gene therapy: applications for molecular medicine, *Trends Mol. Med.*, **7**: 221.

Machida, S., Kondo, M., Jamison, J.A., Khan, N.W., Kononen, L.T., Sugawara, T., Bush, R.A., and Sieving, P.A., 2000, P23H rhodopsin transgenic rat: correlation of retinal function with histopathology, *Invest. Ophthalmol. Vis. Sci.*, **41**: 3200.

Millington-Ward, S., O'Neill, B., Tuohy, G., al Jandal, N., Kiang, A.S., Kenna, P.F., Palfi, A., Hayden, P., Mansergh, F., Kennan, A., Humphries, P., and Farrar, G.J., 1997, Strategems in vitro for gene therapies directed to dominant mutations, *Hum. Mol. Genet.*, **6**: 1415.

Tessitore, A., Parisi, F., Denti, M.A., Allocca, M., Di Vicino, U., Domenici, L., Bozzoni, I., and Auricchio, A., 2006, Preferential silencing of a common dominant rhodopsin mutation does not inhibit retinal degeneration in a transgenic model, *Mol. Ther.*, **14**: 692.

Development of Viral Vectors with Optimal Transgene Expression for Ocular Gene Therapies

Takao Hashimoto

1 Introduction

Various efforts have been dedicated to the development of effective strategies to treat ocular diseases. Investigators have demonstrated that gene therapies using viral vectors are one of the promising technologies. For an ideal therapeutic effect, a variety of vector designs have been tested. Especially, selection of a promoter to drive a transgene is important to obtain adequate level of expression. In this brief chapter, reviewed are the promoters for viral vectors for ocular gene therapies.

2 Promoters for Gene Transduction

Viral constructs for gene therapy are composed of a viral backbone, promoters to drive transgene, and transgenes of interest. Table 1 summarizes the representative transgene expression profiles in ocular tissue by different promoters. Classically, strong constitutive promoters have been used to achieve high expression for maximum efficacy. Most commonly used has been the human cytomegalovirus (CMV) immediate early promoter. It usually drives expression very strongly in the retinal pigment epithelium (RPE). Transduction in other ocular tissues could be achieved by varying viral type, envelope/serotype, and the site and the timing of infection. Other ubiquitous promoters used include those of chicken β-actin (CBA/CAG), and elongation factor 1α (EF1α).

To establish better transduction in the target cells and to minimize possible side effects, targeted gene transduction has been aimed at by taking advantage of tissue specific promoters. Opsin gene promoter has demonstrated to drive expression in photoreceptors and it provides strong and specific expression in the targeted cells. For expression in Muller cells, promoters of glial fibrillary acidic protein (GFAP),

T. Hashimoto
Jules Stein Eye Institute, University of California Los Angeles, CA 90095, U.S.A,
Tel: 310-825-6992, Fax: 425-660-6923
e-mail: gbf00573@nifty.com

R.E. Anderson et al. (eds.), *Recent Advances in Retinal Degeneration*,
© Springer 2008

Table 1 Characteristics of virus, envelope/serotype, promoter and expression profiles for ocular gene therapy

Virus	Env./Sero.	Promoter	Promoter feature	Transgene	Inj.	Cor.	Iris	TM	Lens	GCL	INL	PR	RPE	Other	'Eye'	Sp.	Reference
AAV		CMV	ubiquitous	lacZ	SR					+	+	++	++			m	Ali et al., 1996
AAV		CMV	ubiquitous	lacZ	SR, V					++	+	+	+++			m	Grant et al., 1997
AAV		CMV	ubiquitous	lacZ, GFP	V					+++	+	+		ON		gp	Guy et al., 1999
AAV		CMV	ubiquitous	GFP	SR							++	+++			mk	Bennett et al., 1999
AAV		CMV	ubiquitous	FGF2	SR					+	++	+++	+++			r	Lau et al., 2000
AAV		CMV	ubiquitous	neurturin	V							++				m	Jomary et al., 2001
AAV	2	CMV	ubiquitous	sFlt-1	V		+			+	+	+				m	Bainbridge et al., 2002
AAV		CMV	ubiquitous	CNTF	SR, V										+	m	Bok et al., 2002
AAV	2	CMV	ubiquitous	GFP	SR							++	+			m,r	Shen et al., 2003
AAV	2	CMV	ubiquitous	GFP	SR							+++				m	Bainbridge et al., 2003
AAV	2	CMV	ubiquitous	GFP	V					+	++	++				m	Bainbridge et al., 2003
AAV	2	CMV	ubiquitous	GFP	SR							++	+++			r	Sutanto et al., 2005
AAV		CMV	ubiquitous	PDEβ	SR										+	m	Bennett et al., 1996
Adeno	5	CMV	ubiquitous	antisense	AC	++										r	Lai et al., 2002
Adeno	5	CMV	ubiquitous	PEDF	periocular	periocular								periocular		m	Gehlbach et al., 2003
Lenti	VSVG	CMV	ubiquitous	GFP	SR							(+)	+++			r	Miyoshi et al., 1997
Lenti	VSVG	CMV	ubiquitous	PDEβ	SR						+	+				m	Takahashi et al., 1999
Lenti	VSVG	CMV	ubiquitous	GFP	AC	+++		++								m	Bainbridge et al., 2001
Lenti	VSVG	CMV	ubiquitous	GFP	SR								+++			r	Bainbridge et al., 2001
Lenti	VSVG	CMV	ubiquitous	GFP	SR								+++			r	Bemelmans et al., 2005
Lenti	Mokola	CMV	ubiquitous	GFP	SR								+++			r	Bemelmans et al., 2005
Lenti	VSVG	CMV	ubiquitous	GFP,lacZ	vitro	+++										m,rb,h	Beutelspacher et al., 2005
Lenti	RRVG	CMV	ubiquitous	GFP	SR, V								+++			r	Greenberg et al., 2007
Lenti	VSVG	CMV	ubiquitous	GFP	SR, V								+++			r	Greenberg et al., 2007
Lenti	VSVG	CMV	ubiquitous	MYO7A	SR								++			m	Hashimoto et al., 2007
Adeno		murine CMV	ubiquitous	p35, lacZ	ON				+							r	Kügler et al., 1999
AAV	2	murine CMV	ubiquitous	GFP	V				+							r	Kügler et al., 2003
AAV		CBA/CAG	ubiquitous	RPE65	SR								+++			d	Acland et al., 2001
AAV	2	CBA/CAG	ubiquitous	PEDF, K1K3	SR, V										+	m	Raisler et al., 2002
AAV	2	CBA/CAG	ubiquitous	PEDF, GFP	SR							+++	+++			m	Mori et al., 2002

Table 1 (continued)

Virus	Env./Sero.	Promoter	Promoter feature	Transgene	Inj.	Cor.	Iris	TM	Lens	GCL	INL	PR	RPE	Other	'Eye'	Sp.	Reference
AAV	2	CBA/CAG	ubiquitous	PEDF, GFP	V					++						m	Mori et al., 2002
AAV	2	CBA/CAG	ubiquitous	CNTF	SR,V										+	m	Bok et al., 2002
AAV		CBA/CAG	ubiquitous	BIRC4	V					+++	+			CB		r	Mckinnon et al., 2002
AAV		CBA/CAG	ubiquitous	GFP	V					+++	+					r	Martin et al., 2002
Adeno		CBA/CAG	ubiquitous	FGF2, lacZ	SR								+++			r	Akimoto et al., 1999
Adeno		CBA/CAG	ubiquitous	Smad7, cre	lens				+++							m	Saika et al., 2004
Lenti	VSVG	CBA/CAG	ubiquitous	GFP	SR,V												Greenberg et al., 2007
Lenti	VSVG	PGK	ubiquitous	GFP	SR								+++			r	Bemelmans et al., 2005
Lenti	Mokola	PGK	ubiquitous	GFP	SR								+++			r	Bemelmans et al., 2005
Lenti		PGK	ubiquitous	lacZ	V					+	+		+++			m	Kostic et al., 2003
Lenti	VSVG	PGK	ubiquitous	YFP	vitro	+++										r,s,h	Parker et al., 2007
Lenti	VSVG	SV40	ubiquitous	YFP	vitro	+++										r,s,h	Parker et al., 2007
Lenti	VSVG	MPSV	ubiquitous	YFP	vitro	+++										r,s,h	Parker et al., 2007
Lenti	VSVG	Ubiquitin	ubiquitous	GFP	SR,V								+++			r	Greenberg et al., 2007
Lenti	VSVG	EF1α	ubiquitous	GFP	SR								+++			r	Bemelmans et al., 2005
Lenti	Mokola	EF1α	ubiquitous	GFP	SR								+++			r	Bemelmans et al., 2005
Lenti		EF1α	ubiquitous	lacZ	V					+++	+++	+++	++			m	Kostic et al., 2003
AAV		opsin	PR	Prph2	SR							+++				m	Ali et al., 2000
AAV	2	opsin	PR	CNTF	SR,V										+	m	Bok et al., 2002
AAV	2	opsin	PR	PEDF, K1K3	SR,V										+	m	Raisler et al., 2002
AAV	5	opsin	PR	Rs1h	SR						(+)	+++			+	m	Min et al., 2005
AAV	2	opsin	PR	RPGRIP, GFP	SR							+++				m	Pawlyk et al., 2005
AAV		opsin	PR	PDEβ	V								++			m	Jomary et al., 1997
AAV		opsin	PR	GFRα2	V								++			m	Jomary et al., 2001
Lenti		opsin	PR	lacZ	V							+++				m	Kostic et al., 2003
Lenti	VSVG	opsin	PR	GFP	SR							+++				r	Miyoshi et al., 1997
Lenti	VSVG	opsin	PR	PDEβ	SR							+				m	Takahashi et al., 1999
Lenti	VSVG	opsin	PR	GFP	SR							++	+/-			r	Bemelmans et al., 2005
Lenti	Mokola	opsin	PR	GFP	SR							++	+/-			r	Bemelmans et al., 2005
AAV	2	blue opsin	PR	GFP	SR							+				r	Glushakova et al., 2006

(continued)

Table 1 (continued)

Virus	Env./Sero.	Promoter feature	Promoter	Transgene	Inj.	Cor.	Iris	TM	Lens	GCL	INL	PR	RPE	Other	'Eye'	Sp.	Reference
AAV	5	PR	blue opsin	GFP	SR							+++				r	Glushakova et al., 2006
Lenti	VSVG	Muller	GFAP	GFP	SR, V						++					r	Greenberg et al., 2007
Lenti	VSVG	Muller	CD44	GFP	SR, V						++					r	Greenberg et al., 2007
Lenti	VSVG	Muller	vimentin	GFP	SR, V						++					r	Greenberg et al., 2007
AAV	2	Muller, RPE	CRALBP	PEDF, K1K3	SR, V									+		m	Raisler et al., 2002
AAV	2	GC, EC	PDGF	PEDF, K1K3	SR, V									+		m	Raisler et al., 2002
Adeno	5	TM	Ch3L1	lacZ	vitro			+++								h	Liton et al., 2005
AAV	2	RPE	RPE65	Mertk	SR										+	r	Smith et al., 2003
AAV	2	RPE	cathepsin D	GFP	SR						++	+++				r	Sutanto et al., 2005
AAV	2/4, 2/2	RPE	RPE65	RPE65	SR								+++			d	Le Meur et al., 2007
Lenti	VSVG	RPE	SFFV	Mertk, GFP	SR								+			r	Tschernutter et al., 2005
AAV	2	neuron	synapsin 1	GFP	V					+++	+					r	Kügler et al., 2003
Lenti	VSVG	cornea	E-selection	GFP,lacZ	vitro	+++										m,rb,h	Beutelspacher et al., 2005
Adeno	5	lens	LEP503	lacZ	lens				+							rb,h	Malecaze et al., 2006
Baculo		neuron	CMVE-PDGF	luciferase	V					++		+				r	Li et al., 2005
Lenti	VSVG	RPE, PR	CMVp-MYO7AE	MYO7A, etc.	SR					+			+++			m	Hashimoto et al., 2007

AAV: adeno-associated virus, Adeno: adenovirus, Lenti: lentivirus, Baculo: baculovirus, Env./Sero.: envelope or serotype, VSVG: vesicular stomatitis virus envelope surface glycoprotein, Mokola: lyssavirus Mokola glycoprotein, RRVG: Ross River virus envelope surface glycoprotein, CMV: cytomegalovirus immediate-early promoter, CBA/CAG: chicken β-actin promoter with (CAG) or without (CBA) CMV immediate-early enhancer, PGK: phosphoglycerate kinase 1 promoter, SV40: simian virus type 40 early promoter, MPSV: myeloproliferative sarcoma virus promoter, EF1α: elongation factor 1α, GFAP: glial fibrillary acidic protein, CRALBP: cellular retinaldehyde-binding protein, PDGF: platelet-derived growth factor, Ch3L1: chitinase 3-like 1, SFFV: spleen focus forming virus promoter, CMVE-PDGF: CMV enhancer-PDGF hybrid promoter, CMVp-MYO7AE: partial CMV promoter-MYO7A enhancer hybrid promoter, GFP: green fluorescent protein, FGF2: fibroblast growth factor 2, CNTF: ciliary neurotrophic factor, PDEβ: cyclic guanosine monophosphate-phosphodiesterase β-subunit, PEDF: pigment epithelium-derived factor, MYO7A: myosin 7A, K1K3: Kringle domains 1 through 3 of angiostatin, BIRC4: baculoviral IAP repeat-containing 4, YFP: yellow fluorescent protein, Prph2: peripherin 2, Rs1h: retinoschisin, RPGRIP: retinitis pigmentosa guanosine 5'-triphosphate hydrolase regulator-interacting protein, GFRα2: glial cell line-derived neurotrophic factor family receptor α2, Inj.: injection site, SR: subretinal space, V: vitreous cavity, AC: anterior chamber, vitro: in vitro or ex vivo, lens: lens or lens capsular bag, Cor.: cornea, TM: trabecular meshwork, GCL: ganglion cell layer, INL: inner nuclear layer, PR: photoreceptor cell layer, RPE: retinal pigment epithelium, ON: optic nerve, CB: ciliary body, Transgene Expression +: expression detected, ++: moderate expression detected, +++: strong expression detected, (+): expression detected presumably due to protein transport or diffusion, Sp.: species, m: mouse, gp: guinea pig, mk: monkey, r: rat, rb: rabbit, h: human, d: dog, s: sheep.

CD44, and vimentin are effective. Promoters of RPE65 and cathepsin D can target RPE cells. Other tissue specific promoters have also been used for the transduction in other ocular tissues including the retinal ganglion cells, trabecular meshwork, cornea and lens.

Even with a tissue specific expression, a transgene could deteriorate cellular functions owing to an unacceptable level of transduction (Hashimoto et al., 2007). To alleviate the toxicity and to achieve adequate level of expression, a hybrid promoter may be utilized. By fusing different regulatory fragments, one may be able to modify the expression levels in the targeted cell types (Li et al., 2005; Hashimoto et al., 2007).

3 Summary

Striving for ideal viral constructs by modifying its structure, including promoters, would make the viral gene therapy more promising. Further assessment of the promoters and their expression profiles such as those shown in Table 1 and new designs of hybrid promoters may achieve optimal expression features for ocular gene therapies.

Acknowledgments The author gratefully acknowledges the advice of Drs. X.-J. Yang and D. S. Williams on the work presented at the XII International Symposium on Retinal Degeneration 2006, and the support by the Young Investigator Awards funded by the National Eye Institute, the Foundation Fighting Blindness, and Merck Ophthalmics for attending the meeting.

References

Acland, G. M., et al., 2001, Gene therapy restores vision in a canine model of childhood blindness, *Nat. Genet.* **28**: 92–95.

Akimoto, M., et al., 1999, Adenovirally expressed basic fibroblast growth factor rescues photoreceptor cells in RCS rats, *Invest. Ophthalmol. Vis. Sci.* **40**: 273–279.

Ali, R. R., et al., 1996, Gene transfer into the mouse retina mediated by an adeno-associated viral vector, *Hum. Mol. Genet.* **5**: 591–594.

Ali, R. R., et al., 2000, Restoration of photoreceptor ultrastructure and function in retinal degeneration slow mice by gene therapy, *Nat. Genet.* **25**: 306–310.

Bainbridge, J. W. B., et al., 2001, in vivo gene transfer to the mouse eye using an HIV-based lentiviral vector; efficient long-term transduction of corneal endothelium and retinal pigment epithelium, *Gene Ther.* **8**: 1665–1668.

Bainbridge, J. W. B., et al., 2002, Inhibition of retinal neovascularisation by gene transfer of soluble VEGF receptor sFlt-1, *Gene Ther.* **9**: 320–326.

Bainbridge, J. W. B., et al., 2003, Hypoxia-regulated transgene expression in experimental retinal and choroidal neovascularization, *Gene Ther.* **10**: 1049–1054.

Bemelmans, A.-P., et al., 2005, Retinal cell type expression specificity of HIV-1-derived gene transfer vectors upon subretinal injection in the adult rat: influence of pseudotyping and promoter, *J. Gene Med.* **7**: 1367–1374.

Bennett, J., et al., 1996, Photoreceptor cell rescue in retinal degeneration (*rd*) mice by in vivo gene therapy, *Nat. Med.* **2**: 649–654.

Bennett, J., et al., 1999, Stable transgene expression in rod photoreceptors after recombinant adeno-associated virus-mediated gene transfer to monkey retina, *Proc. Natl. Acad. Sci. U. S. A.* **96**: 9920–9925.

Beutelspacher, S. C., et al., 2005, Comparison of HIV-1 and EIAV-based lentiviral vectors in corneal transduction, *Exp. Eye Res.* **80**: 787–794.

Bok, D., et al., 2002, Effects of adeno-associated virus-vectored ciliary neurotrophic factor on retinal structure and function in mice with a P216L rds/peripherin mutation, *Exp. Eye Res.* **74**: 719–735.

Gehlbach, P., et al., 2003, Periocular injection of an adenoviral vector encoding pigment epithelium-derived factor inhibits choroidal neovascularization, *Gene Ther.* **10**: 637–646.

Glushakova, L. G., et al., 2006, Human blue-opsin promoter preferentially targets reporter gene expression to rat s-cone photoreceptors, *Invest. Ophthalmol. Vis. Sci.* **47**: 3505–3513.

Grant, C. A., et al., 1997, Evaluation of recombinant adeno-associated virus as a gene transfer vector for the retina, *Curr. Eye Res.* **16**: 949–956.

Greenberg, K. P., et al., 2007, Targeted transgene expression in müller glia of normal and diseased retinas using lentiviral vectors, *Invest. Ophthalmol. Vis. Sci.* **48**: 1844–1852.

Guy, J., et al., 1999, Reporter expression persists 1 year after adeno-associated virus-mediated gene transfer to the optic nerve, *Arch. Ophthalmol.* **117**: 929–937.

Hashimoto, T., et al., 2007, Lentiviral gene replacement therapy of retinas in a mouse model for Usher syndrome type 1B, *Gene Ther.* **14**: 584–594.

Jomary, C., et al., 1997, Rescue of photoreceptor function by AAV-mediated gene transfer in a mouse model of inherited retinal degeneration, *Gene Ther.* **4**: 683–690.

Jomary, C., et al., 2001, Epitope-tagged recombinant AAV vectors for expressing neurturin and its receptor in retinal cells, *Mol. Vis.* **7**: 36–41.

Kostic, C., et al., 2003, Activity analysis of housekeeping promoters using self-inactivating lentiviral vector delivery into the mouse retina, *Gene Ther.* **10**: 818–821.

Kügler, S., et al., 1999, Transduction of axotomized retinal ganglion cells by adenoviral vector administration at the optic
nerve stump: an in vivo model system for the inhibition of neuronal apoptotic cell death, *Gene Ther.* **6**: 1759–1767.

Kügler, S., et al., 2003, Differential transgene expression in brain cells in vivo and in vitro from AAV-2 vectors with small transcriptional control units, *Virology* **311**: 89–95.

Lai, C.-M., et al., 2002, Inhibition of corneal neovascularization by recombinant adenovirus mediated antisense VEGF RNA, *Exp. Eye Res.* **75**: 625–634.

Lau, D., et al., 2000, Retinal degeneration is slowed in transgenic rats by AAV-mediated delivery of FGF-2, *Invest. Ophthalmol. Vis. Sci.* **41**: 3622–3633.

Le Meur, G., et al., 2007, Restoration of vision in RPE65-deficient Briard dogs using an AAV serotype 4 vector that specifically targets the retinal pigmented epithelium, *Gene Ther.* **14**: 292–303.

Li, Y., et al., 2005, Neuronal gene transfer by baculovirus-derived vectors accommodating a neurone-specific promoter, *Exp. Physiol.* **90**: 39–44.

Liton, P. B., et al., 2005, Specific targeting of gene expression to a subset of human trabecular meshwork cells using the chitinase 3-like 1 promoter, *Invest. Ophthalmol. Vis. Sci.* **46**: 183–190.

Malecaze, F., et al., 2006, Lens cell targetting for gene therapy of prevention of posterior capsule opacification, *Gene Ther.* **13**: 1422–1429.

Martin, K. R. G., et al., 2002, Gene delivery to the eye using adeno-associated viral vectors, *Methods* **28**: 267–275.

Mckinnon, S. J., et al., 2002, Baculoviral IAP repeat-containing-4 protects optic nerve axons in a rat glaucoma model, *Mol. Ther.* **5**: 780–787.

Min, S. H., et al., 2005, Prolonged recovery of retinal structure/function after gene therapy in an *Rs1h*-deficient mouse model of x-linked juvenile retinoschisis, *Mol. Ther.* **12**: 644–651.

Miyoshi, H., et al., 1997, Stable and efficient gene transfer into the retina using an HIV-based lentiviral vector, *Proc. Natl. Acad. Sci. U. S. A.* **94**: 10319–10323.

Mori, K., et al., 2002, AAV-mediated gene transfer of pigment epithelium-derived factor inhibits choroidal neovascularization, *Invest. Ophthalmol. Vis. Sci.* **43**: 1994–2000.

Parker, D. G. A., et al., 2007, Lentivirus-mediated gene transfer to the rat, ovine and human cornea, *Gene Ther.* **14**: 760–767.

Pawlyk, B. S., et al., 2005, Gene replacement therapy rescues photoreceptor degeneration in a murine model of Leber congenital amaurosis lacking RPGRIP, *Invest. Ophthalmol. Vis. Sci.* **46**: 3039–3045.

Raisler, B. J., et al., 2002, Adeno-associated virus type-2 expression of pigmented epithelium-derived factor or Kringles 1–3 of angiostatin reduce retinal neovascularization, *Proc. Natl. Acad. Sci. U. S. A.* **99**: 8909–8914.

Saika, S., et al., 2004, Transient adenoviral gene transfer of Smad7 prevents injury-induced epithelial-mesenchymal transition of lens epithelium in mice, *Lab. Invest.* **84**: 1259–1270.

Shen, W.-Y., et al., 2003, Practical considerations of recombinant adeno-associated virus-mediated gene transfer for treatment of retinal degenerations, *J. Gene Med.* **5**: 576–587.

Smith, A. J., et al., 2003, AAV-Mediated gene transfer slows photoreceptor loss in the RCS rat model of retinitis pigmentosa, *Mol. Ther.* **8**: 188–195.

Sutanto, E. N., et al., 2005, Development and evaluation of the specificity of a cathepsin D proximal promoter in the eye, *Curr. Eye Res.* **30**: 53–61.

Takahashi, M., et al., 1999, Rescue from photoreceptor degeneration in the *rd* mouse by human immunodeficiency virus vector-mediated gene transfer, *J. Virol.* **73**: 7812–7816.

Tschernutter, M., et al., 2005, Long-term preservation of retinal function in the RCS rat model of retinitis pigmentosa following lentivirus-mediated gene therapy, *Gene Ther.* **12**: 694–701.

Adeno-Associated Viral Vectors and the Retina

John J. Alexander and William W. Hauswirth

1 Prospects for Retinal Gene Therapy

There are a variety of diseases of the retina arising from genetic and non-genetic causes, or a combination of both, that lead to the loss of vision. The retina is a prime location for gene therapy because of its accessibility, immune privileged status (Caspi, 2006), and susceptible cell types. Several strategies have been attempted to rescue retinal disease, including gene replacement (Acland et al., 2001), gene knockdown with both ribozymes (Gorbatyuk et al., 2007) and siRNA (Kiang et al., 2005), and therapeutic gene supplementation (Deng et al., 2005).

While there are a wide range of both viral and non-viral methods to introduce genes into the retina, the review here exclusively describes Adeno-Associated Virus (AAV) and its evolution as a vector. AAV has been extensively studied as a vector for gene therapy in the retina with its safety and toxicology documented (Jacobson et al., 2006a,b). Furthermore, recombinant AAV (rAAV) has received approval from the FDA and the NIH Recombinant DNA Advisory Committee for use in a clinical trial to treat Leber Congenital Amaurosis (LCA).

2 Adeno-associated Virus

AAV was first discovered in the 1960's as a contaminant of adenovirus stocks (Atchison et al., 1965). It is a mammalian ssDNA virus of the family *Parvoviridae*, subfamily *Parvovirinae*, and genus *Dependovirus* (Muzyczka and Berns, 2001), where strands of plus and minus polarity are packaged with equal efficiency and infectivity. The viral DNA contains three promoters, two ORF's, and a polyadenlyation signal, all of which are flanked by palindromic inverted terminal repeats

J.J. Alexander
Department of Molecular Genetics & Microbiology, University of Florida College of Medicine, Gainesville, Florida 32610-0266, Tel: 352-284-4737
e-mail: zander@ufl.edu

R.E. Anderson et al. (eds.), *Recent Advances in Retinal Degeneration*,
© Springer 2008

(ITRs) (Muzyczka and Berns, 2001). Furthermore, AAV has the ability to transduce non-dividing cells and integrate site specifically into what is termed the "AAV S1" sequence within human chromosome 19 (Muzyczka and Berns, 2001). It is estimated that 50% to 96% of the population is seropositive for AAV2 exposure (Warrington and Herzog, 2006); however, AAV is non-pathogenic. AAV has been used as a model system for DNA replication (Berns and Giraud, 1996) and is easily manipulated in vitro because of the small size of the genome and relatively simple organization (Muzyczka and Berns, 2001). Another unique feature of AAV is that it requires a helper virus (such as adenovirus or herpes virus) to replicate (Warrington and Herzog, 2006). Since almost all of the rAAV gene therapy vectors are derived from the prototype serotype AAV2 genome (Choi et al., 2005), more specifically the AAV2 ITRs, efforts to further understand AAV2 continue.

The AAV2 genome is 4,679 base pairs and uses three promoters (p5, p19, and p40) to give rise to four non-structural proteins (Rep78, Rep68, Rep52, and Rep40), and three capsid proteins (VP1, VP2, and VP3). Rep78 and Rep68 are essential regulators for every phase of the AAV life cycle, including integration, while Rep52 and Rep40 are needed for encapsulating mature DNA (Muzyczka and Berns, 2001). The 60 subunit 25 nm capsids are assembled from VP1, VP2, and VP3, in a ratio of 1:1:8, respectively (Huttner et al., 2003). The ITRs consist of 145 bases forming a "hairpin" structure serving as the viral origin of replication (Hauswirth and Berns, 1977), self primers for cellular second strand synthesis, packaging , and are involved in integration. In the absence of a helper virus, an AAV infection can result in site specific integration and latency through a Rep78/68 – ITR – genome interaction. Above all, it is the non-pathogenic and replication deficient nature of AAV makes it an attractive vehicle for gene therapy.

In addition to the classic AAV2 serotype, there have been more than 10 new serotypes classified, and over 100 new isolates identified (Wu et al., 2006). Since many retinal gene therapy experiments utilize capsids of serotypes 1, 2, or 5, their isolation and receptor specificity is important. Types 1 and 2 were originally isolated from adenovirus stocks and type 5 was isolated from a papillomavirus positive condylomatous lesion (Bantel-Schaal and zur Hausen, 1984). Types 2 and 5 are thought to be of human origin, while unclear whether type 1 is of human or simian origin. What mainly sets apart the different serotypes is their affinity for different cell surface receptors for binding, and co-receptors for internalization. The most studied serotype, AAV2, utilizes membrane associated heparan sulfate proteoglycan as its primary receptor, whereas integrins $\alpha_V\beta_5/\alpha_5\beta_1$, hepatocyte growth factor receptor, or human fibroblast growth factor receptor 1 can serve as co-receptor. Serotype 1 appears to bind cells through α-2,3 and α-2,6 sialic acids that are present on N-linked glycoproteins; however, a co-receptor has yet to be identified. Serotype 5 binds to α-2,3-N-linked sialic acid, and platelet-derived growth factor receptor has been identified as a coreceptor. The serotype receptor differences give rise to a wide range and (or) specificity for tissue tropism, something that is exploited using cross packaging techniques in rAAV vectors.

3 Recombinant Adeno-associated Viral Vectors

Deriving a rAAV vector from wild type AAV was first described by Hermonat and Muzyczka in the 1980's (Hermonat and Muzyczka,, 1984). They successfully transduced cultured mouse and human cells with a rAAV carrying the neomycin resistance gene under the control of an SV40 promoter in place of the capsid genes. Their results showed that the recombinant genome not only integrated, but it also expressed the transgene. Based on previous work, they proposed that it would be possible to substitute the entire AAV genome, except for the 145 nucleotide ITRs, with exogenous DNA and use it in the context of "gene therapy." Now, more than 20 years later, what are currently used for rAAV vectors are not much different that what was predicted by Hermonat and Muzyczka. Transgene expression cassettes usually contain the AAV2 ITRs flanking a promoter, intron, splice donor/acceptor, transgene, and poly-A signal that is packaged into the capsid of choice. Since all that is left of the actual virus genome are the ITRs, several systems have been developed to produce and package the different rAAV vectors.

The ability of rAAV to transduce a variety of cell types through cross-packaging or "peudotyping" has led to the identification of serotype tissue tropisms and efficiencies (Wu et al., 2006). A nomenclature has been adopted such that rAAV2/2 refers to serotype 2 ITRs in serotype 2 capsids, and rAAV2/5 would refer to the use of serotype 5 capsids instead. When injected in the subretinal space of the retina both rAAV2/2 and rAAV2/5 can transduce photoreceptors and retinal pigmented epithelial cells (RPE) (Dinculescu et al., 2005), albeit at different efficiencies, and rAAV2/1 is reported to be exclusive to RPE cells (Rolling, 2004); however, there are reports of low level transduction to photoreceptor, muller, and inner nuclear layer cells (Auricchio et al., 2001). When injected in the vitreous, rAAV2/2 results in varying levels of transduction of ganglion cells (Guy et al., 1999), as well as a smaller number of Muller cells perhaps related to retinal injury (Hauswirth, unpublished). In contrast, no appreciable level of transduced cells are observed for rAAV2/1 and rAAV2/5 (Rolling, 2004) when introduced into the vitreous. A notable difference between the two serotypes is that rAAV2/5 has demonstrated a higher transduction efficiency and faster kinetics than rAAV2/2 when injected in the subretinal space (Dinculescu et al., 2005). Additionally, there also appears to be general differences in intracellular trafficking pathways between serotypes 2 and 5 (Wu et al., 2006).

It is now a widely accepted fact that rAAV vectors result in long term, stable, and therapeutic expression of transgenes in the retina (Dinculescu et al., 2005). Several of these studies demonstrate the long term therapeutic efficacy of using rAAV, in particular, those treating LCA and X-linked juvenile retinoschisis (RS). The RS-1 mouse is a model for RS, and when treated with rAAV expressing the wild type human RS gene, the electroretiongram (ERG) and retinal structure improve dramatically and for at least one year (Min et al., 2005). Perhaps the most important success in furthering retinal gene therapy for human use came in 2001 when investigators successfully restored vision to a dog model of LCA (Acland et al., 2001).

The LCA dogs are deficient in RPE65 and have essentially no vision or recordable ERG along with retinal degeneration. In these studies a single subretinal injection of rAAV expressing wild type canine RPE65 was sufficient to restore ERG, preserve retinal structure, and most importantly gain vision (Acland et al., 2001; Acland et al., 2005). This success, along with proven safety in non-human primates (Jacobson et al., 2006b), has paved the way for an LCA clinical trial beginning in 2007.

3.1 rAAV Vector Persistance

Long term expression of transgenes is dependent upon rAAV DNA persistence within cells. While the wild type AAV can integrate into the host genome, the recombinant vectors do not appear to integrate (except in very low frequencies and at random) and persist as episomes. This difference has received much attention because rAAV is now used in a wide range of gene therapy experiments. Wild type AAV uses a complex binding process between the ITRs, the rep binding element (RBE), rep proteins, p5 promoter sequences, and the RBE of the human host AAVS1 sequence for targeted integration (Muzyczka and Berns, 2001). Since almost all vectors used today merely retain the AAV ITRs, efforts to understand the genome persistence of the rAAV vectors are underway. Studies show that after introduction and double strand conversion of rAAV that the DNA is converted from linear to circular, to high molecular weight concatamers, primarily in a head to tail sequence. However, it is interesting to note that experiments using split gene rAAV vectors in the same tissue, but separated by weeks, show that gene expression was reconstituted (Yue et al., 2003). This result is interpreted to mean that single stranded rAAV DNA is not necessary for concatamerization. It appears that intermediates of double stranded linear, circular or concatameric rAAV can interact to form junctions. Current thinking suggests that the episomal rAAV vectors exist in a balance between linear and circular forms, with the circular form dominant (McCarty et al., 2004).

While current research demonstrates that the status of rAAV DNA within cells is predominantly in the episomal form, it is still possible to detect a low frequency of integration in vitro and in vivo. Such integrants would be of concern due to the possibility of an insertion causing a gain or loss of function, and the possibility of oncogenesis. It is unclear from current studies what "low frequency" actually is, because in vitro studies do not accurately represent the quiescent nature of most animal tissues, and in vivo experiments have been difficult to quantify. When analyzing integration, it is possible to examine rAAV junctions with cellular DNA in an attempt to understand the environment of integration. An analysis of current experiments by McCarty et al. suggest that rAAV can be found integrated in actively transcribed regions introduced through non-homologous recombination of ITR and broken chromosome ends, integrated essentially as a "bystander" DNA fragment. Furthermore, rAAV can also integrate into sites of pre-existing chromosomal breaks, leading one to ponder if rearrangements at the site are the product of rAAV integration or from the inaccurate repair of the pre-existing break. It is important to understand that DNA introduced by any means can carry with it the risk of insertional mutagenesis. It is unclear if the "bystander effect" of rAAV integration during repair of these active regions could cause significantly more chromosomal abnormalities than already take place during this process. In this regard, and most importantly, there has been no known association of either wild type or recombinant AAV with malignancies of humans or animals (McCarty et al., 2004).

3.2 Targeting Cell Types in the Retina with rAAV

At the advent of retinal rAAV gene therapy it was common practice to introduce transgenes using ubiquitous promoters such that if a cell type was susceptible to infection it usually expressed the transgene. A popular ubiquitous promoter in early, and current, gene therapy studies is the human cytomegalovirus immediate early promoter/enhancer (CMV). However, one of the drawbacks of this promoter is that it can be subject silencing due to methylation. As an improvement a hybrid of this promoter was created using the CMV enhancer with the chicken β-actin promoter, which does not appear to be subject to silencing. While ubiquitous promoters are a huge benefit in identifying rAAV tropism whether in the retina or elsewhere, it may not be desirable to express a therapeutic transgene in all cell types that take up the rAAV, rather only a subset of cell types. To that end, cell type specific promoters are being evaluated.

Studies evaluating the use of retinal cell type specific promoters have demonstrated the ability to restrict expression to photoreceptors and RPE cells. A version of the proximal mouse rod opsin promoter (−386/+85) was the first to be tested in rAAV2/2 in the retina, and when injected subretinally was sufficient to restrict expression of reporter genes to the photoreceptors (Flannery et al., 1997). Our current, more careful analysis of photoreceptor cell types transduced by a rod opsin promoter-containing vector show that in both mice and rats, although there is a clear preference for rod photoreceptors, there is incomplete subtype-specificity in vivo with transduction of some cones as well (Glushakova and Hauswirth, unpublished). Other studies demonstrated that portions of the human blue cone opsin proximal promoter (−569) predominately targeted cones (Glushakova et al., 2006), and the relative transduction efficiency of AAV5 vector with this promoter driving GFP is 1500:34:1 for S-cones vs. M-cones vs. rods, respectively.

Sections of both the VMD2 (Esumi et al., 2004) and RPE65 (Boulanger et al., 2000) promoters can confine expression of reporter genes to the RPE. The RPE plays a pivotal role in the development and function of the retinal photoreceptors, and, not surprisingly, mutations in RPE genes are the cause of a variety of retinal degenerations. Therefore the RPE-specific expression of the therapeutic genes to restore normal RPE function is an important gene therapy aim. Two well studied RPE specific genes whose mutations cause severe vision defects are VMD2, the bestrophin gene which is responsible for Best's Disease (Sun et al., 2002), and RPE65, which is responsible for one form of LCA (Gu et al., 1997;

Marlhens et al., 1997). Transgenic mouse studies with several VMD2 promoter regions revealed that a −253/+38 bp fragment is minimally sufficient to direct RPE-specific expression in vivo (Esumi et al., 2004). The rodent and human RPE65 genes share several cis-acting elements, an octamer sequence, a nuclear factor one site, and two E-box sites, suggesting a conserved mode of regulation. In transgenic mice the 655/+52 bp fragment of the RPE65 promoter was sufficient to direct high RPE-specific expression, whereas shorter fragments (−297/+52 bp and −188/+52 bp) generated only background activity (Boulanger et al., 2000). Candidate 5'-upstream regions of the human VMD2 and RPE65 genes were tested in AAV1 vectors for their ability to target RPE-specific expression (Glushakova and Hauswirth, unpublished). Both the 585/+38 bp VMD2 promoter and the 814 bp proximal RPE65 promoter in AAV1 limited expression of GFP almost exclusively to the RPE with only an occasional photoreceptor cell also GFP-positive. Thus, there appear to be two current promoter options for targeting RPE expression, the VMD2 and RPE65 promoters. In each case, in combination with AAV serotype 1 vectors, a high level of cell specificity is possible.

Hence the aforementioned studies suggest that promoter targeting coupled with differing AAV serotypes could prove to be a powerful tool for restricting expression of transgenes to specific tissues within the retina.

4 Summary

Recombinant adeno-associated viral vectors have slowly been moving to the forefront of gene therapy experiments. Given the non-pathogenic nature, low immunogenicity, ease of delivery, persistence, and targeting possibilities of rAAV, it is poised to become a major player in retinal gene therapy.

Acknowledgments The authors thank Richard Condit and Lauren Alexander for critically reading the manuscript and for their comments.

Authors' Note Due to page limitations imposed by the publisher, a complete set of references is not included in this review. Upon request to the authors a fully referenced review is available.

References

Acland, G.M., Aguirre, G.D., Bennett, J., Aleman, T.S., Cideciyan, A.V., Bennicelli, J. et al. 2005, Long-term restoration of rod and cone vision by single dose rAAV-mediated gene transfer to the retina in a canine model of childhood blindness. *Mol. Ther.* **12:** 1072–1082.

Acland, G.M., Aguirre, G.D., Ray, J., Zhang, Q., Aleman, T.S., Cideciyan, A.V. et al. 2001, Gene therapy restores vision in a canine model of childhood blindness. *Nat. Genet.* **28:** 92–95.

Atchison, R.W., Casto, B.C., and Hammon, W.M. 1965, Adenovirus-associated defective virus particles. *Science* **149:** 754–756.

Auricchio, A., Kobinger, G., Anand, V., Hildinger, M., O'Connor, E., Maguire, A.M. et al. 2001, Exchange of surface proteins impacts on viral vector cellular specificity and transduction characteristics: the retina as a model. *Hum. Mol. Genet.* **10**: 3075–3081.

Bantel-Schaal, U. and zur Hausen, H. 1984, Characterization of the DNA of a defective human parvovirus isolated from a genital site. *Virology* **134**: 52–63.

Berns, K.I. and Giraud, C. 1996, Biology of adeno-associated virus. *Curr. Top. Microbiol. Immunol.* **218**: 1–23.

Boulanger, A., Liu, S., Henningsgaard, A.A., Yu,S., and Redmond, T.M. 2000, The upstream region of the Rpe65 gene confers retinal pigment epithelium-specific expression in vivo and in vitro and contains critical octamer and E-box binding sites. *J. Biol. Chem.* **275**: 31274–31282.

Caspi, R.R. 2006, Ocular autoimmunity: the price of privilege? *Immunol. Rev.* **213**: 23–35.

Choi, V.W., McCarty, D.M., and Samulski, R.J. 2005, AAV hybrid serotypes: improved vectors for gene delivery. *Curr. Gene Ther.* **5**: 299–310.

Deng, W.T., Yan, Z., Dinculescu, A., Pang, J., Teusner, J.T., Cortez, N.G. et al. 2005, Adeno-associated virus-mediated expression of vascular endothelial growth factor peptides inhibits retinal neovascularization in a mouse model of oxygen-induced retinopathy. *Hum. Gene Ther.* **16**: 1247–1254.

Dinculescu, A., Glushakova, L., Min, S.H., and Hauswirth, W.W. 2005, Adeno-associated virus-vectored gene therapy for retinal disease. *Hum. Gene Ther.* **16**: 649–663.

Esumi, N., Oshima, Y., Li,Y., Campochiaro, P.A., and Zack, D.J. 2004, Analysis of the VMD2 promoter and implication of E-box binding factors in its regulation. *J. Biol. Chem.* **279**: 19064–19073.

Flannery, J.G., Zolotukhin, S., Vaquero, M.I., LaVail, M.M., Muzyczka, N., and Hauswirth, W.W. 1997, Efficient photoreceptor-targeted gene expression in vivo by recombinant adeno-associated virus. *Proc. Natl. Acad. Sci. U. S. A.* **94**: 6916–6921.

Glushakova, L.G., Timmers, A.M., Pang, J., Teusner, J.T., and Hauswirth, W.W. 2006, Human blue-opsin promoter preferentially targets reporter gene expression to rat s-cone photoreceptors. *Invest Ophthalmol. Vis. Sci.* **47**: 3505–3513.

Gorbatyuk, M., Justilien, V., Liu, J., Hauswirth, W.W., and Lewin, A.S. 2007, Preservation of photoreceptor morphology and function in P23H rats using an allele independent ribozyme. *Exp. Eye Res.* **84**: 44–52.

Gu, S.M., Thompson, D.A., Srikumari, C.R., Lorenz, B., Finckh, U., Nicoletti, A. et al. 1997, Mutations in RPE65 cause autosomal recessive childhood-onset severe retinal dystrophy. *Nat. Genet.* **17**: 194–197.

Guy, J., Qi,X., Muzyczka, N., and Hauswirth, W.W. 1999, Reporter expression persists 1 year after adeno-associated virus-mediated gene transfer to the optic nerve. *Arch. Ophthalmol.* **117**: 929–937.

Hauswirth, W.W. and Berns, K.I. 1977, Origin and termination of adeno-associated virus DNA replication. *Virology* **78**: 488–499.

Hermonat, P.L. and Muzyczka, N. 1984, Use of adeno-associated virus as a mammalian DNA cloning vector: transduction of neomycin resistance into mammalian tissue culture cells. *Proc. Natl. Acad. Sci. U. S. A.* **81**: 6466–6470.

Huttner, N.A., Girod, A., Perabo, L., Edbauer, D., Kleinschmidt, J.A., Buning, H., and Hallek, M. 2003, Genetic modifications of the adeno-associated virus type 2 capsid reduce the affinity and the neutralizing effects of human serum antibodies. *Gene Ther.* **10**: 2139–2147.

Jacobson, S.G., Acland, G.M., Aguirre, G.D., Aleman, T.S., Schwartz, S.B., Cideciyan, A.V. et al. 2006a, Safety of recombinant adeno-associated virus type 2-RPE65 vector delivered by ocular subretinal injection. *Mol. Ther.* **13**: 1074–1084.

Jacobson, S.G., Boye, S.L., Aleman, T.S., Conlon, T.J., Zeiss, C.J., Roman, A.J. et al. 2006b, Safety in nonhuman primates of ocular AAV2-RPE65, a candidate treatment for blindness in Leber congenital amaurosis. *Hum. Gene Ther.* **17**: 845–858.

Kiang, A.S., Palfi, A., Ader, M., Kenna, P.F., Millington-Ward, S., Clark, G. et al. 2005, Toward a gene therapy for dominant disease: validation of an RNA interference-based mutation-independent approach. *Mol. Ther.* **12**: 555–561.

Marlhens, F., Bareil, C., Griffoin, J.M., Zrenner, E., Amalric, P., Eliaou, C. et al. 1997, Mutations in RPE65 cause Leber's congenital amaurosis. *Nat. Genet.* **17:** 139–141.

McCarty, D.M., Young, S.M., Jr., and Samulski, R.J. 2004, Integration of adeno-associated virus (AAV) and recombinant AAV vectors. *Annu. Rev. Genet.* **38:** 819–845.

Min, S.H., Molday, L.L., Seeliger, M.W., Dinculescu, A., Timmers, A.M., Janssen, A. et al. 2005, Prolonged recovery of retinal structure/function after gene therapy in an Rs1h-deficient mouse model of x-linked juvenile retinoschisis. *Mol. Ther.* **12:** 644–651.

Muzyczka, N. and Berns, K.I. 2001, Chapter 69, *Fields Virology*. Lippincott Williams & Wilkins.

Rolling, F. 2004, Recombinant AAV-mediated gene transfer to the retina: gene therapy perspectives. *Gene Ther.* **11** Suppl 1: S26–S32.

Sun, H., Tsunenari, T., Yau, K.W., and Nathans, J. 2002, The vitelliform macular dystrophy protein defines a new family of chloride channels. *Proc. Natl. Acad. Sci. U. S. A.* **99:** 4008–4013.

Warrington, K.H., Jr. and Herzog, R.W. 2006, Treatment of human disease by adeno-associated viral gene transfer. *Hum. Genet.* **119:** 571–603.

Wu, Z., Asokan, A., and Samulski, R.J. 2006, Adeno-associated virus serotypes: vector toolkit for human gene therapy. *Mol. Ther.* **14:** 316–327.

Yue, Y. and Duan, D. 2003, Double strand interaction is the predominant pathway for intermolecular recombination of adeno-associated viral genomes. *Virology* **313:** 1–7.

Genetic Supplementation of RDS Alleviates a Loss-of-function Phenotype in C214S Model of Retinitis Pigmentosa

May Nour, Steven J. Fliesler, and Muna I. Naash

1 Introduction

Mutations in the photoreceptor-specific protein, Rds, have been associated with a large number of inherited retinal degenerative diseases. Reports have described the incidence of retinitis pigmentosa, cone-rod dystrophy, diffuse retinal dystrophy, macular degeneration, and central areolar choroidal dystrophy in patients carrying mutations in the RDS gene (Dryja, Hahn, Kajiwara, & Berson, 1997; Ekstrom et al., 1998; Fishman et al., 1997; Fossarello et al., 1996; Jacobson, Cideciyan, Kemp, Sheffield, & Stone, 1996; Nakazawa, Wada, Chida, & Tamai, 1997; Sears, Aaberg, Daiger, & Moshfeghi, 2001; Zhang, Garibaldi, Li, Green, & Zack, 2002). As a membrane glycoprotein located in the disc rim region in the OSs of rods and cones (Connell & Molday, 1990; Molday, Hicks, & Molday, 1987; Travis, Brennan, Danielson, Kozak, & Sutcliffe, 1989), Rds is thought to be necessary for disc assembly, maintenance and renewal (Boesze-Battaglia & Goldberg, 2002; Molday et al., 1987; Wrigley, Ahmed, Nevett, & Findlay, 2000). While current beliefs propose Rds to serve a primarily structural role in OSs, alterations in Rds have strong functional as well as structural implications since this is the region where phototransduction occurs (Ridge, Abdulaev, Sousa, & Palczewski, 2003). Complete absence of the protein in the retinal degeneration slow (rds) mouse (van Nie, Ivanyi, & Demant, 1978) results in a failure of OS formation, an absence of retinal function, and the progression of photoreceptor degeneration (Cohen, 1983; Jansen & Sanyal, 1984; Sanyal, De Ruiter, & Hawkins, 1980; Sanyal & Jansen, 1981). A phenotype of haploinsufficiency has also been reported to associate with the under-expression of Rds (in *rds+/−* animals) and is characterized by malformed and swirl-like OSs, and an early-onset of slow rod degeneration followed by a late-onset and slow cone degeneration (Cheng et al., 1997; Nour, Ding, Stricker, Fliesler, &

M.I. Naash

Cell Biology, University of Oklahoma Health Sciences Center, 940 Stanton L. Young Blvd., Oklahoma City, OK 73104. Steven J. Fliesler, Ophthalmology and Pharmacological & Physiological Science, Saint Louis University School of Medicine, St. Louis, MO, 63104, USA,
Tel: 405-271-2388, Fax: 405-271-3548
e-mail: muna-naash@ouhsc.edu

R.E. Anderson et al. (eds.), *Recent Advances in Retinal Degeneration*,
© Springer 2008

Naash, 2004). In addition to the rds null mutant (Ali et al., 2000; Sarra et al., 2001; Schlichtenbrede et al., 2003), two transgenic mouse models have been generated (Kedzierski, Lloyd, Birch, Bok, & Travis, 1997; Kedzierski et al., 2001), one of which, P216L, has been used to evaluate therapeutic interventions for the treatment of Rds-associated retinal disease (Bok et al., 2002; Liang et al., 2001). However, to date no study has reported both significant functional and structural rescue in any animal model carrying point mutations in the rds gene. In this study, we assessed the feasibility of Rds supplementation to resolve rod defect associated with expression of the C214S mutant of Rds. The C214S mutation causes a loss-of-function defect which primarily affects rods in humans and mice (Saga et al., 1993; Stricker, Ding, Quiambao, Fliesler, & Naash, 2005). To reduce the effect of the mutant protein by competing it out with the wild-type (WT) protein, we generated a transgenic line expressing the WT Rds in both rods and cones driven by the human interphotoreceptor retinoid binding protein (hIRBP) promoter (Nour et al., 2004). A single residue change at the C-terminus was incorporated in the WT transgene to mimic the human sequence that would facilitate specific recognition of the transgene product (Nour et al., 2004). This change is proline to glutamine at position 341 (P341Q), and here the line is named NMP for normal mouse peripherin/*rds*. Structural and functional studies on NMP retinas demonstrated the benign effect of the P341Q modification (Nour et al., 2004). Uniform expression of Rds in rods and cones was achieved by crossing C214S mice with NMP mice. By studying the structure of the double transgenic retinas by histology and the function by electroretinography, we have shown that genetic supplementation of WT Rds is a viable option for loss-of-function mutations in the RDS. As proof-of-principle, this finding provides a basis for the development of future therapeutic approaches. The following represents original material, not previously published or under consideration for publication elsewhere.

2 Materials and Methods

2.1 Generation of Transgenic Mice

The WT Rds with the proline to glutamine substitution has been previously studied in transgenic mice (Nour et al., 2004), where the substitution, used for the specific recognition of the protein by mAb 3B6, caused no aberrant affects on transgenic protein expression or function. Because P341Q seems harmless to Rds structure and function, the C214S transgenic construct used in this study contained this modification. Expression of all constructed transgenes (NMP and C214S) was directed to rods and cones by a 1.3 kb fragment of the human interphotoreceptor retinoid binding protein (hIRBP) promoter. Transgenic mice were identified by polymerase chain reaction (PCR) primers specific to the hIRBP promoter (Forward: 5'-CAGTGTCTGGCATGTAGCAGG) and the coding region of RDS cDNA (Reverse: 5'-GGCTTCCACTTGGCGTACTTG). Transgene product at the protein level generated from one allele of the NMP on the $rds^{-/-}$ background corresponded to 30% of the WT Rds while the C214S transgene showed a transcript level comparable to WT Rds with a trace amount of the mutant protein detected by Western blot analysis (Stricker et al., 2005). Transgenic lines show a rod dominant-defect in C214S (Stricker et al., 2005) while no alteration in retinal phenotype or structure was observed in mice over-expressing Rds (NMP on WT background) (Nour et al., 2004). Both transgenic mouse lines on C57BL/6 genetic backgrounds were crossed to generate single (C214S) and double (C214S/NMP) transgenics on an $rds+/-$ background. Mice were screened for the presence of the RDS mutation as previously described (Cheng et al., 1997).

Animals were maintained under cyclic-light conditions (12 hours dark, 12 hours light, at 20 lux). All experiments were approved by the local Institutional Animal Care and Use Committees and conformed to the National Institutes of Health's *Guide for the Care and Use of Laboratory Animals* and the *ARVO Statement for the Use of Animals in Ophthalmic and Vision Research.*

2.2 Rod and Cone Electroretinography (ERG)

ERG testing was carried out as previously described (Nour, Quiambao, Peterson, Al-Ubaidi, & Naash, 2003). Briefly, for the assessment of rod photoreceptor function, a strobe flash stimulus was presented to the dark-adapted, dilated eyes in a Nicolet ganzfeld (GS-2000) with a 137 cd (sec/m^2) flash intensity. The dark-adapted a-wave amplitude was measured from pre-stimulus baseline to the a-wave trough and the b-wave amplitude measured from the a-wave trough to the b-wave peak. For the evaluation of cone function, a strobe flash stimulus was presented to 5-minute light-adapted, dilated eyes in a Nicolet ganzfeld (GS-2000) with a 77 cd (sec/m^2) flash intensity. The amplitude of the cone b-wave was measured from the trough of the a-wave to the peak of the b-wave. Analysis of variance (ANOVA) and post-hoc statistical tests using Bonferroni's pairwise comparisons were used to determine the significance of differences in ERG responses (GraphPad Prism 3.02, San Diego, CA, USA).

2.3 Electron and Light Microscopy

Enucleated eyes were fixed, processed for embedment in plastic resin, and sectioned as previously described (Ding et al., 2004; Tan et al., 2001). For light microscopy, sections (0.75-μm thickness, stained with 1% Toluidine Blue) were photographed with an Olympus BH-2 photomicroscope (auto-expose mode) using 20X or 60X (oil immersion) DPlanApo objectives. For electron microscopy, ultra-thin (silver-gold) sections were post-stained with lead citrate and uranyl acetate on-grid, and viewed with a JEOL JEM-1200EX electron microscope at an accelerating voltage of 80 KeV.

2.4 Western Blot Analysis

Rabbit polyclonal antibody against residues 331–346 of murine Rds C-terminus was used for detection of Rds as described previously (Ding et al., 2004). Anti-actin antibody (1:250 dilution) (Sigma-Aldrich, St. Louis, MO, USA), was used to control for sample loading. Retinal protein extraction and blot analysis were carried out as previously described (Ding et al., 2004; Li, Ding, O'Brien, Al-Ubaidi, & Naash, 2003).

3 Results

3.1 Functional Rescue of the C214S Mutation in Rds

In order to test the ability of Rds supplementation to resolve retinal degeneration associated with expression of the C214S mutation in Rds, C214S transgenics were crossed to transgenic mice expressing NMP in both rods and cones. Single (C214S) and double transgenic (C214S/NMP) mice, heterozygous for both transgenes, were generated onto an $rds^{+/-}$ genetic background. The $C214S^{+/-}/rds^{+/-}$ genotype mimics the situation in patients, where one correct allele of RDS is accompanied by one mutated allele (Stricker et al., 2005; Saga et al., 1993). The C214S mutation in mice renders a small amount of protein present in retinas, although an abundant amount of mutant RDS mRNA is detected (Stricker et al., 2005).

The cumulative data indicate that retinas of C214S transgenic mice display a loss-of-function defect similar to haploinsufficiency phenotype seen in $rds^{+/-}$ mice as well as retinitis pigmentosa patients carrying the C214S mutation (Stricker et al., 2005; Saga et al., 1993). Representative rod ERG waves demonstrate remarkable restoration in rod function afforded by the supplementation of Rds in double transgenic ($C214S^{+/-}/NMP^{+/-}/rds^{+/-}$) when compared to single transgenic ($C214S^{+/-}/rds^{+/-}$) mice (Fig. 1 A). As early as 1 month of age, $C214S^{+/-}/rds^{+/-}$ mice exhibit a reduction in rod a-wave amplitudes (Fig. 1 A & B). This reduction is comparable to the diminished rod photoreceptor function observed in non-transgenic $rds^{+/-}$ controls (Fig. 1 B). In sharp contrast to the reduced rod photoreceptor response generated by $C214S^{+/-}/rds^{+/-}$ single transgenics, $C214S^{+/-}/NMP^{+/-}/rds^{+/-}$ double transgenic mice showed a statistically significant ($P < 0.001$) improvement in rod a-wave amplitudes at one month and 3 months of age (Fig. 1 B & C).

Interestingly, this functional improvement continued up to 9 months of age, the latest time point tested (Fig. 2D). In terms of cone function, at early ages, haploinsufficiency in Rds has no deleterious impact as shown by $rds^{+/-}$ and $C214S^{+/-}/rds^{+/-}$ responses (Fig. 1A & B). The increased expression of WT Rds in double transgenics ($C214S^{+/-}/NMP^{+/-}/rds^{+/-}$) caused no adverse effects on cone photoreceptor function (Fig. 1A & B). A comparable decline in cone function between single transgenic ($C214S^{+/-}/rds^{+/-}$) and $rds^{+/-}$ mice was

Fig. 1 Rod and cone ERG analysis in C214S transgenics. (A) Representative rod and cone ERG wave forms at 1 month of age (1 mo) show a rescue in rod function in double transgenic $(C214S^{+/-}/NMP^{+/-}/rds^{+/-})$ when compared to single transgenic $(C214S^{+/-}/rds^{+/-})$ mice. No differences are seen in cone wave response. (B) Rod a-wave and cone b-wave averages at 1 month demonstrate a statistically significant $(P<0.001)$ rescue in rod function in double $(C214S^{+/-}/NMP^{+/-}/rds^{+/-})$, compared to single $(C214S^{+/-}/rds^{+/-})$ transgenic mice. At this age, all mice tested generate WT levels of cone ERG response. (C) The statistically significant $(P<0.001)$ improvement in rod function resulting from Rds supplementation in C214S transgenics $(C214S^{+/-}/NMP^{+/-}/rds^{+/-})$ persists even at three 3 months of age (3 mo)

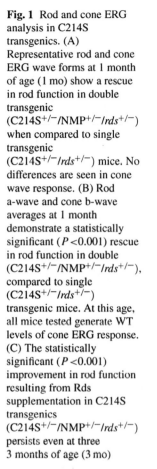

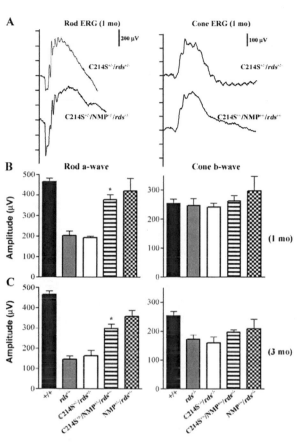

observed at 3 and 9 months of age (Fig. 1 C & Fig. 2). Although double transgenics $(C214S^{+/-}/NMP^{+/-}/rds^{+/-})$ showed slight protection from this age-related decline in cone function (Fig. 1C & Fig. 2, right graph), this level of cone rescue is not statistically significant when compared to WT. $NMP^{+/-}/rds^{+/-}$ controls generated rod and cone ERG responses correlated with total Rds levels (Fig. 1B & C).

3.2 Histological Rescue of the C214S Mutation in Rds

A reduction in Rds level has been shown to cause a disruption in OS alignment and integrity (Cheng et al., 1997; Nour et al., 2004). This haploinsufficiency phenotype has also been seen in $C214S^{+/-}/rds^{+/-}$ retinas at 1 month of age with shorter OSs detected at the light microscopy (Fig. 3A), and typical swirl-like OSs seen at the electron microscopy (Fig. 3B). Genetic supplementation of Rds in $C214S^{+/-}/NMP^{+/-}/rds^{+/-}$ retinas results in a remarkable improvement in both OS

Fig. 2 Rod a-wave and cone b-wave averages at 9 months of age shows a long term rescue in double (C214S$^{+/-}$/NMP$^{+/-}$/rds$^{+/-}$) transgenic mice. ERG wave amplitudes for B and C represent an average of 12–16 eyes for each genotype, and ERG wave amplitudes for D represent 8 eyes for each genotype

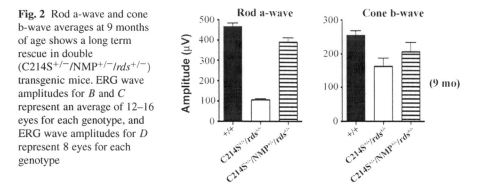

length (Fig. 3A) and integrity (Fig. 3B). This improvement in structural integrity (Fig. 3A & B) correlates with the increase in rod photoreceptor function afforded by the expression of the NMP transgene (Fig. 1A–C).

Under reducing conditions, Western blot analysis with a polyclonal antibody raised against the murine Rds-C-terminus [22] shows a decrease of Rds level in C214S$^{+/-}$/rds$^{+/-}$ retina relative to WT and confirms an increase of total Rds levels in C214S$^{+/-}$/NMP$^{+/-}$/rds$^{+/-}$ retina (Fig. 4). Dimers and higher order oligomers represent partially reduced samples. Actin was used as an internal control and showed comparable levels in all samples examined (Fig. 4).

Fig. 3 Retinal structure in C214S transgenics. (A) Histological evaluation (light microscopy) at 1 month of age reveals an improvement in OS length in C214S$^{+/-}$/NMP$^{+/-}$/rds$^{+/-}$ when compared to C214S$^{+/-}$/rds$^{+/-}$ retinas.(B) Electron microscopy shows amelioration of defects in the alignment and integrity of photoreceptor OSs in double transgenic retinas (C214S$^{+/-}$/NMP$^{+/-}$/rds$^{+/-}$). All tissue sections were evaluated from the superior central region of the retina. Scale bar, 4 μm, (RPE: retinal pigment epithelium; OS: outer segment; IS: inner segment; ONL: outer nuclear layer)

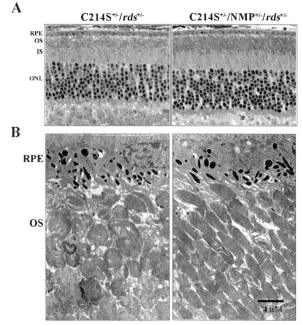

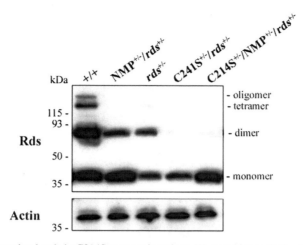

Fig. 4 Rds expression levels in C214S transgenic retinas. Western blot analysis reacted with polyclonal antibody against the murine Rds-C-terminus demonstrates the increase in Rds protein levels in C214S$^{+/-}$/NMP$^{+/-}$/rds$^{+/-}$ relative to C214S$^{+/-}$/rds$^{+/-}$ retinas. Actin immunoblotting shows equal loading in examined samples

4 Discussion

The design of widely applicable therapeutic interventions for Rds-associated retinal diseases has been hindered by multiple factors. These factors include the large number of variable point mutations, the diversity in severity and patterns of disease expression, and the haploinsufficiency phenotype, which dictates a well-regulated level of Rds required for OS morphogenesis. Since over-expression of Rds in the retina is well-tolerated (Nour et al., 2004), gene transfer (or Rds supplementation) logically presents itself as a viable option for resolving defects associated with loss-of-function mutations. However, therapeutic strategies for gain-of-function, dominant mutations have been complicated by the fact that elimination of the mutant protein requires simultaneous transfer of WT Rds in order to prevent haploinsufficiency-related defects. In this study, we provide the first experimental evidence that supports the use of supplementation or gene transfer strategy as a short term and generalized approach for prospective treatment of loss-of-function mutations in Rds. Furthermore, we provide evidence of long-term rescue of photoreceptor structure and function with loss-of-function mutation that is achieved by genetic supplementation of WT Rds.

Patients carrying the C214S mutation in Rds present with retinitis pigmentosa, a rod-dominant functional defect (Saga et al., 1993). In the mouse model, the haploinsufficiency-like phenotype caused by the C214S (loss-of-function) mutation also results in a reduction in rod ERG function stemming from an abnormality in OS structure formation (Stricker et al., 2005). We show that expression of Rds in double transgenics (C214S$^{+/-}$/NMP$^{+/-}$/rds$^{+/-}$) results in long-term resolution of rod functional defects as well as restoration of OS ultrastructural organization.

The replacement of Rds in mice has been demonstrated by two other labs with limited success. First, the Rds transgene expressed exclusively in rods (Opsin-rds) was able to rescue the structure of the *rds* null retina, but only if the transgene was expressed at high levels (Travis, Groshan, Lloyd, & Bok, 1992). This study did not assess any functional rescue of rods afforded by the transgene, nor did the study allow for the investigation of cone structure or function. However, the Opsin-rds transgene established that more than 50% of a WT gene dosage is needed for optimal OS formation. Second, the use of an adeno-associated virus vector containing a rds construct driven by the rhodopsin promoter (AAV-Opsin-rds) was capable of developing tiny rod OS structures and a trace of rod function in cells expressing the viral vector (Ali et al., 2000). Furthermore, the AAV method of delivery (subretinal injection) was not sufficient for expression throughout the entire retina (Sarra et al., 2001). The authors suggest that the unequal distribution of the Rds supplementation coupled with possible apoptotic signals from the untreated cells may have lead to the continued degeneration seen in their treated models. When looking at WT retinas treated with the AAV-Opsin-rds, the authors noted marked photoreceptor loss that was attributed to the delivery procedure, Rds over-expression, or the viral vector (Sarra et al., 2001). In our recent studies involving genetic supplementation in transgenic mice, we did not find over-expression of Rds to be deleterious (Nour et al., 2004), suggesting that the method of delivery of the gene product is crucial. Several therapeutic delivery systems will need to be tested in order to establish optimal expression of the RDS replacement gene as well as minimize possible damaging effects caused by the delivery. The future of gene therapy for the retina is promising with the development of new expression systems such as nanoparticles. When taken together our data provide proof-of-principle for genetic supplementation as a promising treatment for both loss-of-function mutations in Rds. Our use of transgene supplementation is widely applicable and simplifies strategies for therapeutic intervention by providing the fundamental basis for virally- or otherwise-mediated transfer of Rds to the diseased retina.

Acknowledgments The authors thank Barbara Nagel for her technical assistance and Dr. Muayyad R. Al-Ubaidi for his helpful comments on the manuscript. Funding: NEI EY10609 & EY016201 (MIN), EY007361 (SJF), and Core Grant for Vision Research (EY12190); Foundation Fighting Blindness (MIN); an unrestricted departmental grant from Research to Prevent Blindness (SJF); the Norman J. Stupp Charitable Trust (SJF); and the Oklahoma Center for the Advancement of Science and Technology (OCAST) (MIN).

References

Ali, R. R., Sarra, G. M., Stephens, C., Alwis, M. D., Bainbridge, J. W., Munro, P. M., et al., 2000, Restoration of photoreceptor ultrastructure and function in retinal degeneration slow mice by gene therapy. *Nat Genet, 25,* 306–310.

Boesze-Battaglia, K., & Goldberg, A. F., 2002, Photoreceptor renewal: a role for peripherin/rds. *Int Rev Cytol, 217,* 183–225.

Bok, D., Yasumura, D., Matthes, M. T., Ruiz, A., Duncan, J. L., Chappelow, A. V., et al., 2002, Effects of adeno-associated virus-vectored ciliary neurotrophic factor on retinal structure and function in mice with a P216L rds/peripherin mutation. *Exp Eye Res, 74*(6), 719–735.

Cheng, T., Peachey, N. S., Li, S., Goto, Y., Cao, Y., & Naash, M. I., 1997, The effect of peripherin/rds haploinsufficiency on rod and cone photoreceptors. *J Neurosci, 17*, 8118–8128.

Cohen, A. I., 1983, Some cytological and initial biochemical observations on photoreceptors in retinas of rds mice. *Invest Ophthalmol Vis Sci, 24*, 832–843.

Connell, G. J., & Molday, R. S., 1990, Molecular cloning, primary structure, and orientation of the vertebrate photoreceptor cell protein peripherin in the rod outer segment disk membrane. *Biochemistry, 29*, 4691–4698.

Ding, X. Q., Nour, M., Ritter, L. M., Goldberg, A. F., Fliesler, S. J., & Naash, M. I., 2004, The R172W mutation in peripherin/rds causes a cone-rod dystrophy in transgenic mice. *Hum Mol Genet, 13*, 2075–2087.

Dryja, T. P., Hahn, L. B., Kajiwara, K., & Berson, E. L., 1997, Dominant and digenic mutations in the peripherin/RDS and ROM1 genes in retinitis pigmentosa. *Invest Ophthalmol Vis Sci, 38*, 1972–1982.

Ekstrom, U., Ponjavic, V., Abrahamson, M., Nilsson-Ehle, P., Andreasson, S., Stenstrom, I., et al., 1998, Phenotypic expression of autosomal dominant retinitis pigmentosa in a Swedish family expressing a Phe-211-Leu variant of peripherin/RDS. *Ophthalmic Genet, 19*, 27–37.

Fishman, G. A., Stone, E. M., Alexander, K. R., Gilbert, L. D., Derlacki, D. J., & Butler, N. S., 1997, Serine-27-phenylalanine mutation within the peripherin/RDS gene in a family with cone dystrophy. *Ophthalmology, 104*, 299–306.

Fossarello, M., Bertini, C., Galantuomo, M. S., Cao, A., Serra, A., & Pirastu, M., 1996, Deletion in the peripherin/RDS gene in two unrelated Sardinian families with autosomal dominant butterfly-shaped macular dystrophy. *Arch Ophthalmol, 114*, 448–456.

Jacobson, S. G., Cideciyan, A. V., Kemp, C. M., Sheffield, V. C., & Stone, E. M., 1996, Photoreceptor function in heterozygotes with insertion or deletion mutations in the RDS gene. *Invest Ophthalmol Vis Sci, 37*, 1662–1674.

Jansen, H. G., & Sanyal, S., 1984, Development and degeneration of retina in rds mutant mice: electron microscopy. *J Comp Neurol, 224*, 71–84.

Kedzierski, W., Lloyd, M., Birch, D. G., Bok, D., & Travis, G. H., 1997, Generation and analysis of transgenic mice expressing P216L-substituted rds/peripherin in rod photoreceptors. *Invest Ophthalmol Vis Sci, 38*, 498–509.

Kedzierski, W., Nusinowitz, S., Birch, D., Clarke, G., McInnes, R. R., Bok, D., et al., 2001, Deficiency of rds/peripherin causes photoreceptor death in mouse models of digenic and dominant retinitis pigmentosa. *Proc Natl Acad Sci U S A,98*, 7718–7723.

Li, C., Ding, X. Q., O'Brien, J., Al-Ubaidi, M. R., & Naash, M. I., 2003, Molecular characterization of the skate peripherin/rds gene: relationship to its orthologues and paralogues. *Invest Ophthalmol Vis Sci, 44*, 2433–2441.

Liang, F. Q., Aleman, T. S., Dejneka, N. S., Dudus, L., Fisher, K. J., Maguire, A. M., et al., 2001, Long-term protection of retinal structure but not function using RAAV.CNTF in animal models of retinitis pigmentosa. *Mol Ther, 4*, 461–472.

Molday, R. S., Hicks, D., & Molday, L., 1987, Peripherin. A rim-specific membrane protein of rod outer segment discs. *Invest Ophthalmol Vis Sci, 28*, 50–61.

Nakazawa, M., Wada, Y., Chida, Y., & Tamai, M., 1997, A correlation between computer-predicted changes in secondary structure and the phenotype of retinal degeneration associated with mutations in peripherin/RDS. *Curr Eye Res, 16*, 1134–1141.

Nour, M., Ding, X. Q., Stricker, H., Fliesler, S. J., & Naash, M. I., 2004, Modulating expression of peripherin/rds in transgenic mice: critical levels and the effect of overexpression. *Invest Ophthalmol Vis Sci, 45*, 2514–2521.

Nour, M., Quiambao, A. B., Peterson, W. M., Al-Ubaidi, M. R., & Naash, M. I., 2003, P2Y(2) receptor agonist INS37217 enhances functional recovery after detachment caused by subretinal injection in normal and rds mice. *Invest Ophthalmol Vis Sci, 44*, 4505–4514.

Ridge, K. D., Abdulaev, N. G., Sousa, M., & Palczewski, K., 2003, Phototransduction: crystal clear. *Trends Biochem Sci, 28*, 479–487.

Saga, M., Mashima, Y., Akeo, K., Oguchi, Y., Kudoh, J., & Shimizu, N., 1993, A novel Cys-214-Ser mutation in the peripherin/RDS gene in a Japanese family with autosomal dominant retinitis pigmentosa. *Hum Genet, 92*, 519–521.

Sanyal, S., De Ruiter, A., & Hawkins, R. K., 1980, Development and degeneration of retina in rds mutant mice: light microscopy. *J Comp Neurol, 194*, 193–207.

Sanyal, S., & Jansen, H. G., 1981, Absence of receptor outer segments in the retina of rds mutant mice. *Neurosci Lett, 21*, 23–26.

Sarra, G. M., Stephens, C., de Alwis, M., Bainbridge, J. W., Smith, A. J., Thrasher, A. J., et al., 2001, Gene replacement therapy in the retinal degeneration slow (rds) mouse: the effect on retinal degeneration following partial transduction of the retina. *Hum Mol Genet, 10*, 2353–2361.

Schlichtenbrede, F. C., MacNeil, A., Bainbridge, J. W., Tschernutter, M., Thrasher, A. J., Smith, A. J., et al., 2003, Intraocular gene delivery of ciliary neurotrophic factor results in significant loss of retinal function in normal mice and in the Prph2Rd2/Rd2 model of retinal degeneration. *Gene Ther, 10*, 523–527.

Sears, J. E., Aaberg, T. A., Sr., Daiger, S. P., & Moshfeghi, D. M., 2001, Splice site mutation in the peripherin/RDS gene associated with pattern dystrophy of the retina. *Am J Ophthalmol, 132*, 693–699.

Stricker, H. M., Ding, X. Q., Quiambao, A., Fliesler, S. J., & Naash, M. I., 2005, The Cys214->Ser mutation in peripherin/rds causes a loss-of-function phenotype in transgenic mice. *Biochem J, 388*, 605–613.

Tan, E., Wang, Q., Quiambao, A. B., Xu, X., Qtaishat, N. M., Peachey, N. S., et al., 2001, The relationship between opsin overexpression and photoreceptor degeneration. *Invest Ophthalmol Vis Sci, 42*, 589–600.

Travis, G. H., Brennan, M. B., Danielson, P. E., Kozak, C. A., & Sutcliffe, J. G., 1989, Identification of a photoreceptor-specific mRNA encoded by the gene responsible for retinal degeneration slow (rds). *Nature, 338*, 70–73.

Travis, G. H., Groshan, K. R., Lloyd, M., & Bok, D., 1992, Complete rescue of photoreceptor dysplasia and degeneration in transgenic retinal degeneration slow (rds) mice. *Neuron, 9*, 113–119.

van Nie, R., Ivanyi, D., & Demant, P., 1978, A new H-2-linked mutation, rds, causing retinal degeneration in the mouse. *Tissue Antigens, 12*, 106–108.

Wrigley, J. D., Ahmed, T., Nevett, C. L., & Findlay, J. B., 2000, Peripherin/rds influences membrane vesicle morphology. Implications for retinopathies. *J Biol Chem, 275*, 13191–13194.

Zhang, K., Garibaldi, D. C., Li, Y., Green, W. R., & Zack, D. J., 2002, Butterfly-shaped pattern dystrophy: a genetic, clinical, and histopathological report. *Arch Ophthalmol, 120*, 485–490.

Morphological Aspects Related to Long-term Functional Improvement of the Retina in the 4 Years Following rAAV-mediated Gene Transfer in the RPE65 Null Mutation Dog

Kristina Narfström, Mathias Seeliger, Chooi-May Lai, Vaegan, Martin Katz, Elizabeth P. Rakoczy, and Charlotte Remé

1 Introduction

Retinal gene transfer studies performed in our laboratories in groups of 4–42 month-old RPE65 null mutation dogs have shown remarkable functional improvement following a single unilateral subretinal injection of a recombinant adeno-associated virus vector, serotype 2, rAAV2/2, cDNA for dog RPE65 with a cytomegalo virus (CMV) promoter (Narfström et al., 2003a,b, 2005; Ford et al., 2003). The purpose of the present investigation was to further assess long-term therapeutic effects of the gene transfer performed in a group of young RPE65 null mutation dogs and to correlate the functional effects of therapy to morphologic findings up to 4 years following the gene transfer. In addition, retinas of affected dogs were examined for histologic correlates of spots and color changes seen by ophthalmoscopy in both treated and untreated affected dogs.

2 Materials and Methods

Gene transfer surgeries were performed during a 2-year period (2001–2002) in a subgroup of 4–11 month old dogs, derived from an initial pedigree of Swedish Briard-Beagle dogs. Details regarding the procedures and short- and long-term follow-up studies have been reported (Narfström et al., 2003a,b, 2005; Ford et al., 2003). Injections were performed using standard aseptic microsurgical procedures with a two-port entry into the pars plana of the eye, the first port for a light pipe and the second for a hand-drawn glass micropipette. In most cases 100 micro-liters of the rAAV.RPE65 construct was injected subretinally into the right eye and similar volumes of the rAAV.GFP construct into the left eye.

K. Narfström
Department of Veterinary Medicine and Surgery, College of Veterinary Medicine and Department of Ophthalmology, Mason Eye Institute, University of Missouri-Columbia, Columbia, MO, USA, Tel: 573-882-2095, Fax: 573-884-5444
e-mail: narfstromk@missouri.edu

R.E. Anderson et al. (eds.), *Recent Advances in Retinal Degeneration*,
© Springer 2008

Post-operative studies included clinical ophthalmic, behavioural and ERG studies in all treated dogs as previously described (Narfström et al., 2003a). Four affected dogs that had undergone gene transfer were used for angiographic studies 2 years following the gene transfer, using indocyanine green (ICG) and fluorescein (FL) (Seeliger et al., 2006). For this, dogs were anesthetized with Medetomidine and Ketamine, pupils were dilated with 1% Isopto-Atropin, and 2 and 4 ml of ICG and FL, respectively, were injected into the cephalic vein. A Heidelberg SLO was used for fundus visualization and photography throughout the angiography procedure. At variable time periods the 4 affected treated dogs and 2 untreated affected dogs were euthanized and both eyes fixed for light- and electron microscopy. The eyecups were immersion fixed in fresh, cold 2.5% glutaraldehyde in 0.1 M cacodylate buffer. Eyecups were prepared and sectioned using standardized methods for our lab (Narfström et al., 2003a). Plastic sections from three sets of eyes; from two affected dogs, treated 0.8 and 2.5 years previously, and from one affected dog that was not treated were used for light microscopic studies, including morphometric studies performed at the Lions Eye Institute, University of Western Australia. Sections from three sets of eyes; from two affected dogs, treated 3.7 and 4 years previously, and from one dog that was not treated, were sent to the Department of Ophthalmology, University of Zurich, for electron microscopy. For the morphometric studies lipid granules per 80 microns of retina were counted as well as rows of photoreceptor nuclei in 3 serial sections obtained from the following: at the injection site, in the treated area adjacent to the injection site, and in the peripheral area of the fundus. Sections were obtained from similar locations from both eyes. For the ultrastructural studies the treated and untreated eyes were compared, through examination of 12 regions from comparable areas of each eye.

3 Results

ERG responses improved within 4–6 weeks after surgery in all treated dogs. Improved ERG responses were observed throughout the 4-year follow-up period (data not shown). Following the early enhancement of ERG amplitudes, there were successive declines mainly of scotopic low light intensity (rod) responses during the follow-up period, while scotopic high intensity (mixed rod and cone responses) and photopic single flash (cone) responses, as well as 30 Hz flicker responses (cone and inner retinal function) remained better preserved. At termination of the study the ERG responses were still improved (Fig. 1) in comparison to pre-operative responses; barely recordable for both eyes.

Figure 2 shows an example of angiography performed in one of the long-term studied affected treated dogs. A normal vascular pattern was observed in the fundus without leakage from the retinal vasculature. At the injection site, however, marked changes were seen, changes that could not be readily visualized by regular ophthalmoscopy (Fig. 2A). ICG showed a circular area of hypofluorescence (Fig. 2B), while FL showed hyperfluorescence in the same area (Fig. 2C).

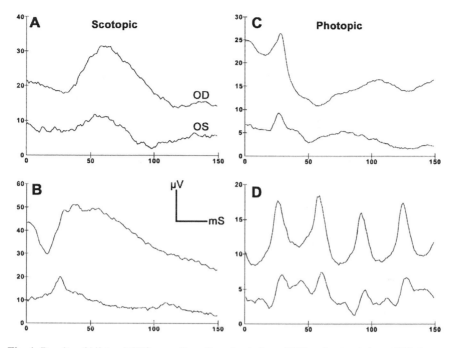

Fig. 1 Results of bilateral ERG recordings from treated eye (OD) and untreated eye (OS) 4 years after subretinal gene transfer in an RPE65 null mutation dog treated at age 11 months. Scotopic recordings were performed after 2 hours of dark adaptation using -2.0 log cd.s/m^2 (A) and 0.6 log cd.s/m^2 (B), respectively, of white light stimuli. After 10 minutes of light adaptation (30cd/m^2) photopic responses were obtained at 0.0 log cd.s/m^2 at 5.1 Hz (C) and 30 Hz (D) respectively

Morphometry showed that the rAAV-RPE65 treatment reduced the RPE lipoid inclusion content specifically in the injected area, shown in Fig. 3A. As seen in Fig. 3B, there was a preservation of photoreceptors in the treatment region adjacent to the injection site of the gene transfer treated eye in comparison to outside the treated area and in comparable areas in the contralateral eye. No major differences

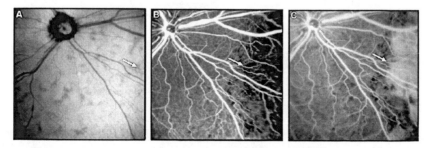

Fig. 2 Fundus of affected treated dog 2 years after subretinal injection of the gene construct in the inferior central part of the fundus, the area shown (arrow) using SLO and infrared light in (A), using Indocyanine Green IV in (B) and Fluorescein IV in (C)

(a)   (b)

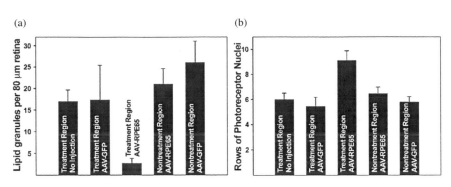

Fig. 3 Morphometry of different fundic regions of treated and fellow eyes of affected dogs that had undergone gene therapy. Lipid granules and rows of photoreceptor nuclei were counted and compared in different regions

were found in amount of inclusion bodies and photoreceptor numbers when areas outside of the injection region were compared for treated and untreated eyes.

Funduscopic studies have shown an increased spotting of the fundus with age both in untreated and in gene transfer treated affected dogs. These spots could be described as irregular dark lesions and whitish, pimple-like specks, as shown in Fig. 4A. Figure 4B shows the ultrastructure of the peripheral non-treated area of the fundus of the treated eye of the same dog from which the image in Fig. 4A was obtained: the eye was enucleated 4 years post-op. The photoreceptor layer is completely degenerated in the most peripheral parts of the fundus, the RPE cells

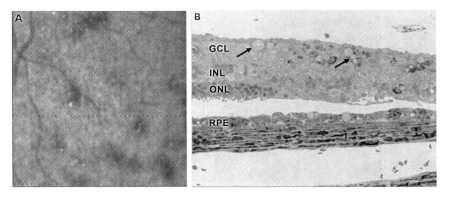

Fig. 4 (A) High magnification, using SLO and infrared light, of the central part of the fundus in the treated area of a dog euthanized 4 years after gene therapy. Note the pigmented spots and the pimple-like whitish specks. (B) 0.5 micron light microscopic section of the same treated eye shown in A. The peripheral retina shows severe degenerative changes with distinctly swollen pigment epithelial cells that contain photoreceptor debris and lipid droplets. The entire outer nuclear layer is missing, the inner retina reveals large pigment laden phagocytic cells (arrow), clinically known as "bone spicules". Original magnification 40X. RPE: Retinal pigment epithelium, ONL: outer nuclear layer, GCL: ganglion cell layer

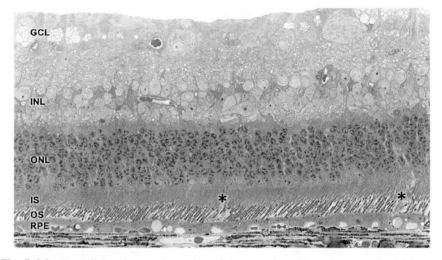

Fig. 5 0.5 micron light microscopic section of the treated area in a dog euthanized 3.7 years after subretinal gene therapy. Photoreceptors appear regularly structured, the pigment epithelium is moderately swollen and contains few lipid droplets and conspicuous nucleoli. Two phagocytic cells appear in the region of outer segments (*). Original mag.: 40X. RPE: Retinal pigment epithelium, OS: outer segments, IS: inner segments, ONL: outer nuclear layer, INL: inner nuclear layer, GCL: ganglion cell layer

are bulging, filled with a multitude of pigment and lipoid laden inclusions. Further, there is migration of large macrophage-like cells to the inner retina. The latter cells are likewise filled with inclusion bodies similar to those observed in the RPE cells. Electron microscopy of the treated region in another dog studied 3.7 years after the gene therapy is shown in Fig. 5. Long and slender photoreceptor outer and inner segments are seen with only slight reduction of the number of outer nuclear layer nuclei. Inner retina is preserved and mainly normal appearing. In the RPE small amounts of lipid droplets are observed.

4 Discussion

Clinically, surgeries in the dogs followed up to 4 years were successful: all regained functional vision 4–6 weeks after surgery. Long-term studies using simultaneous bilateral ERGs showed that improved retinal function was preserved during the entire follow-up period. The differences between dark- and light-adapted ERGs suggest that cone function was preserved better and longer than rod function following RPE65 gene therapy. The successive decline of rod function correlated with the reduced numbers of photoreceptor cell nuclei in the retina found 4 years following the gene therapy. Eventually, the number of photoreceptor nuclei became similar when non-treated regions in both eyes were compared. In the treated eye, specifically in the bleb area, but outside of the direct injection site, ultrastructure showed areas with well preserved photoreceptor cell morphology. In these areas phagosomes were observed in the RPE, indicative of active disc shedding. The well-preserved retina was observed to encircle the specific injection site, in which photoreceptor outer segments were short and stubby, although inner segments were more normal appearing. The focal degenerative changes in the outer segments were most proba- bly due to the trauma induced by the neuroretinal penetration by the injection needle in combination with forceful expression of fluids subretinally. The RPE cells in this area also appeared more flat than normally and slightly changed from their normal cuboidal structure. These findings corroborated the hypo- and hyperfluorescence, using ICG and FL, respectively, observed in the same area in all dogs included in the present study. Focal degenerative changes in RPE cells would cause hyperfluo- rescence using FL angiography. Likewise, an accumulation of degenerative debris in the outer retina, especially in the subretinal space, would cause hypofluorescence using ICG for the evaluation procedure. Severe degenerative changes in the outer retina have been shown to follow more short-term studies of experimental retinal detachments in human, cat and rabbit, respectively (Guerin et al., 1993, Lewis et al., 2002; Ivert et al., 2002). Long-term studies of focal detachments such as those produced through the subretinal gene transfer as performed in the present study has, to the authors' knowledge, not been previously reported. It appears that subretinal injection can have permanent deleterious effects at the injection site. Thus, if the approach to therapy is extended to humans, injection directly under the macula should be avoided.

The area of greatest therapeutic benefit appeared to be restricted to the region of the retina immediately surrounding the injection site. Outside of this region there was progression of the retinal degeneration. With advancing age, migration of giant macrophage-like cells into the inner retina was observed, even in treated eyes. It is possible that these were migrating RPE cells, given their rounded appearance, the latter due to the accumulation of partly pigmented and granular as well as lipoid-like inclusions in these cells. There was, further, a successive degeneration of photore- ceptor cells that occurred, with complete atrophy of photoreceptors in peripheral parts of the retina of the gene transfer treated eye, 4 years after surgery, the dog then approximately 5 years old. This indicates that although there is a long period during which gene transfer can be effective in rescuing retinal function, eventually retinal degenerative changes would make such therapeutic intervention fruitless.

It is clear that it is only a small region, less than the actual injection area that recovers structurally after subretinal gene therapy. However, restoration of the abil- ity of the RPE in this area to synthesize 11-cis retinoids may result in at least partial functional recovery in other parts of the retina. Eleven-cis retinoids, in particular 11-cis retinal, are likely to reach areas of the retina outside of the treatment region via the subretinal space. The production of 11-cis retinal by cells in the area in which transgene expression occurred was apparently large enough to elicit ERG responses up to approximately 50% of those of normal dogs and to provide long- term functional vision. Although restoration of RPE65 gene function in a small area of the RPE may provide 11-cis retinal to a broad region of the retina, RPE cells lacking functional RPE65 still accumulate lipid droplets that may lead to functional impairment of these cells and secondary degeneration of the overlying retina. This degeneration likely accounts for the progressive functional decline in the treated eyes. Therefore, permanent restoration of retinal function by RPE65 gene transfer will likely be restricted to the area of the retina directly overlying regions of the RPE that express the transgene.

Because permanent damage to the retina was observed at the site of subretinal injection, future studies should be directed towards the elucidation of less traumatizing treatment regimes for gene therapy that deliver the transgene to wider areas of the RPE. It is clear from the successful gene transfer studies now performed in three different strains of RPE65 null mutation dogs (Acland et al., 2001, 2006; Narfström et al., 2003a, 2005; Le Meur et al., 2006) that retinal gene therapy is feasible and that long-term alleviation of visual impairment is possible.

Acknowledgments Foundation Fighting Blindness (KN), Research to Prevent Blindness (MK and KN) and, University of Missouri-Columbia Research Board (KN). Leilani Castaner and Ginny Dodam are gratefully acknowledged for technical assistance, Deborah Becker and Howard Wilson for editorial support and assistance with graphics.

References

Acland G.M, Aguirre, G.D., Bennett, J., Aleman, T.S., et al., 2006, Long-term restoration of rod and cone vision by single dose rAAV-mediated gene transfer to the retina in a canine model of childhood blindness, *Mol Therapy*, **12**: 1072–1082.

Acland G.M., Aguirre, G.D., Ray, J., et al., 2001, Gene therapy restores vision in a canine model of childhood blindness, *Nat Genet*, **28**: 92–95.

Ford, M., Bragadottir, R., Rakoczy, P.E., Narfström, K., 2003, Gene transfer in the RPE65 null mutation dog: relationship between construct volume, visual behaviour and electroretinographic (ERG) results, *Doc Ophthalmol*, **107**: 79–86.

Guerin, C.J., Lewis, G.P., Fisher, S.K., Anderson, D.H., 1993, Recovery of photoreceptor outer segment length and analysis of membrane assembly rates in regenerating primate photoreceptor outer segments, *Invest Ophthalmol Vis Sci*, **34**: 175–183.

Ivert, L., Kjeldbye, H., Gouras, P., 2002, Long-term effects of short-term retinal bleb detachments in rabbits. *Graefe's Archive Clin Exp Ophthalmol* **240**: 232–237.

Le Meur, G., Stieger, K., Weber, M., Deschamps, J.Y., et al., 2006, Restoration of vision in RPE65-deficient Briard dogs using an AAV-serotype 4 vector that specifically targets the retinal pigment epithelium, *Gene Therapy* online, doi:10.1038/sj.gt.3302861.

Lewis, G.P., Charteris, D.G., Sethi, C.S., Leitner, W.P., et al., 2002, The ability of rapid retinal reattachment to stop or reverse the cellular and molecular events initiated by detachment, *Invest Ophthalmol Vis Sci*, **43**: 2412–2420.

Narfström, K., Katz, M.L., Bragadottir, R., Seeliger, M., Boulanger, A., Redmoond, R.M., Caro, L., Lai, C-M., Rakoczy, P.E., 2003a, Functional and structural recovery of the retina after gene therapy in the RPE65 null mutation dog, *Invest Ophthalmol Vis Sci*, **44**: 1663–1672.

Narfström, K., Katz, M.L., Bragadottir, R., et al., 2003b, In vivo gene therapy in young and adult RPE65-/- dogs produces long-term visual improvement, *J Hered*, **94**: 31–37.

Narfström, K., Vaegan, Katz, M., Bragadottir, R., Rakoczy, E.P., Seeliger, M., 2005, Assessment of structure and function over a 3-year period after gene transfer in RPE65-/- dog. *Doc Ophthalmol*, **111**: 39–48.

Seeliger, M., Beck, S.C., Pereyra-Munos, N., Dangel, S., et al., 2006, In vivo confocal imaging of the retina in animals models using scanning laser ophthalmoscopy, *Vis Res*, **45**: 3512–3519.

Virus-mediated Gene Delivery to Neuronal Progenitors

Tonia S. Rex

1 Introduction

Virus-mediated gene delivery is a very powerful tool for the treatment of inherited disorders (Bjorklund et al., 2000; Dejneka and Bennett, 2001; Manfredsson et al., 2006). Degenerations due to recessive mutations can be slowed or prevented by gene augmentation in which the wild-type form of the transgene of interest is packaged into a recombinant virus. Neurotrophic or neuroprotective factors can be delivered to tissues of interest by transduction with an appropriate virus. And, in the case of dominant inherited degenerations, a recombinant virus carrying siRNA specific to the mutant transgene could be introduced to the cells of interest to result in decreased production of the dominant negative form of the protein.

The most efficient method known to date for delivery of transgenes is via recombinant viruses. The term recombinant refers to the fact that the replicative (and thus, most of the immunogenic) components of the virus have been removed. This results in a viral particle that can be packaged with a transgene (and promoter) of interest, and used to deliver them to cells. The viruses that have been used include retroviruses (RV), lentivirus (LV), adenovirus (Ad), and adeno-associated virus (AAV).

There are two major hurdles that need to be overcome in regard to gene therapy. The first is activation of an immune response to the virus and/or the transgene. The second is delivery: reaching the target cells; and increasing transduction efficiency in the cells of interest. Both of these challenges might be overcome by delivering to the fetus. By injecting at a stage in development prior to formation of the immune system, it may be possible to avoid an immune response to either the virus or the transgene. Also, it is possible that more cells will be transduced if the progenitors are targeted. Finally, it may be necessary to treat certain congenital inherited degenerations by fetal gene delivery in order to achieve rescue.

T.S. Rex
University of Pennsylvania, 422 Curie Blvd., 3e10 Stellar-Chance Labs, Philadelphia, PA 19104, USA, Tel: 215-898-0163, Fax: 215-573-8083
e-mail: trex@mail.med.upenn.edu

R.E. Anderson et al. (eds.), *Recent Advances in Retinal Degeneration*,
© Springer 2008

The most challenging cells to deliver transgenes to are neurons because of inaccessibility, the post-mitotic nature of the cells, and poor transduction efficiency of the viruses. Initially, gene therapy research was performed using retroviral vectors, which only infect dividing cells. Later, Ad and AAV were used, and were found to transduce mature neurons in vivo. Importantly, AAV is also less immunogenic than the early generations of Ad vectors.

This review will focus on two issues: (1) the immune response to fetal viral gene delivery; and (2) delivery of transgenes to fetal neuronal progenitors using viral vectors. There is also much published work on fetal gene delivery to non-neuronal tissues. However, these studies will not be discussed here.

2 Viral Vectors

RV and LV are RNA viruses that integrate and have a rapid onset of expression. LV, however does not self-inactivate, so it is more advantageous than RV for the generation of transgenic animals (Pfeifer et al., 2002) or for long-term gene expression. Altering the lentiviral envelope changes the cellular specificity of the virus (Auricchio et al., 2001). It may also affect the response of the immune system, since some envelopes are more immunogenic than others. Like LV, Ad also begins gene expression about 2 days after transduction (Bennett et al., 1994; Li et al., 1994). Ad is a double-stranded DNA virus that remains episomal in the transduced cell (it does not integrate into the host cell DNA). Finally, AAV is a ssDNA virus that also remains episomal. The AAV capsid can be changed while maintaining the AAV2 inverted terminal repeats that border the transgene cassette (i.e. the AAV5 capsid can be used to carry the AAV2 genome, creating the hybrid AAV2/5 serotype). The initiation of gene expression varies from 5 days to 5 weeks depending on the AAV serotype used. A comparison of these viral vectors and their transduction patterns after intraocular injections in mouse is shown in Table 1.

Table 1 Viral vectors and retina transduction patterns

Virus	Genetic material	Time of onset	Cell specificity	Cargo capacity	Integrates?	Immunogenicity
AAV	ssDNA	1–4 wks	RPE, PRs, Muller cells, ganglion cells	5kb	No	low
Ad	dsDNA	2 days	RPE, Muller cells	8kb	No	high
LV	RNA	1 week	RPE	8kb	Yes	low

3 Immune Response

A major obstacle to gene therapy is activation of the immune system against either the virus or the transgene. One goal of fetal gene delivery was to circumvent the immune system. However, multiple studies have demonstrated that while fetal exposure to viral vectors does not initiate an immune response, it also does not block one after re-administration of virus into the postnatal mouse (i.e. immune tolerance; see below). This may be good, ultimately, because if the immune response is suppressed towards the viral vector, then a later infection to a wildtype version of the virus also may not elicit an immune response. In the case of neuronal tissue, it may be possible to avoid re-administration by treating the progenitors after much of the cell division has occurred so that the transgene will not be lost. Finally, this issue may be irrelevant in regard to delivery to the immune-protected environment of the central nervous system, although more studies need to be performed.

Direct tests for the induction of tolerance to the virus (and transgene) of interest have been performed. A single fetal injection of virus is followed by re-administration of the same virus in the post-natal mouse, then antibody titers and transgene expression are assessed to analyze the response of the immune system. Lipshutz et al. (2000) injected Ad.luciferase and compared luciferase levels in all experimental groups. A large immune response was elicited after two injections into an adult mouse, but not when the first injection was fetal. However, if the mouse was injected *in utero*, then injected twice after birth, a large immune response was elicited. Jerebtsova et al. (2002) found similar results using either Ad or AAV. An example of the development of immune tolerance to a transgene (not the virus) by viral transduction has been demonstrated, but not by a fetal injection. Fields et al. (2001) delivered Ad.Factor IX to adult mice and then eight weeks later challenged with an injection of AAV.Factor IX. Immune tolerance (i.e. continued presence of transgene) occurred only in one of the strains of mice tested, so it most likely cannot be extrapolated to other species.

Fetal injections of LV, Ad, or AAV result in short-term gene expression (Seppen et al., 2006; Schneider et al., 2002). The loss in expression occurred more slowly than if the injection had been performed post-natal. And, in the lentiviral studies, there was a correlative increase in antibodies to the transgene (Seppen et al., 2006). These results indicate that fetal exposure to viruses does induce an immune response, although at lower levels than an adult injection. In part, the decrease that occurred in the Ad and AAV studies could be explained by the increase in blood volume and therefore the relative dilution of the transgene (Schneider et al., 2002). Even more importantly, the decrease could be due to proliferation of infected cells, which resulted in dilution of the episomal vector. If the dilution effect can be overcome, fetal delivery of transgenes may be a particularly attractive option in degenerations due to the lack of production of the particular transgene. Otherwise, if the treatment were performed in the adult, the therapeutic transgene may elicit an immune response. In fact, this has occurred in some adult patients treated with gene therapy (Manno et al., 2006).

4 Successful Fetal Gene Delivery

Different delivery approaches, viruses, and time points have all been tested and analyzed for the best transduction efficiency with the least harm, i.e. damage or immune response. The results of these studies are discussed below, again focusing purely on the attempt to transduce neuronal precursors.

Thakur et al. (2001) delivered Ad.GFP to the brain of E2-3 chick embryos. Bright fluorescence was present in the area of the injection. There was no obvious negative effect of the procedure. No analyses were performed to identify the cell types that were transduced, or the efficiency of transduction. Stott and Kirik (2006) delivered lenti.GFP or RV.GFP to either the rat lateral ventricle or ganglionic eminence at E14.5–17.5. Unilateral expression was detected in the ganglionic eminence, in contrast, when they injected lenti.GFP, bilateral expression was found. Some of the infected cells developed into glia, but, most of the cells developed into interneurons. Interestingly, more glial cells were GFP-positive when mice were injected at E16. And, conversely, more neurons were GFP-positive when the mice were injected at E14.5. It is unknown why certain cells would be trans-duced better than others at different embryonic time points. Co-delivery of two herpes simplex viral vectors into the brain of E14.5 mice resulted in integration of the β-galactosidase cDNA into the genome of neuronal progenitors (Bowers et al., 2006). Expression levels were highest in the subventricular zone, septofimbrial region, dentate gyrus, hippocampus, and primary and secondary motor cortices. β-galactosidase expression was detected bilaterally, primarily in neurons. Ultimately, cell-type specific promoters will need to be used in this system in order to restrict gene expression to the cells of interest.

Bedrosian et al. (2006) injected viruses carrying EGFP to the E12 mouse otocyst. EGFP was detected in the inner and outer cochlear hair cells of mice injected with LV, AAV2/1, 2/2, or 2/8, but not with AAV2/5, 2/6, 2/7, or 2/9. Transduction with LV resulted in mild hearing loss, but treatment with any of the hyrid AAVs did not affect cochlear structure or function. The most efficient was AAV2/1 which transduced 81% of inner, and 64% of outer cochlear hair cells.

Turner et al. (1990) and Fields-Berry et al. (1992) delivered RV to the fetal rodent retina to confirm clonal mechanisms of retinal cell differentiation. Surace et al. (2003) later injected different serotypes of AAV carrying EGFP into E13–14 mouse retina. AAV2/5 was the most efficient at transducing the retina progenitors, followed by AAV2/2, then AAV2/1. In fact, twice as much EGFP was measured in cells transduced with AAV2/5 than 2/2 (Rex et al., 2005). Fetal infection resulted in a mosaic pattern of EGFP expression in the neural retina. The viruses targeted different sets of retinal progenitors and served as markers to the "birth dates" (i.e. time at which these cells become destined to differentiate into a specific cell type) of these different cells. In the area of transduction, most of the RPE was EGFP-positive, but within the neural retina and depending on the type of virus, there were occasional EGFP-positive cone photoreceptors, Müller cells, horizontal cells, and amacrine cells. No rod photoreceptors or ganglion cells were EGFP-positive. The rod photoreceptors and the ganglion cells have the latest birth-dates of all the retinal neurons.

5 Rescue of Degenerations

There are 1.9 cases of fetal alcohol syndrome per 1000 births in the United States. Exposure of the fetus to alcohol results in neural crest cell death, resulting in decreased frontonasal size, altered facial characteristic, and mental retardation. There is no treatment or cure. Recent studies have indicated that the frontonasal size is also decreased in sonic hedgehog (Shh) knock-out mice. So, Ahigren et al. (2002) attempted to rescue the effects of *in utero* exposure to alcohol by over-expression of Shh. Chick embryos were exposed to Rv.Shh prior to injection of alcohol. The frontonasal size was rescued, with only a slight reduction in the amount of cell death that normally occurs during development. It will be important to test this treatment in other animal models. This is the first example of successful treatment of this disease and is an exciting step forward for the field.

Leber congenital amaurosis (LCA) is a retinal degeneration with an embryonic onset that is due to mutations in several different genes. Ten percent of all cases are due to mutations in Rpe65. Like patients with LCA, the Rpe65$^{-/-}$ mouse also exhibits severe and early vision impairment. Because early intervention may be necessary for complete recovery of visual function, Dejneka et al. (2004) treated Rpe65$^{-/-}$ mice at E14 with AAV2/1.hRpe65. A single subretinal injection transduced about 1/3 of the retina. Electroretinogram (ERG) responses and rhodopsin formation recovered to levels found in normal, control eyes. This was the first demonstration of rescue of a congenital blinding disease by fetal gene delivery, and the first example of rescue in a mouse model of LCA.

The GUCY1B chicken is another model of LCA. The authors delivered lenti.GC1 into the neural tube of E2 chicks, resulting in transduction of 15–40% of the retina, including many photoreceptors. Whole retina thickness was improved in the superior and inferior optic nerve regions, but not in other retinal areas. Full visual behavior recovery was detected in 5 out of 6 animals. In addition, treated animals elicited small responses by ERG. However, a slow progressive retinal degeneration still occurred. The authors explain that this may be due to the low number of transduced photoreceptors since other studies have demonstrated the ability of neighboring dysfunctional cells to negatively impact healthy cells. Therefore, they suggest injecting with a higher titer of virus, in order to introduce more viral particles and increase the number of cells transduced. Alternatively, they suggest co-injecting with a virus carrying a neurotrophic factor in order to block the neighboring cells from undergoing cell death.

6 Future

The potential for gene delivery to neuronal progenitors is very exciting. Neuronal development and differentiation can be studied by transducing progenitors with viruses carrying transgenes of interest. And, congenital degenerations can be treated prior to rewiring of downstream neurons. Novel AAV serotypes are currently being tested and earlier injections into the fetus are being attempted in order to overcome the challenges of low transduction efficiency and slow onset of gene expression. Continued animal studies will illuminate mechanisms and timing of neuronal differentiation and will also provide proof-of-concept for gene therapy of additional forms of neuronal degeneration. While at this point in time, there are many hurdles necessary to overcome in order to extrapolate successful fetal gene therapy to human application, it is possible that some day there will be an acceptable risk:benefit odds for particular early onset neuronal degenerations.

Acknowledgments The author thanks her mentor, Dr. Jean Bennett for her input and support.

References

Ahigren S.C., Thakur V., and Bronner-Fraser M., 2002, Sonic hedgehog rescues cranial neural crest from cell death induced by ethanol exposure, Proc Natl Acad Sci. USA **99**:10476.

Auricchio A., Kobinger G., Anand V., Hildinger M., O'Connor E., Maguire A.M., Wilson J.M., and Bennett J., 2001, Exchange of surface proteins impacts on viral vector cellular specificity and transduction characteristics: the retina as a model, Hum Mol Genet. **10**:3075.

Bedrosian J.C., Gratton M.A., Brigande J.V., Tang W., Landau J., and Bennett J., 2006, In vivo delivery of recombinant viruses to the fetal murine cochlea: Transduction characteristics and long-term effects on auditory function, Mol Ther. **14**:328.

Bennett J., Wilson J., Sun D., Forbes B., and Maguire A., 1994, Adenovirus vector-mediated in vivo gene transfer into adult murine retina, Invest Ophthalmol Vis Sci. **35**:2535.

Bjorklund A., Kirik D., Rosenblad C., Georgievska B., Lundberg C., and Mandel R.J., 2000, Towards a neuroprotective gene therapy for Parkinson's disease: use of adenovirus, AAV and lentivirus vectors for gene transfer of GDNF to the nigrostriatal system in the rat Parkinson model, Brain Res. **886**:82.

Bowers W.J., Mastrangelo M.A., Howard D.F., Southerland H.A., Maguire-Zeiss K.A., and Federoff H.J., 2006, Neuronal precursor-restricted transduction via in utero CNS gene delivery of a novel bipartite HSV amplicon/transposase hybrid vector, Mol Ther. **13**:580.

Dejneka N.S., and Bennett J., 2001, Gene therapy and retinitis pigmentosa: advances and future challenges, Bioessays **23**:662.

Dejneka N.S., Surace E.M., Aleman T.S., Cideciyan A.V., Lyubarsky A., Savchenko A., Redmond T.M., Tang W., Wei Z., Rex T.S., Glover E., Maguire A.M., Pugh Jr. E.N., Jacobson S.G., and Bennett J., 2004, In utero gene therapy rescues vision in a murine model of congenital blindness, Mol Ther. **9**:182.

Fields-Berry S.C., Halliday A.L., and Cepko C.L., 1992, A recombinant retrovirus encoding alkaline phosphatase confirms clonal boundary assignment in lineage analysis of murine retina, Proc Natl Acad Sci. USA **89**:693.

Fields P.A., Armstrong E., Hagstrom J.N., Arruda V.R., Murphy M.L., Farrell J.P., High K.A., and Herzog R.W., 2001, Intravenous administration of an E1/E3-deleted adenoviral vector induces tolerance to factor IX in C57BL/6 mice, Gene Ther. **8**:354.

Jerebtsova M., Batshaw M.L., and Ye X., 2002, Humoral immune response to recombinant adenovirus and adeno-associated virus after in utero administration of viral vectors in mice, Ped Res. **52**:95.

Li T., Adamian M., Roof D.J., Berson E.L., Dryja T.P., Roessler B.J., and Davidson B.L., 1994, In vivo transfer of a reporter gene to the retina mediated by an adenoviral vector, Invest Ophthalmol Vis Sci. **35**:2543.

Lipshutz G.S., Flebbe-Rehwaldt L., and Gaensler K.M.L., 2000, Reexpression following readministration of an adenoviral vector in adult mice after initial *in utero* adenoviral administration, Mol Ther. **2**:374.

Manfredsson F.P., Lewin A.S., and Mandel R.J., 2006, RNA knockdown as a potential therapeutic strategy in Parkinson's disease, Gene Ther. **13**:517.

Manno C.S., Pierce G.F., Arruda V.R., Glader B., Ragni M., Rasko J.J.E., Ozelo M.C., Hoots K., Blatt P., Konkle B., Dake M., Kaye R., Razavi M., Zajko A., Zehnder J., Rustagi P., Nakai H., Chew A., Leonard D., Wright J.F., Lessard R.R., Sommer J.M., Tigges M., Sabatino D., Luk A., Jiang H., Mingozzi F., Couto L., Ertl H.C., High K.A., and Kay M.A., 2006, Successful transduction of liver in hemophilia by AAV-Factor IX and limitations imposed by the host immune response, Nat Med. **12**:342.

Pfeifer A., Ikawa M., Dayn Y., and Verma I.M., 2002, Transgenesis by lentiviral vectors: lack of gene silencing in mammalian embryonic stem cells and preimplantation embryos. Proc Natl Acad Sci. USA **99**:2140.

Rex T.S., Peet J.A., Surace E.M., Calvert P.D., Nikonov S.S., Lyubarsky A.L., Bendo E., Hughes T., Pugh Jr. E.N., and Bennett J., 2005, The distribution, concentration, and toxicity of enhanced green fluorescent protein in retinal cells after genomic or somatic (virus-mediated) gene transfer, Mol Vis. **11**:1236.

Schneider H., Muhle C., Douar A.M., Waddington S., Jiang Q-J., von der Mark K., Coutelle C., and Rascher W., 2002, Sustained delivery of therapeutic concentrations of human clotting factor IX – a comparison of adenoviral and AAV vectors administered *in utero*, J Gene Med. **4**:46.

Seppen J., van Til N.P., van der Rijt R., Hiralall J.K., Kunne C., and Oude Elferink R.P.J., 2006, Immune response to lentiviral bilirubin UDP-glucuronosyltransferase gene transfer in fetal and neonatal rats, Gene Ther. **13**:672.

Stott S.R.W., and Kirik D., 2006, Targeted *in utero* delivery of a retroviral vector for gene transfer in the rodent brain, Eur J Neurosci. **24**:1897.

Surace E.M., Auricchio A., Reich S.J., Rex T., Glover E., Pineles S., Tang W., O'Connor E., Lyubarsky A., Savchenko A., Pugh, Jr. E.N., Maguire A.M., Wilson J.M., and Bennett J., 2003, Delivery of adeno- associated virus vectors to the fetal retina: impact of viral capsid proteins on retinal neuronal progenitor transduction, J Virol. **77**:7957.

Thakur A., Lansford R., Thakur V., Narone J.N., Atkinson J.B., Buchmiller-Crair T., and Fraser S.E., 2001, Gene transfer to the embryo: strategies for the delivery and expression of proteins at 48 to 56 hours postfertilization, J Ped Surg. **36**:1304.

Turner D.L., Snyder E.Y., and Cepko C.L., 1990, Lineage-independent determination of cell type in the embryonic mouse retina, Neuron **4**:833.

Part IV
Animal Models of Retinal Degeneration

Loss of Visual and Retinal Function in Light-stressed Mice

Drew Everhart, Ana Stachowiak, Yumiko Umino, and Robert Barlow

1 Introduction

Extreme light exposure is an environmental factor that can lead to photoreceptor apoptosis and retinal degeneration (Noell and Albrecht, 1971; Reme et al., 1995). Photoreceptor apoptosis is the final cell death pathway in retinal diseases such age-related macular degeneration (AMD) and retinitis pigmentosa (RP). Extreme light stress also accelerates underlying retinal disease in many animal models (Wenzel et al., 2005), providing further evidence for light exposure as an independent risk factor for retinal degeneration. For these reasons, the study of light-induced degeneration in mice may provide a valuable model for uncovering the mechanisms of retinal diseases.

Light-induced photoreceptor damage appears to be rhodopsin mediated. The kinetics of regeneration of the chromophore 11-cis retinal following light exposure dictate the level of an animal's light damage susceptibility (Wenzel et al., 2001). Production of 11-cis retinal following light exposure requires a functional visual cycle or photo-reversal, a process that produces 11-cis retinal from rhodopsin's bleached intermediates when exposed to narrow band blue light. Nonetheless, it appears that bleaching of rhodopsin is a crucial element leading to light-induced damage.

Organisciak et al. (2003) found light damage in rats is dependent on light exposure regimen, light rearing conditions, temperature, diet, and the animal's pigmentation. Genetic makeup also impacts light damage susceptibility. For example, the C57BL/6J mouse strain contains a sequence variation in the RPE65 gene, which results in a Leu450 Met amino acid substitution. This gene mutation is primarily responsible for this mouse strain's high resistance to light damage. This resistance results in part from mutated RPE65's reduced ability to produce 11-cis retinal (Danciger et al., 2000).

D. Everhart
Center for Vision Research, Department of Ophthalmology, Upstate Medical University, 750 East Adams Street, Syracuse, NY 13210, USA, Tel: 315-464-7773, Fax: 315-464-8750
e-mail: everhard@upstate.edu

R.E. Anderson et al. (eds.), *Recent Advances in Retinal Degeneration*,
© Springer 2008

Assessment of the progression of retinal degeneration generally involves measurements of retinal sensitivity using the electroretinogram (ERG) and analysis of retinal anatomy using histological and immunohistochemical techniques. Visual function is rarely assessed. We show here a convenient behavioral method that can readily detect loss of vision induced by light damage.

We report measures of retinal and visual function of a light-stress resistant mouse strain (C57BL/6J) and an albino mouse strain (BALB/c). Following light exposure visual function was measured using a two-alternative choice, optomotor based testing paradigm (Optomotry©; Prusky et al., 2004) and retinal sensitivity was measured via ERG. We find that C57BL/6J mice are markedly resistant to light stress; whereas, BALB/c mice lose retinal and visual function following intermittent white and blue light exposure.

2 Methods

2.1 Animals

C57BL/6J and BALB/c mice were examined. We have previously characterized the retinal anatomy and retinal and visual function of C57BL/6J mice raised under normal lighting conditions (Umino et al., 2006a). We studied the BALB/c strain because others found that this albino strain shows considerable anatomical changes in response to light stress (Wenzel et al., 2001). Thus far, visual function of light-stressed BALB/c mice has not been examined.

The C57BL/6J mice tested in this study were approximately 10-months-old. At this age, they have not experienced loss of visual and retinal function (Umino et al., 2006a). BALB/c albino mice were approximately 3-months-old, an age at which albino mice should not exhibit age-related degeneration of vision. Mice were raised on a 14:10-hour light/dark cycle and were fed Formulab Diet ad libitum in accordance with protocols approved by the Institutional Animal Care and Use Committee at SUNY Upstate Medical University.

2.2 Light Exposure Apparatus and Exposure Regimens

The light exposure apparatus used in this study was kindly loaned to us by Dr. Daniel Organisciak (Wright State University, Dayton, OH). It consists of six circular fluorescent light bulbs surrounding a Plexiglas tube. The Plexiglas tube contains a wire mesh floor and a Plexiglas divider with holes in it to separate the mice being tested. Two mice were simultaneously exposed to light in each experimental trial. The white light intensity was approximately 25,000 lux and the blue light intensity was approximately 400 lux. A wire mesh endcap, fan and a water bottle were placed at each end of the light chamber and food was placed on the wire mesh floor of the apparatus within the tube. The apparatus was isolated from environmental light such that light exposures could be experimentally controlled.

Mice were exposed to various light regimens. Exposures included (1) continuous blue light for 24 hours, (2) intermittent blue light, comprised of 15 minutes periods of light exposure followed by 3 hours 45 minutes of darkness, repeated 6 times in 24 hours, (3) intermittent white light, and (4) 7 days of continuous blue light. In each case, baseline behavioral tests were done prior to light exposures.

2.2.1 Continuous Light Exposure

C57BL/6J mice (n=2) were exposed to intense blue light for 7 consecutive days. Mice were light adapted and pupils were not dilated because the long exposure period. Mice were placed on separate sides of the chamber and their positions alternated every 24-hours. Behavioral tests were performed daily, which involved removing the mice from the exposure chamber for approximately 15 minutes. Mice were also tested 3 days following light exposure. ERGs were performed 1 week following light exposure.

BALB/c albino mice were exposed to 24 hours of blue light (n=2). Prior to exposure, mice were dark-adapted and their pupils were dilated with 1% tropicamide. Visual acuity and contrast sensitivity were tested 3 days following light exposure and ERGs were performed after 1 week.

2.2.2 Intermittent Light Exposure

BALB/c mice were exposed to either intermittent blue or white light (n=2 each). The experiments began at midnight. Mice were dark-adapted but their pupils were not dilated. Each exposure period consisted of 15 minutes of light exposure followed by a period of 3 hours and 45 minutes of darkness. This was repeated 6 times, for a total experimental time of 24 hours. Acuity and contrast were assayed 3 days following exposure and ERGs were recorded one week following exposure.

2.3 Measuring Visual Function

Visual acuity and contrast sensitivity of both strains of mice were measured by observing their optomotor behavior with a computer-controlled threshold measuring system (Umino et al., 2006b). The program (Optomotry©; Cerebral Mechanics, Lethbridge, Alberta, Canada) ran on a dual processor G5 Power Mac computer (Apple, Inc.; Cupertino, CA) controlling four LCD monitors as previously described (Umino et al., 2006a,b). Briefly, a mouse was placed on a pedestal situated in the center of a square array of monitors that displayed a rotating sinusoidal grating. The Optomotry© program controlled the speed, direction of rotation, spatial frequency and contrast of the vertical sinusoidal gratings. The luminance of the monitors was 0.1 cd/m^2 at minimum (black) level and 155 cd/m^2 at maximum (white) level. The observer viewed the mouse on the pedestal via the a video camera but was "blind" to the stimulus. The task of the observer was to choose the direction of pattern rotation based on the animal's behavior, specifically, its reflexive optomotor head movements. In each trial the computer-controlled protocol randomly selected the direction of rotation of the grating, and the experimenter assessed the mouse's behavior for a five-second period after which the observer judged whether the pattern rotated clockwise or counterclockwise. For each response, the observer received an auditory feedback indicating whether the choice was correct or incorrect. The Optomotry© program altered spatial frequency and/or contrast using a staircase paradigm and converged on a threshold of 70% correct responses by the observer.

Mice were tested during the first four hours of their daytime light cycle (14 h light and 10 h dark). Observers were unaware of the genotype, sex, and age of the mice as well as their previously recorded thresholds. Behavioral responses of unexposed mice served as controls. We measured both visual acuity and contrast sensitivity. Acuity was determined at 100% contrast, with spatial frequency increasing or decreasing based on the observer's answers; the drift speed of the rotating grating was 12 degrees/sec. Contrast threshold was tested at a spatial frequency of 0.128 cycles/degree. Contrast sensitivity was the inverse of contrast threshold.

2.4 Measuring Retinal Function

Retinal function was assessed with ERG. Mice were dark-adapted overnight and anesthetized with Nembutal (60 mg/kg). The recorded eye was dilated with tropicamide (1%), and body temperature was monitored and maintained using a rectal probe and a heating pad (37 °C). Corneal moisture was maintained using artificial tears. ERGs were evoked by a series of 10 ms flashes from high intensity LEDs (520 nm, Luxeon III, Future Electronics), and were amplified (Model P15, Grass Instr; 100X gain; 0.1–1000 Hz), digitized at 5000 Hz (Digital 320 A/D Converter, Axon Instr.) and analyzed by pClamp 9.0 Software (Axon Instr.). Light intensities were controlled by an LED Driver (Fourward technologies, Inc) under PC control. Light intensity (Log I=0 in Fig. 2) at the surface of the cornea was 66 cdsm $^{-2}$ (0.9×10^{-5} photons μm $^{-2}$). b-wave amplitudes were measured from the trough of the corneal negative a-wave to the peak of the corneal positive b-wave. Intensity-response data was fitted with the Hill equation. Estimates of photoisomerizations/rod/flash are based on photometric measurements and computations following Lyubarsky and Pugh (1996). ERGs were recorded in response to single flashes allowing sufficient time between flashes for full recovery of sensitivity. Flashes were repeated to achieve a satisfactory signal to noise ratio.

3 Results of Visual and Retinal Function Testing

3.1 Visual Function

BALB/c mice show significant deficits in visual acuity (Fig. 1; Table 1) and contrast sensitivity (Table 2) following 24 hours of intermittent blue or intermittent white light exposure ($P < 0.001$). Acuity was more sensitive to intermittent white light

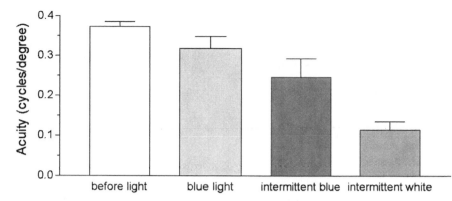

Fig. 1 BALB/c mice display significant losses in visual acuity following 24 hours of exposure to intermittent blue and intermittent white light ($P<0.001$). Included in the graph are the visual acuity of mice exposed to no bright light (white bar, n=51 trials, 6 mice), 24 hours of blue light (light grey bar, n=12 trials, 2 mice), 24 hours of intermittent blue light (dark grey bar, n=16 trials, 2 mice), 24 hours of intermittent white light (grey bar, n=17 trials, 2 mice). Statistics were calculated using one-way ANOVA with Newman-Keuls post hoc test. Bar represents mean ± standard error

than to intermittent blue light ($P<0.01$). 24 hours of continuous blue light did not significantly affect either measure. We did not detect changes in visual acuity or contrast sensitivity of C57BL/6J mice exposed to 7 days of continuous or intermittent blue or white light exposure (data not shown).

3.2 Retinal Function

Losses of retinal function assessed by ERG recordings correlate well with the deficits in visual function uncovered with optomotor behavioral testing. In BALB/c mice we detected a significant difference in the maximum ERG b-wave amplitudes

Table 1 Summary of acuity in BALB/c mice

Acuity (cycles/degree)	Baseline	Blue light	Intermittent blue light	Intermittent white light
Mean	0.37	0.32	0.25	0.11
Standard Error	0.01	0.03	0.02	0.05
95% Confidence	0.35–0.40	0.25–0.38	0.15–0.35	0.07–0.16
Trials	51	12	17	16

Table 2 Summary of contrast sensitivity in BALB/c mice

Contrast sensitivity	Baseline	Blue light	Intermittent blue light	Intermittent white light
Mean	2.31	2.01	1.07	1.10
Standard Error	0.19	0.44	0.10	0.04
95% Confidence	1.93–2.70	1.07–2.95	1.04–1.10	1.01–1.19
Trials	54	17	15	15

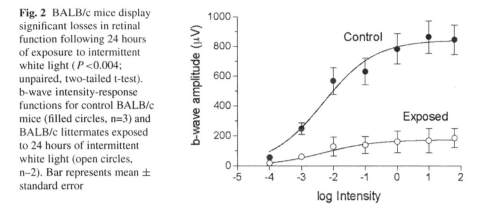

Fig. 2 BALB/c mice display significant losses in retinal function following 24 hours of exposure to intermittent white light ($P < 0.004$; unpaired, two-tailed t-test). b-wave intensity-response functions for control BALB/c mice (filled circles, n=3) and BALB/c littermates exposed to 24 hours of intermittent white light (open circles, n–2). Bar represents mean ± standard error

in mice treated with intermittent white light ($172 \pm 32\mu V$, n=2) versus unexposed animals ($845 \pm 59\mu V$, n=3) ($P < 0.004$). The curve fitting the control mice data was divided by 4.9 to fit the exposed mice data (Fig. 2). Such scaling of the ERG intensity-response functions indicates that intermittent white light exposure altered the gain but not the sensitivity of the retinal responses. Conversely, we did not detect a difference in the C57BL/6J maximum b-wave amplitude following 7 days of continuous blue light, continuous white light, or intermittent white light (data not shown).

4 Discussion

BALB/c mice exhibit losses in visual function as assessed by optomotor behavior and retinal function as assessed by ERG in response to 24 hours of intermittent light exposure. In contrast, 24 hours of continuous blue light was only mildly effective in reducing retinal and visual function in BALB/c mice. At first, this result is perplexing, as mice treated with continuous light are exposed to a much higher greater total photon flux. To reconcile this result, one must consider the mechanism of extreme light damage. Intense intermittent white or blue light exposures provided six periods of complete rhodopsin bleaching in BALB/c mice based on previously published rhodopsin regeneration kinetics (Wenzel et al., 2001). Although continuous light provides a greater total photon flux, it most likely evokes only one complete rhodopsin bleaching event. Thus, in terms of effective "bleaching power" intermittent light is far more powerful and therefore more destructive. The data fully support this assertion, as the most effective exposure paradigm tested was that of intermittent light.

ERG intensity-response functions from control and intermittent light exposed BALB/c mice exhibit similar shapes, but vastly different amplitudes. In fact, the BALB/c treated function plotted in Fig. 2 is simply a scaled down version of the control curve (4.9 times smaller). This is consistent with the currently accepted mechanism of light-induced damage – photoreceptor apoptosis (Wenzel et al., 2005). Loss of photoreceptors reduces the generation of the ERG leading to a simple scaling of ERG amplitudes, which is what we found (Fig. 2).

C57BL/6J mice did not experience losses of visual function or retinal function under any of the extreme light paradigms tested. Tests included 7 days of continuous blue light exposure, 7 days of continuous white light exposure and various intermittent white light exposure paradigms (data not shown). The RPE65 mutation in C57BL/6J mice certainly plays a role, but it may not explain the extremely low light damage susceptibility of these mice. B6;129S(N2) mice have the RPE65 variant, but have at least a ten times higher susceptibility to light damage (Wenzel et al., 2001). Extremely long intermittent light paradigms may lead to damage in C57BL/6J mice, but our test conditions did not.

We find that losses of visual function as assessed by optomotor behavior correlate with losses of retinal function measured with ERG. This may not necessarily be the case, as retinal function could be reduced without comparable loss of visual function. However, it would be much harder to explain losses of visual function without concurrent losses in retinal function if one is studying a retinal based disease. Thus far we have used behavioral testing to detect losses of vision in mildly hypoglycemic Gcgr-/- (Umino et al., 2006a), Isl-/- conditional knockout (Elshatory et al., 2007), and Gnat2^{cpfl3} mice (Alexander et al., 2007). The ability to test individual eyes and specific aspects of vision make optomotor behavior testing attractive for rapidly assaying effects of gene mutations or drug treatments. Behavioral testing of visual function can be performed rapidly and accurately throughout the duration of a study, minimally effecting exposure regimens. This behavioral technique holds great promise for testing the effects of extreme light on visual function.

Acknowledgments We would like to thank Dr. Daniel Organisciak (Wright State University; Dayton, OH) for loan of the light exposure chamber and for helpful suggestions and Rebekah Hafler (SUNY Upstate Medical University; Syracuse, NY) for technical assistance. This work was supported by grants from Fight for Sight (D.E), the National Eye Institute (EY00667) to R.B. and (1F32EY017246) to D.E., NASA, Research to Prevent Blindness, and the Lions of Central NY.

References

Alexander JJ, Umino Y, Chang B, Min SH, Li QH, Everhart D, Timmers AM, Hawes L, Barlow R, Hauswirth WW (2007). Restoration of cone vision in a mouse model of achromotopsia: Cone targeted gene therapy. (Nat Med., submitted).

Danciger M, Matthes MT, Yasamura D, Akhmedov NB, Rickabaugh T, Gentleman S, Redmond TM, La Vail MM, Farber DB (2000). A QTL on distal chromosome 3 that influences the severity of light-induced damage to mouse photoreceptors. Mamm Genome. 11(6):422–7.

Elshatory Y, Everhart D, Deng M, Xie X, Barlow R, Gan L (2007) Islet-1 Controls ON- and OFF- Retinal bipolar cell differentiation and cholinergic phenotype expression (J Neurosci. submitted).

Lyubarsky AL, Pugh EN Jr (1996). Recovery phase of the murine rod photoresponse reconstructed from electroretinographic recordings. J Neurosci. 16(2):563–71.

Organisciak DT, Darrow RM, Barsalou LS (2003). Light-Induced retinal degeneration. Ocular neuroprotection. Ed. L.A. Levin, A. DiPolo. Marcel Dekker, New York, 85–107.

Noell WK, Albrecht R (1971). Irreversible effect on visible light on the retina: role of vitamin A. Science 172(978):72–72.

Prusky GT, Alam NM, Beekman S, Douglas RM (2004). Invest Ophthalmol Visual Sci. 45: 4611–4616.

Reme CE, Weller M, Szczesny P, Munz K, Hafezi F, Reinboth, J, Clausen, M (1995). Degenerative diseases of the retina. New York: Plenum Press. 19–25.

Umino Y, Everhart D, Solessio E, Cusato K, Pan JC, Nguyen TH, Brown ET, Hafler R, Frio BA, Knox BE, Engbretson GA, Haeri M, Cui L, Glenn AS, Charron MJ, Barlow RB (2006a). Hypoglycemia leads to age-related loss of vision. Proc Natl Acad Sci U S A 103:19541–19545.

Umino Y, Frio B, Abbasi M, Barlow R (2006b). A two-alternative, forced choice method for assessing mouse vision. Adv Exp Med Biol. 572:169–172.

Wenzel A, Reme CE, Williams TP, Hafezi F, Grimm C (2001). The RPE65 LeuMet450 variation increases retinal resistance against light-induced degeneration by slowing rhodopsin regeneration. J Neurosci. Jan 1; 21(1):53–58.

Wenzel A, Grimm C, Samardzija M, Reme CE (2005). Molecular mechanisms of light-induced photoreceptor apoptosis and neuroprotection for retinal degeneration. Prog Retin Eye Res. 24(2):275–306.

ERG Responses and Microarray Analysis of Gene Expression in a Multifactorial Murine Model of Age-Related Retinal Degeneration

Goldis Malek, Jeffery A. Jamison, Brian Mace, Patrick Sullivan, and Catherine Bowes Rickman

1 Introduction

Age-related macular degeneration (AMD) is a late-onset neurodegenerative retinal eye disease that manifests as progressive loss of central vision. It is a common disease caused by the interaction of genetic predisposition and exposure to modifiable risk factors. Risk factors identified to date include but are not limited to: advanced age, environmental factors (*e.g.* smoking, diet) (Chua et al. 2006; Guymer and Chong 2006; Seddon et al. 2006; Weale 2006) and genetics (*e.g.* complement factors H & B, *LOC387715*, and apolipoprotein E [*APOE*]) (Klaver et al. 1998; Souied et al. 1998; Schmidt et al. 2002; Edwards Iii et al. 2005; Hageman et al. 2005; Haines et al. 2005; Klein et al. 2005; Conley et al. 2006; Gold et al. 2006). We developed a murine model that closely approximates changes seen in human AMD, by combining advanced age, human *APOE* isoform and a high fat, cholesterol-rich (HF-C) diet, three risk factors associated with the human disease (Malek et al. 2005). We determined that aged *APOE4* mice fed a HF-C diet develop characteristic lesions of AMD including retinal pigment epithelial (RPE)-pigmentary changes, thick lipid-rich diffuse and focal basal deposits and growth factor immunopositive neovascular lesions. These changes were not detected in any of the control, human *APOE3* expressing mice regardless of diet consumed, nor were there any pathologies detected in young *APOE4* animals.

The goal of the current study was to identify altered patterns of retinal and RPE/choroid gene expression in mice with 'AMD' pathology versus normal eyes, based on the hypothesis that these differences will specifically reflect multifactorial AMD-risk factor-induced retinal changes that could identify genes and cellular pathways involved in progression of disease. We also investigated retinal function changes, which were then correlated with morphological changes detected in the retinas of the affected animals.

G. Malek

Department of Ophthalmology, Duke University, Durham NC, USA, Tel: 919-684-0820, Fax: 919-684-3687

e-mail: gmalek@duke.edu

R.E. Anderson et al. (eds.), *Recent Advances in Retinal Degeneration,*
© Springer 2008

2 Gene Expression Profiling

To identify genes affecting the development of, or protection from, AMD-like pathologies in our animal model, microarray based gene expression profiles of retina/RPE/choroid were generated as follows: we used human *APOE* targeted replacement mouse lines, expressing either *APOE3* or *APOE4* that were created by replacing the coding sequences of mouse *apoE* with human *APOE* allele-specific coding sequences (Sullivan et al. 1997). Aged male mice (mean age 80–122 wks) of each genotype (n=3/genotype) were bred and housed conventionally, fed a HF-C diet (35% fat, 20% protein, 45% carbohydrates, 1.25% cholesterol, 0.5% sodium cholate) for 8 weeks or normal chow (4.5% fat, 0.02% cholesterol). Left eyes were prepared for histopathology as described previously (Malek et al. 2005). Right eyes were enucleated, fixed in RNA*later* and stored at −20°C until use. Total RNA was isolated from the retina/RPE/choroid using TriZol-glycogen or Qiagen RNeasy lipid tissue mini kit. Samples were biotin-labeled for hybridization following amplification when necessary. Expression analysis was performed using Operon Mouse Oligo Set, version 3.0 spotted array GeneChips, representing 30,000 genes. Samples were hybridized onto microarray slides and visualized with the GeneChip scanner. Data were normalized and clustered using GeneSpring GX software.

Two RNA based approaches were used to validate the differential gene expression profiles obtained; quantitative real-time PCR of selected genes and large-scale transcript profiling on a novel, high-density microarray profile from Illumina (San Diego, CA). A new cohort of n=6–8/genotype/diet samples (retina/RPE/choroid RNA), was used to probe Illumina mouse Sentrix Beadarrays. This resulted in identification of both a larger number of total and differentially expressed genes. A manuscript detailing the complete Illumina based profiles is in preparation.

3 AMD-Related Pathways

Comparative analysis of the gene expression profiles of *APOE4* mice with AMD pathology versus controls confirmed differential expression of genes previously implicated in the pathogenesis of AMD including inflammatory genes, oxidative stress- and lipid-related genes. Also identified as differentially expressed were extracellular matrix molecules (*e.g. TIMP3, ADAM15*, extracellular matrix protein 1, retinol binding protein, fibronectin), and apoptotic genes (*e.g.* vascular endothelial zinc finger, TNF receptor). Furthermore, retinal synaptic genes, including synapsin, synaptotagmin, and piccolo, which based on preliminary immunohistochemical investigation appear to be disorganized in regions above focal and diffuse sub-RPE deposits in aged, *APOE4* mice fed a HF-C diet, were also differentially expressed (Data not shown). These finding support the hypothesis that these 'diseased' mice share common pathogenic mechanisms with human AMD and provide further insight into the still unknown cholesterol and lipid induced changes in the eye and

Table 1 Candidate genes were prioritized and clustered based on pathways and processes implicated in AMD pathogenesis. Fold change is the statistically significant differential expression between *APOE4* HF-C and normal diet samples, $p < 0.05$

AMD Pathogenic Pathway	Common	Genbank	Description	GO biological process	Fold
Inflammation	Klkb1	M58588	Mouse plasma kallikrein (PK)	inflammatory response, chymotrypsin activity	2.90
	Pfc	X12905	properdin factor, complement	complement activation, alternative pathway	2.01
	Il1f9	AY071843	interleukin 1 family, member 9	immune response, interleukin-1 receptor binding	1.91
	Tollip	AK015062	toll interacting protein	immune response; inflammatory response	1.29
	Cxcl11	AF136449	chemokine (C-X-C motif) ligand 11	chemokine and cytokine activity, immune response	1.20
	Tnfsf11	AB036798	tumor necrosis factor (ligand)	cell differentiation; immune response; TNF receptor binding	1.14
Oxidative Stress	Prnp	M30384	prion protein	copper ion homeostasis; response to oxidative stress	1.95
	Ppp3ca	J04134	protein phosphatase 3	G1/S transition of mitotic cell cycle; calcium transport	1.49
	Hadha	BC027156	hydroxyacyl-CoA dehydrogenase	fatty acid beta-oxidation	1.32
Apoptosis	Madd	Mm.36410	MAP-kinase activating death domain	Regulation of apoptosis	3.00
		Mm.196371	RIKEN cDNA 2610511G16 gene	Positive regulation of apoptosis	1.87
	Dapk1	Mm.24103	Death associated protein kinase 1	Apoptosis and protein amino acid phosphorylation	1.79
	Cul1	Mm.87611	Cullin 1	Apoptosis; cell cycle and proliferation; organogenesis	1.64
	Muc2	Mm.334328	Mucin 2	Induction of apoptosis	1.59
	Casp8ap2	Mm.22279	Caspase 8 associated protein 2	Caspase activation; apoptosis via death domain receptors	1.18
Lipid metabolism	Mvd	AJ309922	mevalonate decarboxylase	cholesterol biosynthesis; isoprenoid biosynthesis; phosphorylation	1.89
	Plcd3	BC031392	phospholipase C, delta 3	intracellular signaling cascade; lipid metabolism; signal transduction	1.67
	Mbtps1	BC011533	transcription factor protease, site 1	cholesterol and lipid metabolism; proteolysis and peptidolysis	1.66
	Pla2g2d	AK004232	phospholipase A2, group IID	lipid catabolism; phospholipase A2 activity	1.54
	Slc27a4	AK036919	fatty acid transporter, member 4	lipid transport; metabolism	1.47

their involvement in AMD. Select differentially expressed genes identified on the Operon microarrays and their AMD-associated pathways are shown in Table 1.

4 Retinal Changes

4.1 Electroretinogram (ERG) Recordings

The ERG recordings were obtained from animals, dark adapted for at least 12 hours. Each animal was anesthetized with a ketamine/xylazine cocktail, pupils were dilated and after the animal stabilized on a 37°C warming pad, ERG tracings were recorded using a silver wire test electrode placed in contact with the eye along with a drop of 2.5% hydroxypropyl methylcellulose. Mice were placed in a photopic stimulator chamber where the animal was exposed to flashes of light (max intensity of $1000 \, cd\text{-}s/m^2$ attenuate in 1 log steps, starting from 0.0005). The a-wave amplitude was measured from baseline to the a-wave trough, and the b-wave amplitude was measured from the a-wave trough to the b-wave peak.

There was a significant reduction in a- and b-wave amplitude in *APOE4* HF-C mice versus mice on the normal diet (Fig. 1). No significant change was seen in the implicit times of the a-waves between the groups. There was a slight increase in the b-wave implicit timing of the *APOE4* HF-C, though this was not statistically significant. Within the *APOE4* HF-C cohort, ERG recordings fell broadly into three groups based on their average a- and b- wave amplitudes; high, med, and low. The degree of histopathological changes observed in affected aged, HF-C fed *APOE4*s varied in each animal in a manner reminiscent of pathologies documented in human

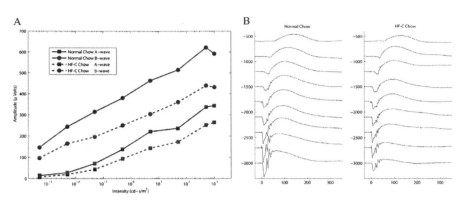

Fig. 1 Graph of intensity of a- and b-waves (A) and sample ERGs (B) from *APOE4* mice aged over 65 weeks and fed a normal or high fat, cholesterol-rich (HF-C) diet

AMD eyes (Malek et al. 2005). Therefore, we wondered whether the heterogeneity in ERG recordings in affected animals would correlate with the morphological changes.

4.2 Morphological Changes

Pathologies in aged APOE4 mice fed and HF-C diet ranged in severity with some animals developing choroidal and retinal neovascularization (~10%), some developing focal and diffuse sub-RPE deposits (~75%) and some maintaining overall

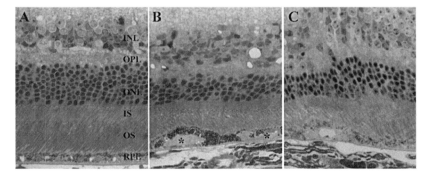

Fig. 2 Light micrographs from one micron plastic sections of posterior retinas of aged *APOE4* expressing mice fed a high fat and cholesterol-rich diet, stained with toludine blue. Retinal pigment epithelium (RPE) contains vacuoles (A). Presence of 'drusen-like' deposits located between the RPE and Bruch's membrane (B; asterisks). Neovascularization confined to a sub-RPE region (C). Note, decreased thickness of the outer nuclear layer (ONL) overlying deposit and neovascularization in panels B and C. Magnification 40X. INL=inner nuclear layer, OPL=outer plexiform layer, IS=inner segments of photoreceptors, OS=outer segments of photoreceptors

Table 2 Measurements of retinal layer thickness and cell counts in aged *APOE4* mice fed and high fat cholesterol-rich diet correlated to ERG a- and b-wave amplitude groups

ERG a and b wave amplitude (group)	Inner plexiform layer (um)	Inner nuclear layer # cells	Outer plexiform layer (um)	Outer nucler layer # cells-central	Outer nucler layer # cells-periphery
High	2.8	1.91	0.78	2.53	4
Med	3.2	1.92	1.01	2.34	3.4
Low	3.1	2.05	1	2.8	3.8

normal retinal morphology (~10%, Fig. 2). Retinal morphometric analysis was performed on plastic embedded tissue cross sections that bisected the optic nerve. Retinal layers were measured and cell numbers were counted in an area adjacent to the optic nerve head and in an area in the far periphery. A total of 10–12 sections were measured and counted and the results were averaged. Local or diffuse sub-RPE deposits were seen in approximately 76% of the mice, belonging to all three functional groups. Based on measurements of thickness of retinal layers and number of cells, there were no significant differences between ERG groups (Table 2). However, in regions immediately adjacent to deposits or neovascularization, some thinning of the outer nuclear layer as well as shortening of the photoreceptor inner and outer segments were documented (Fig. 2B, C).

5 Conclusions

ERG recordings of *APOE4* HF-C mice demonstrate statistically significant decreased a- and b-wave amplitudes. Though gross morphological differences were not seen in the retinal layers, gene expression profiles obtained by microarray analyses suggest that changes may be occurring at a transcriptional and potentially translational level, which warrants further investigation. Several synaptic markers were differentially expressed in the *APOE4* HF-C microarray samples including synaptotagmin, synaptophysin and piccolo. Similar changes have recently been demonstrated in human AMD eyes using these markers (Johnson et al. 2003; Johnson et al. 2005). Changes in synaptic terminals including synaptic retraction occurred in regions overlying drusen in human eyes. Preliminary immunolocalization experiments indicate that this is the case for *APOE4* HF-C mice as well (manuscript in preparation).

Acknowledgments The authors gratefully acknowledge scientific input from Drs. Linc Johnson, Patrick Johnson, and Monte Radeke, technical assistance from Jessica N. Ebright and Peter Saloupis and the following funding agencies: AHAF MDR (CBR), NEI P30 EY005722, A Ruth and Milton Steinbach Award (CBR), Alcon Basic Research Funds (CBR) and Research to Prevent Blindness Core grant.

References

Chua, B., V. Flood, et al. (2006). "Dietary fatty acids and the 5-year incidence of age-related maculopathy." *Arch Ophthalmol* **124**(7): 981–6.

Conley, Y. P., J. Jakobsdottir, et al. (2006). "CFH, ELOVL4, PLEKHA1 and LOC387715 genes and susceptibility to age-related maculopathy: AREDS and CHS cohorts and meta-analyses." *Hum Mol Genet* **15**(21): 3206–18.

Edwards, A. O., R. Ritter Iii, et al. (2005). "Complement factor H polymorphism and age-related macular degeneration." *Science*. **308**: 385–389.

Gold, B., J. E. Merriam, et al. (2006). "Variation in factor B (BF) and complement component 2 (C2) genes is associated with age-related macular degeneration." *Nat Genet* **38**(4): 458–62.

Guymer, R. H. and E. W. Chong (2006). "Modifiable risk factors for age-related macular degeneration." *Med J Aust* **184**(9): 455–58.

Hageman, G. S., D. H. Anderson, et al. (2005). "A common haplotype in the complement regulatory gene factor H (HF1/CFH) predisposes individuals to age-related macular degeneration." *Proc Natl Acad Sci U S A* **102**(20): 7227–32.

Haines, J. L., M. A. Hauser, et al. (2005). "Complement factor H variant increases the risk of age-related macular degeneration." *Science* **308**(5720): 419–21.

Johnson, P. T., M. N. Brown, et al. (2005). "Synaptic pathology, altered gene expression, and degeneration in photoreceptors impacted by drusen." *Invest Ophthalmol Vis Sci* **46**(12): 4788–95.

Johnson, P. T., G. P. Lewis, et al. (2003). "Drusen-associated degeneration in the retina." *Invest Ophthalmol Vis Sci* **44**(10): 4481–88.

Klaver, C. C., M. Kliffen, et al. (1998). "Genetic association of apolipoprotein E with age-related macular degeneration." *Am J Hum Genet* **63**(1): 200–6.

Klein, R. J., C. Zeiss, et al. (2005). "Complement factor H polymorphism in age-related macular degeneration." *Science* **308**(5720): 385–89.

Malek, G., L. V. Johnson, et al. (2005). "Apolipoprotein E allele-dependent pathogenesis: a model for age-related retinal degeneration." *Proc Natl Acad Sci U S A* **102**(33): 11900–5.

Schmidt, S., C. Klaver, et al. (2002). "A pooled case-control study of the apolipoprotein E (APOE) gene in age-related maculopathy." *Ophthalmic Genet* **23**(4): 209–23.

Seddon, J. M., S. George, et al. (2006). "Cigarette smoking, fish consumption, omega-3 fatty acid intake, and associations with age-related macular degeneration: the US twin study of age-related macular degeneration." *Arch Ophthalmol* **124**(7): 995–1001.

Souied, E. H., P. Benlian, et al. (1998). "The epsilon4 allele of the apolipoprotein E gene as a potential protective factor for exudative age-related macular degeneration." *Am J Ophthalmol* **125**(3): 353–59.

Sullivan, P. M., H. Mezdour, et al. (1997). "Targeted replacement of the mouse apolipoprotein E gene with the common human APOE3 allele enhances diet-induced hypercholesterolemia and atherosclerosis." *J Biol Chem* **272**(29): 17972–80.

Weale, R. (2006). "Smoking and age-related maculopathies." *Lancet* **368**(9543): 1235–36.

Oxygen Supply and Retinal Function: Insights from a Transgenic Animal Model

Edda Fahl, Max Gassmann, Christian Grimm, and Mathias W. Seeliger

1 Introduction

Transportation of oxygen to the different retinal layers occurs via two major vascular systems present in the eye. The supply of the outer retina originates in the choroid (choriocapillaris) located beneath the retinal pigment epithelium (RPE). The retinal circulation supplies the inner retina and as shown by Cuthbertson and Mandel (1986), exists in three capillary beds centered on the nerve-fibre layer, the junction of inner plexiform and inner nuclear layer, and the outer plexiform layer. Alder and Cringle (1990) found that a typical PO_2 profile starts at 82 mm Hg at the choroidal side of the retina. With increasing distance of the retinal layers to the choroid the PO_2 value decreases to 2 mm Hg at the balance point of the two circulations and increases up to 15 mm Hg due to the retinal circulation.

Retinal function, commonly measured by electroretinography (ERG), is particularly sensitive to circulatory disturbances. Tazawa and Seaman (1972) nicely demonstrated the rapid decrease and subsequent disappearance of the ERG b-wave in the extracorporeal bovine eye as a result of anoxia, whereas the a-wave was only moderately reduced. This is in line with the origin of the b-wave in the inner retina, which seems to be more sensitive to and more affected by acute anoxia. In contrast, the a-wave originating in the outer retina seems more resistant to anoxia. In vitro experiments with perfused eyes described by Niemeyer (1975) revealed a bi-directional dependency of the b-wave amplitude to changes of oxygen supply: an increased flow leads to a larger b-wave, whereas a decreased flow causes a reduction of the b-wave.

The transgenic mouse line tg6 overexpresses the human erythropoietin (huEpo) gene, leading to a disease phenotype in several tissues as described by Wagner et al. (2001). An important pathophysiologic factor is the development of a hematocrit (the percentage of corpuscular elements in the blood) of about 80%

E. Fahl
Ocular Neurodegeneration Research Group, Centre for Ophthalmology, Institute for Ophthalmic Research, Tuebingen, Germany D-72076, Tel: 49-7071-298-7784, Fax: 49-7071-29-4503
e-mail: edda.fahl@med.uni-tuebingen.de

(i.e. almost twice as high as normal). The blood volume is increased by 75%, whereas blood pressure and cardiac output remain normal. However, features of cardiac dysfunction like increased heart weight and ventricular dilatation can be observed, and the exercise performance is strongly reduced. The life expectance of these mice is reduced to 7.4 months.

In this study, we have investigated the functional and morphological changes to the retina in the tg6 mouse in vivo.

2 Methods

2.1 Animals

All procedures involving animals adhered to the Association for Research in Vision and Ophthalmology statement for the use of animals in ophthalmic and vision research and were conducted with permission of the local authorities.

The tg6 mice used in this study were transgenic for the human Epo and were generated by microinjection of human Epo cDNA as described by Ruschitzka et al. (2000). Mice were 4–6 weeks of age at the time of the study. Assessment of morphology was done in vivo by scanning-laser ophthalmoscopy (SLO), and retinal function was tested by Ganzfeld electroretinography (ERG).

2.2 Scanning-laser Ophthalmoscopy (SLO)

The in vivo confocal imaging technique using SLO has previously been described in detail by Seeliger et al. (2005). The SLO provides valuable information about a number of ocular tissues from cornea through sclera.

In this study, we focussed on the analysis of the retina and the respective vascular systems using the short wavelength range of 514 nm for native imaging and 488 nm (barrier filter 500 nm) for fluorescein angiography.

2.3 Ganzfeld Electroretinography (ERG)

ERGs were obtained according to previously described procedures by Seeliger et al. (2001). Mice were dark-adapted over night before the experiments and their pupils were dilated. Anesthesia was induced by subcutaneous injection of ketamin (66.7 mg/kg) and xylazine (11.7 mg/kg). Silver needle electrodes served as reference (forehead) and ground (tail) electrodes, and gold wire ring electrodes as active electrodes. Methylcellulose was applied to ensure good electrical contact and to keep the eye hydrated during the measurement. The ERG equipment consisted of a Ganzfeld bowl, a DC amplifier, and a PC-based control and recording unit (Toennies Multiliner Vision). ERGs were recorded from both eyes simultaneously. Band-pass filter width was 0.3 to 300 Hz.

In this study, single-flash recordings were obtained both under dark-adapted (scotopic) and light-adapted (photopic) conditions. Stimuli of the scotopic ERG were presented with increasing intensities, reaching from -4 log cd*s/m^2 to 1.5 log cd*s/m^2, divided into 11 steps of 0.5 and 1 log cd*s/m^2. Light-adaptation was performed with a background illumination of 30 cd/m^2 starting 10 minutes before the photopic ERG session, and the stimuli in this session increased from -2 log cd*s/m^2 to 1.5 log cd*s/m^2, divided into 8 steps of 0.5 log cd*s/m^2.

3 Results

3.1 Retinal Vasculature of the tg6-Mouse

The retinal vasculature was studied with native imaging using the green laser (514 nm), and with fluorescence angiography (488 nm laser, barrier filter at 500 nm). In native images obtained with the green laser (Fig. 1), veins can be easily differentiated from arteries. The thin walled veins appear dark because of the strong absorbance of green light by haemoglobin, whereas the arteries look silvery because most of the light is reflected at the interface between the muscular wall and the lumen before it reaches the blood.

Fluorescence angiography (FLA) allows to obtain particularly detailed images of retinal capillaries (Fig. 2). As blood absorption does not play a major role in angiography, the difference between veins and arteries is best visualized as an reduced dye-filled lumen and a more linear shape of arteries.

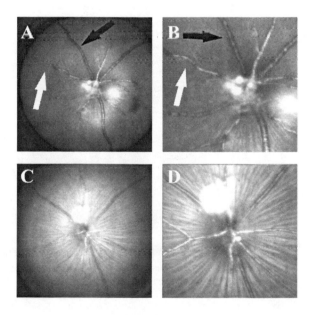

Fig. 1 Native imaging of the fundus of a tg6 mouse (A: full view, B: detail) in comparison to a wildtype mouse (C: full view, D: detail) using a Scanning-Laser Ophthalmoscope. In the tg6 mouse the retinal veins (black arrow) are enlarged and the arteries are tortuous (white arrows)

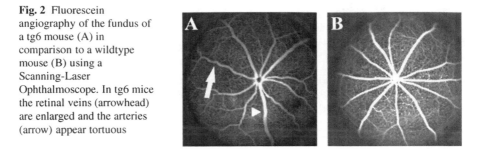

In both native imaging and FLA, the veins of the tg6 mice appear enlarged (Fig. 1A and 1B, black arrow; Fig. 2A, arrowhead) and the arteries show a more tortuous appearance (Fig. 1A and 1B, white arrow; Fig. 2A, arrow) compared to wildtype mice.

3.2 Retinal Function of the tg6-Mouse

Retinal function is commonly assessed with electroretinography, which allows to distinguish between rod and cone system contributions. In the scotopic ERG (Fig. 3, left), responses to light stimuli up to -2 log cd*s/m^2 arise from the rod system only. At higher light intensities, both the rod and cone system contribute to the responses. The photopic ERG is recorded on a static white background to desensitize the rod

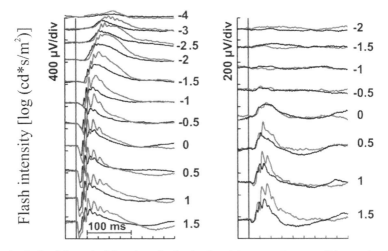

Fig. 3 Analysis of the retinal function of tg6 mice (grey) in comparison to wildtype mice (black) using scotopic (left) and photopic (right) flash intensity series electroretinography (ERG). The overlay of the tg6 and wildtype responses reveals larger amplitudes of the tg6 mouse, accompanied by a slightly prolonged implicit time

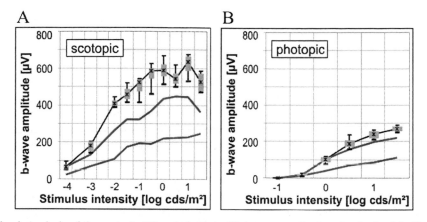

Fig. 4 Analysis of the scotopic (A) and photopic (B) b-wave amplitudes of tg6 mice (black) in comparison to wildtype mice (grey). The tg6 mice reaches larger amplitudes in both, the scotopic and photopic ERG

system by light-adaptation, so that the isolated responses of the cone system can be measured (Fig. 3, right).

In the tg6 mice, both the scotopic and the photopic ERG had larger, supernormal amplitudes, which were accompanied by slightly prolonged implicit times (Fig. 3). In the scotopic ERG, an increased amplitude of the saturated a-wave, which correlates with rod photoreceptor signal size, was observed. The supernormal b-wave amplitude additionally indicated an enhanced signal size by inner retinal ON bipolar cells (Fig. 4).

4 Discussion

The transgenic mouse line tg6 expresses high levels of human erythropoietin. In a previous study, Grimm et al. (2004) found no influence on retinal development and morphology, and also the content and the regeneration of visual pigments were normal. In this study, we provide functional and morphologic evidence for subtle retinal changes concerning the diameter and the tortuosity of vessels and the amplitude of ERG signals. In vivo imaging with the SLO revealed an increased tortuosity of arteries and an enlarged diameter of retinal veins, similar to human hyperviscosity syndromes shown by Mailath et al. (1976); Nagy (1950); Spalton et al. (1994); Rezai et al. (2002), in particular those associated with polycythaemia vera (Nagy, 1950; Spalton et al., 1994). As Ruschitzka et al. (2000) observed nearly doubled values for erythrocytes, hemoglobin, and hematocrit in the tg6 mouse, the vascular changes are most probably the consequence of the enhanced hematocrit together with an increased blood viscosity.

It is well possible that these alterations are rather dynamic in nature, i.e. are caused by the pressure distribution in vivo, and may thus not be accessible histologically. This is supported by the fact that comparable changes in human patients with treatable hyperviscosity syndromes resolved very quickly after the onset of therapy as Rezai et al. (2002) demonstrated.

An interesting question to be resolved in this study was whether the overall result would be retinal ischemia or enhanced oxygen availability. This question was addressed with electroretinography as the ERG is particularly sensitive to the retinal oxygen status. Tazawa and Seaman (1972) nicely showed that mostly b- but also a-wave amplitudes in extracorporeal bovine eyes are strongly dependent on ocular blood flow (and thus oxygen supply): the b-wave decreased rapidly during anoxia, whereas the a-wave decreased only gradually. Niemeyer (1975) further expanded these results by not only decreasing but also increasing normal retinal flow in perfused cat eyes, and found that an increased flow rate, associated with enhanced oxygen availability, increases the b-wave amplitude of the ERG.

Unexpectedly, retinal function in the tg6 mice in both the scotopic and photopic ERG was supernormal in comparison to wildtype mice. The increased amplitude of the a-wave as well as the b-wave in the scotopic ERG indicates that both inner retinal as well as choroidal circulation provided enhanced amounts of oxygen. Our findings thus suggest that the overexpression of huEpo leads to an enhanced oxygen availability to the retina, in line with the in vitro experiments by Niemeyer (1975) mentioned above.

Acknowledgments German Research Council (DFG Se837/4-1, 5-1), EU (IP 'EVI-GenoRet' LSHG-CT-512036, Ministry of Science, Research, and the Arts, Baden-Wuerttemberg, Germany

References

Alder, V. A., and Cringle, S. J. 1990, Vitreal and retinal oxygenation, *Graefe's Arch Clin Exp Ophthalmol. 228: 151–157*

Spalton, D. J., Hatching, R. A., and Hunter, P. A., 1994, *Atlas of Clinical Ophthalmology.* (2nd ed.), London, Philadelphia: Mosby

Cuthbertson, R. A. and Mandel, T. E., 1986, Anatomy of the mouse retina. Endothelial cell-pericyte ratio and capillary distribution, *IOVS. 27(11):1659–1664*

Grimm, C., Wenzel, A., Stanescu, D., Samardzija, M., Hotop, S., Groszer, M., Naash, M., Gassmann, M., and Remé, C., 2004, Constitutive overexpression of human erythropoietin protects the mouse retina against induced but not inherited retinal degeneration, *J Neurosci. 24:5651–5658*

Mailath, L., Nagy, G., Gat, G., and Racz, M., 1976, On the appearance of the eye fundus in polycythaemia vera (author's translation), *Klin Monatsbl Augenheilkd. 169(3):343–348*

Nagy, F., 1950, Changes in the fundus caused by polycythaemia, *Br J Ophthalmol. 34(6):380–384*

Niemeyer, G., 1975, The function of the retina in the perfused eye, *Doc Ophthalmol. 39(1):53–116.*

Rezai, K. A., Patel, S. C., Eliott, D., and Becker, M. A., 2002, Rheumatoid hyperviscosity syndrome: Reversibility of microvascular abnormalities after treatment, *Am J Ophthalmol. 134:130–132*

Ruschitzka, F. T., Wenger, R. H., Stallmach, T., Quaschning, T., de Wit, C., Wagner, K., Labugger, R., Kelm, M., Noll, G., Rülicke, T., Shaw, S., Lindberg, R. L. P., Rodenwaldt, B.,

Lutz, H., Bauer, C., Lüscher, T. F., and Gassmann, M., 2000, Nitric oxide prevents cardiovascular disease and determines survival in polyglobulic mice overexpressing erythropoietin, *Proc Natl Acad Sci USA. 97(21):11609–11613*

Seeliger, M. W., Grimm C., Ståhlberg, F., Friedburg, C., Jaissle, G., Zrenner, E., Guo, H., Remé, C. E., Humphries, P., Hofmann, F., Biel, M., Fariss, R. N., Redmond, T. M., and Wenzel., A., 2001, New views on RPE65 deficiency: the rod system is the source of vision in a mouse model of Leber congenital amaurosis. *Nat Genet. 29(1):70–74.*

Seeliger, M. W., Beck, S. C., Pereyra-Munoz, N., Dangel, S., Tsai, J.-Y., Luhmann, U. F. O., van de Pavert, S. A., Wijnholds, J., Samardzija, M., Wenzel, A., Zrenner, E., Narfstrom, K., Fahl, E., Tanimoto, N., Acar, N., and Tonagel, F., 2005, In vivo confocal imaging of the retina in animal models using scanning laser ophthalmology, *Vis Res. 45:3512–3519.*

Tazawa, Y., and Seaman, A. J., 1972, The electroretinogram of the living extracorporeal bovine eye. The influence of anoxia and hypothermia, *Invest Ophthalmol. 11(8):691–698.*

Wagner, K. F., Katschinski, D. M., Hasegawa, J., Schumacher, D., Meller, B., Gembruch, U., Schramm, U., Jelkmann, W., Gassmann, M., and Fandrey, J., 2001, Chronic inborn erythrocytosis leads to cardiac dysfunction and premature death in mice overexpressing erythropoietin, *Blood. 98(2):536–542.*

Characterization of Gene Expression Profiles of Normal Canine Retina and Brain Using a Retinal cDNA Microarray

Gerardo L. Paez, Barbara Zangerl, Kimberly Sellers, Gregory M. Acland, and Gustavo D. Aguirre

1 Introduction

Microarrays have been useful in the simultaneous analysis of transcript levels of thousands of genes in different physiological states of an organism, tissue or cell (Shalon et al., 1996; Schena et al., 1996). Construction of microarrays is most efficient when information is utilized from annotated genomes or expressed sequence tags (ESTs), and has led to new insights into animal development, cancer, infectious diseases and aging (Yoshida et al., 2002; Whitney et al., 1999; Alizadeh et al., 2000). A major limitation of the technique is the analysis of sequences represented on the array. This disadvantage is particularly problematic when analyzing highly specialized tissues such as the retina due to the repertoire of uniquely or preferentially expressed genes contributing to its structure and function. In the case of "orphan" species, commercial arrays are either not available or targeted to a broader research community and under represent the tissue of interest. The current available canine microarray is based on transcripts representing 11 non-retina tissues and gene predictions not supported by experimental data (Affymetrix Genechip® Canine Genome Array, Santa Clara, CA. USA). To obtain insight into intrinsic processes of the canine and human retina, great efforts are directed towards the identification and characterization of transcripts with functional relevance to this tissue (Swaroop and Zack, 2002; Chowers et al., 2003; Buraczynska et al., 2002; Zangerl et al., 2006). Despite these advances, a remaining challenge is to obtain an expression map of the canine retina/RPE transcriptome, further facilitating the identification of retinal susceptibility genes but, most importantly, offering an invaluable resource for functional genomics studies.

To overcome discussed limitations and drive the development of the canine retina transcriptome, we selected ∼4,500 genes from a normalized canine retinal EST database (Paez et al., 2006). These were used to construct a canine retinal cDNA

G.L. Paez
Department of Clinical Studies Philadelphia, School of Veterinary Medicine,
University of Pennsylvania Philadelphia. PA 19104, Tel: 215-898-7479, Fax: 215-573-2162
e-mail: gpaez@vet.upenn.edu

R.E. Anderson et al. (eds.), *Recent Advances in Retinal Degeneration*,
© Springer 2008

microarray for expression profiling of genes that are of interest in studies of normal development and function, and pathological conditions of the retina. As the brain and retina have a common embryological origin, a common brain pool was initially validated as reference sample for comparing expression profiles in multiple samples from animals with different molecularly defined retinal diseases, and at different stages of the disorder. The overall aim of this study is to identify retina specific gene expression patterns that will maximize the use in a variety of PRA dog models (Aguirre and Acland, 2006).

2 Material and Methods

Total RNA was isolated using Trizol reagent (Invitrogen) and further purified by Rneasy mini kit (Qiagen, Valencia, CA). Purity and RNA quality were evaluated by absorbance at 260nm and by denaturing formaldehyde agarose gel electrophoresis. High quality RNAs with A260/280 ratio over 1.8 and intact 28S and 18S RNA bands were used for microarray analysis.

To generate a RNA reference sample for microarray hybridizations, we pooled equal amounts of total RNA from the occipital, temporal and frontal brain lobes to achieve a homogeneous pool of transcripts. The pooled RNA was divided into aliquots ($2\mu g/\mu l$) and stored at $-80°C$ until use. For the purpose of this work 4 hybridization groups have been established. Each hybridization group contained five (for normal retina) or three (for frontal, occipital and temporal lobes respectively) unrelated samples labeled with Cy5 hybridized against the reference sample (labeled with Cy3).

For microarray production, 3,355 clones represented in the EST library as singlets were immediately chosen for printing. 1,014 contigs were reviewed individually. A representative clone was chosen for each of 894 contigs, while another 120 are represented by two clones to assure complete coverage of the obtained sequence.

Scanned images were processed using Genepix Pro version 4.1 software (Axon Instruments, Inc. USA). The main quantities of interest produced by the image analysis method (segmentation and background correction) are the (R, G) fluorescence intensity pairs for each gene on each array (where R=red for Cy5 and G=green for Cy3). Loess normalization was performed in order to remove systematic variation that occurs in every microarray experiment. An "MA plot", as described in Dudoit et al. (2002) is used to represent the (R, G) data, where M=$\log_2 R/G$ and A=$\log \sqrt{(RxG)}$. We apply loess normalization over the entire chip and loess normalization stratified by block followed by additional scaling via maximum likelihood estimation (MLE) or median absolute deviation (MAD).

Each hybridization was annotated according to MIAME (Minimal Information About a Microarray Experiment) standards with the GeneSpring version 7.1 software (Silicon Genetics, Agilent Technologies). Principal component analysis (PCA) was performed on a complete microarray dataset consisting of log-transformed expression values for each individual replicate. Genes preferentially expressed were identified by SAM. Northern blot analysis was used to confirm expression patterns.

3 Results

We applied a loess normalization stratified by block (sub-grid normalization), and also considered alternative normalization approaches including a general loess normalization on the entire array (global normalization), and sub-grid loess normalizations followed by either a MLE or MAD scaling procedure. We considered these variants of the loess normalization to ascertain the appropriateness and sufficiency of the sub-grid procedure with regard to our data (Table 1). There does not appear to be a substantial difference in the number of genes falling in any region of interest between the different normalization procedures, arguing against the use of additional variance scaling. From the above results, we feel that the sub-grid normalization approach is reasonable. By comparing the results of the different normalizations, however, we concluded that the added scaling via MLE or MAD did not demonstrate substantial changes in the gene detection results, while a global normalization overlooked much of the spatial dependencies addressed via the sub-grid normalization. Thus, the sub-grid normalization as performed in GeneSpring was reasonable and applied to the data generated by this study.

The SAM algorithm was used to identify statistically significant differences in expression. Using SAM with a FDR of 10%, 13.2% of the 3070 valid spots were found to hybridize strongly with the retina cDNA targets, implying that 405 genes on the microarray are preferentially expressed in the normal retina. Of the remaining 2665 valid spots, 2213 genes are shared between normal retina and the brain pool reference tissue, and 452 genes were preferentially expressed in the brain. Table 3 shows a subset of novel and known genes differentially expressed in retina and brain, respectively.

Table 1 Contingency table results for each of the datasets showing how many genes/spots lad in each subregion on the associated scatter plot. The differentially expressed genes did not affect the Loess normalization curve significantly. MLE, loess normalization stratified by block followed by additional scaling via maximum likelihood estimation; MAD, median absolute deviation

Counts for loess normalization over the entire chip		
0	6	16
2	4254	2
40	7	0
Counts for loess normalization stratified by blocks		
0	8	11
4	4233	7
38	26	0
Counts for loess normalization + MLE scaling		
0	18	7
13	4213	11
29	36	0
Counts for loess normalization + MAD scaling		
0	12	11
5	4215	7
37	40	0

To complete the gene expression profile between normal retina and brain regions, the array dataset was analyzed using PCA (Fig. 1). PCA revealed retina replicates and the three brain regions clustered independently, and there was a large degree of separation between them. The overall clustering pattern formed from PCA, additionally, showed no differences in retinal gene expression in animals from different litters, or between males and females (Fig. 1). To confirm the microarray results, we selected five genes for northern analysis based on their microarray expression profiles. Two show preferential expression in retina (*NEUROD4*, DR010030A20H09), two in brain (*SYN2*, *SPP1*), and one was equally expressed in retina and brain

Table 2 Retina enriched genes

Gene	Unigene	Retina/Brain
SAG	Hs308	37
	Cfa. 7077	
GNB1	Hs 648519	36.5
	Cfa.3191	
PDC	Hs. 580	36
	Cfa.1202	
FJL39155	Hs. 20103	31.5
RHO	Hs. 247565	27.5
	Cfa. 7396	
EST	Hs.150406	26
PDE6B	Hs. 59872	25
	Cfa. 3793	
ROM1	Hs 281564	24.5
EST		23
RDH8	Hs 272405	21

Table 3 Brain enriched genes

Gene	Unigene	Retina/Brain
PLP1	Hs. 1787	−25
	Cfa.3274	
SPP1	Hs. 313	−20
SPARCL1	Hs. 1424	−17
NISCH	Hs. 435290	−16
LMO4	Hs. 436792	−11
SNY2	Hs. 445503	−9
GPM6A	Hs. 75819	−8
DDEF1	Hs. 106015	−6.5
	Cfa. 10191	
NRN1	Hs. 103291	−6.5
SNAP25	Hs. 167317	−6

List of the top 10 brain and retina enriched genes in a retina brain comparison. The corresponding Unigen cluster number, expression ratios and function are listed. Hs. *Homo sapiens*, Cfa. *Canis familiaris*

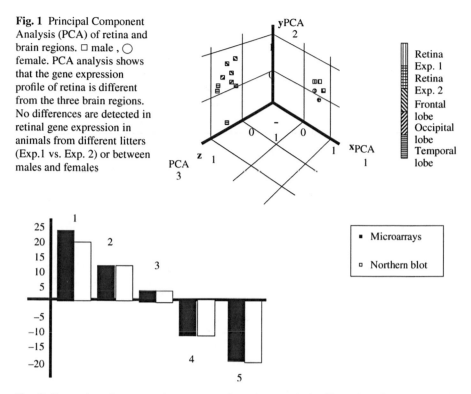

Fig. 1 Principal Component Analysis (PCA) of retina and brain regions. □ male , ○ female. PCA analysis shows that the gene expression profile of retina is different from the three brain regions. No differences are detected in retinal gene expression in animals from different litters (Exp.1 vs. Exp. 2) or between males and females

Fig. 2 Comparison between microarrays and northern analysis. The selected gees tested in microarrays and northern blot gave comparable results. 1- DR010030A20H09, 2- NEUROD4: Neurogenic differentiation 4; 3- DR010024A20G01 4- SYN2: Synapsin II; 5- SPP1: Secreted phosphoprotein 1

(DR010024A20G01). We found that the northern blots showed the same patterns of expression in retina and brain as predicted by the microarray data (Fig. 2).

4 Discussion

As an initial step in evaluating the microarray, we have examined gene expression pattern differences between normal retina and the brain pool tissue reference sample. As expected, known photoreceptor genes were expressed in retina, demonstrating the specificity of the hybridization. Over a third of the differentially expressed clones were ESTs, representing potentially novel genes that are enriched or even specific to retina or brain (Zhao, 2003).

Many genes important to neural activity were differentially expressed, such as ion channels (transport class) and cytoskeletal proteins (structural class). Genes involved in more general processes, such as energy generation, also showed retina or brain preferential expression. Compared to the total number of genes with preferential expression, we found higher frequencies of proliferation and cell death genes expressed in the brain than retina, and nucleic acid processing genes in retina than brain.

Principal component analysis was done to compare the expression profiles within and across the tissue samples. It is clear that, despite the common embryonic origin of retina and brain tissues, there are two different gene expression profiles corresponding to retina and brain regions, respectively. PCA also reveals strong similarities in each of the replicates for a given tissue, showing the sensitivity and robustness of the custom cDNA microarray. In regards to the retina, we did not observe significant differences in gene expression profiles between 16 week old dogs of different gender, different breeds, or different litters. These results can now be extended to examine the gene expression profiles of different models at different stages of the disease.

References

Aguirre, G.D. and Acland, G.M. Models, mutants and man: Searching for unique phenotypes and genes in the dog model of inherited retinal degeneration. *The Dog and its Genome.* Cold Spring Harbor 2006; chapter 16, 291–325.

Alizadeh M, Gelfman CM, Bench SR, Hjelmeland LM. Expression and splicing of FGF receptor mRNAs during APRE-19 cell differentiation in vitro. *Invest Ophthalmol Vis Sci.* 2000; 41(8):2357–62.

Buraczynska M, Mears AJ, Zareparst S, Farjo R, Filippova E, Yuan Y, MacNee SP, Hughes B, Swaroop A. Gene expression profile of native human retinal pigment epithelium. *IOVS* 2002; 43(9):603–607.

Chowers I, Liu D, Farkas, RH, Gunatilaka TL, Hackman AS, Bernstein SL, Campochiaro PA, Parmigiani G, Zack DJ. Gene expression variation in the adult human retina. *Human Molecular Genetics* 2003; 12(22):2881–2893.

Dudoit S, and Fridlyand J. A prediction-based resampling method for estimating the number of clusters in a dataset. *Genome Biol.* 2002 Jun 25; 3(7): RESEARCH0036. Epub 2002 June 25.

Paez GL, Sellers KF, Band M, Acland GM, Zangerl B, Aguirre GD. Characterization of gene expression profiles of normal canine retina and brain using a retinal cDNA microarray. *Mol Vis* 2006 Sep 7; 12:1048–1056.

Schena M, Shalon D, Heller R, Chai A, Brown PO, Davis RW. Parallel human genome analysis: microarray-based expression monitoring of 1000 genes. *Proc Natl Acad Sci U S A.* 1996; 1; 93(20):10614–9.

Shalon D, Smith SJ, Brown PO. A DNA microarray system for analyzing complex DNA samples using two-color fluorescent probe hybridization. *Genome Res* 1996; 6(7):639–645.

Swaroop A, Zack. DJ Transcriptome analysis of the retina. *Genome Biology* 2002; 3(8): 1022.1–1022.4.

Whitney LW, Becker KG, Tresser NJ, Caballero-Ramos CI, Munson PJ, Prabhu VV, Trent JM, McFarland HF, Biddison WE. Analysis of gene expression in mutiple sclerosis lesions using cDNA microarrays. *Ann Neurol* 1999; 46(3):425–428.

Yoshida S, Yashar BM, Hiriyanna S, Swaroop A. Microarray analysis of gene expression in the aging human retina. *Invest Ophthalmol Vis Sci.* 2002; 43(8):2554–2560.

Zangerl B, Sun Q, et al. Development and characterization of a normalized canine retinal cDNA library for genomic and expression studies. *IOVS* 2006 Jun; 47(6):2632–2638.

Zhao Y, Hong DH, Pawlyk B, Yue G, Adamian M, Grynberg M, Godzik A, Li T. The retinitis pigmentosa GTPase regulator (RPGR)- interacting protein: subserving RPGR function and participating in disk morophogenesis. *Proc Natl Acad Sci USA.* 2003 Apr 1; 100(7):3965–70. Epub 2003 Mar 21.

Toward a Higher Fidelity Model of AMD

Brian J. Raisler, Miho Nozaki, Judit Baffi, William W. Hauswirth,
and Jayakrishna Ambati

1 Introduction

Age-related macular degeneration (AMD) is the leading cause of acquired blindness
in the elderly population of industrialized countries (Klein et al., 1997; Vingerling
et al., 1995; Leibowitz et al., 1980). Characterized clinically in two stages; 'dry'
AMD consists of deposition of drusen under the RPE, particularly in the macular region, while 'wet/exudative' AMD consists of formation of new, invasive
blood vessels originating from the choriodal vascular bed. Dry AMD can lead to
vision loss due to geographic atrophy and photoreceptor loss, but most patients
with drusen do not suffer loss of vision. Exudative AMD is the less common
form, but is by far the greater cause of vision loss. Retina scarring and macular
edema due to poorly formed and leaky choriodal vessels contribute to visual loss in
advanced AMD.

1.1 Multiple Risk Factors

AMD is recognized as a multifactoral disease; many contributing factors are
involved including both genetic and environmental elements. Risk factors for
developing AMD include increased age, sunlight exposure, smoking, and dietary
contributions all of which may be mediating disease progression by increased
oxidative stress. Oxidative stress has been identified as a risk factor for AMD
and may act through mitochondrial (Beatty et al., 2000). As counterpoint to the
increased oxidative damage causing increased risk of AMD progression, a diet
rich in anti-oxidants and protective lutein and xeazanthin yields a decreased risk of
AMD (AREDS, 2001). Genetic correlations point toward inflammatory pathways
having a role in AMD disease progression. Polymorphisms occurring in genes for

B.J. Raisler
Department of Ophthalmology, University of Kentucky, Lexington, Kentucky, 40356,
Tel: 859-323-9787, Fax: 859-257-9700
e-mail: raisler@uky.edu

R.E. Anderson et al. (eds.), *Recent Advances in Retinal Degeneration*,
© Springer 2008

complement factor H (CFH) (Edwards et al., 2005; Hageman et al., 2005; Haines et al., 2005; Klein et al., 2005; Magnusson et al., 2006), factor B (Gold et al., 2006), the LOC387715 locus (Rivera et al., 2005), HTRA1(Dewan et al., 2006; Yang et al., 2006), and complement component 2 (Gold et al., 2006) have each been identified as major risk factors for AMD. In particular, the high risk for AMD associated with the 402H allele of complement factor H coupled with findings of complement components in both human drusen and in the drusen-like deposits of macrophage deficient mice indicates that inflammatory processes are central to the disease state. We can conclude that at least two pathways, inflammation and oxidative stress, have major roles in contributing to AMD pathogenesis.

1.2 The Role of Macrophages

One of the primary factors involved in progression to drusen deposition in AMD appears to be a malfunction in macrophage recruitment and activity. Macrophages normally act as scavengers to remove cellular debris and prevent the buildup of toxic components beneath the RPE. If this mechanism is disrupted or reduced later in life, accumulations of metabolic by-products can reach damaging levels and lead to early stages of AMD characterized by drusen deposition geographic atrophy. As this process continues, there may be a shift in macrophage function from physiologically useful scavenging to pathological upregulation of pro-angiogenic factors and establishment of CNV. Early in the process loss of macrophage activity may limit the scavenging of by-products of oxidative stress. Later AMD may be mediated in part through an inflammatory mechanism involving macrophage production of various cytokines including VEGF, TNFα, IL-6, and IL-1β. Understanding the shift from 'helpful' macrophage function of removing sub-RPE accumulations, to 'harmful' macrophage inflammatory actions is key to successfully applying our knowledge to better patient care.

The focus of our current research involves the mouse knockout strains Ccr2 -/- and Ccl2 -/- that are deficient in macrophage recruitment, as they lack either the receptor or cognate ligand respectively that is required for macrophage signaling. These mice exhibit bilateral drusen like accumulation beneath their RPE that begins later in life and mirrors the progression of human AMD (Ambati et al., 2003). As in human AMD, a certain percentage of mice with drusen-like deposits spontaneously progress to CNV. This is considered to be higher fidelity model of AMD than the more typically used method of laser-induced rupture of Bruch's membrane to induce CNV. The drawback, of course, being the longer time-line required to establish a drusen-like phenotype and the lack of uniformity in progression to exudative CNV. Still, this model directly relates to the role of macrophage deficiency and therefore provides an excellent platform for testing hypotheses relating this interesting area of AMD pathology.

Table 1 Proteomic analysis of Ccl2-/- and wild-type RPE/Choriod samples

Wild-type		Ccl2-/-	
Oxidative stress	mediators of oxidative Stress	Oxidative stress	Mediators of oxidative stress
β and γ-crystallin	α-crystallin A Chaperone	β and γ-crystallin	Absent
	Superoxide dismutase		
	Peroxiredoxins 5 and 6		
Anti-apoptosis	Pro-apoptosis	Anti-apoptosis	Pro-apoptosis
Cystatin B	Absent	Absent	Adenosine A3 receptor
			Cathepsin D & Z precursors
Cytoskeletal disruption		Cytoskeletal disruption	
Absent		Actin-depolymerizing factors	
		Tubulin A chaperone	

1.3 Preliminary Studies

Proteomic analysis of RPE/Choriod samples from 9 month age-matched Ccl2-/- and wild-type mice showed a pattern of oxidative damage and dys-regulation of apoptosis (Table 1). Our analysis revealed a pattern of β and γ-crystallins that are indicative of oxidative stress was present in both the wild-type and the macrophage deficient Ccl2-/- mice. However, conspicuously absent in the Ccl2-/- mice were mediators of oxidative damage found in the wild-type samples: α-crystallin A chaperone protein, superoxide dismutase (SOD), and peroxiredoxins 5 and 6. Similarly, the differential on apoptotic factors demonstrated that pro-apoptotic factors such as adenosine A3 receptor and precursors to Cathepsin D and Cathepsin Z were present only in the Ccl2-/- samples. The anti-apoptotic protein Cystatin B was found solely in the wild-type sample. Also present only in the Ccl2-/- samples were indications of cytoskeletal disruption, including actin-depolymerizing factors and tubulin-A chaperone proteins. This pattern of oxidative stress indicates that macrophage function may be crucial to mediating the effects of age-related accumulation of oxidative damage as theorized above.

2 Gene Therapy

As AMD is a chronic disease, some have suggested that a long-term therapeutic strategy involving expression of an anti-angiogenic factor like PEDF (Rasmussen et al., 2001; Mori et al., 2002; Saishin et al. , 2005), inhibitors of matrix remodeling like TIMP-2 (Murata et al., 2000), or interfering with the expression of pro-angiogenic pathways involving VEGF signaling (Cashman et al. , 2006; Eter et al., 2006; Wada et al., 1999). Vector selection for therapeutic genes has included retroviral constructs which seem to home to areas of CNV in the laser photocoagulation model (Murata et al., 1998). Adenoviral vectors have been used for expression of genes or methods of interfering with gene products and offer a brief, controlled period of expression. Recombinant adeno-associated viral (rAAV) vectors offer the longest term expression and the ability to transfect dividing and non-dividing cells.

2.1 Experimental Design

As a means of studying the effects of macrophage function in the aged Ccl2-/-mice, we used a gene therapy approach to restore macrophage signaling. The mice were divided into two groups after fundoscopic examination to classify whether they exhibited drusen-like sub-RPE deposits. The mice without drusen at the time of initial examination were deemed a 'prevention' group (n=9). Mice which had drusen were placed in the 'regression' group (n=9). The hypothesis is that restoration of macrophage signaling would allow clearance of the sub-RPE deposits in eyes where such deposits were already present (regression) or reduce or eliminate the deposits in eyes currently without drusen-like deposits. Each group was treated in the same way; rAAV vector expressing Ccl2 (AAV-Ccl2) was injected subretinally into one eye. The contralateral eye was injected with a control vector expressing GFP (AAV-GFP). In this pilot study, the genes were under the control of the ubiquitously expressing chicken beta-actin, cytomegalovirus promoter (CBA-CMV) to achieve maximal levels of the target construct.

2.2 Experimental Results

After a period of 6 weeks to allow for maximal vector expression, the fundus of each mouse was examined again for drusen-like deposits, and for autofluorescence. In the prevention group, all control eyes that were injected with AAV-GFP had progressed to a drusen-positive phenotype (Fig. 1a). Eyes where macrophage signaling had been restored by the AAV-CCL2 vector did not exhibit sub-RPE deposits (Fig. 1b). Even more significant were the results from the regression group of mice. As expected the control eyes showed no reduction in the degree of persistent drusen (Fig. 1c). The AAV-CCL2 treated eyes had a uniform and substantial reduction in drusen-like deposits (Fig. 1d).

During a sub-retinal injection, a portion of the retina can temporarily detach. This area of detachment corresponds well with the area of maximal AAV transduction. The clearing of deposits observed in the regression group occurred in the same area that was detached during the subretinal injections in these eyes. In some eyes within the regression group, persistant deposits could be observed at the periphery of the retina. Presumably, macrophages were not recruited to these areas, and little or no phagocytosis of deposits had occurred.

In order to confirm that macrophages were being recruited to AAV-Ccl2 treated eyes, a subset of eyes (n=4) was analyzed by flow cytometry. Eyes were enucleated and the posterior segment dissected, carefully separating the choriod from the neural retina. Macrophages were defined as F4/80$^+$CD11c$^-$ staining cells. The number of macrophages as a percentage of total cells was calculated for the choroid and retina separately. The percentage of macrophages increases specifically in the choroid of AAV-Ccl2 treated eyes (Fig. 2). This confirms that macrophage signaling has been restored and that it is likely that these macrophages are functioning to remove sub-RPE deposits.

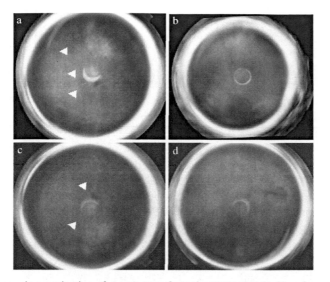

Fig. 1 Funduscopic examination of mouse eyes from the prevention (a, b) and regression (c, d) experimental groups. Eyes treated with AAV-GFP had established drusen-like deposits at 6 weeks post injection as indicated by arrowheads (a), while eyes injected with AAV-Ccl2 had not progressed to the drusen phenotype (b). In eyes were drusen were already present at the time of injection, AAV-GFP failed to clear deposits (c) while AAV-Ccl2 cleared deposits in the area of the injection

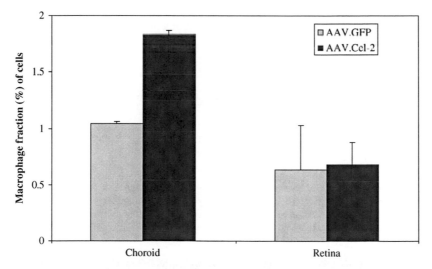

Fig. 2 Macrophages as a percent of total cell number were analyzed by flow cytometry. Recruitment of macrophages to the choroid was clearly increased in eyes injected with AAV-Ccl2 when compared with their contralateral control eye injected with AAV-GFP. No difference was observed in the neural retina

3 Future Directions

While it is encouraging that a gene therapy approach was capable of resolving the drusen-like phenotype in the eyes of aged Ccl-2 mice, much work remains to be done. It is not clear whether clearing of these deposits would translate to reduced incidence of spontaneous CNV later in life. This holds true both for the Ccl-2 mouse model and for AMD patients. While drusen are a common clinical hallmark of AMD, some patients of Asian ethnic background progress to exudative AMD without ever having presented clinically with drusen. In patients with drusen, if the drusen was reduced or eliminated, would this delay or prevent disease progression? The answer is not simple or clear. It would be informative to study mice treated with this gene therapy approach for a longer period of time to determine whether CNV is also reduced as a result of sub-RPE deposit clearance. This would be an arduous study to undertake due to the Ccl2 -/- slow progression to the drusen phenotype, and the relatively low percentage of drusen-positive mice that later progress to spontaneous CNV.

These preliminary results indicate the ability of a single, sub-retinal injection of AAV-Ccl2 to restore macrophage signaling in Ccl2 -/- mice, the preferential recruitment of macrophages to the choroid, and the clearance of drusen-like deposits. It would be illuminating to examine these treated eyes by immunohistochemistry to look for other hallmark proteins that have been identified in human drusen and in Ccl2 -/- deposits. Funduscopic examination may not tell the whole story. Perhaps complement components, as markers of inflammatory processes, or oxidatively modified proteins are still present in the sub-RPE space.

Lastly, it is unlikely that any clinical application of gene therapy would move forward using the ubiquitous CBA-CMV promoter to drive expression. Fortunately much more elegant designs using promoters targeted to a specific cellular sub-set or inducible promoter systems that can be turned 'on' or 'off' at need are now readily available.

Acknowledgments This work was supported in part by NIH grants EY15422 and 5T32DC000065 and by Research to Prevent Blindness.

References

AREDS Report no. 8. (2001) A randomized, placebo-controlled, clinical trial of high-dose supplementation with vitamins C and E, beta carotene, and zinc for age-related macular degeneration and vision loss. *Arch. Ophthalmol.* **119**, 1417–1436.

Ambati J., Anand A., Fernandez S., Sakurai E., Lynn B.C., Kuziel W.A., Rollins B.J., & Ambati B.K. (2003) An animal model of age-related macular degeneration in senescent Ccl-2- or Ccr-2-deficient mice. *Nat. Med.* **9**, 1390–1397.

Beatty S., Koh H., Phil M., Henson D., & Boulton M. (2000) The role of oxidative stress in the pathogenesis of age-related macular degeneration. *Surv. Ophthalmol.* **45**, 115–134.

Cashman S.M., Bowman L., Christofferson J., & Kumar-Singh R. (2006) Inhibition of choroidal neovascularization by adenovirus-mediated delivery of short hairpin RNAs targeting VEGF as a potential therapy for AMD. *Invest Ophthalmol. Vis. Sci.* **47**, 3496–3504.

Dewan A., Liu M., Hartman S., Zhang S.S., Liu D.T., Zhao C., Tam P.O., Chan W.M., Lam D.S., Snyder M., Barnstable C., Pang C.P., & Hoh J. (2006) HTRA1 promoter polymorphism in wet age-related macular degeneration. *Science* **314**, 989–992.

Edwards A.O., Ritter R., III, Abel K.J., Manning A., Panhuysen C., & Farrer L.A. (2005) Complement factor H polymorphism and age-related macular degeneration. *Science* **308**, 421–424.

Eter N., Krohne T.U., & Holz F.G. (2006) New pharmacologic approaches to therapy for age-related macular degeneration. *BioDrugs.* **20**, 167–179.

Gold B., Merriam J.E., Zernant J., Hancox L.S., Taiber A.J., Gehrs K., Cramer K., Neel J., Bergeron J., Barile G.R., Smith R.T., Hageman G.S., Dean M., & Allikmets R. (2006) Variation in factor B (BF) and complement component 2 (C2) genes is associated with age-related macular degeneration. *Nat. Genet.* **38**, 458–462.

Hageman G.S., Anderson D.H., Johnson L.V., Hancox L.S., Taiber A.J., Hardisty L.I., Hageman J.L., Stockman H.A., Borchardt J.D., Gehrs K.M., Smith R.J., Silvestri G., Russell S.R., Klaver C.C., Barbazetto I., Chang S., Yannuzzi L.A., Barile G.R., Merriam J.C., Smith R.T., Olsh A.K., Bergeron J., Zernant J., Merriam J.E., Gold B., Dean M., & Allikmets R. (2005) A common haplotype in the complement regulatory gene factor H (HF1/CFH) predisposes individuals to age-related macular degeneration. *Proc. Natl. Acad. Sci. U.S.A.* **102**, 7227–7232.

Haines J.L., Hauser M.A., Schmidt S., Scott W.K., Olson L.M., Gallins P., Spencer K.L., Kwan S.Y., Noureddine M., Gilbert J.R., Schnetz-Boutaud N., Agarwal A., Postel E.A., & Pericak-Vance M.A. (2005) Complement factor H variant increases the risk of age-related macular degeneration. *Science* **308**, 419–421.

Klein R., Klein B.E., Jensen S.C., & Meuer S.M. (1997) The five-year incidence and progression of age-related maculopathy: the Beaver Dam eye study. *Ophthalmology* **104**, 7–21.

Klein R.J., Zeiss C., Chew E.Y., Tsai J.Y., Sackler R.S., Haynes C., Henning A.K., SanGiovanni J.P., Mane S.M., Mayne S.T., Bracken M.B., Ferris F.L., Ott J., Barnstable C., & Hoh J. (2005) Complement factor H polymorphism in age-related macular degeneration. *Science* **308**, 385–389.

Leibowitz H.M., Krueger D.E., Maunder L.R., Milton R.C., Kini M.M., Kahn H.A., Nickerson R.J., Pool J., Colton T.L., Ganley J.P., Loewenstein J.I., & Dawber T.R. (1980) The Framingham eye study monograph: An ophthalmological and epidemiological study of cataract, glaucoma, diabetic retinopathy, macular degeneration, and visual acuity in a general population of 2631 adults, 1973–1975. *Surv. Ophthalmol.* **24**, 335–610.

Magnusson K.P., Duan S., Sigurdsson H., Petursson H., Yang Z., Zhao Y., Bernstein P.S., Ge J., Jonasson F., Stefansson E., Helgadottir G., Zabriskie N.A., Jonsson T., Bjornsson A., Thorlacius T., Jonsson P.V., Thorleifsson G., Kong A., Stefansson H., Zhang K., Stefansson K., & Gulcher J.R. (2006) CFH Y402H confers similar risk of soft drusen and both forms of advanced AMD. *PLoS. Med.* **3**, e5.

Mori K., Gehlbach P., Yamamoto S., Duh E., Zack D.J., Li Q., Berns K.I., Raisler B.J., Hauswirth W.W., & Campochiaro P.A. (2002) AAV-mediated gene transfer of pigment epithelium-derived factor inhibits choroidal neovascularization. *Invest Ophthalmol. Vis. Sci.* **43**, 1994–2000.

Murata T., Cui J., Taba K.E., Oh J.Y., Spee C., Hinton D.R., & Ryan S.J. (2000) The possibility of gene therapy for the treatment of choroidal neovascularization. *Ophthalmology* **107**, 1364–1373.

Murata T., Hangai M., Ishibashi T., Spee C., Gordon E.M., Anderson W.F., Hinton D.R., & Ryan S.J. (1998) Retrovirus-mediated gene transfer to photocoagulation-induced choroidal neovascular membranes. *Invest Ophthalmol. Vis. Sci.* **39**, 2474–2478.

Rasmussen H., Chu K.W., Campochiaro P., Gehlbach P.L., Haller J.A., Handa J.T., Nguyen Q.D., & Sung J.U. (2001) Clinical protocol. An open-label, phase I, single administration, dose-escalation study of ADGVPEDF.11D (ADPEDF) in neovascular age-related macular degeneration (AMD). *Hum. Gene Ther.* **12**, 2029–2032.

Rivera A., Fisher S.A., Fritsche L.G., Keilhauer C.N., Lichtner P., Meitinger T., & Weber B.H. (2005) Hypothetical LOC387715 is a second major susceptibility gene for age-related macular degeneration, contributing independently of complement factor H to disease risk. *Hum. Mol. Genet.* **14**, 3227–3236.

Saishin Y., Silva R.L., Saishin Y., Kachi S., Aslam S., Gong Y.Y., Lai H., Carrion M., Harris B., Hamilton M., Wei L., & Campochiaro P.A. (2005) Periocular gene transfer of pigment epithelium-derived factor inhibits choroidal neovascularization in a human-sized eye. *Hum. Gene Ther.* **16**, 473–478.

Vingerling J.R., Dielemans I., Hofman A., Grobbee D.E., Hijmering M., Kramer C.F., & de Jong P.T. (1995) The prevalence of age-related maculopathy in the Rotterdam Study. *Ophthalmology* **102**, 205–210.

Wada M., Ogata N., Otsuji T., & Uyama M. (1999) Expression of vascular endothelial growth factor and its receptor (KDR/flk-1) mRNA in experimental choroidal neovascularization. *Curr. Eye Res.* **18**, 203–213.

Yang Z., Camp N.J., Sun H., Tong Z., Gibbs D., Cameron D.J., Chen H., Zhao Y., Pearson E., Li X., Chien J., Dewan A., Harmon J., Bernstein P.S., Shridhar V., Zabriskie N.A., Hoh J., Howes K., & Zhang K. (2006) A variant of the HTRA1 gene increases susceptibility to age-related macular degeneration. *Science* **314**, 992–993.

The Potential of Ambient Light Restriction to Restore Function to the Degenerating P23H-3 Rat Retina

Krisztina Valter, Diana K. Kirk, and Jonathan Stone

1 Introduction

Reviewing, in 1999, the non-genetic factors that regulate retinal degeneration, we (Stone et al., 1999) hypothesized that the loss of vision during degeneration results only partly from photoreceptor death. Significant visual loss results, we argued, from loss of performance in surviving photoreceptors, and might be reversible. To test the idea, we first demonstrated that, in the rhodopsin-mutant P23H-3 transgenic rat, the retina is hypersensitive to modest levels of ambient light, which accelerate photoreceptor death, shorten outer segments and degrade the ERG more severely than in non-degenerative controls (Walsh et al., 2004). A comparable hypersensitivity to ambient light has since been reported in a rhodopsin-mutant degeneration which occurs naturally in the dog (Cideciyan et al., 2005). We then showed that the reduction of the a-wave and the shortening of outer segments, induced by ambient light in the P23H-3 retina, can be reversed by reducing ambient light levels. (Jozwick et al., 2006).

The idea that restricting the exposure of the retina to light might slow the retinal degenerations goes back over 100 years (Johnson, 1901) (cited in (Berson, 1971)). In humans suffering retinal degeneration, however, results of light restriction have been mixed, Berson (1971) reporting no effect , while Pe'er and Meron (reviewed in (Stone et al., 1999)) reported slowing of visual field loss in 10 of 14 patients. In animal models (the RCS rat (Dowling and Sidman, 1962; Kaitz, 1976), the P23H transgenic mouse (Naash et al., 1996) and rat (Bicknell et al., 2002), and in the rhodopsin-mutant dog (Cideciyan et al., 2005); reviewed in (Paskowitz et al., 2006)), light restriction slows retinal degeneration robustly. The idea that light restriction might reverse the loss of retinal function is more recent.

This study explores light-restriction-induced functional recovery in two ways. First, we have tested whether restriction of ambient light is effective in infancy, when

K. Valter
CNS Stability and Degeneration Group and ARC Centre of Excellence in Vision Science, Research School of Biological Sciences, The Australian National University, Tel: 02 6125 1095, Fax: 02 6125 0758
e-mail: valter@rsbs.anu.edu.au

R.E. Anderson et al. (eds.), *Recent Advances in Retinal Degeneration,*
© Springer 2008

the degeneration is most rapid (Walsh et al., 2004), as well as young adulthood; and, second, we have traced the recovery over a much longer period (3 months). Results confirm the hypersensitivity of the P23H-3 retina to modest ambient light, show that the protective and restorative effects of light restriction can be induced in both infancy and adulthood, and show that, over time, the restoration of the a-wave of the ERG reaches an amplitude equal to scotopic controls and almost 3-fold greater than mesopic controls. This is a much greater increase than we were able to demonstrate previously (Jozwick et al., 2006), over a shorter recovery period. We are separately studying the mechanism of the recovery, to determine the contributions of photoreceptor death rates, outer segment regrowth and cone recovery.

2 Methods

All procedures were in accord with the ARVO Statement for the use of Animals in Ophthalmic and Vision Research, and with the requirements of the Australian National University Animal Ethics Committee.

2.1 Strains Studied

Transgenic rats containing the P23H mutation on the rhodopsin gene were used (Line 3, from Beckman Laboratories, University of California, San Francisco). P23H-3 homozygous animals were established as a breeding colony. The animals used in the present experiments were heterozygotes, the offspring of mating P23H-3 homozygotes with Sprague-Dawley controls.

2.2 Experimental Design

All animals were raised in cyclic ambient light (12h light, 12h dark) with the light phase at either 5 lux (mesopic conditions) or 40 lux (mesopic conditions. Animals were exposed to 4 variants of these two conditions. One group (scotopic controls) was raised to P120 in scotopic conditions. One group (mesopic controls) was raised to P120 in mesopic conditions. One group (scotopic/mesopic) was raised to P30 in scotopic conditions and was then moved to mesopic conditions until P40, P60, P80, P100 or P120. One group (mesopic/scotopic) was raised to P30 in mesopic conditions and was then moved to scotopic conditions until P40, P60, P80, P100 or P120.

2.3 Recording the ERG

The dark-adapted flash-evoked electroretinogram (ERG) was recorded, as described previously (Walsh et al., 2004). Animals were dark-adapted overnight, and prepared in dim red illumination. After a re-adaptation period of 10 minutes, the ERG was

Fig. 1 Flash-evoked, dark adapted ERG data from P23H-3 rats. (A) Responses from P23H-3 rats aged P100 to a standard flash. The responses were recorded from a rat raised in mesopic conditions, and from a rat raised to P30 in mesopic conditions and then in scotopic conditions. The asterisks mark the peak of the a-wave, which is determined principally by rods. (B) The amplitude of the dark-adapted a-wave, as a function of age, for 4 rearing conditions. The key findings of this study are shown by the M/S data points. In animals raised in mesopic (M) conditions, the ERG at P30 was small. In animals raised in mesopic conditions and then moved to scotopic (S) conditions (the M/S group), the amplitude of the a-wave increased, almost doubling in amplitude. By P120 the a-wave in the M/S group was 2–3 larger than in the M (mesopic throughout) group. The error bars show SEMs

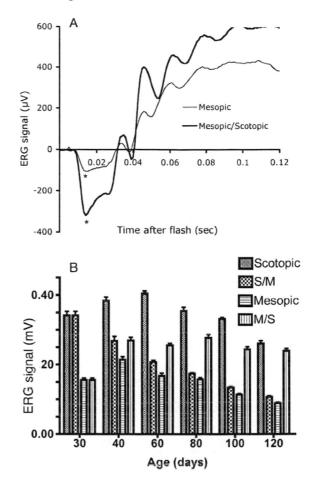

recorded in response to a standard flash of 20×10^3 photoisomerisaton/rod/sec. This flash is approximately 2 log units dimmer than saturating. Responses were recorded to the same flash given at 3 minute intervals for an hour. Only responses recorded when body temperature was in the range of $37\pm0.5°C$ were included. For each animal, 8–10 responses fitting these criteria were recorded, the a-waves measured and their mean calculated. A minimum of 6 animals were recorded at each time point in each group. For each time point, the mean and standard deviation of these means were calculated, and are shown in Fig. 1.

3 Results

3.1 Mesopic Rearing Degrades the ERG

The amplitude of the ERG varied with both age and ambient light. In scotopic conditions, a-wave amplitude increased from $\sim350\mu V$ at P30 to $\sim400\mu V$ at P60, and then declined to $250\mu V$ at P120. In mesopic conditions the a-wave at P30 was $\sim150\mu V$ and by P120 had declined to $\sim100\mu V$ (60% less than scotopic). The mesopia-induced degradation of the a-wave was thus substantial and sustained. Comparing scotopic and mesopic groups, the difference in amplitude is strongly significant at all ages.

3.2 Mesopic Exposure After Scotopic Rearing Degrades the a-Wave

When animals raised in scotopic conditions to P30 were exposed to mesopic conditions, the a-wave fell steadily in amplitude. By P60, mean amplitude was $\sim200\mu V$, 50% below the age-matched scotopic value; by P120, its amplitude had fallen to $107\mu V$, a reduction of $\sim60\%$. Again the timing and form of the ERG were similar in scotopic and mesopic conditions; ambient exposure affected the amplitude of all components. The mesopia-induced reduction in a-wave amplitude is strongly significant at all ages except P30, where the data is shared between the two groups.

3.3 The Mesopia-Induced Degradation of the ERG is Largely Reversible

When animals raised to P30 in mesopic conditions were exposed to scotopic conditions, the a-wave increased (Fig. 1) reaching $250\mu V$ at P40 and maintaining this value to the latest age studied, P120. The value at P120 matched the scotopic reared value and was 2.5-fold greater than the mesopic-reared value at this age. Comparing mesopic and mesopic/scotopic groups statistically, the increase in a-wave amplitude associated with light reduction is strongly significant at all ages, excluding P30, where the data is shared between the two groups.

3.4 Scotopic Rearing Does Not Increase the Vulnerability of the Retina

We tested whether scotopic rearing to P30 makes the retina more vulnerable to damage by mesopic light. The question arises because previous workers. (Penn and Anderson, 1991) reported that scotopic-reared retinas are more vulnerable to light damage than retinas raised in brighter conditions. In the present paradigm, the degradation of the a-wave induced by mesopia in the scotopic-reared retina was substantial and progressive, but was no worse than in mesopic-reared controls. Comparing mesopic and scotopic/mesopic groups, the differences in a-wave amplitude was statistically significant between P30 and P60. From P80 to P120 the difference between the groups become non-significant.

4 Discussion

Perhaps the most important element of the present results is evidence that restricting ambient light to scotopic levels can significantly increase the amplitude of the a-wave in P23H-3 rats. This builds on our earlier report. (Jozwick et al., 2006) that ERG loss in the P23H-3 rat is partially reversible by light restriction. That study reported a 30% increase over a period of 5w; this study demonstrates much larger increases over a period of 90d, at the end of which the a-wave is almost 3-fold larger than in mesopic-reared controls. Additional observations show that mesopia-induced degradation of the a-wave can be reduced or reversed by light restriction both during infancy (before P30), and from P30 into young adulthood (P120).

4.1 Clinical Relevance

The ability of the a-wave in a rhodopsin-mutant degeneration such as the P23H transgenic to regain amplitude is of interest clinically, for it suggests that similar recovery may be possible in rhodopsin-mutant forms of human retinal degeneration. To date, restoration of visual function to the surviving retina has not been considered a realistic goal in the treatment of the retinal degenerations, without cellular transplantation or genetic therapy. Significant recovery may, the present results suggest, be a realistic goal for some forms of degeneration, by the manipulation of non-genetic factors, in the present work ambient light.

The present experiments were designed to test two other clinical parameters, age and treatment-induced risk. Concerning age, present results show that the ERG of young adults is maximal where ambient light is kept to scotopic levels throughout rearing, but can regain significant amplitude even when restriction is not begun until after the critical period of photoreceptor development (approximately P15 to P30 in the rat (Maslim et al., 1997; Walsh et al., 2004)). Concerning treatment-induced risk, our results suggest that early light restriction does not predispose the P23H-3 retina to damage induced by raised ambient illumination. Both results, to the extent that they prove relevant to human retinal degenerations, encourage the trial of light management for comparable human conditions.

4.2 Why has the Potential of Light Restriction Gone Unrecognized?

Encouraging results in rodent models go back several decades to work on the RCS rat, in which it was shown that dark-rearing slows the degeneration (Dowling and Sidman, 1962; Kaitz, 1976), and that the damaging effect of light is rhodopsin-mediated (Kaitz and Auerbach, 1978). Initially disappointing results in humans (Berson, 1971) and growing understanding of the genetic basis of many forms of retinal degenerations, may have led to neglect of the idea. With the reality of restriction-induced a-wave recovery documented, previously (Jozwick et al., 2006) and here, further study is encouraged to assess the clinical value of the observations.

4.3 Is Re-Growth of the Erg Likely to be Strain-Specific?

The mutations which cause photoreceptor degeneration are diverse (Dryja and Berson, 1995) and it is already clear that light restriction will help all forms of the disease (Paskowitz et al., 2006). Nevertheless, normal (non-degenerative) rat retina shows the major trends shown in Figure 1 for the degenerative P23H-3 strain. Bright ambient illumination reduces the ERG and the effect is largely, but not completely, reversible (Jozwick et al., 2006). This reduction and restoration of the ERG have been related to an underlying shortening and re-growth of outer segments, and to an accompanying reduction and increase in rhodopsin levels in the retina, in the photostasis phenomenon (Penn and Williams, 1986; Penn, 1998; Williams, 1998). Mutations which cause photoreceptor degeneration occur on a 'normal' background, making it unlikely that the recovery of retinal function shown here will be specific to the P23H-3 strain, or to rhodopsin mutants.

4.4 Mechanisms of Re-growth of ERG

We are currently exploring mechanisms which underlie the light-restriction-induced regrowth of the ERG, with the working hypothesis that the a-wave increases in amplitude in response to light restriction because the outer segment grows longer, as proposed previously. (Jozwick et al., 2006), with a corresponding increase in rhodopsin content and dark current. Other mechanisms need to be considered, however, especially the down regulation of stress-induced factors such as FGF-2 and CNTF, which are known to reduce the a-wave (Gargini et al., 1999; Valter et al., 2005).

Acknowledgments This work was supported by grants from Retina Australia, the Australian Research Council and the National Health and Medical Research Council.

References

Berson E (1971) Light deprivation for early retinitis pigmentosa. Arch Ophthalmol 85: 521 529.
Bicknell IR, Darrow R, Barsalou L, Fliesler SJ, Organisciak DT (2002) Alterations in retinal rod outer segment fatty acids and light-damage susceptibility in P23H rats. Mol Vis 8: 333–340.
Cideciyan AV, Jacobson SG, Aleman TS, Gu D, Pearce-Kelling SE, Sumaroka A, Acland GM, Aguirre GD (2005) In vivo dynamics of retinal injury and repair in the rhodopsin mutant dog model of human retinitis pigmentosa. Proc Natl Acad Sci U S A 102: 5233–5238.
Dowling J, Sidman R (1962) Inherited retinal dystrophy in the rat. J Cell Biol 14: 73 109.
Dryja T, Berson EL (1995) Retinitis pigmentosa and allied diseases. Implications of genetic heterogeneity. Invest Ophthalmol Vis Sci 36: 1197–1200.

Color Plates

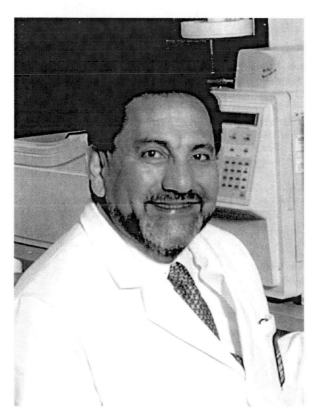

Color Plate 1 Nicolas G. Bazan, M.D., Ph.D.

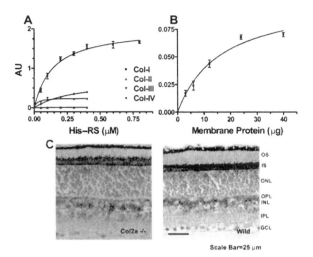

Color Plate 2 Purified recombinant RS binds more avidly to Type I collagen than to collagen Types II, III, and IV. Increasing amounts of purified His-RS (A) or mice retinal membrane fractions (B) were incubated with collagen coated plates and the amount of bound RS was measured by ELISA using anti-RS antibody. (C) Immunohistochemical labeling of RS (brown staining) in 2 month old Col2a1 mutant and wild type mice retina using anti-RS antibody and goat anti-rabbit conjugated HRP (horseradish peroxidase)

Color Plate 3 Immunoblots of WT, GC1-/-, GC2-/- and GCdko retina lysates probed with (left panel) anti-rhodopsin, anti-rod Tα, anti-rod PDE, anti-GCAP1, anti-GCAP2 antibodies; (right panel) anti-cone Tα, anti-cone arrestin, and anti-GRK1 antibodies. Internal controls with β-actin demonstrate approximately equal loading levels

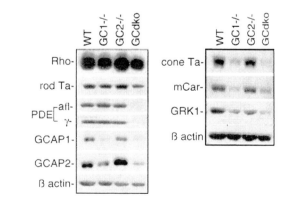

Gargini C, Belfiore MS, Bisti S, Cervetto L, Valter K, Stone J (1999) The impact of basic fibroblast growth factor on photoreceptor function and morphology. Invest Ophthalmol Vis Sci 40: 2088–2099.

Johnson G (1901) Contributions to the comparative anatomy of the mammalian eye chiefly based on ophthalmoscopic examination. Phil Trans Roy Soc London 194.

Jozwick C, Valter K, Stone J (2006) Reversal of functional loss in the P23H-3 rat retina by management of ambient light. Exp Eye Res 83: 1074–080.

Kaitz M (1976) Protection of the dystrophic retina from susceptibility to light stress. Invest Ophthalmol 15: 153–156.

Kaitz M, Auerbach E (1978) Action spectrum for light-induced retinal degeneration in dystrophic rats. Vision Res 19: 1041–1044.

Maslim J, Valter K, Egensperger R, Hollander H, Stone J (1997) Tissue oxygen during a critical developmental period controls the death and survival of photoreceptors. Invest Ophthalmol Vis Sci 38: 1667–1677.

Naash M, Peachey N, Yi Li Z, Gryczan C, Goto Y, Blanks J, Milam A, Ripps H (1996) Light-induced acceleration of photoreceptor degeneration in transgenic mice expressing mutant rhodopsin. Invest Ophthalmol Vis Sci 37: 775–782.

Paskowitz DM, LaVail MM, Duncan JL (2006) Light and inherited retinal degeneration. Br J Ophthalmol 90: 1060–1066.

Penn J, Anderson R (1991) Effects of light history on the rat retina. Prog Ret Res 11: 75–98.

Penn JS (1998) Early studies of the photostasis phenomenon. In: Photostasis and Related Phenomenon. Plenum Press, New York, pp 1–16.

Penn JS, Williams TP (1986) Photostasis: regulation of daily photon-catch by rat retinas in response to various cyclic illuminances. Exp Eye Res 43: 915–28.

Stone J, Maslim J, Valter-Kocsi K, Mervin K, Bowers F, Chu Y, Barnett N, Provis J, Lewis G, Fisher S, Bisti S, Gargini C, Cervetto L, Merin S, Pe'er J (1999) Mechanisms of photoreceptor death and survival in mammalian retina. Prog Ret Eye Res 18: 689–735.

Valter K, Bisti S, Gargini C, Di Loreto S, Maccarone R, Cervetto L, Stone J (2005) Time course of neurotrophic factor upregulation and retinal protection against light-induced damage after optic nerve section. Invest Ophthalmol Vis Sci 46: 1748–1754.

Walsh N, Van Driel D, Lee D, Stone J (2004) Multiple vulnerability of photoreceptors to mesopic ambient light in the P23H transgenic rat. Brain Res 1013: 197–203.

Williams TP (1998) Light history and photostastis. In: Photostasis and Related Phenomena. Plenum Press, New York, pp 17–32.

Part V
Molecular Genetics and Candidate Genes

Mutations in Known Genes Account for 58% of Autosomal Dominant Retinitis Pigmentosa (adRP)

Stephen P. Daiger, Lori S. Sullivan, Anisa I. Gire, David G. Birch, John R. Heckenlively, and Sara J. Bowne

1 Introduction

Inherited retinal diseases such as autosomal dominant retinitis pigmentosa (adRP) are strikingly complex, with mutations in many different genes causing the same disease, with many different mutations in each gene, and with different clinical consequences resulting from the same mutation, even within the same family. For example, mutations in sixteen genes are known to cause adRP and an additional two adRP genes have been mapped but not identified yet (Table 1). This raises two questions: what fraction of adRP cases are accounted for by mutations in known genes, and what accounts for the remaining cases?

To answer these questions we applied a step-wise screening process to a cohort of well-characterized adRP families, now numbering 215 (Sullivan et al., 2006a). Methods included sequencing of known genes, detection of deletions using MLPA (multiplex ligation-dependent probe amplification) (Sullivan et al., 2006b), linkage mapping against known loci, and genome-wide linkage mapping. By this combination of approaches we detected mutations in 58% of the families (largely Americans of European origin). Approximately 3% of these families have large deletions that cannot be detected by conventional PCR-based methods, and linkage testing against known loci revealed several additional mutations that were not detected earlier. Thus some of the remaining families are likely to have large deletions or other "hidden" mutations in known genes. However, linkage testing also confirms the existence of new adRP genes.

Being able to find the cause of adRP in all or nearly all affected individuals is a difficult but achievable goal, perhaps within the next decade (Daiger et al., 2007). This information is of immediate value to patients and families, and is a necessary precursor to gene and mutation-specific therapies.

S.P. Daiger
Human Genetics Center, School of Public Health, and Dept. of Ophthalmology, The Univ. of Texas, Houston, TX, USA, Tel: 713-500-9829, Fax: 713-500-0900
e-mail: stephen.p.daiger@uth.tmc.edu

R.E. Anderson et al. (eds.), *Recent Advances in Retinal Degeneration,*
© Springer 2008

Table 1 Genes known to cause adRP, references in RetNet, (RetNet, 2007)

	Symbol	Protein	Location
	a. Known adRP genes		
1.	PRPF3 (RP18)	pre-mRNA splicing factor 3	1q21.2
2.	SEMA4A	semaphorin 4A	1q22
3.	RHO	rhodopsin	3q22.1
4.	GUCA1B	guanylate cyclase activating protein 1B	6p21.1
5.	RDS	peripherin 2	6p21.2
6.	RP9 (PAP1)	pim-1 kinase associated protein	7p14.3
7.	IMPDH1 (RP10)	inosine monophosphate dehydrogenase 1	7q32.1
8.	RP1	RP1 protein	8q12.1
9.	ROM1	rod outer membrane protein 1	11q12.3
10.	NRL	neural retina leucine zipper	14q11.2
11.	NR2E3	nuclear receptor subfamily 2 group E3	15q23
12.	PRPF8 (RP13)	pre-mRNA splicing factor 8	17p13.3
13.	CA4 (RP17)	carbonic anhydrase 4	17q23.2
14.	FSCN2	retinal fascin homolog 2	17q25
15.	CRX	cone-rod homeobox transcription factor	19q13.32
16.	PRPF31 (RP11)	pre-mRNA splicing factor 31	19q13.42
	b. Mapped autosomal genes		
1.	RP33		2cen-q12.1
2.	RP31		9p22-p13
	c. Dominant-acting X-linked gene		
1.	RPGR (RP3)	retinitis pigmentosa GTPase regulator	Xp11.4

2 Methods

We tested a panel of affected individuals from 215 adRP families for mutations in most of the known dominant RP genes (Table 1) (Sullivan et al., 2006a) and unpublished]. To be included in the study a family had to have a diagnosis of adRP by a knowledgeable clinical specialist, and either (a) three affected generations with affected females, or (b) two affected generations with male-to-male transmission. The latter requirement was to reduce the likelihood of including families with X-linked RP. This possibility arises because some mutations in the X-linked gene RPGR affect female "carriers", thus the disease in these families may be misinterpreted as adRP (Mears et al., 2000; Rozet et al., 2002; Vervoort et al., 2000).

The cohort of adRP patients was screened (largely by DNA sequencing) for mutations in the protein coding regions and intron-exon junctions of all adRP genes or gene regions causing at least 1% of cases. ORF15, the "hot spot" for mutations in RPGR, was also tested in families without male-to-male transmission. Determining whether a novel, rare variant is pathogenic was done using several computational and genetic tools (Grantham et al., 1974; Ng, 2003; Ramensky et al., 2002; Reese et al., 1997).

In subsequent studies, we tested several of the remaining families for linkage to genetic markers within or close to the known adRP genes and to RPGR [(Sullivan et al., 2006b) and unpublished]. This was done to uncover mutations that might have been missed by sequencing or to locate genes that have been mapped but not identified yet. In one large family we found linkage to the PRPF31 gene, even though careful re-sequencing failed to disclose a DNA change. Further testing revealed that affected members of the family have a complex deletion and insertion in PRPF31. This rearrangement was not detected earlier because only the non-deleted, homologous chromosome was sequenced, that is, the deletion is "invisible" to sequencing. We then tested the remaining families for deletions in PRPF31 using multiplex ligation-dependent probe amplification (MLPA)(Schouten et al., 2002; Sullivan et al., 2006b).

Finally, two large families without mutations in known genes were tested for genome-wide linkage using the ABI 5 cM microsatellite panel (n=811) (Sullivan et al., 2005) and unpublished]. Multipoint linkage analysis was done using the LINKAGE package (Lathrop et al., 1984).

3 Results

3.1 Mutations in Known Dominant RP Genes Account for 58.6% of adRP Families

To determine the genes and mutations causing retinopathy in the 215 families in the adRP cohort we tested affected probands for mutations predicted to cause at least 1% of adRP cases. Subsequently, families without mutations detected by sequencing were subjected to linkage testing against STRP (short tandem repeat polymorphism) marker sets within or contiguous to known adRP loci, if sufficient family members were present (Sullivan et al., 2006b). In those cases were linkage testing indicated a known gene, that gene was tested more extensively in affected family members.

By these approaches, we identified single-nucleotide substitutions and small indels as the likely cause of adRP in 55.8% of the cohort families (Table 2 and Fig. 1). Pathogenicity of novel variants was confirmed by segregation within families and bioinformatic analyses [(Sullivan et al., 2006a) and unpublished].

In addition, linkage mapping and SNP (single-nucleotide polymorphism) exclusion in one large adRP family revealed a complex chromosomal rearrangement in the PRPF31 (RP11) gene not detectable by sequencing. Based on this finding we designed MLPA probe sets spanning the PRPF31 locus and tested for deletions and copy number variants in other families in the cohort. In total, we identified deletions and rearrangements in the PRPF31 gene in six (2.8%) additional families (Fig. 2) [(Sullivan et al., 2006b) and unpublished].

3.2 Several adRP Genes are Rare Causes of adRP or are Misidentified

We found no mutations in four of the genes, CA4, FSCN2, NRL and RP9 (PAP1). Based on published evidence, mutations in CA4, FSCN2 and NRL are real but rare causes of adRP. In contrast, we believe that the gene associated with the RP9 locus,

Table 2 Mutations in the adRP cohort, N = 215 [(Sullivan et al., 2006a,b) and unpublished]

Gene	No. families	% total
CA4	0	0.0
CRX	2	0.9
FSCN2	0	0.0
IMPDH1	6	2.8
NR2E3	3	1.4
NRL	0	0.0
PRPF3 (RP18)	2	0.9
PRPF8 (RP13)	6	2.8
PRPF31 (RP11)	17	7.9
RDS	18	8.4
RDS-ROM1 digenic	1	0.5
RHO	60	27.9
ROM1	0	0.0
RP1	8	3.7
RP9	0	0.0
RPGR	3	1.4
TOTALS	126	58.6

PAP1, is not the cause of this disease. We and others failed to find mutations; in addition, we discovered that one of the reported disease-causing mutations is probably a paralogus variant, that is, the result of PCR amplification of two nearly identical

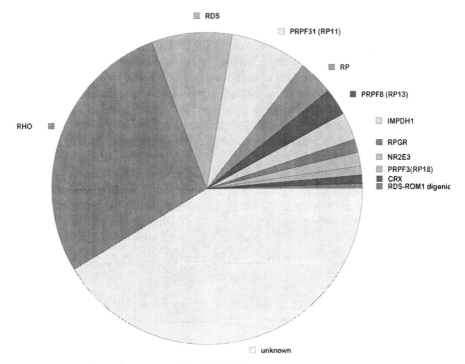

Fig. 1 Percent of mutations per gene in adRP families

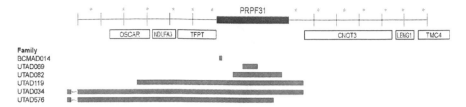

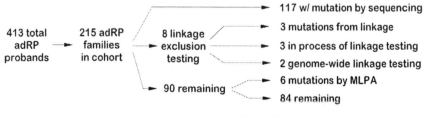

Fig. 2 PRPF31 deletions in six adRP families. Stars indicate SNPs, bars indicate deleted regions

gene copies. For this reason, we believe that the gene at the RP9 locus has not been identified yet.

3.3 Family History and Phenotypes are Useful for Prioritizing Genes to Test

We considered whether the pedigree and phenotype are useful predictors of the underlying gene. In three circumstances they are. First, families in which females are consistently less severely affected than males, and without male-to-male transmission, are more likely to have an RPGR mutation. Second, skipped generations are more common with mutations in PRPF31 than in other adRP genes. Third, symptoms of RDS mutations are much more varied than mutations in other genes, ranging from RP, to choroidal atrophy, to complex maculopathies (Felbor et al., 1997; Kajiwara et al., 1993; Sears et al., 2001). Otherwise, there are numerous phenotypic differences among individuals with different mutations, but there is so much clinical variability that these differences are not pathognomonic.

3.4 Linkage Mapping Indicates Additional adRP Loci

Of the 215 adRP families enrolled in these studies, we identified disease-causing mutations in 126 using a variety of methods (Fig. 3). Of the remaining families, two are large enough for genome-wide linkage mapping and were tested for linkage

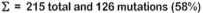

413 total adRP probands → 215 adRP families in cohort

8 linkage exclusion testing

90 remaining

- ► 117 w/ mutation by sequencing
- ► 3 mutations from linkage
- ► 3 in process of linkage testing
- ► 2 genome-wide linkage testing
- ► 6 mutations by MLPA
- ► 84 remaining

Σ = 215 total and 126 mutations (58%)

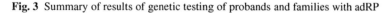

Fig. 3 Summary of results of genetic testing of probands and families with adRP

to the ABI 5 cM STR marker set. Linkage mapping in these families suggests the existence of novel adRP loci [(Sullivan et al., 2005) and unpublished].

4 Conclusions

Mutations in known adRP genes account for at least 58% of adRP cases. "Common" mutations among the total account for at least 35% of cases, but novel mutations are found in the remainder. Thus screening adRP patients for known mutations and for mutations in selected regions of adRP genes can detect a large fraction of disease-causing variants, but additional methods, including MPLA and linkage, are also required. These prevalences are based largely on Americans of European origin and Europeans; other populations have different "common" mutations and different prevalences.

Deletions and copy number variants in PRPF31, not detectable by sequencing, account for 2.8 % of cases. Some of these deletions are very large, encompassing flanking genes. Deletions in other genes may also cause adRP.

Digenic RDS-ROM1 and X-linked dominant mutations in RPGR affect 0.5% and 1.5%, respectively, of "dominant" RP families. For diagnostic and counseling purposes it is very important to consider alternate modes of inheritance in adRP families.

Identifying the underlying disease-causing mutation in families with adRP is an essential step in diagnosis, counseling and, eventually, treatment (Daiger et al., 2007).

Acknowledgments Supported by grants from the Foundation Fighting Blindness, the William Stamps Farish Fund, the Gustavus and Louise Pfeiffer Research Foundation, and the Hermann Eye Fund; and by NIH grants EY007142, EY014170, and EY005235.

References

Daiger, S. P., Bowne, S. J., and Sullivan, L. S., 2007, Perspective on genes and mutations causing retinitis pigmentosa, Arch. Ophthalmol. **125**: 151–158.

Felbor, U., Schilling, H., and Weber, B. H., 1997, Adult vitelliform macular dystrophy is frequently associated with mutations in the peripherin/*RDS* gene, Hum. Mutat. **10**: 301–309.

Grantham, R., 1974, Amino acid difference formula to help explain protein evolution, Science **185**: 862–864.

Kajiwara, K., Sandberg, M. A., Berson, E. L., and Dryja, T. P., 1993, A null mutation in the human peripherin/RDS gene in a family with autosomal dominant retinitis punctata albescens, Nat. Genet. **3**: 208–212.

Lathrop, G. M., Lalouel, J. M., Julier, C., and Ott, J., 1984, Strategies for multilocus linkage analysis in humans, Proc. Natl. Acad. Sci. USA **81**: 3443–3446.

Mears, A. J., Hiriyanna, S., Vervoort, R., Yashar, B., Gieser, L., Fahrner, S., Daiger, S. P., Heckenlively, J. R., Sieving, P. A., Wright, A. F., and Swaroop, A., 2000, Remapping of the

RP15 locus for X-linked cone-rod degeneration to Xp11.4-p21.1, and identification of a de novo insertion in the RPGR exon ORF15, Am. J. Hum. Genet. **67**: 1000–1003.

Ng, P. C., and Henikoff, S., 2003, SIFT: Predicting amino acid changes that affect protein function, Nucleic Acids Res. **31**: 3812–3814.

Ramensky, V., Bork, P., and Sunyaev, S., 2002, Human non-synonymous SNPs: server and survey, Nucleic Acids Res. **30**: 3894–3900.

Reese, M. G., Eeckman, F. H., Kulp, D., and Haussler, D., 1997, Improved splice site detection in Genie, J. Comput. Biol. **4**: 311–323.

Rozet, J. M., Perrault, I., Gigarel, N., Souied, E., Ghazi, I., Gerber, S., Dufier, J. L., Munnich, A., and Kaplan, J., 2002, Dominant X linked retinitis pigmentosa is frequently accounted for by truncating mutations in exon ORF15 of the RPGR gene, J. Med. Genet. **39**: 284–285.

Schouten, J. P., McElgunn, C. J., Waaijer, R., Zwijnenburg, D., Diepvens, F., and Pals, G., 2002, Relative quantification of 40 nucleic acid sequences by multiplex ligation-dependent probe amplification, Nucleic Acids Res. **30**: e57.

Sears, J. E., Aaberg, T. A., Sr., Daiger, S. P., and Moshfeghi, D. M., 2001, Splice site mutation in the peripherin/RDS gene associated with pattern dystrophy of the retina, Am. J. Ophthalmol. **132**: 693–699.

Sullivan, L. S., Bowne, S. J., Birch, D. G., Hughbanks-Wheaton, D., Heckenlively, J. R., Lewis, R. A., Garcia, C. A., Ruiz, R. S., Blanton, S. H., Northrup, H., Gire, A. I., Seaman, R., Duzkale, H., Spellicy, C. J., Zhu, J., Shankar, S. P., and Daiger, S. P., 2006a, Prevalence of disease-causing mutations in families with autosomal dominant retinitis pigmentosa (adRP): a screen of known genes in 200 families, Invest. Ophthalmol. Vis. Sci. **47**: 3052–3064.

Sullivan, L. S., Bowne, S. J., Seaman, C. R., Blanton, S. H., Lewis, R. A., Heckenlively, J. R., Birch, D. G., Hughbanks-Wheaton, D., and Daiger, S. P., 2006b, Genomic rearrangements of the PRPF31 gene account for 2.5% of autosomal dominant retinitis pigmentosa, Invest. Ophthalmol. Vis. Sci. **47**: 4579–4588.

Sullivan, L. S., Bowne, S. J., Shankar, S. P., Blanton, S. H., Heckenlively, J. R., Birch, D. G., Wheaton, D. H., Pelias, M. Z., and Daiger, S. P., 2005, Linkage mapping in families with autosomal dominant retinitis pigmentosa (adRP), Invest. Ophthalmol. Vis. Sci. **46**: E-Abstract 2293.

Vervoort, R., Lennon, A., Bird, A. C., Tulloch, B., Axton, R., Miano, M. G., Meindl, A., Meitinger, T., Ciccodicola, A., and Wright, A. F., 2000, Mutational hot spot within a new RPGR exon in X-linked retinitis pigmentosa, Nat. Genet. **25**: 462–466.

Genetics of Age-related Macular Degeneration

Albert O. Edwards

There have been major advances over the past two years in identifying genetic risks for age-related macular degeneration (AMD). The complexity of genetic association and genetic epidemiology studies and differences in the conclusions and data reported from various laboratories make it difficult for the general scientific reader to understand the significance and limitations of these advances. Thus, the scientific foundations and limitations of these genetic studies are not widely understood. The general scientific reader needs an approach to recognize spurious genetic association from those that are real and to understand what genetic association studies can teach us about AMD and where we need to be cautious. The purpose of this article is to provide an overview of the genetics of AMD and explain how to approach a genetic association study.

1 Genetic Risks for AMD

Reported genetic risks for AMD include genes with confirmed sequence variation increasing the risk of AMD in most studies, variants that have been partially reproducible, and those that have not been replicated, either because they are recent reports or could not be replicated (Table 1).

Genes with confirmed sequence variation include complement factor H (CFH) on chromosome 1q31 (Edwards et al., 2005; Haines et al., 2005; Klein et al., 2005). The Y402H polymorphism in this gene has a minor allele frequency of 40% and is highly associated with AMD. The LOC387715/PRSS11 locus on chromosome 10q26 contains multiple sequence variants associated with AMD, including an Ala69Ser polymorphism in LOC387715 with a minor allele frequency of 30%; the precise variant or variants explaining the association is not yet understood as discussed below (Jakobsdottir et al., 2005; Rivera et al., 2005). Finally, the factor

A.O. Edwards

Mayo Clinic, Department of Ophthalmology, 200 First Street SW, Rochester, MN 55905.
Supported by the NEI, FFB, and RPB, Tel: (507) 284-2787, Fax: (507) 284-4612
e-mail: edwards.albert@mayo.edu

Table 1 DNA sequence variants reported to increase the risk of AMD grouped by reproducibility and frequency of variant

Genes with sequence variants confirmed in all studies
- Complement factor H (Tyr402His) with MAF = 40%
- LOC387715/PRSS11 (Ala69Ser) with MAF = 30%
- BF/C2 protective variants (e.g., Lue9His) with MAF = 3%

Genes with variants confirmed in some studies
- APOE4 with MAF = 10%
- VEGF (multiple variants)

Genes with unconfirmed variants
- ERCC6, CX3CR1, LRP6, VLDLR, IL1A, CRP, HLA, MMP-9

Genes reported to have rare variation associated with AMD
- Fibulin 3, Fibulin 5, ABCA4

Genes reported, but not reproduced
- PON1, SOD2, CST3, ACE, FBLN6, TLR4

B/C2 locus (BF/C2) contains variants on chromosome 6 that alter the risk of AMD (Gold et al., 2006). Other variation has been reported to increase the risk of AMD, but less support for the association exists and they will not be discussed in this article.

1.1 Genetic Association Studies

Genetic association studies may include affected cases and related controls (e.g., sib-pairs, including either an affected or unaffected sib), or unrelated, unaffected controls. In the case in which one ascertains unrelated cases and controls, genetic association studies are fundamentally similar to other case-control studies. To perform a genetic association study, one must first ascertain a sample of cases and controls from the population of interest. Careful attention should be paid to the definitions of phenotype (diagnosis or quantification of disease) and, in particular its absence. The cases and controls should be from as similar groups as possible, with the exception of the complex trait being studied. Population stratification or admixture (e.g., concluding that a variant is associated with disease when the variant actually is associated with an unobserved difference in ethnicity between cases and controls) is always a possibility in association studies based on unrelated individuals. These concerns need to be address with good study design or within the statistical analysis. Input from an epidemiologist or statistician should be considered prior to starting the project.

Second, polymorphisms are selected and genotyped in the population or cohort; these polymorphisms are typically single nuclei-type polymorphisms or SNPs. The SNPs are often selected based on possible functional significance (e.g., coding polymorphism) or their presence near a gene with the expectation that they will be close enough to a nearby polymorphism altering the risk of disease to also be associated with disease (see next paragraph). The SNPs are usually selected manually taking into consideration the extent of linkage disequilibrium across the gene (see next paragraph), but software is available to optimize and streamline the process

(Xu et al., 2005). The minor allele frequency should be sufficiently common to enable statistical power in the population being studied; it is important to look at the allele and genotype counts in addition to measures of statistical power when small numbers of observations are expected.

One reason why genetic association studies are a powerful means for refining the location of a disease variant or discovering novel variants is linkage disequilibrium(Daly et al., 2001). Linkage disequilibrium refers to the observation that polymorphisms may be inherited more frequently together than would be expected by chance. For example, if two polymorphisms are located near each other and are in linkage disequilibrium, they will be inherited together more than the 50% expected by random inheritance (segregation). Some polymorphisms are in such tight linkage disequilibrium that they serve as proxies for each other and provide the same information. Depending on the region of the genome being studied, a single SNP can provide information over several hundred to many thousands of base-pairs. For example, in each of three AMD loci described above (CFH, 10q26, and BF/C2) the linkage disequilibrium is extensive, making it difficult to identify the exact polymorphisms explaining the association with disease. The greater the linkage disequilibrium, the easier it is to identify association because fewer SNPs are needed over a large region to detect the association, but the harder it is to refine the association. This process can be further complicated by the presence of multiple different risk variants in the same locus (see discussion of CFH below).

The third step is to validate the genotyping assay, for example, by confirming Hardy-Weinberg equilibrium (i.e., the genotypes frequencies roughly follow p2, (1–p)2 and 2p(1–p) were p represents the frequency of the common allele) and reviewing the original datafile for the accuracy of the allele calls. In the fourth step, one performs a statistical test of association, using one of the many available approaches. For quantitative phenotypes, often analysis of variance (ANOVA) or linear regression is performed. In the cases of a binary phenotype (e.g., affection status), allelic tests or genotype test are often performed with Chi-square test or tests for trend (Crochran-Armtigage Trend test, logistic regression). Regardless of type of phenotype, tests of genetic assocation are used to assess if a genotype or allele is significantly associated with the phenotype.Regardless of the specific statistical test employed, their purpose is to provide an estimate of obtaining the significant result by chance. They cannot be used to determine which of the various SNPs might explain the association with disease because other variables such as allele frequency influence the p-values. Increasing statistical significance does not equate to increasing chance of causality, a fallacy frequently observed in the literature. In addition to the p-value not implying causative findings, testing of multiple genetic variants increases the chance of a type I error (i.e., false-positive). Hence, care should be taken when interpreting p-values from statistical tests. We next need to know if there is one SNP or multiple SNPs that are associated with disease. This question is answered by using a multilocus statistical method or statistical test that conditions the effect of one SNP to assessthe effect of another SNP. The end result of these analyses are to determine which if any SNPs across a region/gene independently contribute to altered disease risk.

The fifth step is to define the segments of DNA in the population (i.e., the haplotypes) carrying the risk variant explaining the association with disease. Over short regions, the DNA strands tend to segregate as intact segments or blocks. Recombination is not randomly distributed along the chromosome and this give rise to the haplotype blocks and linkage disequilibrium. We can use the blocks or haplotypes to define the segments of DNA segregating in the population that increase the risk of disease. These methods allow us to determine if there is additional information beyond that provided by specific individual SNPs studied. If the haplotypes associated with disease to not contribute additionally to disease risk, it is likely that only the SNPs explain the association with disease. If the haplotypes remain associated with disease risk, there may be other variants associated with disease within the haplotype block being studies, or even within an adjacent haplotype block (see CFH discussion below). DNA sequencing ("resequencing") or other genomic techniques (e.g., deletion detection methods) are needed in this situation to identify the other variants associated with disease.

The sixth step is to replicate the results in other populations or cohorts. Although this step is often overlooked, it is essential to avoid reporting spurious results(Todd, 2006). One must be fastidious in avoiding multiple subgroup analysis and data-mining to avoid spurious results. While protein-based functional studies are important, they cannot substitute for robust statistical analysis, careful haplotype and re-sequencing studies, and, replication in additional populations.

1.2 Genetic Association Studies on 1q31 and 10q26 for AMD

In this section, examples of genetic association studies performed for AMD are reviewed. The regulation of complement activation (RCA) locus on chromosome 1q31 and the chromosome 10q26 locus will be discussed.

1.2.1 RCA Locus

The regulation of complement activation locus spans 400,000 base pairs on chromosome 1q31. This region of chromosome 1q was first identified by the author and colleagues in a large family from Oregon and called the ARMD1 locus(Klein et al., 1998). It was subsequently confirmed in multiple sib-pair and small family studies (Majewski et al., 2003; Seddon et al., 2003; Weeks et al., 2000; Weeks et al., 2001; Weeks et al., 2004). In 2005, our group and two others published simultaneously genetic association studies in *Science* refining this ARMD1 locus to RCA region on chromosome 1q31 (Edwards et al., 2005; Haines et al., 2005; Klein et al., 2005). The RCA locus contains 7 genes (Rodriguez de Cordoba et al., 2004). The first of these is the gene encoding complement factor H (CFH). CFH is followed by five CFH-like genes which arose through ancestral duplications. On the terminal region of this 400,000 base-pair locus is the factor 13B gene. There is extensive linkage disequilibrium across this entire region. In the initial studies, the major risk appeared to be centralized on a 20,000 base-pair segment centered on the gene encoding complement factor H. There were many risk variants identified, some of which had higher P-values than the Y402H coding variant eventually thought to provide the best biological basis of the association with AMD. In our study, we were unable to identify any haplotypes that showed independent association with AMD (Edwards et al., 2005). The other groups that published in 2005 also did not report any association with AMD independent of Y402H (Hageman et al., 2005; Haines et al., 2005; Klein et al., 2005). However, Klein and colleagues reported approximately 3% of haplotypes associated with AMD did not carry the Y402H polymorphism (Klein et al., 2005). Hageman and colleagues found two protective haplotypes; however, both of those haplotypes contain the protective Y402 allele, and the statistical independence of the haplotypes was not reported (Hageman et al., 2005). Based on the observation that the 402H polymorphism was present on all or most risk haplotypes and that no protective haplotypes contained the 402H variant, it was felt that the this coding amino acid polymorphism was the best candidate for explaining the association with AMD. However, the much higher P-values in SNPs distal to Y402H remained unexplained, and this observation was not easily explained away by allele frequency or other variables. In 2006, Li et al. (2006) and colleagues reported five independent SNPs out of over 80 that they studied which contributed statistically independent information. The major effect was a haplotype that contained the Y402H variant and could be partially explained by it. There was also a haplotype present in 8% of the total population that appeared to be independent of Y402H that was also a risk haplotype. They found two common protective haplotypes but their independence was unclear. Li and colleagues also stated in their conclusions that multiple rare haplotypes altering disease risks existed. The results suggested that there was additional variation in the regulation of complement activation locus that increased the risk of macular degeneration beyond 402H. Maller and colleagues, around the same time in 2006, confirmed these findings (Maller et al., 2006). They found that 1 out of 63 SNPs that they studied was independent of Y402H using logistic regression. This SNP, rs1410996, remained significant with a P value of 2.7×10^{-15} after conditioning on the Y402H polymorphism (rs1061170). They also found that the protective allele (Y402) was present on two independent haplotypes, as observed or suggested by others.

Hughes and colleagues in 2006 performed a similar study and also found that there were two independent protective haplotypes in a region distal to the complement factor H gene. They demonstrated through resequencing and other techniques that one of these haplotypes carried a deletion of the CFHR3 and CFHR1 genes and demonstrated that the proteins from these genes were absent in the serum. It is likely that this observation explains the two protective haplotypes observed by others.

In summary, the regulation of complement activation locus contains a large block of genomic DNA approximately 20,000 base pairs in length which is very highly associated with age-related macular degeneration. This region demonstrates extensive linkage disequilibrium thus making the specific disease variants difficult to pinpoint. However, extensive re-sequencing has failed to demonstrate a more attractive variant than Y402H to explain most of the risk. There are currently functional studies ongoing which may help understand how this polymorphism could contribute to macular degeneration. There are also two independent and common haplotypes that increase the risk of AMD. The basis of the second risk haplotype remains unexplained, while the first is due to Y402H. There are two independent and common haplotypes decreasing disease risk, one of which is most likely explained by the absence of the Y402H variant and the other by a genomic deletion of two CFH-like genes. Interestingly, the risk associated with AMD at the RCA locus is independent of other genes, smoking, and disease subtype in most studies. This suggests that the CFH risk variants increase the chance of getting the maculopathy that characterizes AMD and is not specific for the complications of AMD such as geographic atrophy or exudation.

1.2.2 Chromosome 10q26 Locus

Studies of the chromosome 10q26 locus show themes similar to those we observed with the regulation of complement activation (RCA) locus discussed above. Jakobsdottir and colleagues (Jakobsdottir et al., 2005) followed by Rivera and colleagues (Rivera et al., 2005) in 2005 first demonstrated the association of this locus with AMD. The region contains two known genes and one hypothetical gene. From centromeric to telomeric they are the PLEKHA1 gene, the LOC387715 hypothetical gene, and the PRSS11 serine protease gene. PRSS11 is also referred to as HTRA1. These genes are located on a segment of DNA approximately 100 KB in length with extensive linkage disequilibrium. One group was unable to determine which of the three genes contained SNPs explaining the association with AMD in the population studied (Jakobsdottir et al., 2005). The other group reported that PLEKHA1 SNPs did not contribute to AMD risk independent of LOC387715(Rivera et al., 2005). In particular, both groups identified rs10490924 which codes for an Ala69Ser coding polymorphism within an open reading frame of the hypothetical gene LOC387715. The association was confined to a 60 kilobase block of DNA that contained the PLEKHA1, LOC387715, and the 5-prime region of PRSS11. In 2006, the first group looked at the Ala69Ser variation in the cardiovascular health study and AREDS populations; they found that this variation increased the risk of AMD while PLEKHA1 variations did not (Conley et al., 2006). Maller and colleagues (Maller et al., 2006) in 2006 found evidence for association with three other SNPs after conditioning on Ala69Ser and 100% linkage disequilibrium between Ala69Ser and other SNPs in the region including one SNP in PRSS11. This suggested that the Ala69Ser and SNPs in complete disequilibrium with it may not explain the entire effect. Schmidt and colleagues (Schmidt et al., 2006) in 2006 felt that the Ala69Ser polymorphism best explained the linkage and association in this region. They found no other SNPs that contributed to the risk of AMD after conditioning on Ala69Ser. However, they did not perform genotyping of SNPs within the PRSS11 promoter region. Recently, two papers were published in *Science* in October of 2006 which suggested that promoter polymorphisms in the PRSS11 locus best explained the association with AMD (Dewan et al., 2006; Yang et al., 2006). One paper argued that because the P-value of a PRSS11 promoter SNP was greater (80-fold) than the Ala69Ser in LOC387715, the promotor SNP was most likely to be the causative variant. As noted earlier, P-values are not reliable markers of causality conclusions because other variables can influence them. There was no report of conditional analysis, thus, these data would not help us distinguish between the many SNPs in this region. The other paper argued that because LOC387715 was removed from some genomic database, it was not a real gene and therefore the Ala69Ser polymorphism may be a surrogate marker. The linkage disequilibrium between Ala69Ser and the PRSS11 promoter SNP (rs112638) is greater than 99%. While this conclusion may be correct, the published genetic studies cannot prove this argument at this time. No conditional analysis was reported in the paper, and therefore, this conclusion also does not demonstrate which of the many SNPs in this short segment DNA explain the association with AMD. Although, these two papers presented preliminary expression studies, the functional observations need to be further studied. Furthermore, as noted earlier, functional studies are a useful but not infallible substitute for robust genetic methods in identifying the variation explaining the association with AMD.

In summary, as of October 2006 which of the many variations in the short segment of DNA encompassing LOC387715 and the PRSS11 promoter is the best candidate for increasing the risk of AMD is unknown. Interestingly, the risk allele/haplotype was found in a significantly higher proportion of cases with exudation or geographic atrophy in most studies. Some have argued that this may mean that the 10q26 risk variant(s) specifically increases the risk of late AMD. While this may be the case, it certainly also increases the risk of early AMD, i.e., the maculopathy that characterizes AMD.

Interestingly, the reported interaction with smoking by Schmidt and colleagues (Schmidt et al., 2006) in 2005 was not confirmed by Conley and colleagues in 2006 (Conley et al., 2006). This potentially interesting genotype-phenotype interaction requires further study.

2 Conclusion

As can be seen from this short overview of the chromosome 1q31 and 10q26 regions, the dissection of genetic risks for complex disorders is an exciting but challenging arena. Three regions have consistently shown coding variation that increases the risk of AMD including the regulation of activation complement locus, the 10q26 locus, and the BF/C2 locus on chromosome 6. Variation in these regions increases the risk of AMD independent of each other, suggesting that they act independently to increase the risk of AMD. This overview has illustrated the extensive genetic studies that are required to identify the precise genomic variation given rise to changes in disease risk. Because of the extensive linkage disequilibrium in some regions of the genome, it may remain difficult to genetically distinguish between which of the many variants along the segment of DNA explain the association with disease. Although not discussed earlier, it is important to note that several other loci have been identified in linkage studies, and likely contain major variants altering the risk of AMD. Further, no exhaustive search for moderate to minor risk variants (e.g., relative risks below that which can be detected in a sib-pair or medium sized family study) has been reported. Although, we have identified three important risk regions for AMD, others remain to be found and will likely be discovered over the next few years both within and outside of currently reported chromosomal regions associated with AMD. High density genome-wide association studies in multiple populations should be performed to advance our understanding of AMD.

References

Conley, Y. P., Jakobsdottir, J., Mah, T., Weeks, D. E., Klein, R., Kuller, L., Ferrell, R. E., and Gorin, M. B., 2006, CFH, ELOVL4, PLEKHA1 and LOC387715 genes and susceptibility to age-related maculopathy: AREDS and CHS cohorts and meta-analyses, *Hum Mol Genet* **15**: 3206–18.

Daly, M. J., Rioux, J. D., Schaffner, S. F., Hudson, T. J., and Lander, E. S., 2001, High-resolution haplotype structure in the human genome, *Nat Genet* **29**: 229–32.

Dewan, A., Liu, M., Hartman, S., Zhang, S. S., Liu, D. T., Zhao, C., Tam, P. O., Chan, W. M., Lam, D. S., Snyder, M., Barnstable, C., Pang, C. P., and Hoh, J., 2006, HTRA1 promoter polymorphism in wet age related macular degeneration, *Science* **314**: 989–92.

Edwards, A. O., Ritter, R., 3rd, Abel, K. J., Manning, A., Panhuysen, C., and Farrer, L. A., 2005, Complement factor H polymorphism and age-related macular degeneration, *Science* **308**: 421–24.

Gold, B., Merriam, J. E., Zernant, J., Hancox, L. S., Taiber, A. J., Gehrs, K., Cramer, K., Neel, J., Bergeron, J., Barile, G. R., Smith, R. T., Hageman, G. S., Dean, M., and Allikmets, R., 2006, Variation in factor B (BF) and complement component 2 (C2) genes is associated with age-related macular degeneration, *Nat Genet* **38**: 458–62.

Hageman, G. S., Anderson, D. H., Johnson, L. V., Hancox, L. S., Taiber, A. J., Hardisty, L. I., Hageman, J. L., Stockman, H. A., Borchardt, J. D., Gehrs, K. M., Smith, R. J., Silvestri, G., Russell, S. R., Klaver, C. C., Barbazetto, I., Chang, S., Yannuzzi, L. A., Barile, G. R., Merriam, J. C., Smith, R. T., Olsh, A. K., Bergeron, J., Zernant, J., Merriam, J. E., Gold, B., Dean, M., and Allikmets, R., 2005, A common haplotype in the complement regulatory gene factor H (HF1/CFH) predisposes individuals to age-related macular degeneration, *Proc Natl Acad Sci U S A* **102**: 7227–7232.

Haines, J. L., Hauser, M. A., Schmidt, S., Scott, W. K., Olson, L. M., Gallins, P., Spencer, K. L., Kwan, S. Y., Noureddine, M., Gilbert, J. R., Schnetz-Boutaud, N., Agarwal, A., Postel, E. A., and Pericak-Vance, M. A., 2005, Complement factor H variant increases the risk of age-related macular degeneration, *Science* **308**: 419–21.

Jakobsdottir, J., Conley, Y. P., Weeks, D. E., Mah, T. S., Ferrell, R. E., and Gorin, M. B., 2005, Susceptibility genes for age-related maculopathy on chromosome 10q26, *Am J Hum Genet* **77**: 389–407.

Klein, M. L., Schultz, D. W., Edwards, A., Matise, T. C., Rust, K., Berselli, C. B., Trzupek, K., Weleber, R. G., Ott, J., Wirtz, M. K., and Acott, T. S., 1998, Age-related macular degeneration. Clinical features in a large family and linkage to chromosome 1q, *Arch Ophthalmol* **116**: 1082–88.

Klein, R. J., Zeiss, C., Chew, E. Y., Tsai, J. Y., Sackler, R. S., Haynes, C., Henning, A. K., Sangiovanni, J. P., Mane, S. M., Mayne, S. T., Bracken, M. B., Ferris, F. L., Ott, J., Barnstable, C., and Hoh, J., 2005, Complement factor H polymorphism in age-related macular degeneration, *Science* **308**: 385–89.

Li, M., Atmaca-Sonmez, P., Othman, M., Branham, K. E., Khanna, R., Wade, M. S., Li, Y., Liang, L., Zareparsi, S., Swaroop, A., and Abecasis, G. R., 2006, CFH haplotypes without the Y402H coding variant show strong association with susceptibility to age-related macular degeneration, *Nat Genet* **38**: 1049–54.

Majewski, J., Schultz, D. W., Weleber, R. G., Schain, M. B., Edwards, A. O., Matise, T. C., Acott, T. S., Ott, J., and Klein, M. L., 2003, Age-related macular degeneration – a genome scan in extended families, *Am J Hum Genet* **73**: 540–50.

Maller, J., George, S., Purcell, S., Fagerness, J., Altshuler, D., Daly, M. J., and Seddon, J. M., 2006, Common variation in three genes, including a noncoding variant in CFH, strongly influences risk of age-related macular degeneration, *Nat Genet* **38**: 1055–59.

Rivera, A., Fisher, S. A., Fritsche, L. G., Keilhauer, C. N., Lichtner, P., Meitinger, T., and Weber, B. H., 2005, Hypothetical LOC387715 is a second major susceptibility gene for age-related macular degeneration, contributing independently of complement factor H to disease risk, *Hum Mol Genet* **14**: 3227–36.

Rodriguez de Cordoba, S., Esparza-Gordillo, J., Goicoechea de Jorge, E., Lopez-Trascasa, M., and Sanchez-Corral, P., 2004, The human complement factor H: functional roles, genetic variations and disease associations, *Mol Immunol* **41**: 355–67.

Schmidt, S., Hauser, M. A., Scott, W. K., Postel, E. A., Agarwal, A., Gallins, P., Wong, F., Chen, Y. S., Spencer, K., Schnetz-Boutaud, N., Haines, J. L., and Pericak-Vance, M. A., 2006, Cigarette smoking strongly modifies the association of LOC387715 and age-related macular degeneration, *Am J Hum Genet* **78**: 852–64.

Seddon, J. M., Santangelo, S. L., Book, K., Chong, S., and Cote, J., 2003, A genomewide scan for age-related macular degeneration provides evidence for linkage to several chromosomal regions, *Am J Hum Genet* **73**: 780–90.

Todd, J. A., 2006, Statistical false positive or true disease pathway? *Nat Genet* **38**: 731–33.

Weeks, D. E., Conley, Y. P., Mah, T. S., Paul, T. O., Morse, L., Ngo-Chang, J., Dailey, J. P., Ferrell, R. E., and Gorin, M. B., 2000, A full genome scan for age-related maculopathy, *Hum Mol Genet* **9**: 1329–49.

Weeks, D. E., Conley, Y. P., Tsai, H. J., Mah, T. S., Rosenfeld, P. J., Paul, T. O., Eller, A. W., Morse, L. S., Dailey, J. P., Ferrell, R. E., and Gorin, M. B., 2001, Age-related maculopathy: an expanded genome-wide scan with evidence of susceptibility loci within the 1q31 and 17q25 regions, *Am J Ophthalmol* **132**: 682–92.

Weeks, D. E., Conley, Y. P., Tsai, H. J., Mah, T. S., Schmidt, S., Postel, E. A., Agarwal, A., Haines, J. L., Pericak-Vance, M. A., Rosenfeld, P. J., Paul, T. O., Eller, A. W., Morse, L. S., Dailey, J. P., Ferrell, R. E., and Gorin, M. B., 2004, Age-related maculopathy: a genomewide scan with continued evidence of susceptibility loci within the 1q31, 10q26, and 17q25 regions, *Am J Hum Genet* **75**: 174–89.

Xu, H., Gregory, S. G., Hauser, E. R., Stenger, J. E., Pericak-Vance, M. A., Vance, J. M., Zuchner, S., and Hauser, M. A., 2005, SNPselector: a web tool for selecting SNPs for genetic association studies, *Bioinformatics* **21**: 4181–86.

Yang, Z., Camp, N. J., Sun, H., Tong, Z., Gibbs, D., Cameron, D. J., Chen, H., Zhao, Y., Pearson, E., Li, X., Chien, J., Dewan, A., Harmon, J., Bernstein, P. S., Shridhar, V., Zabriskie, N. A., Hoh, J., Howes, K., and Zhang, K., 2006, A variant of the HTRA1 gene increases susceptibility to age-related macular degeneration, *Science* **314**: 992–93.

Retinal Phenotype of an X-Linked Pseudo-usher Syndrome in Association with the G173R Mutation in the *RPGR* Gene

Alessandro Iannaccone, Mohammad I. Othman, April D. Cantrell, Barbara J. Jennings, Kari Branham, and Anand Swaroop

1 Introduction

Retinitis pigmentosa (RP) is the most common hereditary retinal degeneration, affecting approximately 1:3,500 individuals (Iannaccone, 2005). X-linked recessive RP (XLRP) accounts for about 10–20% of cases and, typically, causes one of the most severe forms of RP (Iannaccone, 2005). To date, two of the genes responsible for XLRP have been cloned, *RP2* (Schwahn et al., 1998) and the retinitis pigmentosa GTPase regulator, *RPGR* (Meindl et al., 1996; Roepman et al., 1996). Mutations in the *RPGR* gene account for the majority of cases of XLRP (Breuer et al., 2002).

Classical RP is characterized by night blindness at onset and progressive peripheral visual field constriction. Deterioration of central vision can ultimately occur in many patients. These symptoms are accompanied by degenerative and pigmentary changes of the retinal tissue that are detectable during fundus exam and by abnormalities in the electrical retinal response to flashes of light, the electroretinogram (ERG). ERG abnormalities are typically present before any retinal change becomes clinically visible.

Systemic manifestations often accompany RP, configuring specific syndromes. Among these symptoms, one of the most common one is hearing loss. As reviewed elsewhere (Iannaccone, 2005), there is a host of RP syndromes associated with hearing loss, Usher syndrome being the most common one. The differential diagnosis of these hearing loss-associated syndromes can be challenging, and clinically distinct subtypes of Usher syndrome also exist (Smith et al., 1994; Iannaccone, 2003; Iannaccone, 2005). Usher syndrome is, by definition, inherited as an autosomal recessive trait, and is due to mutations in numerous genes (Iannaccone, 2005). Unlike this, Usher syndrome phenocopies with an autosomal dominant and an X-linked recessive mode of inheritance have been identified reviewed in

A. Iannaccone

Hamilton Eye Institute, Department of Ophthalmology, University of Tennessee Health Science Center, 930 Madison Avenue, Suite 731, Memphis, TN 38163, USA, Tel: 901-448-7831, Fax: 901-448-5028

e-mail: aiannacc@utmem.edu

R.E. Anderson et al. (eds.), *Recent Advances in Retinal Degeneration*,
© Springer 2008

(Iannaccone et al., 2003; Koenekoop et al., 2003; Zito et al., 2003; Iannaccone et al., 2004). To date, the latter ones have all been ascribed to mutations affecting the RCC1-like domain of the *RPGR* gene. Systemic manifestations in some families include not only hearing loss but also recurrent respiratory tract infections (Iannaccone et al., 2003; Zito et al., 2003; Iannaccone et al., 2004), and we have provided evidence that RPGR expression can be detected immunohistochemically in all of the tissues in which these manifestations occur (Iannaccone et al., 2003).

Herein we report in detail the retinal phenotype of a family characterized by XLRP, otitis media, upper respiratory tract infections, and hearing loss, resulting from a missense mutation of the *RPGR* gene. This family exemplifies the full range of manifestations thus far appreciated within this RPGR-associated syndrome (OMIM #300455), and the data reported herein provide novel and more detailed information about the characteristics of the retinal disease associated with this mutation. Furthermore, the availability of functional data in affected children offers us the opportunity to provide insight in the early stage phenotypic effects of this specific mutation. Further details about this family have been reported elsewhere (Iannaccone et al., 2003).

2 Material and Methods

Five subjects from this six-generation family were examined (Fig. 1) and whole blood samples were collected from seven subjects to extract genomic DNA for molecular characterization. The proband, (subject VI:1 in the pedigree) was initially referred for suspected Usher syndrome, but further ascertainment of this family revealed, in addition to phenotypic systemic characteristics that appeared in conflict with the standard diagnostic criteria for Usher syndrome (Smith et al., 1994;

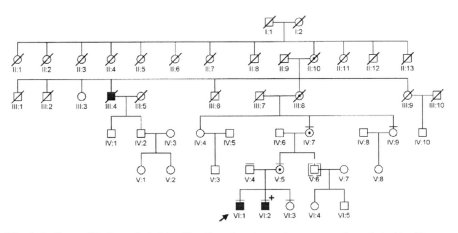

Fig. 1 Pedigree. Black symbols identify affected males and target round symbols identify carrier females. Bars above symbols identify subjects that contributed blood samples. Modified from Iannaccone et al., (2003)

Iannaccone, 2003; Iannaccone, 2005), that an X-linked pattern of inheritance was more likely. This led to the evaluation of the brother of the proband (subject VI:2), their mother (subject V:5) and maternal grandmother (subject IV:7), which corroborated this suspicion. Ensuing screening for mutations in the *RPGR* gene revealed a G to C nucleotide substitution at position 576 (G576C) of the *RPGR* gene in the hemizygous state in the affected males (subjects VI:1 and VI:2) and in the heterozygous state in an asymptomatic obligate carrier (subject V:5) and in a symptomatic carrier (subject IV:7). Molecular testing further demonstrated the absence of this mutation in the father, the probands' sister, and the maternal aunt, all of whom had no signs of disease. The G576C nucleotide change is predicted to result in a glycine (non-polar amino acid) to arginine (charged amino acid) change at position 173 (G173R), which is a highly conserved amino acid within the RCC1-like homology domain of RPGR.

All patients were evaluated clinically, visual acuity was measured with ETDRS charts, and representative fundus features were documented photographically as appropriate. Whenever possible, functional testing included automated (dark- and light-adapted) monochromatic perimetry according to the criteria by Jacobson et al., Goldmann kinetic perimetry, and flash electroretinograms (ERGs). The latter ones were obtained under anesthesia induced via i.v. Propofol in the two affected male children identified in this family. All procedures were in compliance with the Declaration of Helsinki and were approved by the Institutional Review Board of the University of Tennessee Health Science Center. Informed consent was obtained from all subjects or their legal guardians, as applicable, for all research studies conducted in the course of this investigation.

3 Results

3.1 Affected Males

The proband (VI:1), who we first examined at age 10, became symptomatic at age 6 with visual field and at age 8 with night blindness and light aversion. His brother (VI:2) was examined at age 7, at which time he remained asymptomatic. Both male children had a history of recurrent ear and sinus infections since being 1 year old, and had both been diagnosed with hearing loss shortly before our examination. Other details about the systemic manifestations experienced by these children have been reported elsewhere (Iannaccone et al., 2003; Zito et al., 2003; Iannaccone et al., 2004).

Upon clinical examination, both male children exhibited mild myopia and, despite the lack of complaint of reduced visual acuity, neither one of them could not be corrected to better than 20/32 in their better seeing eye. Fundus examination of the peripheral retina of affected males in this family was characterized by a finely punched-out appearance but no bone spicules (Iannaccone et al., 2003; Zito et al., 2003; Iannaccone et al., 2004). The functional phenotype exhibited by these

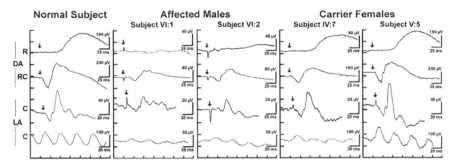

Fig. 2 Comparison of normal flash ERGs (left) to those of affected males and molecularly confirmed female carriers. R = rod-driven ERG; RC = rod/cone-driven (mixed) ERG; C = cone-driven ERGs. DA = dark-adapted. LA = light-adapted. Please note the difference in amplitude scales for subjects VI:1, VI:2, and IV:7

young patients was that of a rod>cone pattern of dysfunction, but with partial preservation of rod ERGs and persistence of recordable responses in both cases (Fig. 2).

Visual fields (Fig. 3) were full in size but depressed in peripheral sensitivity, with areas to the I4e targets limited to the central 5° around fixation. This pattern of concentric depression of visual field isopter sizes was associated with significant losses in both rod and cone sensitivities. The pattern of rod- and cone-mediated losses exhibited large regional differences across the visual field (Fig. 3). Of note,

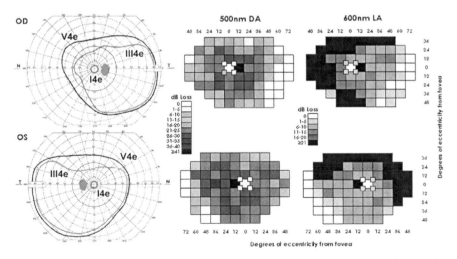

Fig. 3 Goldmann visual fields (left) and grayscale automated monochromatic perimetry plots obtained under dark-adapted (DA) conditions to 500 nm stimuli (rod-mediated sensitivity loss plots) and under light-adapted (LA) conditions to 600 nm stimuli on a white background (L/M cone-mediated sensitivity loss plots) for the right (OD, top) and left (OS, bottom) eyes of subject VI:1. The size to the V4e target (black isopter) was essentially normal, whereas constriction of the peripheral isopters to the III4e and especially the I4e targets (grey isopters) was evident. Rod (500 nm) and L/M cone (600 nm) sensitivity losses varied considerably

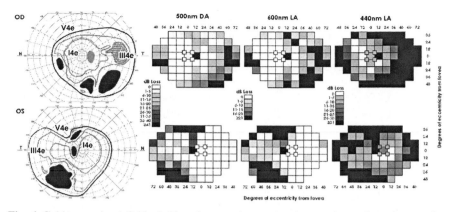

Fig. 4 Goldmann visual fields (left) and grayscale automated monochromatic perimetry plots obtained under dark-adapted (DA) conditions to 500 nm stimuli (rod-mediated sensitivity loss plots) and under light-adapted (LA) conditions to 600 nm stimuli on white background (L/M cone-mediated sensitivity loss plots) and to 440 nm stimuli on yellow background (S-cones) for the right (OD, top) and left (OS, bottom) eyes of subject IV:7. Patches of absolute and relative scotomas were evident, paralleled by areas of sensitivity losses at corresponding loci at all wavelengths. More severe and more widespread dysfunction was seen for S-cones

normal rod- and cone-mediated sensitivities were identified in the macular region, corresponding to the area of preservation of the I4e target, and in the far periphery. In the remainder of the visual field, dissociation in the severity of rod- (i.e., ≤ 1.0 log unit) and L/M cone-mediated (i.e., ≥ 2.0 log unit) sensitivity losses at corresponding loci was also observed

3.2 Female Carriers

Female carriers were either entirely symptom-free subjectively and disease-free to visual function testing (subject V:5), or showed late-onset mild patchy and asymmetric RP with corresponding regional cone>rod areas of dysfunction (subject IV:7, Fig. 4) and cone>rod amplitude losses to ERG testing (Fig. 2). In subject IV:7, monochromatic perimetry revealed that S-cones were significantly more severely affected than L/M-cones. Systemic manifestations were seen also in carriers (Iannaccone et al., 2003).

4 Discussion

Males carrying the G173R *RPGR* mutation have early-onset sizable reduction in both rod- and cone-mediated function, although rod function can still be measured and displays regional variability. These findings indicate that, at least in association with this specific mutation, rod function is still partially preserved in *RPGR*-associated phenotypes within the first decade of life. On the other hand, although cone function remains overall better preserved than that of rods, cone disease can be already severe within the retina of children with the G173R mutation, and can exceed that of rods at corresponding loci. This suggests that rods and cones may undergo degeneration in the presence of this mutation as a result of events intrinsic to each cell type and, quite possibly, independent of one another. This is different than what is observed, e.g., in many rhodopsin mutants, in which cone disease tends to follow rod disease (Cideciyan et al., 1998; Iannaccone et al., 2006). This observation underscores the important function that RPGR has not only in rods but also in cones. It remains to be determined if this pattern of rod-cone dissociation is observed also in other *RPGR*-associated phenotypes.

Female carriers presented with late-onset, cone>rod disease. Comparison between light-adapted thresholds conducted at 440 nm (S-cones) vs. 600 nm (L/M cones) revealed that S-cones are significantly more affected than L/M-cones, with very few loci with normal thresholds to 440 nm stimuli, even when many corresponding loci retained entirely normal L/M-cone function. This also suggests that S-cones may be more vulnerable to defective RPGR function than L/M-cones. We could not obtain 440 nm thresholds in males to verify whether this pattern would occur also in males, or whether it may be unique to females, who have an opposite (i.e., cone>rod) pattern of dysfunction.

The existence of families affected with complex phenotypes resembling closely yet distinct from Usher syndrome has now been well documented. This *RPGR*-linked syndrome can be associated only with mild to moderate sensorineural hearing loss, as is the case of genuine Usher syndrome type II; with recurrent upper respiratory tract infections; or both (reviewed in Iannaccone et al., 2003, 2004).

Mutations affecting the RPGR RCC1-like domain account for all families with *RPGR*-linked pseudo-Usher phenotypes reported to date, and likely for earlier reports of a possible X-linked (type-IV) Usher syndrome (Davenport et al., 1978; Gorlin et al., 1979; Grondhal, 1987; Tamayo et al., 1991; Baldellou Vázquez et al., 1993). It cannot be presently excluded that more severe instances of hearing loss, possibly also congenital in nature, may also occur, mimicking Usher syndrome type I. Based on our findings, we propose that males with presumed Usher syndrome who test negative for mutations in Usher genes should be carefully evaluated for the possible presence of any of the aforementioned systemic manifestations and screened for mutations in the *RPGR* gene.

Acknowledgments Supported by: RPB, New York, NY (unrestricted grants to UTHSC and UM Depts. Ophthalmology, and individual awards to AI, MMJ and AS); NEI grants EY07961 and EY07003 (AS); and FFB, Hunt Valley, MD (AS).

References

Baldellou Vázquez, A., et al., 1993, Síndrome De Usher De Posible Herencia Ligada Al Cromosoma X., *An. Esp. Pediatr.* **39**:462–464.
Breuer, D. K., et al., 2002, A Comprehensive Analysis of *RPGR* and *RP2* Genes in 233 Families with X-Linked Retinitis Pigmentosa., *Am. J. Hum. Genet.* **70**:1545–1554.

Cideciyan, A. V., et al., 1998, Disease Sequence from Mutant *Rhodopsin* Allele to Rod and Cone Photoreceptor Degeneration in Man, *Proc. Natl. Acad. Sci. USA* **95**:7103–7108.

Davenport, S. L. H., et al., 1978, Usher Syndrome in Four Hard-of-Hearing Siblings, *Pediatrics* **62**:578–583.

Gorlin, R. J., et al., 1979, Usher's Syndrome Type III, *Arch. Otolaryngol.* **105**:353–354.

Grondhal, J., 1987, Estimation of Prognosis and Prevalence of the Retinitis Pigmentosa and Usher Syndrome in Norway., *Clin. Genet.* **31**:255–264.

Iannaccone, A., 2003, Usher Syndrome: Correlation between Visual Field Size and Maximal ERG Response b-Wave Amplitude., In: LaVail, M. M., Hollyfield, J. G., and Anderson, R. E., *Retinal Degenerations: Mechanisms and Experimental Therapy*, Plenum Publishers, New York, **533**: 123–131.

Iannaccone, A., 2005, The Genetics of Retinal and Optic Nerve Diseases, *Comp. Ophthalmol. Update* **5**:39–62.

Iannaccone, A., et al., 2003, Clinical and Immunohistochemical Evidence for an X Linked Retinitis Pigmentosa Syndrome with Recurrent Infections and Hearing Loss in Association with an *RPGR* Mutation, *J. Med. Genet.* **40**:e118.

Iannaccone, A., et al., 2006, Retinitis Pigmentosa Associated with Rhodopsin Mutations: Correlation between Phenotypic Variability and Molecular Effects, *Vision Res.* **46**:4556–4567.

Iannaccone, A., et al., 2004, Increasing Evidence for Syndromic Phenotypes Associated with *RPGR* Mutations, *Am. J. Ophthalmol.* **137**:785–786.

Koenekoop, R. K., et al., 2003, Novel *RPGR* Mutations with Distinct Retinitis Pigmentosa Phenotypes in French-Canadian Families, *Am. J. Ophthalmol.* **136**:678–687.

Meindl, A., et al., 1996, A Gene (RPGR) with Homology to the RCC1 Guanine Nucleotide Exchange Factor is Mutated in X-Linked Retinitis Pigmentos (RP3), *Nat. Genet.* **13**:35–42.

Roepman, R., et al., 1996, Positional Cloning of the Gene for X-Linked Retinitis Pigmentosa 3: Homology with the Guanine-Nucleotide-Exchange Factor RCC1, *Hum. Mol. Genet.* **5**: 1035–1041.

Schwahn, U., et al., 1998, Positional Cloning of the Gene for X-Linked Retinitis Pigmentosa 2, *Nat. Genet.* **19**:327–332.

Smith, R. J. H., et al., 1994, Clinical Diagnosis of the Usher Syndromes. Usher Syndrome Consortium, *Am. J. Med. Genet.* **50**:32–38.

Tamayo, M. L., et al., 1991, Usher Syndrome: Results of a Screening Program in Colombia, *Clin. Genet.* **40**:304–311.

Zito, H., et al., 2003, *RPGR* Mutation Associated with Retinitis Pigmentosa, Impaired Hearing and Sino-Respiratory Infections, *J. Med. Genet.* **40**:609–615.

Mutation in the PYK2-Binding Domain of PITPNM3 Causes Autosomal Dominant Cone Dystrophy (CORD5) in Two Swedish Families

Linda Köhn, Konstantin Kadzhaev, Marie S. I. Burstedt, Susann Haraldsson, Ola Sandgren, and Irina Golovleva

1 Introduction

Progressive cone or cone-rod dystrophies (CORDs) characterized by a defective cone function demonstrate abnormalities in cone-mediated electroretinogram (ERG) components. The presenting symptoms are defective color vision, impaired central visual acuity and sensitivity to light (Small and Gehrs, 1996; van Ghelue et al., 2000). The inheritance patterns for CORDs are autosomal dominant, autosomal recessive and X-linked (Michaelides et al., 2005a). The preservation of rod function in CORDs can differ both between and within families and depends on the disease causing mutation within a gene (Small and Gehrs, 1996; Michaelides et al., 2005b).

A variant of autosomal dominant cone dystrophy was mapped to 17p12-p13 in a Swedish family (Balciuniene et al., 1995) (CORD5, MIM 600977). Two other studies, one from the UK and one from the USA also showed linkage of dominant cone dystrophy to 17p (Small et al., 1996; Kelsell et al., 1997). The disorder in the British family, designated as CORD6 (MIM 601777) was caused by mutations in the *GUCY2D* gene (Kelsell et al., 1998). In the USA family, the disease mapped to 17p12-p13 was later reported to be caused by the same mutation as in the British CORD6 family, and therefore, it was concluded that CORD5 and CORD6 is the same disease (Small 1996; Udar et al., 2003). However, in CORD5 patients of Swedish origin there were no indications of *GUCY2D* mutations (van Ghelue et al., 2000).

Besides *GUCY2D*, another gene, *AIPL1* (MIM 604392) at 17p13 is associated with autosomal dominant CORD (Sohocki et al., 2000). Other variants of autosomal dominant CORDs are caused by mutations in *RIM1* (6q14) (MIM 606629), peripherin/*RDS* (MIM 179605) (6p21.2), *GUCA1A* (6p21.1) (MIM 600364) and *CRX* (19q13) (MIM 602225) genes.

Here, we report on fine mapping of the CORD5 locus and a mutation in *PITPNM3* associated with CORD5 in two Swedish families.

I. Golovleva
Medical and Clinical Genetics, Department of Medical Biosciences, Umeå University, S-901 85 Umeå, Sweden, Tel: 46 907856820, Fax: 46 90 128163
e-mail: Irina.Golovleva@vll.se

2 Materials and Methods

DNA from 80 individuals belonging to two multi-generation Swedish families (151 and 152, Fig. 1) and originating from the same geographical area in Northern Sweden were used for linkage analysis and mutation screening.

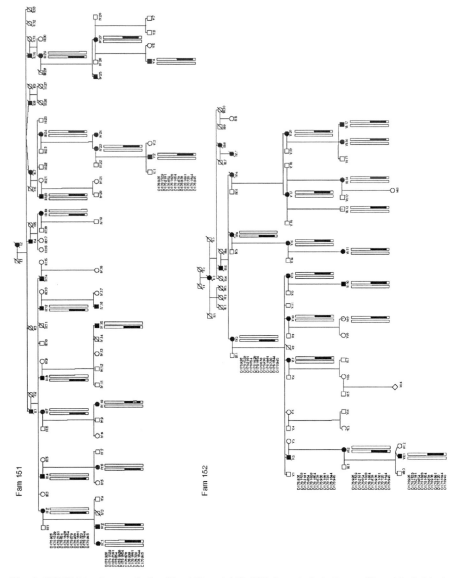

Fig. 1 CORD5 haplotypes in families 151 and 152. Filled symbols indicate affected individuals, while empty symbols indicate unaffected. Symbols with? had unknown disease status. Only haplotypes shared by affected individuals in both families are boxed

Twelve microsatellite markers in the proximity to D17S938 situated approximately 2 cM apart were used for genotyping. The raw data collected on a 3730 xl DNA analyzer were analyzed with ABI Prism GeneMapper Software v3.0 (Applied Biosystems).

Two-point linkage analyses were done using the FASTLINK implementation of the LINKAGE program package. CORD5 was analyzed as an autosomal dominant trait, with a disease allele frequency of 0.01 using five age-dependent liability classes (Balciuniene et al., 1995).

For bidirectional sequencing of *PITPNM3* (MIM 608921), coding and adjacent intronic sequences of 19 exons were amplified from genomic DNA. Primers designed with Primer3 software (http://frodo.wi.mit.edu/cgi-bin/primer3/primer3_www.cgi) can be found in Köhn *et al* (2007).The sequencing reactions were separated on a 3730 xl DNA analyzer (Applied Biosystems). Sequences were compared with a reference sequence of the *PITPNM3* gene (ENSG00000091622) available on the http://www.ensembl.org.

3 Results

3.1 Linkage and Haplotype Analysis

Fine mapping of the CORD5 locus revealed significant LOD scores at $\theta = 0$ for D17S945 to D17S1828 with a maximum of 12.67 at D17S938 (Fig. 2A, Table 1). The reconstructed haplotypes in both families (Fig. 1) confirmed segregation of CORD5 with markers D17S678, D17S938, D17S1881, D17S720 and D17S1844. In family 151 the CORD locus was limited by one recombination event for D17S945 in three affected individuals and in family 152 recombination events at D17S1828 and D17S1854 were detected. Thus, the CORD5 locus was narrowed down from 26.9 cM to 14.3 cM including flanking markers. In this region at least three genes of interest were present: *AIPL1*, an aryl-hydrocarbon interacting protein-like 1; *GUCY2D*, guanylate cyclase 2D, both known to be mutated in cone rod dystrophy and Leber congenital amaurosis; and *PITPNM3*, a membrane associated phosphatidylinositol transfer protein 3, a human homologue of the *Drosophila* retinal degeneration B (*rdgB*). *AIPL1* and *GUCY2D* were excluded by SSCP and direct sequencing.

3.2 Mutation Analysis

The human *rdgB* homolog, *PITPNM3* contains 20 exons and encodes a protein belonging to the phosphatidyl-inosytol transfer protein (PITP) family. *PITPNM3* was proposed to be a gene causing retinal degenerations (Lev et al., 1999; Lev, 2001) based on linkage of several retinal disorders to 17p12-p13. Sequence analysis of 19 exons revealed a transversion c.1878G>C (NM_031220) in exon 14 resulting

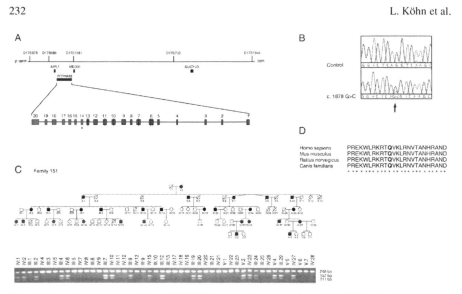

Fig. 2 Genomic structure of the *PITPNM3* gene and segregation of Q626H with CORD5. A – schematic representation of the genomic region in proximity to the D17S938 marker. Exon 2 in *PITPNM3* encodes a Ca^{+2}-binding domain, six transmembrane domains spread over exons 6, 7, 10, 11, 12 and exons 14 to 20 encode PYK2-binding domain. The PITP domain characteristic for this family is missing in PITPNM3. Q626H in exon 14 is marked with an asterisk. B – c.1878G>C (p.Q626H) detected by direct sequencing. C – segregation of CORD5 and the Q626H mutation in family 151. Filled symbols indicate affected individuals, while empty symbols indicate unaffected. D – partial protein sequence alignment of PYK-2 binding domain between mammalian PITPNM3 (http://www.ebi.ac.uk/clustalw/). Position 626 is marked in bold

in substitution of a glutamine at position 626 by a histidine (p.Q626H) (Fig. 2B). PCR-RFLP analysis using *Mae*II endonuclease showed consistent segregation of the Q626H in all affected individuals in family 151 (Fig. 2C).

Three individuals from family 152 with unknown disease history shared the same haplotype as all affected individuals (Fig. 1) and also had the Q626H mutation.

Table 1 Two-point LOD scores between markers on chromosome 17p13 and CORD5

MARKER	POSITION[a]		LOD SCORE AT θ =						
	cM	Mb	0.0	0.01	0.05	0.1	0.2	0.3	0.4
D17S926	0.63	0.58	−1.33	2.67	4.47	4.83	4.25	2.96	1.36
D17S1529	2.81	0.99	−1.70	2.25	4.07	4.45	3.95	2.76	1.28
D17S2181	4.52	1.49	−2.86	−1.49	−0.20	0.29	0.56	0.50	0.29
D17S654	6.63	1.86	−1.53	2.48	4.40	4.81	4.26	2.99	1.43
D17S1828	10.34	3.76	3.26	4.52	4.73	4.42	3.43	2.23	0.99
D17S1854	13.10	5.61	3.59	3.60	3.48	3.16	2.28	1.28	0.39
D17S678	15.65	5.97	11.68	11.48	10.68	9.63	7.38	4.90	2.24
D17S938	16.50	6.19	12.67	12.44	11.52	10.33	7.81	5.10	2.29
D17S1881	16.81	6.47	6.96	6.84	6.32	5.66	4.24	2.73	1.18
D17S720	20.00	7.64	5.40	5.52	5.44	5.01	3.79	2.38	0.98
D17S1844	21.35	8.56	12.05	11.83	10.96	9.83	7.44	4.88	2.19
D17S945	27.40	9.76	5.60	7.32	7.49	7.01	5.51	3.64	1.56

[a] marker location is based on the human genome assembly Build 35

Shared haplotypes and presence of the Q626H mutation in both families indicate that these families have a common descent (Fig. 1).

The Q626H mutation was absent on 322 control chromosomes of ethnically matched healthy individuals and in 140 individuals affected with autosomal dominant or recessive forms of retinitis pigmentosa. Residue 626 in PITPNM3 is located in a PYK2-binding domain (Lev et al., 1999), which is evolutionary conserved in mammals (Fig. 2D).

4 Discussion

Presence of the Q626H mutation in Swedish CORD5 patients, its absence on healthy chromosomes and the fact that PITPNM3 is a *Drosophila* retinal degeneration homologue causing light-induced retinal degeneration and severely impaired ERG (Harris and Stark, 1977) indicate a potential pathogenic role of the *PITPNM3* gene.

In humans PITPNM3 is expressed in the brain, spleen and ovary (Lev et al., 1999). pl-RdgB, a zebrafish homologue, is mainly expressed in inner segments of cone photoreceptors (Elagin et al., 2000), while in rat retina PITPNM3 is found through all cell layers but mainly in Muller cells (Tian and Lev, 2002).

Members of the PITP- family contain a phosphatidylinositol transfer domain (PIT), an acidic region/Ca^{+2} binding domain, six transmembrane domains, the DDHD and a C-terminal. PITPs participate in phospholipase C-mediated inositol signaling, ATP-dependent Ca^{+2}– activated secretion, lipid metabolism, trafficking from Golgi-membranes and exocytosis (Lev, 2004). An importance of a PIT domain was shown in *rdgB* mutant flies with light-dependent retinal degeneration which was rescued by transfer of the PIT-domain (Milligan et al., 1997). However, transgenic expression of zebrafish pl-RdgB lacking a PIT domain in Drosophila *rdgB²* null mutant improved photoreceptor survival but did not show any effect on ERG (Elagin et al., 2000) suggesting that PIT-domain is necessary for light response and function of others protein domains prevents photoreceptors degeneration.

Recently it was shown that the C-terminal region of the PITPNM3 is necessary for the interaction with protein tyrosine kinase PYK2 (Lev et al., 1999; Lev, 2004). We showed that the Q626H mutation in PITPNM3 is located in PYK-2 binding domain, therefore one obvious expectation might be that the mutation abolishes or modifies the interaction with PYK2 in humans. Further screening for additional *PITPNM3* mutations in both familiar and isolated cases and studies on model organisms carrying the Q626H mutation will clarify the mechanisms by which mutations in the PYK-2-binding domain result in defective vision.

In summary, this study adds one more gene on 17p, which causes retinal degeneration. We provide evidence that CORD5 in Swedish patients is a distinct clinical entity and describe the first disease causing mutation within the PYK2 – binding domain in the PITP family.

Acknowledgments This study was supported by grants from Visare Norr and University Hospital of Umeå.

References

Balciuniene, J., Johansson, K., Sandgren, O., Wachtmeister, L., Holmgren, G., and Forsman, K., 1995, A gene for autosomal dominant progressive cone dystrophy maps to chromosome 17p12-p13, *Genomics.* **30**:281.

Elagin, V.A., Elagina, R. B., Doro, C. J., Vihtelic, T. S., and Hyde, D. R., 2000, Cloning and tissue localization of a novel zebrafish RdgB homolog that lacks a phospholipid transfer domain, *Vis Neurosci.* **17**:303.

van Ghelue, M., Eriksen, H. L., Ponjavic, V., Fagerheim, T., Andreasson, S., Forsman-Semb, K., Sandgren, O., Holmgren, G., and Tranebjaerg, L., 2000, Autosomal dominant cone-rod dystrophy due to a missense mutation (R838C) in retinal guanylate cyclase gene (RETGC-1) is associated with considerable variation, *Ophthalmol Genet.* **21**:197.

Harris, W. A., and Stark, W. S., 1977, Hereditary retinal degeneration in Drosophila melanogaster, A mutant defect associated with the phototransduction process, *J Gen Physiol.* **69**:261.

Kelsell, R. E., Evans, K., Gregory, C. Y., Moore, A. T., Bird, A. C., and Hunt, D. M., 1997, Localization of a gene for dominant cone-rod dystrophy (CORD6) to chromosome 17p, *Hum Molec Genet.* **6**:597.

Kelsell, R. E., Gregory-Evans, K., Payne, A. M., Perrault, I., Kaplan, J., Yang, R. B., Garbers, D. L., Bird, A. C. A., Moore, T., and Hunt, D. M., 1998, Mutations in the retinal guanylate cyclase (RETGC-1) gene in dominant cone-rod dystrophy, *Hum Molec Genet.* **7**:1179.

Köhn, L., Kadzhaev, K., Burstedt, M. S. I., Haraldsson, S., Hallberg, B., Sandgren, O., and Golovleva, I., 2007, Mutation in the PYK2-binding domain of PITPNM3 causes autosomal dominant cone dystrophy (CORD5) in two Swedish families, *Eur J Hum Genet.* **15**:664.

Lev, S., Hernandez, J., Martinez, R., Chen, A., Plowman, G., and Schlessinger, J., 1999, Identification of a novel family of targets of PYK2 related to Drosophila retinal degeneration B (rdgB) protein, *Mol Cell Biol.* **19**:2278.

Lev, S., 2001, Molecular aspects of retinal degenerative diseases, *Cell Mol Neurobiol.* **21**(6): 575–589.

Lev, S., 2004, The role of the Nir/rdgB protein family in membrane trafficking and cytoskeleton remodeling, *Exp Cell Res.* **297**:1.

Michaelides, M., Holder, G. E., Hunt, D. M., Fitzke, F. W., Bird, A. C., and Moore, A. T., 2005a, A detailed study of the phenotype of an autosomal dominant cone-rod dystrophy (CORD7) associated with mutation in the gene for RIM1, *Br J Ophthalmol.* **89**:198.

Michaelides, M., Holder, G. E., Bradshaw, K., Hunt, D. M., and Moore, A. T., 2005b, Cone-rod dystrophy, intrafamilial variability, and incomplete penetrance associated with the R172W mutation in the peripherin/RDS gene, *Ophthalmol.* **112**:1592.

Milligan, S. C., Alb, J. G., Elagina, R. B., Bankaitis, V. A., and Hyde, D. R., 1997, The phosphatidylinositol transfer protein domain of Drosophila retinal degeneration B protein is essential for photoreceptor cell survival and recovery from light stimulation, *J Cell Biol.* **139**:351.

Small, K. W., and Gehrs K, 1996, Clinical study of a large family with autosomal dominant progressive cone degeneration, *Am J Ophthalmol.* **121**:1.

Small, K. W., Syrquin, M., Mullen, L., and Gehrs, K., 1996, Mapping of autosomal dominant cone degeneration to chromosome 17p, *Am J Ophthalmol.* **121**:13.

Sohocki, M. M., Perrault, I., Leroy, B. P., Payne, A. M., Dharmaraj, S., Bhattacharya, S. S., Kaplan, J., Maumenee, I. H., Koenekoop, R., Meire, F. M., Birch, D. G., Heckenlively, J. R., and Daiger, S. P., 2000, Prevalence of AIPL1 mutations in inherited retinal degenerative disease, *Mol Genet Metab.* **70**:142.

Tian, D., and Lev, S., 2002, Cellular and developmental distribution of human homologues of the Drosophilia rdgB protein in the rat retina, *Invest Ophthalmol Vis Sci.* **43**:1946.

Udar, N., Yelchits, S., Chalukya, M., Yellore, V., Nusinowitz, S., Silva-Garcia, R., Vrabec, T., Hussles Maumenee, I., Donoso, L., and Small, K. W., 2003, Identification of GUCY2D gene mutations in CORD5 families and evidence of incomplete penetrance, *Hum Mutat.* **21**:170.

Identification and Characterization of Genes Expressed in Cone Photoreceptors

Mehrnoosh Saghizadeh, Novrouz B. Akhmedov, and Debora B. Farber

1 Introduction

Most human hereditary retinal degenerations can be classified as rod-cone degenerations (such as retinitis pigmentosa), cone-rod degenerations (exemplified by some cone dystrophies), and diseases affecting cones exclusively (i.e., cone degenerations)(Krill, 1977; Hamel, 2007; Simunovic and Moore, 1998). In these disorders the disease process is often difficult to analyze because its time-course is slow (many years) and tissues for morphologic, biochemical or molecular biology studies are not always available. Use of animal models of retinal degeneration and advanced biotechnology have helped to elucidate the cause of some of these diseases and the mechanisms by which mutated genes lead to blindness. In general, when there is widespread degeneration of rods, regardless of the selective or not selective expression of the gene product in these cells, there is a concomitant loss of cones. In contrast, molecular defects affecting cone photoreceptors result in diseases either manifesting subsequent loss of rod-mediated vision or just loss of cones without progressive and generalized involvement of rods. Since cones, like rods, have their own unique set of genes and proteins, it is still not clear why mutations in any of the rod or cone-specific genes can lead to degeneration of the other type of photoreceptor.

Cone dystrophies are usually associated with a panretinal loss of cones that often affects the macula resulting in loss of central vision and day blindness. Although cone gene products have a major contribution to vision, only few genes expressed in cones have been studied in detail. A complete understanding of cone-associated retinal diseases will be achieved only after the function of most of the uncharacterized genes in cone cells has been elucidated. This is why for many years we have been interested in the isolation and characterization of genes expressed in cone photoreceptors. To carry out this task, we initially took advantage of the adult *cd*

M. Saghizadeh
Jules Stein Eye Institute, David Geffen School of Medicine and Molecular Biology Institute, UCLA, Los Angeles, California 90095, Tel: 310-206-6935, Fax: 818-986-7400
e-mail: nooshs@ucla.edu

R.E. Anderson et al. (eds.), *Recent Advances in Retinal Degeneration,*
© Springer 2008

dog retina that is devoid of cones but has the complete rod cell population. Cone degeneration (*cd*) is an autosomal recessive disorder that occurs naturally and was originally found in the Alaskan Malamute dog (Aguirre and Rubin, 1974). This disease is caused by a deletion in the cone cyclic nucleotide-gated channel β subunit gene (CNGB3) (Sidjanin et al., 2002).

2 Strategy and Methods

Retinal mRNAs from adult, cone-less *cd* dogs were subtracted from normal dog retinal mRNAs using two rounds of representational difference analysis (Akhmedov et al., 2002). We then took the output of RDA and shotgun cloned it into a plasmid vector to create a mini-library in a bacterial host. Approximately 2000 cDNA clones generated from the subtracted library were arrayed on microarray chips after amplification of inserts from individual colonies with vector-specific primers. The arrayed target cDNAs were hybridized with the Cy3- and Cy5-labeled original amplicons from normal and adult *cd* dog retinas, and subsequently screened by repetitive probing with mixtures of the inserts that had the brightest signal after hybridization with the initial amplicons (Saghizadeh et al., 2003). This screening created a non-redundant set of clones. Eighty of these clones were differentially expressed. After sequencing, BLAST analyses were performed utilizing the National Center for Biotechnology Database (www.ncbi.nlm.nih.gov/BLAST) and the Institute for Genomic Research (www.tigr.com.).

2.1 Microarray Screening Identified Several Potentially Cone-Expressed cDNAs

Out of the 80 sequenced clones, we identified several that have been described as cone-specific (i.e., 3 clones for different regions of cone opsin cDNA, 4 clones for the different subunits of cone transducin and 3 clones for different regions of α' subunit of cone PDE cDNA), and several that did not correspond to any known gene (8 clones, Table 1) or to genes that had not been described as present in the retina (27 clones, i.e., VPS35 and PTDSR). The rest corresponded to mitochondrial genome fragments. Northern blots and real-time RT-PCR were used to confirm the differential expression of the isolated cDNAs.

3 Preliminary Characterization Of Unknown cDNAs

The 8 differentially expressed clones from Table 1 were used as probes on Northern blots of total RNA from dog retinas. Only three clones (12B7, 21D1 and 4A1) showed detectable signals after one-week exposure (Fig. 1). It is possible that the other 5 clones were less abundant than 12B7, 21D1 and 4A1; at the time we also

Table 1 Unknown dog cDNAs identified as expressed in cone photoreceptors after microarray screening of the RDA-subtracted pool of cDNAs

cDNA clone	Mapped to human Chr.	Human database hit
12B7	14	None
21D1	9	KIAA1896
4A1	–	No hit
15A15	22	ZBED4
8H5	13	CUL4A
13D8	–	No hit
5E1	X	MBTPS2

thought that they could be pseudogenes. 12B7 was expressed specifically in normal retina and was not present in brain, heart, kidney, liver, muscle, or spleen (Fig. 1A). Two transcripts for 12B7 of approximately 7.0 kb and 3.5 kb were observed in normal retinas. The larger transcript and a smaller than 3.5 kb transcript were present in *cd* dog retinal RNA, (Fig. 1A). 21D1 was preferentially expressed in retina with a transcript approximately 3.0 kb long (Fig. 1B). This transcript was in much lower amount in *cd* than in normal retina (Fig. 1B). 4A1 was expressed in normal and *cd* dog retina and also in all dog tissues investigated. The size of the transcript hybridized to the 4A1 cDNA probe was approximately 1.8 kb.

In collaboration with The Institute for Genomic Research (Tigr), human orthologs of both the 21D1 and 15A15 clones were identified as predicted genes. 12B7 and 8H5 were mapped to human chromosome 14 and 13, respectively. The latter was found to encode a known gene, Cullin 4A (GenBankTM accession number AF077188). Similarly, 5E1 mapped to human chromosome X, and was found to encode the known gene, MBTPS2. Clones 13D8 and 4A1 could not be mapped to any human chromosome.

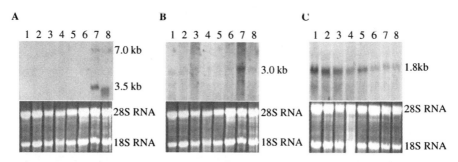

Fig. 1 Northern blots of dog RNAs hybridized with cDNA fragments corresponding to three isolated clones. 30 µg of total RNA from multiple normal dog tissues and *cd* dog retina were electrophoresed on a 1.2% agarose gel containing formaldehyde, transferred to Hybond N+ and hybridized at 68°c with radiolabeled cDNA probes. (A) Expression of 12B7 mRNA. (B) The same blot was stripped and probed with a radiolabeled 21D1 cDNA fragment. (c) Different blot showing the expression of 4A1 mRNA. Lanes: 1, brain; 2, heart; 3, liver; 4,kidney; 5, lung; 6, testis; 7, normal retina; 8, *cd* retina

Therefore, preliminary characterization of unknown cDNAs and computer analysis of their primary sequences led us to choose the cDNA candidates for further investigation.

4 Characterization of Mouse 21D1

4.1 Molecular Cloning

The clone originally obtained was a part of the 5' dog archive sequence, intronic to the cDNA sequence, and it had 94% homology to a human sequence and 95% homology to a mouse sequence. *21D*1 was mapped to human chromosome 9 and mouse chromosome 2. The complete 21D1 mouse cDNA, including the coding region and 3' and 5' UTRs, was obtained by 5' and 3' RACE using oligo-dT-primed mouse retinal first-strand cDNA and gene-specific sequences. The 2970–bp cDNA comprises an open reading frame of 1506 bp, a 367-bp 5'-UTR, and a 1097-bp 3'-UTR.

4.2 Northern Blot Analysis and Developmental Studies of Mouse 21D1 mRNA

Using RT-PCR, a 700 bp probe from the coding region of the 21D1 mouse sequence was subcloned. Northern blots of mRNAs from different mouse tissues hybridized to this 21D1 cDNA probe showed a transcript of the same size of dog 21D1 mRNA, approximately 3.0 kb long in retina and larger than 3.0 kb in other tissues. This mRNA was abundantly expressed in retina and brain, in lesser amounts in liver and testis and was present at low levels in kidney, lung, and muscle and barely detected in heart (Fig. 2A). Northern blots of retinal mRNAs from mice at different times during postnatal development showed that 21D1mRNA expression increased from birth and peaked at 15-21 day (Fig. 2B). Interestingly, the developmental increase in 21D1 mRNA expression correlates with the time of differentiation, growth and elongation of outer segments of photoreceptor cells. This observation suggests that 21D1 may be expressed in visual cells.

4.3 Computer Analysis of the 21D1 Primary Sequence

Search of the protein database with the deduced amino acid sequence of the original dog 21D1 clone revealed its homology with the human KIAA1896 protein and the mouse peroxisomal Ca2+-dependent solute carrier-like protein. However, after cloning the full-length mouse cDNA from retina, we found that the first 73 amino acids of the predicted protein corresponding to the 21D1 cDNA had no homology with other proteins in the database. The amino-terminal-half of the 21D1 predicted

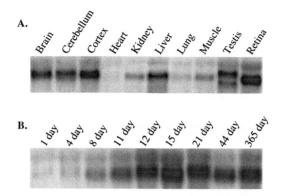

Fig. 2 Northern blots of mRNAs from mouse tissues probed with a 21D1 cDNA fragment. Each lane contains 30 µg of total RNA. (A) Multiple mouse tissues. Note the size difference of the transcript in retina compared to those in other tissues. (B) Developmental expression of 21D1 mRNA in mouse retina. Ethidium bromide staining of the gels was used to demonstrate the equal loading of mRNA in each lane (not shown)

protein contains three conserved Ca2+ elongation factor (EF)-hand binding loops and the carboxyl-terminal-half has conserved-domain similarity with proteins of the mitochondrial solute carrier family. While carrying out these studies, a novel member of the mitochondrial Ca2+-dependent solute carrier protein subfamily was reported to be present in liver, MCSC (Mashima et al., 2003). This protein has 99% identity with the 21D1 predicted protein. However, the first 73 amino acids of 21D1 have no homology with MCSC.

4.4 21D1, A New Mouse Variant of the MCSC Sub-family

Members of the mitochondrial carrier family (MC) that exist exclusively in eukaryotes (del Arco and Satrustegui, 2004) are integral proteins of the mitochondrial inner membrane and facilitate the transport of metabolites, nucleotides and cofactors between the cytosol and mitochondria. Calcium-binding mitochondrial carriers (CaMCs) are a subfamily of the MC family. They have an N-terminal extension harboring four EF-hand binding motifs, and a carrier domain at the C terminus that has all the characteristic features of carrier domains in the MC family. Two groups of proteins belong to the CaMC subfamily. They differ in the length of their N-terminal region; proteins with the long N-terminal region are called CaMC and proteins with the short N-terminal region, SCaMC (Fig. 3). The human *SCaMC-2* gene has four variants generated by the use of alternative promoters. These variants differ in the length and amino acid sequence of exon 1. 21D1 is the mouse ortholog of the human variant c of SCaMC-2 that is expressed abundantly in brain (Fig. 3). Therefore, we designated our protein MCSC-c. Comparison of the genomic structures of MCSC and the MCSC-c variant (Fig. 4) showed that exons 2–10 are identical in both, but exon 1 in each gene is from different regions of chromosome 2. Since the start

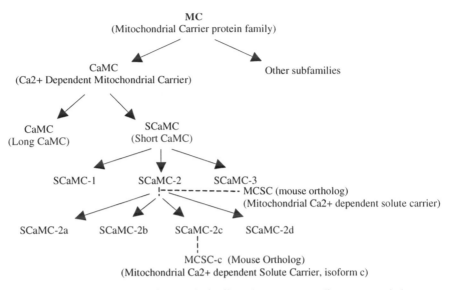

Fig. 3 Human mitochondrial carrier protein family and two corresponding mouse orthologs

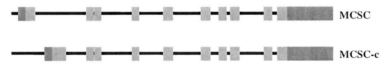

Fig. 4 Genomic organization of MCSC and the MCSC-c variant. Dark gray boxes are the 5' or 3'-UTRs and light gray boxes are the 10 exons that form the mRAN coding region

codon of these two variants is present in exon 1, the mRNA 5' UTRs as well as the N-terminal sequences of both resulting proteins are different.

5 Characterization of the Human 15A15 Clone

5.1 Computer Analysis of the 15A15 Primary Sequence

The sequence of the 15A15 dog clone that we originally obtained (260 bp) showed 89% homology to the coding region of a human predicted gene, ZBED4. This predicted gene is located on human chromosome 22 and mouse chromosome 15, is 34.5 kb long in human and 29.8 kb in mouse and has 2 exons in both species. The ZBED4 cDNA sequence predicts a protein formed by 1171-amino acids that contains four BED type zinc finger domains and a hATC type dimerization domain near the C terminus.

5.2 Molecular Cloning of ZBED4

Using RT-PCR, a 713-bp probe from the 3' coding region of the mouse sequence was obtained. This fragment was subcloned and used for Northern blot hybridization. In addition, the complete coding region of ZBED4 was amplified from mouse retina mRNA using the appropriate primers, and the isolated cDNA was subcloned into an expression vector for subcellular localization studies.

5.3 Northern Blot Analysis

Northern blots of mouse retinal and brain mRNAs hybridized to the corresponding ZBED4 cDNA probe showed a major transcript of 5.3 kb, which is consistent with the molecular size estimated for *ZBED4* mRNA (Fig. 5).

5.4 Localization of ZBED4 to Human Cone Photoreceptor Cells

Immunohistochemistry studies using a polyclonal ZBED4 antibody and human retinal sections localized ZBED4 to the nuclei and inner segments of cone photoreceptors (Fig. 6). These results were confirmed with double immunostaining of human sections with anti-ZBED antibody and rhodamine-conjugated peanut agglutinin, which binds to the matrix surrounding cone photoreceptors, but not to that surrounding rods (data not shown).

5.5 Subcellular Localization of ZBED4

Immunostaining studies using Y79 retinoblastoma cells and anti-ZBED4 antibody showed the nuclear localization of ZBED4 (Fig. 7). This localization was also seen when Y79 retinoblastoma cells transfected with an expression vector containing the

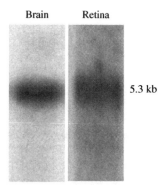

Fig. 5 Northern blots of mouse mRNAs from retina and brain probed with a radiolabeled 15A15 (ZBED4) cDNA fragment. Each lane contains 2 μg of mRNA

Fig. 6 Localization of the
ZBED4 protein in human
retina. Human retinal sections
were incubated with a
polyclonal antibody to a
ZBED4 peptide (that we
generated in rabbit), followed
by reaction with
FITC-conjugated goat
anti-rabbit antibody. Arrow
shows nuclei and arrowhead
shows cone inner segment
staining. Magnification 400X

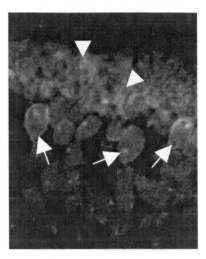

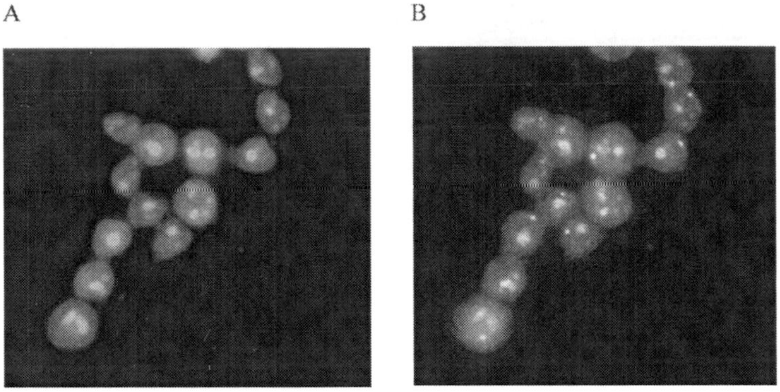

A   B

Fig. 7 Subcellular localization of the ZBED4 protein in Y79 retinoblastoma cells. Y79 retinoblastoma cells incubated with anti-ZBED4 antibody show the enogenous localization of ZBED4 to nuclei of these cells A. DAPI staining of nuclei. B. Anti-ZBED4 antibody staining

complete coding region of ZBED4 attached to the Xpress epitope were reacted with anti-Xpress antibody: the conjugated ZBED4-Xpress protein was detected in the nuclei (data not shown).

6 Discussion

Microarray screening of our subtracted cDNA pool (retinal cDNAs from *cd* dog subtracted from those of normal dog retina) helped us to identify several uncharacterized cDNAs expressed in cone photoreceptors. After preliminary studies on several of these cDNAs and computer analysis of their primary sequences, we chose a couple cDNAs for further investigation.

We report here the identification in retina of a new variant of mouse mitochondrial carrier solute carrier, MCSC-c. This protein belongs to the Ca2+-dependent mitochondrial transporter subfamily and is encoded by an mRNA that has a different exon 1 than the liver MCSC mRNA (see Fig. 4). The N-terminal of the MCSC-c protein has no homology to that of MCSC. These variants may have different functional characteristics or sensitivity to Ca+2, which could explain their tissue or cell specificity.

Several studies have established that 60–65% of retinal mitochondria are located in the inner segments of photoreceptors (Hoang et al., 2002; Kageyama and Wong-Riley, 1984). These cells have 2- to 3-fold greater oxygen consumption and higher cytochrome c oxidase (CO) activity than the cells of the inner retina (Chen et al., 1989). It has also been shown that rod and cone mitochondria have fundamental substructural and functional differences (Perkins et al., 2003). Cone inner segments contain 2-fold more mitochondria and create more CO activity than rod inner segments. Therefore, cones utilize complementary mechanisms to compensate for their differences with rods in bioenergetic processes. These include: increased number of mitochondria, increased cristae surface membrane area and probably, the presence of specific proteins or variants of functional proteins in the outer or inner membrane of their mitochondria with different functional sensitivities.

Variations in the N-terminal half of the human SCaMC-2 splice variants result in different number of EF-hand domains in the proteins. It has been reported that the splice isoforms of UCP5 and phosphate carrier proteins (another carrier protein family) differ in their functional characteristics (Fiermonte et al., 1998). It is possible that absence of a specific EF-hand motif in different variants of SCaMC-2 or in MCSC and MCSC-c provides a mechanism for Ca2+ signaling diversification. Furthermore, different N-terminal variants arising from tissue or cell-specific promoter usage may also provide additional mechanisms to modulate sensitivity to Ca2+.

Another cDNA that we identified after substractive hybridization and microarray screening of normal and cone-less mRNAs is 15A15. This cDNA encodes a novel 1171-amino acid protein, ZBED4. Primary sequence analysis of ZBED4 revealed characteristic features of a nuclear regulatory protein. It contains four zinc finger BED domains that have the $Cx_2Cx_nHx_{3-5}[H/C]$ signature in the amino-terminal-half, and a hATC dimerization domain in the carboxyl-terminal-half. Interestingly, two nuclear receptor-interacting modules (LXXLL) are present in the ZBED4 amino acid sequence, suggesting its possible direct or indirect interaction with nuclear hormone receptors. The hATC dimerization domain of ZBED4 also makes this protein a member of the human hAT transposase family. It has been reported that the hATC domain is very conserved among proteins of this family and functions in self-association, an essential feature required for nuclear accumulation and DNA binding (Yamashita et al., 2007).

Expression of ZBED4 is limited to cone photoreceptors and completely absent from rods in human retina, as determined by immunocytochemistry (Fig. 6). Furthermore, ZBED4 is present in cell nuclei, as shown by co-localization of transfected ZBED4 with the nuclear marker DAPI. Considering the specific features of the ZBED4 primary sequence: that ZBED fingers bind to DNA, that hATC domains usually facilitate accumulation of proteins in nuclei and that LXXLL motifs bind to nuclear hormone receptors, we hypothesize that ZBED4 may be directly or indirectly involved as a co-activator or co-repressor in the regulation of transcription of cone-specific genes.

Acknowledgments This work was supported by NIH R01 grant EY 08285 to DBF, NIH training grant EY07062 (MS) and a grant from the Foundation Fighting Blindness (DBF). We thank Dr. Alex Yuan for his help in the preparation of this chapter. Mehrnoosh Saghizadeh was the recipient of an RD2006 Young Investigator Award.

References

G. D. Aguirre and L. F. Rubin, Pathology of hemeralopia in the Alaskan malamute dog, *Invest Ophthalmol.* **13**(3), 231–35 (1974).

N. B. Akhmedov, V. J. Baldwin, B. Zangerl, J.W. Kijas, L. Hunter, K. D. Minoofar, C. Mellersh, E. A. Ostrander, G. M. Acland, D. B. Farber and G. D. Aguirre, Cloning and characterization of the canine photoreceptor specific cone-rod homeobox (CRX) gene and evaluation as a candidate for early onset photoreceptor diseases in the dog, *Mol Vis.* **8**, 79–84 (2002).

A. del Arco and J. Satrustegui, Identification of a novel human subfamily of mitochondrial carriers with calcium-binding domains, *J Biol Chem.* **279**(23), 24701–13 (2004).

E. Chen, P. G. Soderberg and B. Lindstrom, Activity distribution of cytochrome oxidase in the rat retina. A quantitative histochemical study, *Acta Ophthalmol.* **67**(6), 645–51 (1989).

G. Fiermonte, V. Dolce and F. Palmieri, Expression in Escherichia coli, functional characterization, and tissue distribution of isoforms A and B of the phosphate carrier from bovine mitochondria. *J Biol Chem.* **273**(35), 22782–87 (1998).

C. P. Hamel, Cone rod dystrophies, *Orphanet J Rare Dis.* **2**,7 (2007).

Q. V. Hoang, R. A. Linsenmeier, C. K. Chung and C. A. Curcio, Photoreceptor inner segments in monkey and human retina: mitochondrial density, optics, and regional variation, *Vis Neurosci.* **19**(4), 395–407 (2002).

G. H. Kageyama and M.T. Wong-Riley, The histochemical localization of cytochrome oxidase in the retina and lateral geniculate nucleus of the ferret, cat, and monkey, with particular reference to retinal mosaics and ON/OFF-center visual channels, *J Neurosci.* **4**(10), 2445–59 (1984).

A. E. Krill, Rod-cone dystrophies, In: *Krill's Hereditary Retinal and Choroidal Diseases,* edited by A. E. Krill and D. B. Archer, (Harper & Row, Hagerstown, 1977), pp. 479–644.

H. Mashima, N. Ueda, H. Ohno, J. Suzuki, H. Ohnishi, H. Yasuda, T. Tsuchida, C. Kanamaru, N. Makita, T. Iiri, M. Omata and I. Kojima, A novel mitochondrial Ca2+-dependent solute carrier in the liver identified by mRNA differential display, *J Biol Chem.* **278**(11), 9520–27 (2003).

G. A. Perkins, M. H. Ellisman and D. A. Fox, Three-dimensional analysis of mouse rod and cone mitochondrial cristae architecture: Bioenergetic and functional implications, *Mol Vis.* **9**, 60–73 (2003).

M. Saghizadeh, D. J. Brown, J. Tajbakhsh, Z. Chen, M. C. Kenney, D. B Farber and S. F. Nelson, Evaluation of techniques using amplified nucleic acid probes for gene expression profiling, *Biomol Eng.* **20**(3), 97–106 (2003).

D. J. Sidjanin, J. K. Lowe, J. L. McElwee, B. S. Milne, T. M. Phippen, I. Sargan, G. D. Aguirre, G. M. Acland and E. A. Ostrander, Canine *CNGB3* mutation established cone degeneration as orthologous to the human achromatopsia locus *ACHM3*, *Hum Mol Genet.* **11**(16), 1823–33 (2002).

M. P. Simunovic and A.T. Moore, The cone dystrophies, *Eye.* **12**(pt 3b), 553–65 (1998).

D. Yamashita, H. Komori, Y. Higuchi, T. Yamaguchi, T. Osumi and F. Hirose, Human DNA replication-related element binding factor (hDREF) self-association via hATC domain is necessary for its nuclear accumulation and DNA binding, *J Biol Chem.* **282**(10), 7563–75 (2007).

Clinical and Genetic Characterization of a Chinese Family with CSNB1

Ruifang Sui, Fengrong Li, Jialiang Zhao, and Ruxin Jiang

1 Introduction

Human congenital stationary night blindness (CSNB) is a group of non-progressive retinal dystrophies characterized by night blindness from birth and other symptoms such as myopia, hyperopia, reduced visual acuity and occasionally accompanied by nystagmus, and optic disc hypoplasia (Heonand and Musarella, 1994). CSNB can be inherited on autosomal dominant, autosomal recessive and X-linked recessive mode. According to the clinical and genetic studies, X-linked recessive CSNB (XLCSNB) can be divided into two subtypes: complete (CSNB1; MIM 310500) and incomplete (CSNB2; MIM 300710). The distinction between the two subtypes of XLCSNB is in electroretinogram (ERG) and in genetic basis. CSNB1 is characterized by the complete absence of the rod b-wave, but almost normal cone amplitudes, while CSNB2 is associated with a reduced rod activity and a significantly abnormal cone ERG. The disease gene responsible for CSNB2 (*CACNA1F*) at Xp11.23 encodes a retina-specific L-type calcium channel α-subunit. CSNB1 results from mutations in the *NYX* (nyctalopin on chromosome X) gene at Xp11.4 (Miyake et al., 1986; Bech Hansen et al., 1998). We describe a Chinese family with multiple individuals affected with reduced vision and high myopia, which has been misdiagnosed as "pathologic myopia and amblyopia". Clinical and genetic investigation indicated a phenotype of CSNB1. Linkage analysis for the family mapped this phenotype to Xp11.4. Sequencing of *NYX* identified one novel mutation.

R. Sui

Department of Ophthalmology, Peking Union Medical College Hospital, Beijing 100730, China,
Tel: 86-1065296358, Fax: 86-1065296565
e-mail: hrfsui@yahoo.com

R.E. Anderson et al. (eds.), *Recent Advances in Retinal Degeneration*,
© Springer 2008

2 Materials and Methods

2.1 Family and Clinical Data

The proband was a seven-year old boy suffered from bad vision. His visual acuity was 20/200 at right eye (OD) and 20/100 at left eye (OS). The best corrected visual acuity (BCVA) with refraction −5.00–0.75×70 was 20/60 (OD) and with refraction −4.50–1.00×90 was 20/50 (OS). He has been diagnosed as "pathologic myopia and amblyopia". His male relatives have similar eye problems. The clinical characteristics of this family were evaluated using a comprehensive ophthalmologic examination including refraction, Snellen visual acuity, slit-lamp, and funduscopic examinations. Recordings of ERGs for selected members were conducted in consistent with ISCEV standards. ERG responses are compared with those of age-matched controls. All investigations followed the tenets of the Declaration of Helsinki, and informed consent was obtained from the subjects after an explanation of the study's purpose.

2.2 Linkage Analysis

Genomic DNA was extracted from leukocytes from 5mL of peripheral blood of all participants. Genotyping was performed using 5'-fluorescently labeled microsatellite markers at Xp11.4. Genotyping data were collected by using GeneMapper 3.0 and analyzed by Genotyper 2.5. Linkage analysis by calculating two-point lod score was performed using LINKAGE 5.2 software suite. This family was analyzed as an X-linked recessive trait with full penetrance and a disease allele frequency of 0.001. Haplotypes were generated by Cyrillic 2.1 program and confirmed by inspection.

2.3 Mutation Screening

Six primer pairs were designed to amplify the two coding exons and the adjacent introns sequences of the *NYX* gene (primer pairs and conditions are available in request). After purification, amplicons were sequenced on both strands using both forward and reverse primers on an ABI 377 Genetic Analyzer. Sequencing results from affected and unaffected individuals as well as *NYX* consensus sequences from the NCBI Human Genome Database were imported into the ChromasPro program and then aligned to identify variations.

3 Results

3.1 Pedigree Analysis

This four generation Chinese family with 28 individuals lived in the east China (Fig. 1). Twenty one members participated in this study (Table 1). Pedigree analysis

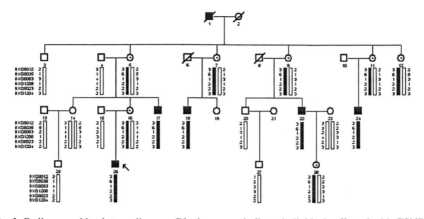

Fig. 1 Pedigree and haplotype diagram. Black squares indicate individuals affected with CSNB1. Circles with a central black dot indicate carriers. Black bars represent the disease allele inherited from ancestor. White bars represent normal allele. Arrow indicates proband

elucidated that: (1) all affected individual was male; (2) no father-son transmission; (3) none of the parents of affected individual was affected. These features strongly suggest that the condition is inherited as an X-linked recessive trait. Females (ID 5,7,9,11,12,16) with affected sons and daughter (ID 28) with affected father must be obligate carriers.

Table 1 Clinical data of available individuals in this CSNB family

Pt ID	Sex	Year of birth	Refractive error Right eye	Left eye	Infected Status
3	M	1935	+1.00–0.50×3	+0.75–0.75×106	Unaffected
4	M	1945	+0.25–0.25×88	+0.75–0.25×91	Unaffected
5	F	1947	+1.00–0.50×103	+1.00–0.75×86	Obligate Carrier
7	F	1938	+1.75–0.75×90	+5.25–4.75×102	Obligate Carrier, left pterygium
9	F	1945	+1.00	+0.75+0.25×170	Obligate Carrier
11	F	1950	+0.25	+0.50	Obligate Carrier
12	F	1954	–10.75–1.25×86	+0.25–0.50×100	Obligate Carrier
13	M	1964	–0.5	–0.5–0.5×170	Unaffected
14	F	1968	Plano-0.50×92	–0.50	Unaffected
15	M	1971	–0.25–0.25×92	–0.25–0.25×103	Unaffected
16	F	1971	–0.5–0.75×86	Plano-0.50×111	Obligate Carrier
17	M	1974	–9.25–1.25×97	–8.00–1.75×102	Affected
18	M	1972	–10.00–2.50×117	–12.50–1.75×88	Affected
20	M	1971	– 0.50–1.00×82	+0.25–0.75×107	Unaffected
22	M	1967	–7.50–3.50×111	–9.50–3.50×90	Affected, Exotropia & nystagmus
23	F	1972	–0.25–0.50×2	Plano-0.50×9	Unaffected
24	M	1977	–13.25–2.25×92	–13.25–1.50×77	Affected
25	M	1990	–1.25–0.5×97	–1.75–0.5×130	Unaffected
26	M	1995	–5.75–0.75×97	–5.00–1.25×118	Affected (proband)
27	M	1996	–0.50–0.50×171	–0.75–0.25×6	Unaffected
28	F	1995	Plano-0.50×97	Plano	Obligate Carrier

3.2 Clinical Results

The manifest refraction was –9.00 D or lower (spherical equivalent) in affected GFP-positive when the mice were injected at E14.5. It is unknown why certain cells would be adults, with BCVA less than 20/25. Funduscopic observation of all affected individuals revealed myopic fundus changes typical of high myopia with optic nerve head crescent and "tigroid" appearance of posterior retina. Such fundus changes and high myopia were not observed in unaffected individuals and obligate carriers except one who had high myopic changes in one eye (ID 12). The axial length of the proband was 25.22 mm (OD) and 24.97 mm (OS) at 8 years old. One (ID 17) in five patients complained of impaired night vision and there was no suggestion of a night vision problem in the rest.

3.3 Electroretinogram

ERG recordings under ISCEV of the proband and his uncle (ID 17) demonstrated that the rod ERG was absent; the mixed rod-cone response elicited by a single bright flash had a negative configuration with normal a-wave amplitude and reduced b-wave amplitude; the OPs were absent; the cone and 30Hz flicker ERGs appear nearly normal except the a-wave of the cone ERG has a plateau-like flat bottom. The ERG results of the proband's mother revealed no abnormality (Fig. 2).

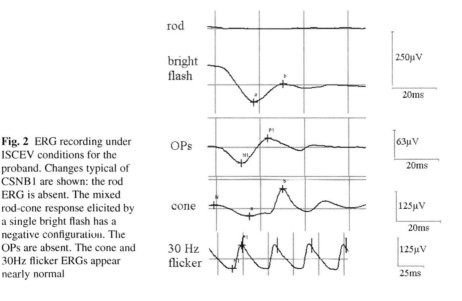

Fig. 2 ERG recording under ISCEV conditions for the proband. Changes typical of CSNB1 are shown: the rod ERG is absent. The mixed rod-cone response elicited by a single bright flash has a negative configuration. The OPs are absent. The cone and 30Hz flicker ERGs appear nearly normal

Table 2 Two-Point linkage analysis between CSNB1 and markers on Xp11.4

Marker	cM	LOD Score at θ					
		0.0	0.1	0.2	0.3	0.4	0.5
DXS8012	42.21	1.62	1.38	1.12	0.80	0.43	0.00
DXS8035	43.83	2.23	1.91	1.54	1.11	0.60	0.00
DXS8083	46.54	2.22	1.90	1.52	1.10	0.59	0.00
DXS1208	50.83	2.22	1.88	1.50	1.07	0.57	0.00
DXS8023	51.78	0.00	0.00	0.00	0.00	0.00	0.00
DXS1204	52.50	0.43	0.36	0.20	0.11	0.11	0.00

3.4 Linkage Analysis

Two point linkage analysis yielded positive lod scores with five of the six selected markers on Xp11.4 (DXS8012, DXS8035, DXS8083, DXS1208, DXS1204), with DXS8035 showing the highest lod score of 2.23 for at theta=0 (Table 2). Haplotypes of markers in this region support the linkage results. The haplotype "361223" was co-segregated with affected family member (Fig. 1).

3.5 Mutation Analysis

Mutation screening by direct sequencing in affected male identified a novel A-to-C transversion in exon 2, resulting in a change ACG of Threonine to Proline at codon 258. Obligate carriers carried a heterozygous A-to-C. Neither normal subject of the family nor 110 ethnically matched controls show this mutation (Fig. 3).

4 Discussion

CSNB is a genetically and clinically heterogeneous nonprogressive retinal disorder. Ten loci with ten genes have been implicated in CSNB, including GNAT1, PDE6B,

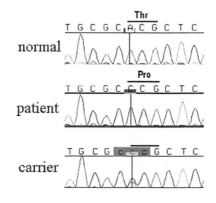

Fig. 3 Sequence results of the NYX gene fragments in normal controls, patients and carriers. At cDNA 772 Adenosine is changed to Cytosine, the encoded amino acid is changed from Threonine to Proline. All female carriers are heterozygous

RHO, GRK1, GRM6, RDH5, SAG, CACNA1F, NYX, and RPGR. Based fundamentally on the ERG findings, XLCSNB can be divided into complete (CSNB1) characterized by absent rod system function and incomplete (CSNB2) with evidence of rod function.

X-linked CSNB is not readily identified clinically owing to the lack of specificity of the main clinical features. Patients with complete X-linked CSNB usually have high myopia with a tigroid-appearing fundus and tilted myopic disc and some patients have mild nystagmus. In this report, all affected males had high myopia but only one complained of night-blindness. Miyake reported (Miyake, 2006a) that 15/49 complete XLCSNB and 1/41 incomplete XLCSNB patients had history of impaired night vision. Therefore, clinicians must be cautious when diagnosing CSNB relying on history of night blindness. In our electrically illuminated night-time environment, people can be unaware of loss of night vision because night-time activities are typically done with sufficient light. Another contributing factor of misdiagnosis of CSNB is its absence of a clinical identifiable structural abnormality. However, the shape of ERGs is extremely uniform for CSNB1 patients with the scotopic b-wave evoked by dim flashes and the early oscillatory potential wavelets unrecordable and the photopic system nearly normal. The correct diagnosis of CNSB1 is not easy unless ERG performed. Carrier states of CSNB1 with selectively reduced Ops have been reported (Miyake, 2006b), the obligate carrier (ID 16) in this study didn't show ERG anomalies. One eye with high myopia in one obligate carrier (ID 12) may be associated with special X inactivation.

Two causative genes for XLCSNB have been identified through positional cloning. *CACNA1F* (encoding a calcium channel α1-subunit) is mutated in CSNB2 patients and is localized in Xp11.23 (Bech-Hansen et al., 1998; Strom et al., 1998). The gene responsible for CSNB1, *NYX* encodes a protein of 481 amino acids containing an N-terminal signal peptide and a C-terminal GPI anchor. The central part of the polypeptide encodes 11 consecutive LRRs (Leucine Rich Repeats), which are flanked by N- and C-terminal cysteine-rich LRRs (Bech-Hansen et al., 2000; Pusch et al., 2000). According to the cysteine pattern (C'CxC(9x)C), nyctalopin belongs to the class II small leucine-rich proteoglycans (Zeitz et al., 2003). LRRs are suggested to mediate protein-protein interaction (Kobe and Deisenhofer, 1994).

The role of *NYX* in the pathogenesis of CSNB1 is not clear. CSNB1 is characterized by the absence of post-receptor rod-mediated function (Miyake et al., 1986). This information suggests a defect in synaptic transmission between photoreceptor and second-order neurons. The presence of a subnormal photopic ON response suggests an additional effect on the cone photoreceptor-ON bipolar pathway but no apparent effect on the cone OFF bipolar response. Defective *NYX* gene product prevents detectable signal transmission through ON rod bipolar cells, but there is a residual transmission through rod–cone gap junctions in CSNB1, possibly through the OFF cone pathway (Scholl et al., 2001). Recently, Morgans et al. demonstrated that the nyctalopin was associated with the synapses of both rod and cone terminals and with rod bipolar cell terminals of mammalian retina. This supports a role for nyctalopin in the synaptic transmission and/or synapse formation in the retina (Morgans et al., 2006).

Fig. 4 3D structure of
nyctalopin. The novel
mutation T258P was shown
with asterisk

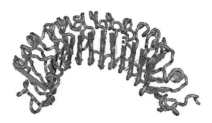

In this study, we confirm the diagnosis of CSNB1 in a Chinese family by combined clinical and genetic investigation. A novel T258P mutation was identified related to this phenotype. Including this one, 40 mutations in *NYX* have been reported among CSNB1 patients (www.hgmd.org). More than 50% of them are missense mutations and 80% missense mutations present in LRR. Each LRR is thought to form a β-sheet and an α-helix. The mutation we found is in the 9th LRR, which is a β-sheet by 3D protein structure modeling using Cn3D (Fig. 4). The substitution is predicted to interfere the formation of β-sheet that would possibly disturb the structural stability and function of nyctalopin.

Acknowledgments We thank all patients and family members for their participation. This study was supported in part by the National 863 Plan of China (2002BA711A08 to R.S.) and Beijing science and technology project (H020220020510 to R.S.)

References

Bech-Hansen N.T., Naylor M.J., Maybaum T.A., Pearce W.G., Koop B., Fishman G.A., Mets M., Musarella M.A., and Boycott K.M., 1998, Loss-of-function mutations in a calcium-channel alpha-1-subunit gene in Xp11.23 cause incomplete X-linked congenital stationary night blindness, Nat. Genet. **19**: 264.

Bech-Hansen N.T., Naylor M.J., Maybaum T.A., Sparkes R.L., Koop B., Birch D.G., Bergen A.A., Prinsen C.F., Polomeno R.C., Gal A., Drack A.V., Musarella M.A., Jacobson S.G., Young R.S., and Weleber R.G., 2000, Mutations in NYX, encoding the leucine-rich proteoglycan nyctalopin, cause X-linked complete congenital stationary night blindness, Nat. Genet. **26**: 319.

Heon E., and Musarella M.A., 1994, Congenital stationary night blindness. In: Molecular genetics of inherited eye disorders, edited by A.F. Wright and B. Jay, (Harwood Academic, Switzerland), pp. 277–301.

Kobe B., and Deisenhofer J., 1994, The leucine-rich repeat: a versatile binding motif, Trends Biol. Sci. **19**: 415.

Miyake Y., Yagasaki K., Horiguchi M., Kawase Y., and Kanda T., 1986, Congenital stationary night blindness with negative electroretinogram: a new classification, Arch. Ophthalmol. **104**: 1013.

Miyake Y., 2006a Initial complaints of patients, In: Electrodiagnosis of retinal diseases, edited by Y. Miyake, (Springer, Japan), pp. 94.

Miyake Y., 2006b Carrier State of X-linked CSNB, In: Electrodiagnosis of retinal diseases, edited by Y. Miyake, (Springer, Japan), pp. 104.

Morgans C.W., Ren G., and Akileswaran L., 2006, Localization of nyctalopin in the mammalian retina. Euro. J. Neurosci. **23**: 1163.

Pusch C.M., Zeitz C., Brandau O., Pesch K., Achatz H., Feil S., Scharfe C., Maurer J., Jacobi F.K., Pinckers A., Andreasson S., Hardcastle A., Wissinger B., Berger W., and Meindl A., 2000, The complete form of X-linked congenital stationary night blindness is caused by mutations in a gene encoding a leucine-rich repeat protein, Nat. Genet. **26**: 324.

Scholl H.P., Langrova H., Pusch C.M., Wissinger B., Zrenner E., and Apfelstedt-Sylla E., 2001, Slow and fast rod ERG Pathways in Patients with X-Linked Complete Stationary Night Blindness Carrying Mutations in the *NYX* Gene, Invest. Ophthalmol. Vis. Sci. **42**: 2728.

Strom T.M., Nyakatura G., Apfelstedt-Sylla E., Hellebrand H., Lorenz B., Weber B.H., Wutz K., Gutwillinger N., Ruther K., Drescher B., Sauer C., Zrenner E., Meitinger T., Rosenthal A., and Meindl A., 1998, An L-type calcium-channel gene mutated in incomplete X-linked congenital stationary night blindness, Nat. Genet. **19**: 260.

Zeitz C., Scherthan H., Freier S., Feil S., Suckow V., Schweiger S., and Berger W., 2003, NYX (Nyctalopin on Chromosome X), the gene mutated in congenital stationary night blindness, encodes a cell surface protein, Invest. Ophthalmol. Vis. Sci. **44**: 4184.

10q26 Is Associated with Increased Risk of Age-Related Macular Degeneration in the Utah Population

D. Joshua Cameron, Zhenglin Yang, Zhongzhong Tong, Yu Zhao, Alissa Praggastis, Eric Brinton, Jennifer Harmon, Yali Chen, Erik Pearson, Paul S. Bernstein, Gregory Brinton, Xi Li, Adam Jorgensen, Sara Schneider, Daniel Gibbs, Haoyu Chen, Changguan Wang, Kimberly Howes, Nicola J. Camp, and Kang Zhang

1 Introduction

Age-related macular degeneration (AMD) includes a wide range of phenotypes. Early AMD is mainly characterized by the presence of soft dusen in the macula without visual loss, while advanced AMD is characterized by geographic atrophy (GA or dry AMD) and neovascular AMD (wet AMD) with visual loss. Despite the rising prevalence of AMD as a result of increasing life expectancy, its underlying etiology is poorly understood and there is no specific therapy. Nutritional supplements and antagonists of vascular endothelial growth factor (*VEGF*) have been reported to halt the progression of visual loss in wet AMD (Bressler et al., 1988). Wet AMD is usually associated with an aggressive form of visual loss due to choroidal neovascularization (CNV).

Previous reports by several groups have identified a significant association between a common missense variant (Y402H) and non-coding variants in *CFH* and AMD in the United States (Edwards et al., 2005; Fisher et al., 2005; Hageman et al., 2005; Haines et al., 2005; Klein et al., 2005; Li et al., 2006; Maller et al., 2006) and Europe (Fisher et al., 2005; Souied et al., 2005; Despriet et al., 2006; Magnusson et al., 2006; Postel et al., 2006; Sepp et al., 2006; Simonelli et al., 2006). Recently, it was reported that rs10490924 in LOC387715 is the second major locus for AMD located at 10q locus (Conley et al., 2005; Rivera et al., 2005; Haddad et al., 2006; Maller et al., 2006; Schmidt et al., 2006). In this study we performed an association study incorporating SNP data for LOC387715 and PLEKHA1 at 10q26 and for CFH at 1q31.3 in the Utah AMD cohort. Our results support previous findings that

D.J. Cameron
Department of Ophthalmology and Visual Sciences, Moran Eye Center and Program in Human Molecular Biology and Genetics, University of Utah School of Medicine, Salt Lake City, UT 84132, Tel: 801-363-2433
e-mail: joshua.cameron@utah.edu

R.E. Anderson et al. (eds.), *Recent Advances in Retinal Degeneration*,
© Springer 2008

10q26, excluding regions of PLEKHA,is the second major locus for wet AMD in Utah populations, and that the associations found were independent, yet additive to the risk conferred from CFH.

2 Methods

This study was approved by the Institutional Review Board of the University of Utah. All subjects provided informed consent prior to participation in the study. AMD patients were recruited in Utah at the Moran Eye Center of University of Utah, as were normal age-matched controls with eye examinations (individuals age 60 years or older with no drusen or RPE changes). All participants went through a standard examination protocol and visual acuity measurements. Grading was carried out using a standard grid classification suggested by the International ARM Epidemiological Study Group for the age-related maculopathy (ARM) and age-related macular degeneration group (Bird et al., 1995). All abnormalities in the macula were characterized according to type, size and number of drusen as well as presence of hyperpigmentation and hypopigmentation, and advanced AMD.

The Utah cohort of 260 wet AMD was genotyped and allele frequencies were compared to 297 age and ethnicity matched normal controls. Direct DNA sequencing was performed on an ABI 3100 genetic analyzer (Applied Biosystems, Foster City, CA) to genotype the Utah cohort by lab personnel blinded to case/control status.

The chi-squared test for trend for the additive model over alleles was performed to assess evidence for association for each variant separately. Odds Ratios (OR) and 95% confidence intervals (CI) were also calculated to estimate risk size for the heterozygotes and homozygotes for the risk alleles. Single locus analyses were followed by conditional association analyses based on the most significant SNP findings, to establish whether the less significant findings at 10q26 were simply due to linkage disequilibrium (LD). For risk genotypes identified, we calculated population attributable risks (PAR) using the Levin formula (Levin, 1953).

Two-locus analyses were performed for the CFH Y402H variant at 1q31 and the principal variant identified for 10q26. Conditional association analysis of the principal 10q variant, based on the genotype at CFH Y402H was performed. A global two locus (9×2) contingency table, enumerating all 9 two-locus genotype combinations was constructed. Odds ratios and 95% CIs, comparing each genotypic combination to the baseline of homozygosity for the common allele at both loci, were calculated. A forward stepwise logistic regression procedure was used to formally test for epistasis (interaction of the two loci) under a log-additive model.

3 Results

Table 1 shows the association results for LOC387715 rs10490924, *PLEKHA1* rs2421016, and *PLEKHA1* rs4146894 at 10q26, where each variant was analyzed separately. In addition, the single locus results for CFH Y402H are shown. All

Table 1 Association results for three SNPs at 10q26.13 and CFH in wet AMD Cases and Controls

Gene	Marker	Risk allele	Frequency in wet AMD (n = 260)	Control (n = 297)	P Value	ORhet CI	ORhom CI
LOC387715	rs10490924	T	0.423	0.247	1.0×10^{-9}	1.7 (1.18, 2.44)	7.09 (3.67, 13.70)
PLEKHA1	rs2421016	T	0.558	0.459	8.7×10^{-4}	1.82 (1.24, 2.66)	2.21 (1.39, 3.53)
PLEKHA1	rs4146894	T	0.573	0.454	4.7×10^{-5}	1.76 (1.22, 2.53)	2.32 (1.55, 3.46)
CFH	rs1061170	C	0.569	0.426	1.1×10^{-6}	1.62 (1.06, 2.49)	3.56 (2.12, 5.97)

results were highly significant, with rs10490924 associated with the highest risk ($p=1.0\times10^{-9}$) and the largest difference in allele frequency for the risk allele (T: 39.7% versus 24.7%, $P=4.5\times10^{-9}$). A clear dose effect for the risk allele, T, was observed, with individuals heterozygous for rs10490924 showing a 1.70-fold increased risk (95% CI: 1.18, 2.44) and a 7.09-fold increased risk with TT homozygotes (95% CI: 3.67, 13.70), to develop wet AMD (Table 1). The PAR for this locus is estimated to be 39%. Details for the association with CFH in the Utah cohort were previously reported (Magnusson et al., 2006).

In agreement with previous reports (Conley et al., 2005; Rivera et al., 2005), we found a major association for 10q26 at LOC387715 rs10490924. To investigate this further, we performed two separate association analyses for *PLEKHA1* rs2421016 and *PLEKHA1* rs4146894 conditional on genotype at LOC387715 rs10490924. No significant association was found for either PLEKHA1 SNP conditional on genotypes GG or TT at LOC388715 rs10490924. There is substantial and highly significant LD between rs10490924 and rs2421016 (D' = 0.53, p = 1.2×10^{-17}) and rs4146894 (D' = 0.53, p = 2.4×10^{-18}) in AMD cases, and this appears to drive associations. However, some marginal significance is still observed for both PLEKHA1 variants when LOC388715 rs10490924 is GT. Such a result is consistent with a disease haplotype upon which all three variants lie.

We constructed a putative disease haplotype using multiple SNPs spanning this region. An extended disease haplotype TTTACT defined by SNPs rs4146894, rs2421016, rs10490924, rs3750847, rs2014307, rs2248799 showed the strongest

Table 2 Conditional association for rs10490924 on genotype at *CFH* rs1061170

CFH Genotype	Sample size (case/control)	Risk Allele at rs10490924	P Value	ORhet CI	ORhom CI
CFH rs1061170 = TT	45/85	T	2.1×10^{-3}	3.16 (1.43,6.96)	4.55 (1.08,19.25)
CFH rS1061170 = TC	134/156	T	1.4×10^{-5}	1.92 (1.16,3.17)	5.90 (2.46,14.15)
CFH rs1061170 = CC	81/43	T	2.0×10^{-2}	0.79 (0.36,1.74)	14.00 (1.75,111.77)

Table 3 Two locus odds ratios

	rs10490924 = GG		rs10490924 = GT		rs10490924 = TT	
	n	OR	n	OR	n	OR
rs1061170 = TT	14	1.0	26	3.16 (1.43,6.96)	5	4.55 (1.08,19.25)
rs1061170 = CT	45	1.93 (0.96, 3.86)	64	3.70 (1.86,7.35)	25	11.38 (4.22,30.69)
rs1061170 = CC	33	5.72 (2.56,12.81)	26	4.51 (1.98,10.29)	22	80.14 (9.92,647.61)

association (chi = 76.466, p = 2.2 × 10–18). This haplotype spanned 80 kilobases and encompassed three genes: *PLEKHA1, LOC388715, and PRSS11/HTRA1*. These results are consistent with the true underlying varaint lying on this haplotype.

We analyzed and compared the one of the principal variants at 10q26 (LOC388715 rs10490924) with the CFH Y402H variant. Table 2 shows the three separate association analyses for rs10490924 conditional on the three genotypes at CFH Y402H. All results maintained significance, despite a large reduction in sample size for each subset analysis. In particular, significance was maintained for the individuals that carry risk alleles at CFH at 1q31. In all cases, the risk estimates indicate that homozygotes for TT are at an increased risk over that of heterozygotes.

To further investigate the interaction of CFH and rs10490924, we analyzed the data in a logistic regression framework and allowed for an interaction term. A forward-stepwise procedure was used. As expected, both CFHY402H and LOC387715 rs10490924 risk allele T were entered in to the model and were significant (p = 2.4×10^{-6} and p = 9.5×10^{-13}, respectively). However, the inter-action term was not entered, and when forced into the model, there was no significant evidence for any interaction between the loci (p=0.829). In Table 3 the nine two-locus genotype combinations for LOC388715 rs10490924 and CFH Y402H have been identified and estimates for risk (OR and 95% CI) are given for each two-locus genotypic combination compared to the double wild-type (GG/TT for rs10490924/CFH Y402H).

4 Discussion

The discovery of a locus at 10q26, LOC387715, recently proposed to be the second major gene contributing to the common form of AMD is another major advance towards understanding genetic risk and pathogenesis of AMD. Using conditional associations, we have confirmed that LOC38715 rs10490924 is one of the primary variants that tags the association evidence at 10q26 for wet AMD. Further, our data are consistent with that risk being independent of that for CFH at 1q31. However, it should be noted that limited power may have impeded our ability to test for more subtle interactions between the two loci. The first of these findings, via conditional analyses suggest that a large part of the single locus association significance found for the PLEKHA1 variants (Table 1) is due to linkage disequilibrium (LD) with LOC388715 rs10490924 and further that rs10490924 does not fully explain all of the 10q26 association evidence. Both observations taken together illustrate that rs10490924 certainly shows strong association evidence for 10q26, but that it is likely tagging the true underlying causal variant, which, by virtue of our first finding, can not to be either of the PLEKHA1 variants studied. Futher support of this notion came from the evidence that an extended disease haplotype TTTACT captures the disease risk even better than rs10490924. Together, these results suggest the true disease variant most likely resides on this haplotype.

Since the completion of this study, we along with others have shown that a SNP, rs11200638, in the promoter region of HTRA1 is significantly associated with both dry and wet AMD (Dewan et al., 2006; Yang et al., 2006; Cameron et al., 2007). This region falls within the disease haplotype described above and has the strongest association signal. Furthermore, when conditioned to the LOC387715 SNP rs10490924, rs11200638 remains significant in dry AMD, whereas the opposite is not the case (Cameron et al., 2007). Along with preliminary functional data showing that HTRA1 expression is elevated in association with the disease variant rs11200638 (Dewan et al., 2006; Yang et al., 2006), the genetic association results point to rs11200638 as being the causal variant for AMD in the 10q26 region.

Acknowledgments We thank the participating AMD patients and their families. We acknowledge the following grant support to KZ: NIH (R01EY14428, R01EY14448, P30EY014800 and GCRC M01-RR00064), Foundation Fighting Blindness, the Ruth and Milton Steinbach Fund, Ronald McDonald House Charities, the Macular Vision Research Foundation, Grant Ritter Fund, American Health Assistance Foundation, the Karl Kirchgessner Foundation, Val and Edith Green Foundation, and the Simmons Foundation; to ZY: Knights Templar Eye Research Foundation; to NC: K07 (NCI CA98364).

References

Bird, A. C., N. M. Bressler, et al. (1995). "An international classification and grading system for age-related maculopathy and age-related macular degeneration. The International ARM Epidemiological Study Group." *Surv Ophthalmol* 39(5): 367–74.

Bressler, N. M., S. B. Bressler, et al. (1988). "Age-related macular degeneration." *Surv Ophthalmol* 32(6): 375–413.

Cameron, D. J., Z. Yang, et al. (2007). "HTRA1 Variant confers similar risks to geographic atrophy and neovascular age-related macular degeneration." *Cell Cycle* 6(9): 1122–1125.

Conley YP, T. A., J. Jakobsdottir, D.E. Weeks, T. Mah, R.E. Ferrell, M.B. Gorin, (2005). "Candidate gene analysis suggests a role for fatty acid biosynthesis and regulation of the complement system in the etiology of age-related maculopathy." *Human Molecular Genetics* 14: 1991–2002.

Despriet, D. D., C. C. Klaver, et al. (2006). "Complement factor H polymorphism, complement activators, and risk of age-related macular degeneration." *Jama* 296(3): 301–9.

Dewan, A., M. Liu, et al. (2006). "HTRA1 promoter polymorphism in wet age-related macular degeneration." *Science* 314(5801): 989–92.

Edwards, A. O., R. Ritter, 3rd, et al. (2005). "Complement factor H polymorphism and age-related macular degeneration." *Science* 308(5720): 421–24.

Fisher, S. A., G. R. Abecasis, et al. (2005). "Meta-analysis of genome scans of age-related macular degeneration." *Hum Mol Genet* 14(15): 2257–64.

Gold, B., J. E. Merriam, et al. (2006). "Variation in factor B (BF) and complement component 2 (C2) genes is associated with age-related macular degeneration." *Nat Genet* 38(4): 458–62.

Haddad, S., C. A. Chen, et al. (2006). "The genetics of age-related macular degeneration: a review of progress to date." *Surv Ophthalmol* **51**(4): 316–63.

Hageman, G. S., D. H. Anderson, et al. (2005). "A common haplotype in the complement regulatory gene factor H (HF1/CFH) predisposes individuals to age-related macular degeneration." *Proc Natl Acad Sci U S A* **102**(20): 7227–32.

Haines, J. L., M. A. Hauser, et al. (2005). "Complement factor H variant increases the risk of age-related macular degeneration." *Science* **308**: 419–421.

Klein, R. J., C. Zeiss, et al. (2005). "Complement factor H polymorphism in age-related macular degeneration." *Science* **308**: 385–389.

Levin, M. L. (1953). "The occurrence of lung cancer in man." *Acta Unio Int Contra Cancrum* **9**(3): 531–41.

Li, M., P. Atmaca-Sonmez, et al. (2006). "CFH haplotypes without the Y402H coding variant show strong association with susceptibility to age-related macular degeneration." *Nat Genet* **38**(9): 1049–54.

Magnusson, K. P., S. Duan, et al. (2006). "CFH Y402H confers similar risk of soft drusen and both forms of advanced AMD." *PLoS Med* **3**(1): e5.

Maller, J., S. George, et al. (2006). "Common variation in three genes, including a noncoding variant in CFH, strongly influences risk of age-related macular degeneration." *Nat Genet* **38**(9): 1055–59.

Postel, E. A., A. Agarwal, et al. (2006). "Complement factor H increases risk for atrophic age-related macular degeneration." *Ophthalmology* **113**: 1504–1507.

Rivera, A., S. A. Fisher, et al. (2005). "Hypothetical LOC387715 is a second major susceptibility gene for age-related macular degeneration, contributing independently of complement factor H to disease risk." *Hum Mol Genet* **14**(21): 3227–36.

Schmidt, S., M. A. Hauser, et al. (2006). "Cigarette smoking strongly modifies the association of LOC387715 and age-related macular degeneration." *Am J Hum Genet* **78**(5): 852–64.

Sepp, T., J. C. Khan, et al. (2006). "Complement factor H variant Y402H is a major risk determinant for geographic atrophy and choroidal neovascularization in smokers and nonsmokers." *Invest Ophthalmol Vis Sci* **47**(2): 536–40.

Simonelli, F., G. Frisso, et al. (2006). "Polymorphism p.402Y>H in the complement factor H protein is a risk factor for age-related macular degeneration in an Italian population." *Br J Ophthalmol* **90**: 1142–1145.

Souied, E. H., N. Leveziel, et al. (2005). "Y402H complement factor H polymorphism associated with exudative age-related macular degeneration in the French population." *Mol Vis* **11**: 1135–40.

Yang, Z., N. J. Camp, et al. (2006). "A variant of the HTRA1 gene increases susceptibility to age-related macular degeneration." *Science* **314**(5801): 992–93.

Part VI
Diagnostic, Clinical, Cytopathological and Physiologic Aspects of Retinal Degeneration

Carboxyethylpyrrole Adducts, Age-related Macular Degeneration and Neovascularization

Kutralanathan Renganathan, Quteba Ebrahem, Amit Vasanji, Xiaorong Gu, Liang Lu, Jonathan Sears, Robert G. Salomon, Bela Anand-Apte, and John W. Crabb

1 Introduction

Choroidal neovascularization (CNV) in late stage age-related macular degeneration (AMD) involves abnormal vessel growth from the choriocapillaris through Bruch's membrane and the retinal pigment epithelium (RPE) and accounts for more than 80% of the severe debilitating vision loss in all AMD patients. The molecular mechanisms associated with AMD pathogenesis and the development of CNV remain poorly understood. We hypothesize that oxidative protein modifications are primary catalysts in AMD pathogenesis and play a role in the development of CNV (Crabb et al., 2002). Oxidative damage has long been suspected of contributing to AMD (Beatty et al., 2000), supported by indirect evidence that smoking increases the risk of AMD (Seddon et al., 1996) and that antioxidant vitamins and zinc can slow disease progression for select individuals (AREDS, 2001). Our proteomic study of drusen established a direct link between oxidative damage and AMD by demonstrating elevated carboxyethylpyrrole (CEP) adducts in AMD Bruch's membrane (Crabb et al., 2002). CEP protein adducts are uniquely generated from oxidation of docosahexaenoate (DHA)-containing lipids and DHA accounts for approximately 80 mol% of the polyunsaturated lipids in photoreceptor outer segments (Fliesler and Anderson, 1983). CEP adducts are also significantly elevated in plasma from AMD donors, as are CEP autoantibodies(Gu et al., 2003), both of which may have utility as biomarkers for monitoring AMD therapeutic efficacies. The high levels of CEP-adducts in AMD are likely associated with the high levels of DHA in photoreceptors, the fact that DHA is the most oxidizable fatty acid in humans, and the high photooxidative stress in the retina (Fig. 1).

Genetic evidence now supports an association between AMD susceptibility and variants in genes encoding complement factor H, factor B, complement component 2 and a heat shock serine protease (Edwards et al., 2005; Gold et al., 2006) (Dewan et al., 2006; Hageman et al., 2005; Haines et al., 2005; Jakobsdottir et al., 2005;

K. Renganathan
Cole Eye Institute, Department of Chemistry, Case Western Reserve University, Cleveland, Ohio,
Tel: 216-445-0425, Fax: 216-445-3670

R.E. Anderson et al. (eds.), *Recent Advances in Retinal Degeneration*,
© Springer 2008

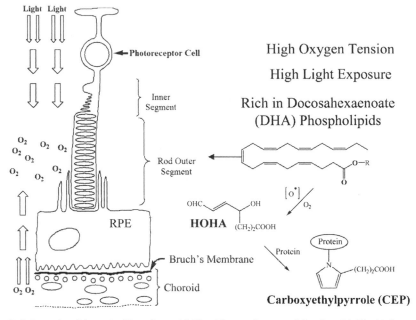

Fig. 1 Schematic of the retinal interface with Bruch's membrane and the choroid. The high oxygen tension and light exposure in the retina facilitate the oxidative fragmentation of DHA-containing lipids and formation of CEP protein adducts from the reactive lipid fragment HOHA (4-hydroxy-7-oxohept-5-enoic acid)

Klein et al., 2005; Rivera et al., 2005; Yang et al., 2006). These associations implicate inflammatory processes in the pathophysiology of AMD and oxidative protein modifications may be the central catalysts or initiators of such processes. Additional evidence implicating oxidative damage in AMD pathogenesis comes from recent animal studies. Aged mice exhibiting the apo-lipoprotein E4 genotype develop AMD – like pathologies, including CNV, when fed a high cholesterol diet (Malek et al., 2005). In addition, mice deficient in the antioxidant enzyme superoxide dismutase 1 (SOD1) develop drusen, thickened Bruch's membrane and CNV (Imamura et al., 2006). Targeted disruption of SOD2 in the RPE generates pathological changes in the outer retina resembling AMD as well as increased levels of CEP adducts in the RPE (Lewin et al., 2007). Here we review recent results showing that CEP oxidative protein modifications stimulate neovascularization in vivo and possibly contribute to CNV in late stage AMD (Ebrahem et al., 2006).

2 Cep Induces Neovascularization

The chick chorioallantoic membrane (CAM) assay and the rat corneal micropocket assay were used to evaluate the angiogenic potential of CEP-modified human serum albumin (CEP-HSA) and/or a CEP-modified dipeptide (Ebrahem et al., 2006). In the CAM assay, CEP-HSA (0.17 μg) containing methylcellulose discs induced sprouting of new blood vessels while unmodified HSA (0.5 μg) did not. Vascular endothelial growth factor was used as a positive control and the angiogenic response of 0.17 μg CEP-HSA was similar to the half maximal response of VEGF at a dose of 20 ng in the CAM assay. In the corneal micropocket assay, hydron/sucralfate pellets containing CEP-HSA (1 μg) or CEP-dipeptide (37 ng) were implanted 1 mm from the limbus of rat cornea and found to stimulate limbal blood vessel growth towards the pellet while unmodified HSA (1 μg) or dipeptide (41 ng) did not. Statistically significant increases in peak vessel extensions were observed in response to CEP-HSA ($\sim$2.7 fold) or CEP-dipeptide ($\sim$3.1 fold) when compared with the unmodified parent molecules. To further test the specificity of the angiogenic response, the assay was repeated with pellets containing premixed anti-CEP monoclonal antibody and CEP-HSA. Monoclonal anti-CEP antibody almost completely neutralized the formation of new blood vessels from CEP-HSA implants in the corneal micropocket assay. Control mouse antibodies did not show inhibition of CEP-HSA mediated corneal neovascularization.

3 CNV in Mice is Exacerbated by CEP

CEP adducts are concentrated in AMD Bruch's membrane, between the blood bearing choroid and RPE, and possibly contribute to CNV in AMD. To explore this possibility, mice with laser-induced rupture of Bruch's membrane were given a sub-retinal injection of phosphate buffered saline, mouse serum albumin (MSA), CEP-MSA, or VEGF and analyzed 2 weeks later for CNV. Quantitative image analysis revealed that CEP-MSA significantly amplified the CNV area when compared with injections of PBS or unmodified MSA and was similar to that obtained with injections of VEGF (Ebrahem et al., 2006). Sub-retinal injections of CEP-MSA, MSA, or VEGF in the absence of laser injury did not induce CNV.

4 CEP Induced Angiogenesis may be Independent of VEGF

The angiogenic potential of CEP adducts was first questioned because other oxidative protein modifications, namely advanced glycation end products (AGEs), stimulate neovascularization in vivo (Okamoto et al., 2002) and induce VEGF secretion in vitro (Hirata et al., 1997; Hoffmann et al., 2000). We used the corneal micropocket assay and an RPE cell culture assay to evaluate whether CEP-induced angiogenesis might involve vascular endothelial growth factor (VEGF) pathways. Pellets containing premixed anti-VEGF + CEP-HSA or anti-VEGF + VEGF were evaluated in the micropocket assay and VEGF antibody was found to only partially inhibit CEP-HSA induced neovascularization in vivo while completely inhibiting the VEGF induced response (Ebrahem et al., 2006). To determine whether CEP adducts influence VEGF secretion, RPE cells were treated in vitro with CEP-dipeptide or CEP-HSA and ELISA was used to quantify VEGF secretion into the growth media

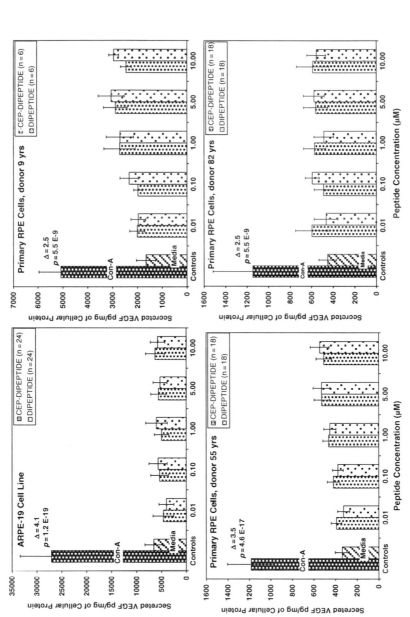

Fig. 2 CEP dipeptide does not increase secretion of VEGF in RPE cells. Human primary RPE cells from donors of 9, 55 or 82 years and ARPE-19 cells were treated with CEP-dipeptide or dipeptide at the indicated concentrations. After 18 hours, VEGF in the conditioned medium was assayed multiple times as indicated by n (in replicates of 6 per independent experiment). Error bars represent standard deviation. Concanavalin A (Con-A) was used as a positive control for VEGF stimulation. (Reproduced from Ebrahem et al., 2006 with copyright permission)

(Fig. 2). Neither human primary RPE cells or the human ARPE19 cell line treated with 0.1–10 μM CEP-dipeptide demonstrated increased VEGF in the growth media relative to the unmodified dipeptide or media alone (Ebrahem et al., 2006). ARPE19 cells treated with CEP-HSA also exhibited no increase in VEGF secretion.

5 Conclusions

We have shown that CEP adducts induce neovascularization in the CAM and corneal micropocket assays and exacerbate laser-induced CNV in mice. These results coupled with the elevated levels of CEP adducts in AMD tissues strongly suggest that CEP may play a role in the development of CNV in late stage AMD. Our results are consistent with studies showing that AGEs also accumulate with age in Bruch's membrane (Handa et al., 1999) and CNV membranes (Ishibashi et al., 1998) (Handa et al., 1999; Wu, 1993) and can stimulate the proliferation of choroid endothelial cells, the expression of MMP-2 and VEGF and angiogenesis in vivo (Okamoto et al., 2002). The molecular mechanism by which CEP induces angiogenesis are not known but appear to be different from those proposed for AGEs. VEGF neutralizing antibody only partially blocked CEP induced angiogenesis in vivo and VEGF secretion was not stimulated in RPE cell by CEP-dipeptide or CEP-HSA, suggesting that CEP angiogenic mechanisms may use VEGF independent pathways. Notably, anti-VEGF treatment modalities for CNV are under clinical evaluation (Gragoudas et al., 2004; Rosenfeld et al., 2005). CEP neutralization modalities may offer complementary therapies for the inhibition of CNV in AMD.

Acknowledgments This work was supported in part by US National Institute of Health EY016490, CA106415, EY015638, EY06603, EY014239, GM21249, Foundation Fighting Blindness Center Grant, AHA Grant in Aid, Research to Prevent Blindness (RPB) Challenge Grant and Ohio BRTT 05-29. JWC is a RPB Senior Scientific Investigator. We are grateful to Dr. Janice Burke and Christine Skumatz (Medical College of Wisconsin, Milwaukee, WI) for primary human RPE cells.

References

AREDS (2001). "A randomized, placebo-controlled, clinical trial of high-dose supplementation with vitamins c and e, beta carotene, and zinc for age-related macular degeneration and vision loss: Areds report no. 8." *Arch Ophthalmol* **119**: 1417.

Beatty, S., H. Koh, M. Phil, D. Henson and M. Boulton (2000). "The role of oxidative stress in the pathogenesis of age-related macular degeneration." *Surv Ophthalmol* **45**: 115.

Crabb, J. W., M. Miyagi, X. Gu, K. Shadrach, K. A. West, H. Sakaguchi, M. Kamei, A. Hasan, L. Yan, M. E. Rayborn, R. G. Salomon and J. G. Hollyfield (2002). "Drusen proteome analysis: An approach to the etiology of age-related macular degeneration." *Proc Natl Acad Sci U S A* **99**: 14682.

Dewan, A., M. Liu, S. Hartman, S. S. Zhang, D. T. Liu, C. Zhao, P. O. Tam, W. M. Chan, D. S. Lam, M. Snyder, C. Barnstable, C. P. Pang and J. Hoh (2006). "Htra1 promoter polymorphism in wet age-related macular degeneration." *Science* **314**: 989.

Ebrahem, Q., K. Renganathan, J. Sears, A. Vasanji, X. Gu, L. Lu, R. G. Salomon, J. W. Crabb and B. Anand-Apte (2006). "Carboxyethylpyrrole oxidative protein modifications stimulate neovascularization: Implications for age-related macular degeneration." *Proc Natl Acad Sci U S A* **103**: 13480.

Edwards, A. O., R. Ritter, 3rd, K. J. Abel, A. Manning, C. Panhuysen and L. A. Farrer (2005). "Complement factor h polymorphism and age-related macular degeneration." *Science* **308**: 421.

Fliesler, S. J. and R. E. Anderson (1983). "Chemistry and metabolism of lipids in the vertebrate retina." *Prog Lipid Res* **22**: 79.

Gold, B., J. E. Merriam, J. Zernant, L. S. Hancox, A. J. Taiber, K. Gehrs, K. Cramer, J. Neel, J. Bergeron, G. R. Barile, R. T. Smith, G. S. Hageman, M. Dean and R. Allikmets (2006). "Variation in factor b (bf) and complement component 2 (c2) genes is associated with age-related macular degeneration." *Nat Genet* **38**: 458.

Gragoudas, E. S., A. P. Adamis, E. T. Cunningham, Jr., M. Feinsod and D. R. Guyer (2004). "Pegaptanib for neovascular age-related macular degeneration." *N Engl J Med* **351**: 2805.

Gu, X., S. G. Meer, M. Miyagi, M. Rayborn, J. G. Hollyfield, J. W. Crabb and R. G. Salomon (2003). "Carboxyethylpyrrole proein adducts and autoantibodies, biomarkers for age-related macular degeneration." *J. Biol. Chem.* **278**: 42027.

Hageman, G. S., D. H. Anderson, L. V. Johnson, L. S. Hancox, A. J. Taiber, L. I. Hardisty, J. L. Hageman, H. A. Stockman, J. D. Borchardt, K. M. Gehrs, R. J. Smith, G. Silvestri, S. R. Russell, C. C. Klaver, I. Barbazetto, S. Chang, L. A. Yannuzzi, G. R. Barile, J. C. Merriam, R. T. Smith, A. K. Olsh, J. Bergeron, J. Zernant, J. E. Merriam, B. Gold, M. Dean and R. Allikmets (2005). "A common haplotype in the complement regulatory gene factor h (hf1/cfh) predisposes individuals to age-related macular degeneration." *Proc Natl Acad Sci U S A* **102**: 7227.

Haines, J. L., M. A. Hauser, S. Schmidt, W. K. Scott, L. M. Olson, P. Gallins, K. L. Spencer, S. Y. Kwan, M. Noureddine, J. R. Gilbert, N. Schnetz-Boutaud, A. Agarwal, E. A. Postel and M. A. Pericak-Vance (2005). "Complement factor h variant increases the risk of age-related macular degeneration." *Science* **308**: 419.

Handa, J. T., N. Verzijl, H. Matsunaga, A. Aotaki-Keen, G. A. Lutty, J. M. te Koppele, T. Miyata and L. M. Hjelmeland (1999). "Increase in the advanced glycation end product pentosidine in bruch's membrane with age." *Invest Ophthalmol Vis Sci* **40**: 775.

Hirata, C., K. Nakano, N. Nakamura, Y. Kitagawa, H. Shigeta, G. Hasegawa, M. Ogata, T. Ikeda, H. Sawa, K. Nakamura, K. Ienaga, H. Obayashi and M. Kondo (1997). "Advanced glycation end products induce expression of vascular endothelial growth factor by retinal muller cells." *Biochem Biophys Res Commun* **236**: 712.

Hoffmann, S., R. Masood, Y. Zhang, S. He, S. J. Ryan, P. Gill and D. R. Hinton (2000). "Selective killing of rpe with a vascular endothelial growth factor chimeric toxin." *Invest Ophthalmol Vis Sci* **41**: 2389.

Imamura, Y., S. Noda, K. Hashizume, K. Shinoda, M. Yamaguchi, S. Uchiyama, T. Shimizu, Y. Mizushima, T. Shirasawa and K. Tsubota (2006). "Drusen, choroidal neovascularization, and retinal pigment epithelium dysfunction in sod1-deficient mice: A model of age-related macular degeneration." *Proc Natl Acad Sci U S A* **103**: 11282.

Ishibashi, T., T. Murata, M. Hangai, R. Nagai, S. Horiuchi, P. F. Lopez, D. R. Hinton and S. J. Ryan (1998). "Advanced glycation end products in age-related macular degeneration." *Arch Ophthalmol* **116**: 1629.

Jakobsdottir, J., Y. P. Conley, D. E. Weeks, T. S. Mah, R. E. Ferrell and M. B. Gorin (2005). "Susceptibility genes for age-related maculopathy on chromosome 10q26." *Am J Hum Genet* **77**: 389.

Klein, R. J., C. Zeiss, E. Y. Chew, J. Y. Tsai, R. S. Sackler, C. Haynes, A. K. Henning, J. P. SanGiovanni, S. M. Mane, S. T. Mayne, M. B. Bracken, F. L. Ferris, J. Ott, C. Barnstable and J. Hoh (2005). "Complement factor h polymorphism in age-related macular degeneration." *Science* **308**: 385.

Lewin, A. S., V. Justilien, J. Pang, W. W. Hauswirth, J. W. Crabb, N. Renganathan, S. R. Kim and J. R. Sparrow (2007). "Modeling early stages of age-related macular degeneration (amd) by inducing oxidative stress in the rpe " *Invest Opthalmol Vis Sci, E-abstract 5055*.

Malek, G., L. V. Johnson, B. E. Mace, P. Saloupis, D. E. Schmechel, D. W. Rickman, C. A. Toth, P. M. Sullivan and C. B. Rickman (2005). "Apolipoprotein e allele-dependent pathogenesis: A model for age-related retinal degeneration." *Proc Natl Acad Sci U S A* **102**: 11900.

Okamoto, T., S. Tanaka, A. C. Stan, T. Koike, M. Kase, Z. Makita, H. Sawa and K. Nagashima (2002). "Advanced glycation end products induce angiogenesis in vivo." *Microvasc Res* **63**: 186.

Rivera, A., S. A. Fisher, L. G. Fritsche, C. N. Keilhauer, P. Lichtner, T. Meitinger and B. H. Weber (2005). "Hypothetical loc387715 is a second major susceptibility gene for age-related macular degeneration, contributing independently of complement factor h to disease risk." *Hum Mol Genet* **14**: 3227.

Rosenfeld, P. J., S. D. Schwartz, M. S. Blumenkranz, J. W. Miller, J. A. Haller, J. D. Reimann, W. L. Greene and N. Shams (2005). "Maximum tolerated dose of a humanized anti-vascular endothelial growth factor antibody fragment for treating neovascular age-related macular degeneration." *Ophthalmology* **112**: 1048.

Seddon, J. M., W. C. Willett, F. E. Speizer and S. E. Hankinson (1996). "A prospective study of cigarette smoking and age-related macular degeneration in women." *J Am Med Assoc* **276**: 1141.

Wu, J. T. (1993). "Advanced glycosylation end products: A new disease marker for diabetes and aging." *J Clin Lab Anal* **7**: 252.

Yang, Z., N. J. Camp, H. Sun, Z. Tong, D. Gibbs, D. J. Cameron, H. Chen, Y. Zhao, E. Pearson, X. Li, J. Chien, A. Dewan, J. Harmon, P. S. Bernstein, V. Shridhar, N. A. Zabriskie, J. Hoh, K. Howes and K. Zhang (2006). "A variant of the htra1 gene increases susceptibility to age-related macular degeneration." *Science* **314**: 992.

A Possible Impaired Signaling Mechanism in Human Retinal Pigment Epithelial Cells from Patients with Macular Degeneration

Piyush C. Kothary and Monte A. Del Monte

1 Introduction

The human retinal pigment epithelial (hRPE) cells form a monolayer of polarized cells in the posterior segments of human eyes. They play an important role in the flow of nutrients from the choroid to the neural retina. They normally are mitotically inactive in adult human eyes. Pathological proliferation in later life has been implicated in the pathogenesis of age related macular degeneration (AMD) (Hamdi and Kenney, 2003; Tezel et al., 2004; Zarbin, 2006)

AMD is a frequent cause of reduced vision among the patients with diabetes (Voutilainen-Kaunisto et al., 2000). Voutilainen-Kaunisto et al. (2000) has also shown that visual acuity deteriorates rapidly in AMD patients with diabetes than non-diabetic patients. Insulin is a mitogen for hRPE cells (Campochiaro et al., 1991). Exogenous insulin is required to treat patients with diabetes. This insulin therapy may result in transient increase in diabetic retinopathy (Lu et al., 1999). This led us to examine the effect of insulin on the proliferation and signaling mechanism in hRPE cells obtained from patients with AMD.

2 Methods

2.1 Chemicals

Insulin was purchased from Sigma Chemicals, St. Louise, MO. Anti-pERK1-2 was purchased from R & D Systems, Minneapolis, MN. 3H-thymidine and 14C-Methionine were purchased from Amersham Corporation, Arlington Heights, IL. Ham's F-12 nutrient medium, Dulbecco's minimum essential media (DMEM), Hank's balanced salt solution, fetal bovine serum (FBS), penicillin and streptomycin

P.C. Kothary
Kellogg Eye Center, University of Michigan, Ann Arbor,
MI 48105-0714, Tel: 734-936-9254, Fax: 734-647-0228
e-mail: kotha@umich.edu

and trypsin were purchased from GIBCO BRL, Gaithersburg, MD. PD98059 was purchased from Cell Signaling Technology, Beverly, MA.

2.2 Establishment and Maintenance of hRPE Cell Cultures

Primary cultures of hRPE cells were established from human eyes obtained from a patient with AMD and three without AMD as described previously (Kusaka et al., 1998). Briefly, the anterior segment, vitreous and the retina of human eyes were surgically removed. The posterior segments were then washed with balanced salt solution, filled with papain (0.623 mg/ml in cystein/EDTA) and incubated for one hour at 37°C. The Papain was aspirated and replaced with Ham's F-12 nutrient medium containing 15% FBS, 100 U/ml penicillin, 100 mg/ml streptomycin and 0.075% (wt/vol) sodium bicarbonate (medium-1). The loosely adherent hRPE cells were detached by gentle brushing and hydrostatic pressure with a sterile Pasteur pipet. The cells were plated in 16-mm Primaria plates and incubated at 37°C in a 95% air/5% $CO2$ incubator. The medium was changed every three days until the cells were confluent. Primary cultures were then washed with Hank's balanced salt solution and subcultured by trypsinization with 0.5g/100 ml trypsin and 0.2g/100 ml EDTA in Hank's normal salt solution (Sigma T-3924) at 37°C for 10 minutes. The cell suspension was centrifuged at 500 xg and replated. The morphology of cells was examined daily by phase-contrast microscopy. For maintenance of cell lines, cells were plated in 75-mm flask at density of 50,000 cells/flask. The medium was changed every three days until the cells were ready for trypsinization. Cells were counted by hemocytometer and viability was assessed by trypan blue exclusion test.

2.3 Cellular Proliferation

Cellular proliferation of cultured hRPE cells was measured by tritiated thymidine incorporation (3H-thy) and direct cell counting by hemocytometer. Briefly, hRPE cells at passage 4–8 were trypsinized and plated in 16-mm wells of 24-well plates at 1 x 10,000 cells per well in medium-1. Experimental reagents were added for 48 hours when the cells became confluent. Sixteen hours prior to the termination time of experiment, cells were pulsed with 2 mCi/ml of 3H-thymidine (specific activity 25 Ci/mmol, Amesham Life Science, Arlington Heights, IL). The cells were washed three times with PBS (pH 7.4) and two times with ice-cold 5% trichloroacetic acid. One milliliter of 0.1 M NaOH, containing 0.1% SDS was added to 9.5 ml of scintillation fluid and counted in a Beckman scintillation counter.

2.4 Immunoprecipitation Assay

To measure intracellular pERK1/2 synthesis, hRPE cells were labeled by 14-C-Methionine and then treated with insulin in the presence and absence of the

MAP kinase inhibitor, PD98059, using the method described previously (Bitar et al., 1996; Kothary et al., 2006). hRPE cells were then lysed with zwittergent 3–12 and precipitated with phosphorylated ERK1/2 (pERK 1/2) specific antibody. PD98059 is a specific inhibitor of mitogen-activated protein kinase (Davis et al., 2000; Alessi et al., 1995; Kothary et al., 2005).

2.5 Statistical Analysis

All values represent the % mean of control. Differences between two groups of data were tested by Student's 't' test. A $p < 0.05$ was used to assess significant differences between two groups.

3 Results

Insulin (0–5 µg/ml) stimulated proliferation of hRPE cells from normal human eyes as determined by the trypan exclusion method as well as 3H-thy incorporation. However, no stimulation of proliferation was noted in hRPE obtained from a patient with AMD (Fig. 1 and 2).

As shown in Fig. 3 and 4, PD98059 significantly inhibited insulin stimulated 3H-thy incorporation and cell proliferation in hRPE from normal counts. However, PD98059 had no significant effect on hRPE cell growth in the presence of insulin in hRPE from the AMD patient as determined by 3H-thymidine incorporation or cell number.

Insulin (5 µg/ml) stimulated 14C-pERK 1/2 synthesis in hRPE cells from eyes obtained of non-AMD patients. However, no stimulation of 14C-pERK 1/2 Synthesis was noted in hRPE obtained from the AMD patient (Fig. 5).

As shown in Fig. 6, PD98059 significantly inhibited 14C-pERK 1/2 synthesis (1654.3±498 vs. 1269.3±339, CPM±SEM, n=6, $p < 0.05$) in hRPE cells obtained from non-AMD patients. However, PD98059 had no effect (stimulation or inhibition) on 14C-pERK 1/2 synthesis in presence of insulin in the AMD patient.

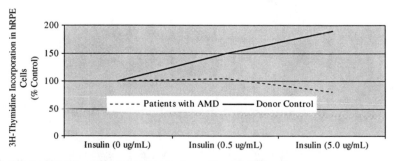

Fig. 1 Effect of insulin on 3H-thymidine incorporation of hRPE cells

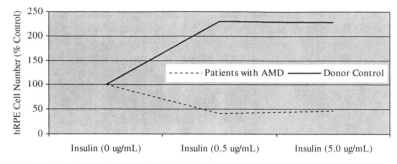

Fig. 2 Effect of insulin on the growth of hRPE cells

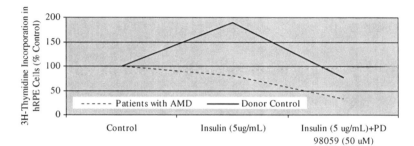

Fig. 3 Effect of PD 98059 on insulin-stimulated 3H-thydimine incorporation of hRPE cells

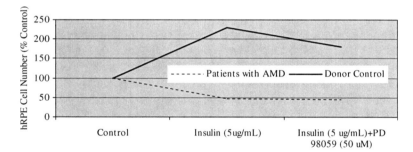

Fig. 4 Effect of PD 98509 on insulin-stimulated growth of hRPE cells

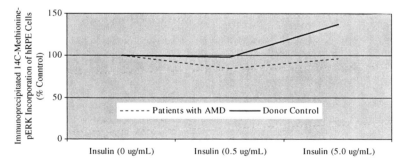

Fig. 5 Effect of insulin on 14C-methionine-pERK 1/2 synthesis in hRPE cells

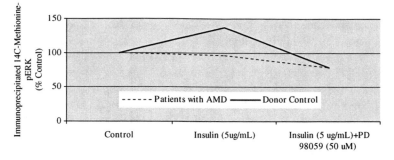

Fig. 6 Effect of PD 98059 on insulin-stimulated 14C-methionine-pERK 1/2 synthesis in hRPE cells

4 Discussion

The biochemical studies presented here demonstrate that cell proliferation and signal protein synthesis in hRPE cells obtained from the eyes of an AMD patient are abnormal when compared with hRPE obtained from the eyes of non-AMD patients. Unlike hRPE obtained from non-AMD normal control eyes, insulin did not stimulate cell proliferation, measured by direct cell counting using the trypan blue exclusion method, in hRPE cells obtained from the eyes of a patient with AMD. This insulin stimulated increase in hRPE proliferation in normal eyes is consistent with previously published data (Campochiaro et al., 1991). In addition, we have shown that increasing concentrations of insulin did not stimulate 3H-thymidine incorporation in hRPE cells obtained from the eyes of a patient with AMD when compared with hRPE obtained from the eyes from non-AMD normal controls. This suggests that insulin does not induce DNA synthesis in hRPE cells from patients with AMD.

The involvement of growth factors in hRPE cell proliferation has been extensively studied (Kothary and Del Monte, 2004; Kothary and Del Monte, 2005; Mascarelli et al., 2001). Insulin is a mitogen for hRPE cells (Campochiaro et al., 1991). However, very little is known about the signaling and molecular mechanism of action of insulin and other growth factors in hRPE cells from patients with AMD. Recently, we documented the role of phosphorylated ERK 1/2 as a signaling molecule in the proliferation of hRPE cells obtained from the eyes of non-AMD patients (Kothary et al., 2005). Since the neural retina in the macular area degenerates in AMD and the hRPE plays an important role in maintenance of the neural retina, we compared the pERK 1/2 synthesis in hRPE cells obtained from the eyes of AMD and non-AMD patients.

Insulin did not significantly change pERK 1/2 synthesis in hRPE cells obtained from the eyes of the AMD patient. However, there was an insulin dose-dependent increase in pERK 1/2 synthesis in hRPE cells obtained from non-AMD controls. The participation of pERK 1/2 in insulin action is suggested by Khoo et al. (2003), who demonstrated regulation of insulin gene transcription by ERK1 and ERK2 in pancreatic beta cells.

Hecquet et al. (2002) has shown that (1) fetal bovine serum initially activates the downstream Kinase: MAP kinase/ERK kinase (MEK), which in turn activates pERK 1/2 and (2) PD98059 inhibits MEK in hRPE cells. In our studies, PD98059 inhibited insulin stimulated 3H-thymidine incorporation as well as pERK 1/2 synthesis in hRPE cells obtained from the eyes of non-AMD patients, but had no effect on 3H-thymidine incorporation or pERK 1/2 synthesis in the presence of insulin in hRPE cells obtained from AMD eyes. This suggests that the ERK signaling mechanism may be impaired in hRPE from AMD patients thereby affecting DNA synthesis and cell function. Further studies of the exact kinase signaling abnormality in hRPE cells from patients with AMD and strategies to restore these signals may result in the development of new ways to treat age-related macular degeneration.

Acknowledgments The authors thank Sohil Patel and Jeeyong Kim for their assistance in preparing this chapter. This research was funded by the Skillman Foundation.

References

Alessi, D. R., Cuenda, A., Cohen, P., Dudley, D. T., Saltiel, A. R., 1995, PD 098059 is a specific inhibitor of the activation of mitogen-activated protein kinase kinase in vitro and in vivo, *J Biol Chem* **270(46)**:27489–94.

Bitar, K. N., Kothary, S., Kothary, P. C., 1996, Somatostatin inhibits bombesin-stimulated Gi-protein via its own receptor in rabbit colonic smooth muscle cells, *J Pharm Exp Therapeutics* **276**:714–19.

Campochiaro P. A., Hackett S. F., and Conway, B. P., 1991, Retinoic acid promotes density-dependent growth arrest in human retinal pigment epithelial cells, *IOVS* **32**:65–72.

Davis, S. P., Reddy, H., Caivano, M., et al., 2000, Specificity and mechanism of action of some commonly used protein kinase inhibitors, *Biochem J* **351**:95–105.

Hamdi, H. K., Kenney, C., 2003, Age-related macular degeneration: a new viewpoint, *Front Biosci* **8**:e305–14. Review.

Hecquet, C., Lefevre, G., Valtink, M., Engelmann, K., Mascarelli, F., 2002, Activation and role of MAP kinase-dependent pathways in retinal pigment epithelial cells: ERK and RPE cell proliferation, *Invest Ophthalmol Vis Sci* **43(9)**:3091–98.

Khoo, S., Griffen, S. C., Xia, Y., Baer, R. J., German, M. S., Cobb, M. H., 2003, Regulation of insulin gene transcription by ERK1 and ERK2 in pancreatic beta cells, *J Biol Chem* **278(35)**:32969–7.

Kothary, P. C., Britton, A., Lewis, N., Patel, V., Rivers, D., and Del Monte, M. A., 2005, ERK-pathway inhibitor and proliferative eye disease. Presented at International Drug Discovery Science and Technology, Shanghai, China.

Kothary, P. C., Del Monte, M. A., 2004. Growth factors, and their receptors and inhibitors with a special focus on human retinal pigment epithelial cells and the eye, In: *Recent Res Devel Biochem*, Edited by S. G. Pandalai, Transworld Research Network, Trivandrum, Kerala, India, pp. 99–116.

Kothary, P. C., Del Monte, M. A., 2005, High glucose modulates growth factor action in human retinal pigment epithelial cells, In: *Recent Res Devel*, Edited by S. G. Pandalai, Transworld Research Network, Trivandrum, Kerala, India, pp. 1–16.

Kothary, P. C., Lahiri, R., Kee, L., Sharma, N., Chun, E., Kuznia, A., and Del Monte, M. A., 2006, In: *Retinal Degenerative Diseases*, Edited by J. G. Hollyfield, R. E. Anderson and M. M. LaVail. Springer, New York, pp. 513–518.

Kusaka, K., Kothary, P. C., Del Monte, M. A., 1998, Modulation of basic fibroblast growth factor effect by retinoic acid in cultured retinal pigment epithelium, *Current Eye Research* **17(5)**: 524–30.

Lu, M., Amano, S., Miyamoto, K., Garland, R., Keough, K., Qin, W., Adamis A. P., 1999, Insulin-induced vascular endothelial growth factor expression in retina, *IOVS* **40**:3281–86.

Mascarelli, F., Hecquet, C., Guillonneau, X., Courtois, Y., 2001, Control of the intracellular signaling induced by fibroblast growth factors (FGF) over the proliferation and survival of retinal pigment epithelium cells: example of the signaling regulation of growth factors endogenous to the retina, *Journal de la Societe de Biologie* **195(2)**:101–6.

Tezel, T. H., Bora, N. S., Kaplan, H. J., 2004, Pathogenesis of age-related macular degeneration, *Trends Mol Med* **10(9)**:417–20.

Voutilainen-Kaunisto, R. M., Terasvirta, M. E., Uusitupa, M. I., and Niskanen, L. K. 2000, Age-related macular degeneration in newly diagnosed type 2 diabetic patients and control subjects: a 10-year follow-up on evolution, risk factors, and prognostic significance, *Diabetes Care* **23**:1672–78.

Zarbin, M. A., 2006, Progressive RPE atrophy around disciform scars, *Br J Ophthalmol* **90(4)**: 396–97.

Expression and Cell Compartmentalization of EFEMP1, a Protein Associated with *Malattia Leventinese*

Adam Kundzewicz, Francis Munier, and Jean-Marc Matter

1 Introduction

Malattia Leventinese holds its name from the beautiful Leventine Valley in Ticino, Southern Switzerland, from which all the Swiss families touched by this disease come from. It is an autosomal, dominant retinal dystrophy, first described by ophthalmologists in 1925 (Vogt, 1925). A characteristic hallmark of *Malattia Leventinese*, extracellular, amorphous deposits known as drusen, between the retinal pigment epithelium (RPE) and Bruch's membrane (Doyne, 1899), are also an early hallmark of age related macular degeneration (AMD), which accounts for approximately 50% of registered blindness in the developed world (Bressler et al., 1988). *Malattia Leventinese* exhibits features more consistent with AMD than any other heritable macular disorder so it is easy to understand why it should be considered as a burning issue, specially when taking into consideration the fact that the population affected by AMD is expected to nearly double in the next 25 years. What distinguishes *Malattia Leventinese* from other types of AMD is a radial pattern of drusen (Stone et al., 1999). In few cases of *Malattia Leventinese* drusen were only observed around the optic nerve head (Forni et al., 1962). Patients are usually asymptomatic until the age of 30 to 40 years and there is a high variability of the disease phenotype. At a later stage of the disease *Malattia Leventinese* exhibits a variety of clinical and histopathological features, including decreased visual acuity, geographic athropy, pigmentary changes and choroidal neovascularisation (Piguet et al., 1995).

Malattia Leventinese has been mapped to chromosome 2 (Heon et al., 1996) and associated with a single missense mutation (R345W) in a widely expressed gene of rather unknown function called *EFEMP1* (*S1-5*, fibulin *3*, *FBNL3*) for EGF-containing fibrillin-like extracellular matrix protein 1 (Stone et al., 1999), first

A. Kundzewicz
Department of Ophthalmology, School of Medicine, University of Geneva, 22 Rue Alcide Jentzer, 1211 Geneva 14, Switzerland, Tel: 41763472742, Fax: 41216268888
e-mail: Adam.Kundzewicz@unil.ch

R.E. Anderson et al. (eds.), *Recent Advances in Retinal Degeneration,*
© Springer 2008

isolated from fibroblasts of a patient with Werner syndrome, a premature ageing disease (Lecka-Czernik et al., 1995).

This mutation is believed to interfere with the secretion of EFEMP1, resulting in the accumulation of misfolded protein between RPE and Bruch's membrane (Marmorstein et al., 2002). Although mutated protein accumulates in a region directly overlaying drusen, it doesn't appear to be its major component (Marmorstein et al., 2002).

Human *EFEMP1* cDNA encodes a putative protein of 387 to 493 amino acids, with a predicted molecular mass of 43 to 55 kDa, depending on a splice variant. There are five predicted splice variants (Fig. 1), but only the shortest (43.1 kDa) and the longest (54.6 kDa) are expressed in substantial amounts at the protein level (Lecka-Czernik et al., 1995). EFEMP1 contains 5 to 6 EGF-like, calcium binding domains and is highly conserved among humans and rodents, but this homology is restricted to the EGF-like domains. Single Arg-Trp mutation associated with *Malattia Leventinese* alters the last, calcium binding EGF-like domain of EFEMP1 and it is very similar to number of fibrillin mutations. Fibrillins are found throughout the connective tissue as integral components of extended fibrils, which occur both isolated or in conjunction with elastin. Out of over 500 published fibrillin mutations leading to disease phenotypes many are missense mutations affecting one of the conserved cysteine residues of the EGF domains. Many of these mutations result in Marfan syndrome, a heritable disorder of the connective tissue that affects different organ systems, including the skeleton, lungs, eyes, heart and blood vessels (Dietz et al., 1991, 1992). EFEMP1 shows a strong homology (around 35% identity) to members of the fibrillin family (Ikegawa et al., 1996). Single mutation associated with *Malattia Leventinese* is thought to cause an abnormal accumulation of this protein between the RPE and Bruch membrane, what might create a physical barrier between the RPE and the choroidal blood vessels, which might result in accumulation of all set of other molecules, leading to a drusen formation (Marmorstein, 2004).

EFEMP1 mutation, present in *Malattia Leventinese*, affects an EGF-like, calcium binding domain of the protein. Many mutations known to result in Marfan

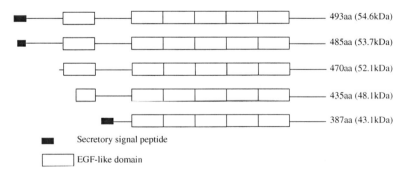

Fig. 1 Modular structure of the putative EFEMP1 proteins. Only the longest (54.6kDa) and the shortest (43.1kDa) variants are predicted to be expressed in substantial amounts at the protein level (Lecka-Czernik et al., 1995)

syndrome are predicted to disrupt calcium binding, so calcium binding by fibrillin seems to play an important role. It can be crucial for protein-protein interaction, stabilization of the molecule, protection against proteolysis and maturation of a proform of fibrillin. Single mutation in EGF-like, calcium binding domain of EFEMP1 might disrupt potential protein-protein interactions and results in misfolding and accumulation of EFEMP1. Protein-protein interactions through EGF-like domains are well known, for example Notch-Serrate proteins interact that way during development of the nervous system in *Drosophila melanogaster* (Rebay et al., 1991). This type of interactions is also known from the vertebrates (Notch/Delta signalling pathway). There is a possibility that EFEMP1 accumulates because of inability to bind its normal secretion partner. It has been recently discovered, that EFEMP1 binds tissue inhibitor of metalloproteinases-3 (TIMP-3), a matrix-bound inhibitor of matrix metalloproteinases (Klenotic et al., 2004). It is known, that mutations in the Timp-3 gene cause Sorsby fundus dystrophy (SFD), other hereditary macular degenerative disease (Langton et al., 2000).

EFEMP1 has been recently named fibulin 3 (Giltay et al., 1999) and qualified to the family of fibulins, extracellular matrix proteins (Argraves et al., 2003; Timpl et al., 2003). Six know members, including FBLN3 (EFEMP1), has been characterized from mammalian species. All of them share an elongated structure and many calcium-binding sites, owing to the presence of tandem arrays of epidermal growth factor-like domains. The structure of most of the fibulins can be modified by alternative messanger RNA splicing. They are hypothesized to function as intramolecular bridges that stabilize the organization of extracellular matrix structures (Argraves et al., 2003). The involvement of mutant fibulins in the development of macular degeneration has been confirmed lately by the identification of mutations in FBLN 5 and 6 in subsets of patients with AMD (Schultz et al., 2003; Stone et al., 2004) .

EFEMP1 is known to be a secreted protein, but the retinal cells that express its gene have not yet been identified. Our goal was to localize the *EFEMP1* transcripts in different types of human retinal cells. We also wanted to analyze the compartmentalization of the wild type and mutated EFEMP1 proteins.

2 EFEMP1 Displays an Unexpected Expression Pattern in Diseased Human Retina

We have cloned *EFEMP1* genes (mutated and wild type) into pBluescript vector and performed *in situ* hybridization on human retinas. This technique allows specific nucleic acid sequences to be detected in morphologically preserved cells or tissue sections. In combination with immunohistochemistry it can relate microscopic topological information to gene activity at the DNA, mRNA, and protein level. In order to obtain probes for *in situ* hybridization we have performed *in vitro* transcription with T3 or T7 polymerase to produce sense or antisense probes. Sense probes served as a negative control as they cannot hybridize with *EFEMP1* mRNA. *In vitro* transcription was conducted in presence of radioactive compound — ^{35}S. Radioactive riboprobes were synthesized and hydrolyzed to finally produce fragments of around 150 base pairs, which were then used for hybridization. The length of a probe is usually a compromise between the strength of the signal (long probe) and the penetration into the tissue (short probe).

To determine expression patterns of the *EFEMP1* gene, *in situ* hybridization studies were carried out on pre-treated paraffin sections of normal and *Malattia Leventinese* (ML) human retinas. We have used melanoma affected eyes as a control for all experiments. In normal eye *EFEMP1* transcripts were localized mainly in the retinal ganglion cells and the photoreceptors. In the diseased human eyes, transcripts were principally found in the RPE accompanied with drastic morphological changes of this tissue. This upregulation is not specific for the ML eye except in the ciliary body. *In situ* hybridization studies revealed specific localization of *EFEMP1* transcripts in ML and control human retinas. Despite being a widely expressed gene, *EFEMP1* pattern shows tissue specificity and differs between normal and diseased eyes. To compare the level of *EFEMP1* gene expression between different regions of RPE in ML eye, laser capture microdissections (LCM) were combined with RNA isolation and real-time PCR. Significant differences were observed between different regions of RPE in ML eye.

Fusion proteins containing wild type and mutated (R345W) *EFEMP1* (the shortest and the longest splice variants) with C-terminal GFP or flag peptide under the control of CMV promoter were constructed in order to determine cellular localization of the protein. Plasmids were transfected into VERO (African green monkey kidney) and ARPE-19 (human RPE) cells. While long variants of the protein showed an uniform, cytoplasmic localization, short variants were localized within the vacuoles and the cells expressing the transgenes died few hours after transfection. Western-blot analysis showed that the long variant of the protein is stable and gives a strong signal whereas the short variant is degraded. These observation led us to conclusions, that the short variant of EFEMP1 (43 kDa) probably doesn't exist in substantial amounts at the protein level. We have been unable to detect any striking difference in cell compartmentalization between the wild type and the mutated EFEMP1 during these studies.

Both abnormal expression of the *EFEMP1* gene and mutation and accumulation of EFEMP1 protein (inside or outside the cells) might contribute to the *Malattia Leventinese* pathology.

References

Argraves, W. S., Greene, L. M., Cooley, M. A., and Gallagher, W. M., 2003, Fibulins: physiological and disease perspectives, *EMBO reports.* 4:12

Bressler, N. M., Bressler, S. B., and Fine, S. L., 1988, Age-related macular degeneration, *Surv. Ophtalmol.* 32:375

Dietz, H. C., Cutting, C. R., Pyeritz, R. E., Maslen, C. L., Sakai, L. Y., Corson, G. M., Puffenberger, E. G., Hamosh, A., Nanthakumar, E. J., Curristin, S. M., Stetten, G., Meyers, D. A., and Francomano, C. A., 1991, Marfan syndrome caused by a recurrent *de novo* missense mutation in the fibrillin gene, *Nature.* 352:337

Dietz, H. C., Saraiva, J. M., Pyeritz, R. E., Cutting, G. R., and Francomano, C. A., 1992, Clustering of fibrillin (FBN1) missense mutation in Marfan syndrome patients at cysteine residues in EGF-like domains, *Hum. Mutat.* **1**:5

Doyne, R. W., 1899, Peculiar condition of choroiditis occurring in several members of the same family, *Trans. Ophthalmol. Soc. UK.* **19**

Forni, S., Babel, J., 1962, Etude clinique et histologique de la malattia leventinese: affection appartenant en groupe des dégénérescences hyalines du pole postérieur, *Ophtalmologica.* **143**

Giltay, R., Timpl, R., and Kostka, G., 1999, Sequence, recombinant expression and tissue localization of two novel extracellular matrix proteins, fibulin-3 and fibulin-4, *Matrix Biol.* **18**:5

Heon, E., Piguet, B., Munier, F., Sneed, S. R., Morgan, C. M., Forni, S., Pescia, G., Schorderet, D., Taylor, C. M., Streb, L. M., Wiles, C. D., Nishimura, D. Y., Sheffield, V. C., and Stone, E. M., 1996, Linkage of autosomal dominant radial drusen (malattia leventinese) to chromosome 2p16-21, *Arch. Ophthalmol.* **114**:2

Ikegawa, S., Toda, T., Okui, K., and Nakamura, Y., 1996, Structure and chromosomal assignment of the human S1-5 gene (FBNL) that is highly homologous to fibrillin, *Genomics.* **35**:3

Klenotic, P. A., Munier, F. L., Marmorstein, L. Y., and Anand-Apte, B., 2004, Tissue inhibitor of metalloproteinases 3 (TIMP-3) is a binding partner of epithelial growth factor-containing fibulin-like extracellular matrix protein 1 (EFEMP1), *J. Biol. Chem.* **279**:29

Langton, K. P., McKie, N., Curtis, A., Goodship, J. A., Bond, P. M., Barker, M. D., and Clarke, M., 2000, A novel tissue inhibitor of metalloproteinases-3 mutation reveals a common molecular phenotype in Sorsby's fundus dystrophy, *J. Biol. Chem.* **275**:35

Lecka-Czernik, B., Lumpkin, C. K. J., and Goldstein, S., 1995, An overexpressed gene transcript in senescent and quiescent human fibroblasts encoding a novel protein in the epidermal growth factor-like repeat family stimulates DNA synthesis, *Mol. Cell. Biol.* **15**:1

Marmorstein, L. Y., Munier, F. L., Arsenijevic, Y., Schorderet, D. F., McLaughlin, P. J., Chung, D., Traboulsi, E., and Marmorstein, A.D., 2002, Aberrant accumulation of EFEMP1 underlies drusen formation in Malattia Leventinese and age-related macular degeneration, *Proc. Natl. Acad. Sci. USA.* **99**:20

Marmorstein, L. Y., 2004, association of EFEMP1 with malattia leventinese and age-related macular degeneration: a mini-review, *Ophtalmic Genet.* **25**:3

Piguet, B., Haimovici, R., and Bird, A. C., 1995, Dominantly inherited drusen represent more than one disorder: a historical review, *Eye.* **9**:34

Rebay, I., Fleming, R. J., Fehon, R. G., Cherbas, L., Cherbas, P., and Artavanis-Tsakonas, S., 1991, Specific EGF repeats of Notch mediate interactions with Delta and Serrate: implications for Notch as a multifunctional receptor, *Cell.* **67**:4

Schultz, D. W., Klein, M. L., Humpert, A. J., Luzier, C. W., Persun, V., Schain, M., Mahan, A., Runckel, C., Cassera, M., Vittal, V., Doyle, T. M., Martin, T. M., Weleber, R. G., Francis, P. J., and Acott, T. S., 2003, Analysis of the ARMD1 locus: evidence that a mutation in HEMICENTIN-1 is associated with age-related macular degeneration in a large family, *Hum. Mol. Genet.* **12**:24

Stone, E. M., Lotery, A. J., Munier, F. M., Héon, E., Piguet, B., Guymer, R. H., Vandenburgh, K., Cousin, P., Nishimura, D., swiderski, R. E., Silvestri, G., Mackey, D. A., Hageman, G. S., Bird, A. C., Sheffield, V. C., and Schorderet, D. F., 1999, A single EFEMP1 mutation associated with both Malattia Leventinese and Doyne honeycomb retinal dystrophy, *Nature Genet.* **22**:2

Stone, E. M., Braun, T. A., Russel, R. S., Kuehn, M. H., Lotery, A. J., Moore, P. A., Eastman, C. G., Casavant, T. L., and Sheffield, V. C., 2004, Missense variations in the fibulin 5 gene and age-related macular degeneration, *N Engl J Med.* **351**:4

Timpl, R., Sasaki, T., Kostka, G., and Chu, M. L., 2003, Fibulins: a versatile family of extracellular matrix proteins, *Nature Rev. Mol. Cell Biol.* **4**:6

Vogt, A., 1925, Die Ophthalmoskopie im Rotfreien Licht. In Handbuch der Gesammten Augenheikunde. Untersuchungsmethoden., Verlag von Wilhelm Engelman, Berlin, pp. 1–118.

Role of ELOVL4 in Fatty Acid Metabolism

Vidyullatha Vasireddy, Majchrzak Sharon, Norman Salem, Jr,
and Radha Ayyagari

1 Introduction

Stargardt like macular dystrophy (STGD3) is an inherited form of early onset autosomal dominant macular degeneration. Pathophysiology of STGD3 is associated with the loss of central vision and RPE atrophy. Accumulation of lipofuscin was observed with the progression of the disease (Stone et al., 1994; Griesinger et al., 2000). Mutations in a novel gene, elongation of very long chain fatty acid-4 (*ELOVL4*) were found to be associated with STGD3 (Zhang et al., 2001).

ELOVL4 is homologous to the ELO family of proteins that play a role in fatty acid metabolism in yeast (Tvrdik et al., 2000). Human ELOVL4 protein has 314 amino acids with a putative dilysine (KXKXX) endoplasmic reticulum retention signal at the C-terminus. So far a 5 bp-deletion mutation and two additional mutations, all resulting in truncation of the protein have been identified in the *ELOVL4* gene (Bernstein et al., 2001; Maugeri et al., 2004). The 5 bp deletion mutation in the exon 6 of *ELOVL4* causes a frame shift, leading to the loss of 51 amino acids and a premature truncation of the protein (Zhang et al., 2001). Co-expression of mutant and wild type ELOVL4 in COS-7 cells revealed that the mutant protein interacts with the wild type, forming higher molecular weight aggregates (Grayson and Molday, 2005; Vasireddy et al., 2005).

To better understand the mechanism underlying the pathology of STGD3, we generated and characterized two mouse models: a knock-in mouse model carrying the *Elovl4* 5-bp deletion ($Elovl4^{+/del}$) and an *Elovl4* knock-out mouse model. $Elovl4^{+/del}$ were viable and developed progressive photoreceptor degeneration, while the heterozygous *Elovl4* knock-out mice had normal retinal function (Raz-Prag et al., 2006; Vasireddy et al., 2006). The homozygous knock-out mice and the 5-bp deletion knock-in mice carrying the deletion in the homozygous state $(Elovl4^{del/del})$ died within a few hours after birth due to an defect in the

R. Ayyagari
Ophthalmology and Visual Sciences, W. K. Kellogg Eye Center, University of Michigan, Ann Arbor, Tel: 313-647-6345, Fax: 313-936-7231
e-mail: ayyagari@umich.edu

epidermal barrier (Vasireddy et al., 2007). Through studies on these mice,we have demonstrated that ELOVL4 is essential for the synthesis of epidermal very long-chain FA (VLFA), and is required for generating omega-O-acylceramides, which are essential for the formation of epidermal permeability barrier (Vasireddy et al., 2007). Subsequently, these observations were confirmed by studies reported by other investigators (Cameron et al., 2007; McMahon et al., 2007).

In the mouse, expression of *Elovl4* has been observed in retina, brain, whole skin, and testis (Mandal et al., 2004). Similar to retina and skin, brain tissue is also known to have a unique unsaturated fatty acid composition. In the skin, lack of functional ELOVL4 resulted in depletion of fatty acids with chain length longer than C28, however, the function of ELOVL4 in brain and ocular tissue is not known. To study the effect of an absence of functional ELOVL4 on brain and eye, we analyzed the fatty acid composition of these tissues from homozygous *Elovl4* 5-bp deletion knock-in mice and compared with the litter mate controls.

2 Materials and Methods

2.1 Animal Maintenance and Tissue Collection

Design of the construct and generation of $Elovl4^{+/del}$ has been described elsewhere (Vasireddy et al., 2006). Experiments were conducted in accordance with the Statement for the Use of Animals in Ophthalmic and Vision Research and protocols used were approved by the Animal Care and Use Committee of the University of Michigan. All the animals were maintained in a 12-hour dark and light cycle. For the present studies, P0 pups were dissected on day 0. Total eye balls and brain were collected, weighed and stored at -80°C until fatty acid analysis was performed. Tail samples were collected for genotyping of the animals.

2.2 Extraction and Analysis of Fatty Acid Profiles

To determine the effect of *Elovl4* 5-bp deletion mutation on fatty acid composition in the eye and brain, the levels of saturated and unsaturated fatty acids in these tissues from P0 pups of $Elovl4^{del/del}$ mice (N=10) were determined and compared with wild type littermate controls (N=10). The tissues were weighed and lipid extraction was performed according to the Bligh and Dyer method (Bligh and Dyer, 1959). Butylated hydroxytoluene (BHT) was added to each sample, along with the internal standard 22:3n-3 methyl ester. Retinas were subsequently transmethylated using the BF$_3$-methanol method of Morrison and Smith (Morrison and Smith, 1964) as modified by Salem et al (Salem et al., 1996), with the co-solvent hexane (Salem et al., 1996). The methyl ester samples were analyzed by gas chromatography as previously described (Salem et al., 1996).

2.3 Statistical Analysis

Data of eye ball fatty acids are presented as the mean ± standard deviation (SD) and the Fatty acid profiles of the brain and diet are presented as mean± Standard Error (SE). Comparisons of means between two experimental groups were performed using the two tailed, independent Student's t test. To compare the mean among more than two different groups, Analysis of variance (ANOVA) was used.

3 Results

The *Elovl4* 5-bp deletion knock in mice with homozygous and heterozygous genotypes were born in an expected Mandalian ratio. Pups carrying the different genotypes were indistinguishable at birth. Total eye balls and brains were collected from new born pups for fatty acid analysis.

Comparison of the fatty acid profile of the eye balls of P0 pups from mice carrying the 5-bp deletion in the homozygous state and litter mate heterozygous pups and wild type controls showed a significant alteration in the levels of several n–3 fatty acids including 20:5 n–3 ($P = 0.006$), 22:5n–3 ($P<0.01$), 24:5 n–3 ($P = 0.003$) and 24:6 n–3 ($P = 0.046$) (Table 1). The levels of 20:5 n–3, 22:5 n–3, 24:5 n–3 and 24:6 n–3 FA were found to be decreased in *Elovl4* $^{del/del}$ pups when compared with the Wt controls as well as *Elovl4* $^{+/del}$ pups. Where as the levels of these FA were found to be increased in *Elovl4* $^{+/del}$ animals when compared with the Wt animals. However, there was no significant alteration in the levels of 22:6n–3 in the eye balls of these pups. Although the exact role of ELOVL4 in the fatty acid metabolism in these tissues is not known, the altered fatty acid levels indicate a possible role of ELOVL4 in long chain fatty acid metabolism in ocular tissue.

The fatty acid profile of brain tissue did not show significant alteration in the levels of the saturated, monounsaturated or polyunsaturated fatty acids in *Elovl4* $^{del/del}$ animals when compared with the Wt controls (Table 2).

4 Discussion

The present study is designed to investigate the effect of the lack of a functional ELOVL4 on the fatty acid composition of the brain, and eye balls, using mice carrying the 5-bp deletion in the homozygous state. In mammals, fatty acids consisting up to 16 carbon atoms (C16) are synthesized by fatty acid synthase complex. Significant amounts of these synthesized fatty acids and the dietary fatty acids are further elongated to long chain fatty acids and to very long chain fatty acids (VLFA). Formation of VLFA takes place in the ER by membrane bound elongases. Six Elovls (ELOVL1-6), which are proposed play a role in the condensation step of the fatty acid chain elongation have been identified. *Elovl1* was observed to be involved in the synthesis of saturated C26 fatty acids

Table 1 Fatty acid profiles of the eye balls of *Elovl4* $^{del/del}$ and *Elovl4* $^{+/del}$ pups in comparison to Wt controls

	Wild Type		*Elovl4* $^{+/del}$		*Elovl4* $^{del/del}$		
Variable (ug/mg)	Mean	SD	Mean	SD	Mean	SD	raw-p
FA 14:0	0.0953	0.0171	0.1246	0.02349	0.11735	0.0296	0.073
FA 16:0-DMA	0.1385	0.0249	0.1628	0.04038	0.16348	0.04206	0.397
FA 16:0	1.8433	0.2050	2.1737	0.32792	1.9802	0.59809	0.35
FA 18:0DMA	0.05290	0.0064	0.0548	0.0189	0.063028	0.01502	0.341
FA 18:0	1.0516	0.1288	1.3168	0.25902	1.23221	0.23385	0.097
FA 20:0	0.0175	0.0022	0.02761	0.00738	0.020944	0.00652	0.01
FA 22.0	0.0174	0.0020	0.02397	0.00764	0.02162	0.00411	0.087
FA 24:0	0.01919	0.0039	0.02658	0.01064	0.025699	0.0094	0.27
Total Saturates	3.2358	0.3653	3.9111	0.65843	3.62456	0.84579	0.194
FA 20:3 n9	0.0565	0.0117	0.07849	0.023936	0.077043	0.02238	0.118
FA 16:1	0.2845	0.0477	0.32355	0.071913	0.34655	0.06859	0.202
FA 18:1 DMA	0.0507	0.0101	0.05928	0.023845	0.05872	0.01341	0.599
FA 18:1 n9	1.5125	0.1892	1.79343	0.32556	1.71183	0.32111	0.211
FA 18:1 n7	0.4491	0.0554	0.54779	0.11132	0.541559	0.11062	0.15
FA 20:1 n9	0.03596	0.0038	0.05188	0.012379	0.046012	0.01253	0.038
FA 24:1 n9	0.03131	0.0054	0.041	0.01432	0.03744	0.0097	0.257
Total mono unsaturates	2.364	0.2857	2.8169	0.53923	2.74212	0.52135	0.199
FA 18:2 n6	0.2551	0.0712	0.3038	0.07939	0.25887	0.0734	0.321
FA 20:2 n6	0.0161	0.0054	0.02288	0.00767	0.01704	0.00437	0.053
FA 20:3 n6	0.0502	0.0084	0.06376	0.01052	0.056	0.01593	0.125
FA 20:4 n6	0.7981	0.1177	0.9808	0.18782	0.94385	0.18756	0.14
FA 22:4 n6	0.1389	0.0133	0.16337	0.02666	0.17301	0.03579	0.085
FA 22:5 n6	0.0533	0.0045	0.05582	0.009867	0.05849	0.0107	0.551
FA24:4 n6	0.0211	0.0202	0.01769	0.00767	0.01765	0.01047	0.832
FA 24:5 n6	0.0211	0.0030	0.02239	0.003764	0.026317	0.00591	0.068
Total n6	1.3541	0.1963	1.6306	0.31694	1.55124	0.30898	0.204
FA 20:5 n3	**0.0212**	**0.0093**	**0.02808**	**0.00671**	**0.016215**	**0.00725**	**0.006**
FA 22:5N3	**0.06368**	**0.0208**	**0.09675**	**0.018469**	**0.058957**	**0.02042**	**5E-04**
FA 22:6n3	0.05439	0.1050	0.6541	0.07428	0.58235	0.13003	0.126
FA 24:5 n3	**0.0021**	**0.0009**	**0.0027**	**0.0006**	**0.001577**	**0.00051**	**0.003**
FA 24:6 N3	**0.0134**	**0.0030**	**0.01428**	**0.00163**	**0.01168**	**0.00231**	**0.046**
Total n–3	0.6443	0.1316	0.7816	0.08642	0.6708	0.1449	0.064
Total FA	9.4473	1.5393	11.9534	2.52552	10.9316	2.0218	0.097

and sphingolipid formation (Salem et al., 1996; Tvrdik et al., 2000). *Elovl2* was hypothesized to have a role in PUFA synthesis. Both mouse and human *Elovl2* were shown to elongate arachidonic acid (20:4n–6), eicosapentaenoic acid (20:5n–3), docosatetraenoic acid (22:4n–6) and docosapentaenoic acid (22:5n–3). Ablation of *Elovl3* also showed an impaired epidermal permeability barrier and synthesis of VLCFA in the skin (Westerberg et al., 2004) *Elovl5*, is involved in the elongation of various polyunsaturated long-chain fatty acids of C18–C20 (Leonard et al., 2002). *Elovl6* has been reported to be involved in the elongation of saturated fatty acids with 12–16 carbons to C18 and may not participate in the

Table 2 Brain Fatty acid profiles of Elovl4 del/del pups in comparison to the Wt littermate controls. Data are expressed as the mean ± sem ug/mg tissue wet weight

Fatty acid	Wild type		Elovl4 del/del	
	Mean	SE	Mean	SE
14:0	0.40	0.05	0.38	0.01
16:0DMA	0.23	0.04	0.24	0.02
16:0	4.92	0.68	4.76	0.25
18:0DMA	0.12	0.02	0.13	0.01
18:0	2.78	0.37	2.70	0.13
20:0	0.03	0.005	0.03	0.005
22:0	0.04	0.008	0.04	0.004
24:0	0.03	0.004	0.04	0.007
Total Saturates	8.54	1.16	8.31	0.42
Monounsaturates				
16:1DMA	0.31	0.08	0.64	0.27
16:1n7	0.44	0.06	0.44	0.02
18:1DMA	0.03	0.005	0.04	0.004
18:1n9	2.34	0.32	2.34	0.12
18:1n7	0.60	0.08	0.63	0.04
20:1n9	0.08	0.009	0.10	0.012
24:1n9	0.06	0.007	0.07	0.013
Total Monounsaturates	3.84	0.51	4.24	0.46
n–6 Polyunsaturates				
18:2n6	0.17	0.03	0.16	0.02
20:2n6	0.06	0.03	0.03	0.00
20:3n6	0.11	0.01	0.09	0.01
20:4n6	2.03	0.31	1.94	0.11
22:4n6	0.51	0.07	0.50	0.03
22:5n6	0.19	0.02	0.21	0.02
Total n–6	3.07	0.45	2.93	0.18
n–3 polyunsaturates				
22:5n3	0.12	0.02	0.10	0.01
22:6n3	2.59	0.34	2.51	0.13
Total n–3	2.71	0.36	2.61	0.13
Total FA (μg/mg wet weight)	19.8	2.6	19.6	1.4

elongation of fatty acids with chain lengths longer than C18 (Moon et al., 2001). These observations indicate that the ELOVL family of proteins participates in fatty acid elongation in mammals similar to the Elo group of enzymes in yeast.

Although *Elovl4* was initially discovered as a gene associated with Stargardt-like macular degeneration (Zhang et al., 2001), significant amount of *Elovl4* expression was observed in non-ocular tissues, like brain and skin. (Mandal et al., 2004). The high expression of ELOVL4 in the retina leads to the speculation that it might be involved in the elongation steps required for the synthesis of docosahexaenoic acid (22:6n–3) the major long-chain fatty acid present in the retina (Zhang et al., 2001).

Depletion of very long-chain fatty acids with chain length longer than C26, OH-ceramides and glycosyl-ceramides was observed in the skin of mice lacking functional ELOVL4 suggesting a role for ELOVL4 in the synthesis of FAs with chain length longer than C26 (Vasireddy et al., 2007). The retinal FA profile of mice carrying the 5-bp deletion Elvol4 mutation in the heterozygous state showed a significant decrease in the levels of 20:5n–3 ($P<0.028$), 22:5 n–3 ($P<0.04$), 24:6 n3 ($P<0.005$). Consistent with these results, a significant decrease in the 20:5 n–3($P<0.02$), 22:5 n–3 ($P<0.01$), 24:5 n–3 ($P<0.01$), 24:6 n–3 ($P<0.01$) fatty acid levels was observed in the eye balls of Elovl4 $^{del/del}$ pups compared to the age matched littermate wild type controls (Table 1). This data clearly indicates a role for ELOVL4 in long-chain fatty acid metabolism in the ocular tissue. The analysis of fatty acid profiles in the retina and eye balls of heterozygous and homozygous 5-bp deletion knock-in mice respectively did not include very long chain fatty acids and ceramides. Therefore, the effect of the absence of functional ELOVL4 on these classes of fatty acids in the ocular tissue is not known.

The analysis of the fatty acid profiles of the brain of Elovl4 $^{del/del}$ pups did not show significant alteration in the levels of saturated, mono-unsaturated and polyunsaturated fatty acids. In the brain tissue, in addition to ELOVL4 gene, Elovl1, Elovl3, Elovl4, Elovl5 are expressed and the level of expression of Elovl4 was found to be less than the expression of Elovl1 and Elovl6. The unaltered long chain fatty acid profiles of brain tissue from Elovl4 $^{del/del}$ pups also indicate that the ELOVL4 may not be the major fatty acid elongase in the brain. The brain fatty acid profiles of mice carrying the Elovl4 Y270X mutation in the homozygous state were also reported to be not significantly different from the control mice (Cameron et al., 2007). These results are consistent with our observation on the brain lipid profile of 5-bp deletion knock in mice.

Though the general function of the Elovl genes is partially understood, very little is known about the role of fatty acids of specific chain length in cellular and developmental processes. Although the altered key epidermal FA profiles of Elovl4$^{del/del}$ mice and Elovl4 deficient mice are now identified, we are still at an early stage in understanding the biological function of ELOVL4 and its specific role in the regulation of fatty acid chain elongation. The analysis of the epidermal fatty acids of Elovl4$^{del/del}$ showed an alteration in the VLFA and ceramide metabolism. We do not know whether similar alterations will be observed in the eyes and brain of Elovl4 $^{del/del}$ pups. The present study was not designed to evaluate the levels of VLFAs or ceramides in the retina and brain. Hence, additional studies are needed to establish the role of Elovl4 in fatty acid metabolism of the brain and eye balls of these pups. Further detailed analysis of the VLFA profiles in these pups may aid in the understanding of the effect of ELOVL4 mutation on VLFA metabolism.

Acknowledgments The authors would like to thank Austra Liepa (University of Michigan) for generation and maintenance of the animals. This work was supported by grants to RA from NIH (R01EY13198) and the Foundation Fighting Blindness; a research grant to RA, core grant to the University of Michigan, Department of Ophthalmology (P30EY007003) and Vision Research (P30EY07060). The project was supported in part by the Intramural Research Program of the National Institutes of Health, NIAAA.

References

Bernstein PS, Tammur J, Singh N, Hutchinson A, Dixon M, Pappas CM, Zabriskie NA, Zhang K, Petrukhin K, Leppert M, Allikmets R (2001) Diverse macular dystrophy phenotype caused by a novel complex mutation in the ELOVL4 gene. Invest Ophthalmol Vis Sci 42:3331–3336

Bligh EG, Dyer WJ (1959) A rapid method of total lipid extraction and purification. Can J Biochem Physiol 37:911–917

Cameron DJ, Tong Z, Yang Z, Kaminoh J, Kamiyah S, Chen H, Zeng J, chen Y, Luo L, Zhang K (2007) Essential role of Elovl4 in very long chain fatty acid synthesis, skin permeability barrier function, and neonatal survival. Int J Biol Sci Feb 6:111–119

Grayson C, Molday RS (2005) Dominant negative mechanism underlies autosomal dominant Stargardt-like macular dystrophy linked to mutations in ELOVL4. J Biol Chem 280: 32521–32530

Griesinger IB, Sieving PA, Ayyagari R (2000) Autosomal dominant macular atrophy at 6q14 excludes CORD7 and MCDR1/PBCRA loci. Invest Ophthalmol Vis Sci 41:248–255

Leonard AE, Kelder B, Bobik EG, Chuang LT, Lewis CJ, Kopchick JJ, Mukerji P, Huang YS (2002) Identification and expression of mammalian long-chain PUFA elongation enzymes. Lipids 37:733–740

Mandal MN, Ambasudhan R, Wong PW, Gage PJ, Sieving PA, Ayyagari R (2004) Characterization of mouse orthologue of ELOVL4: genomic organization and spatial and temporal expression. Genomics 83:626–635

Maugeri A, Meire F, Hoyng CB, Vink C, Van Regemorter N, Karan G, Yang Z, Cremers FP, Zhang K (2004) A novel mutation in the ELOVL4 gene causes autosomal dominant Stargardt-like macular dystrophy. Invest Ophthalmol Vis Sci 45:4263–4267

McMahon A, Butovich IA, Mata NL, Klein M, Ritter R, 3rd, Richardson J, Birch DG, Edwards AO, Kedzierski W (2007) Retinal pathology and skin barrier defect in mice carrying a Stargardt disease-3 mutation in elongase of very long chain fatty acids-4. Mol Vis 13: 258–272

Moon YA, Shah NA, Mohapatra S, Warrington JA, Horton JD (2001) Identification of a mammalian long chain fatty acyl elongase regulated by sterol regulatory element-binding proteins. J Biol Chem 276:45358–45366

Morrison WR, Smith LM (1964) Preparation of fatty acid methyl esters and dimethylacetals from lipids with boron fluoride – Methanol. J Lipid Res 53:600–608

Raz-Prag D, Ayyagari R, Fariss RN, Mandal MN, Vasireddy V, Majchrzak S, Webber AL, Bush RA, Salem N, Jr., Petrukhin K, Sieving PA (2006) Haploinsufficiency is not the key mechanism of pathogenesis in a heterozygous Elovl4 knockout mouse model of STGD3 disease. Invest Ophthalmol Vis Sci 47:3603–3611

Salem N, Jr., Reyzer M, Karanian J (1996) Losses of arachidonic acid in rat liver after alcohol inhalation. Lipids 31 (Suppl):S153–156

Stone EM, Nichols BE, Kimura AE, Weingeist TA, Drack A, Sheffield VC (1994) Clinical features of a Stargardt-like dominant progressive macular dystrophy with genetic linkage to chromosome 6q. Arch Ophthalmol 112:765–772

Tvrdik P, Westerberg R, Silve S, Asadi A, Jakobsson A, Cannon B, Loison G, Jacobsson A (2000) Role of a new mammalian gene family in the biosynthesis of very long chain fatty acids and sphingolipids. J Cell Biol 149:707–718

Vasireddy V, Jablonski MM, Mandal MN, Raz-Prag D, Wang XF, Nizol L, Iannaccone A, Musch DC, Bush RA, Salem N, Jr., Sieving PA, Ayyagari R (2006) Elovl4 5-bp-deletion knock-in mice develop progressive photoreceptor degeneration. Invest Ophthalmol Vis Sci 47: 4558–4568

Vasireddy V, Uchida Y, Salem N, Kim SY, Mandal MN, Reddy GB, Bodepudi R, Alderson NL, Brown JC, Hama H, Dlugosz A, Elias PM, Holleran WM, Ayyagari R (2007) Loss of functional ELOVL4 depletes very long-chain fatty acids (>=C28) and the unique {omega}-O-acylceramides in skin leading to neonatal death. Hum Mol Genet 16:471–482

Vasireddy V, Vijayasarathy C, Huang J, Wang XF, Jablonski MM, Petty HR, Sieving PA, Ayyagari R (2005) Stargardt-like macular dystrophy protein ELOVL4 exerts a dominant negative effect by recruiting wild-type protein into aggresomes. Mol Vis 11:665–676

Westerberg R, Tvrdik P, Unden AB, Mansson JE, Norlen L, Jakobsson A, Holleran WH, Elias PM, Asadi A, Flodby P, Toftgard R, Capecchi MR, Jacobsson A (2004) Role for ELOVL3 and fatty acid chain length in development of hair and skin function. J Biol Chem 279:5621–5629

Zhang K, Kniazeva M, Han M, Li W, Yu Z, Yang Z, Li Y, Metzker ML, Allikmets R, Zack DJ, Kakuk LE, Lagali PS, Wong PW, MacDonald IM, Sieving PA, Figueroa DJ, Austin CP, Gould RJ, Ayyagari R, Petrukhin K (2001) A 5-bp deletion in ELOVL4 is associated with two related forms of autosomal dominant macular dystrophy. Nat Genet 27:89–93

Organization and Molecular Interactions of Retinoschisin in Photoreceptors

Camasamudram Vijayasarathy, Yuichiro Takada, Yong Zeng,
Ronald A. Bush, and Paul A. Sieving

1 Introduction

Retinoschisin (RS), the product of the *RS1* gene on the X-chromosome (Xp22), is a 24 kDa secreted protein which is expressed exclusively in the retina (Reid et al., 1999; Sauer et al., 1997) and pineal gland (Takada et al., 2006). In the retina, photoreceptors, bipolar cells, and ganglion cells synthesize RS (Takada et al., 2004). The structural features and functional implications of the 224 amino acid RS sequence include a N-terminus signal peptide (amino acids 1–23) and a 157 amino acid (amino acids 68–217) discoidin domain (Reid et al., 1999; Sauer et al., 1997). The signal peptide guides the secretion of mature RS across the plasma membrane and is cleaved off during the translocation process (Molday, 2007). Discoidin domains, which are highly conserved across species and found on the extracellular cell surface, are known to be involved in cell adhesion and signaling (Reid et al., 1999). Based on this structural feature, RS is believed to function as an adhesive protein in preserving the structural and functional integrity of the retina (Weber et al., 2002). A spectrum of missense mutations occurring throughout the *RS1* gene was found to interfere with one of the several steps in RS biosynthesis and secretion pathway (Molday, 2007; Wang et al., 2006). The loss of function mutations lead to a form of macular disruption and degeneration in males known as X-linked retinoschisis (XLRS) (Sikkink et al., 2006). XLRS patients exhibit a split or schisis and cystic-like spaces within the retinal layers that lead to early and progressive loss of vision. While there is no established treatment for XLRS, a recent study reported a reduction in foveal cysts and improvement in vision in XLRS patients who were treated with a topical form of dorzolamide, a carbonic anhydrase inhibitor (Apushkin and Fishman, 2006). Further, the feasibility of gene therapy as an approach to treating retinoschisis was also demonstrated in mouse model of XLRS (Molday, 2007; Zeng et al., 2004). Although these studies have advanced our current understanding of RS

Paul A. Sieving
National Eye Institute, National Institutes of Health, Bethesda, MD 20892, USA,
Tel: 301-496-2234, Fax: 301-496-9972
e-mail: pas@nei.nih.gov

and XLRS, the precise molecular details of RS function still remain unknown. In an effort toward understanding the molecular basis of RS function, we carried out a biochemical characterization and ultrastructural localization of RS in intact murine retina.

1.1 Isoforms of RS

RS represents a rare example of a naturally occurring signal sequence cleavage at more than one site in vivo and a secretory protein being found in two mature isoforms (Vijayasarathy et al., 2006). The flexibility of signal peptidase to process RS signal sequence at two cleavage sites (between amino acids 21–22 and 23–24) is the basis for the occurrence of Leu 22–224 and Ser 24–224 isoforms of RS and the cleavage at both the sites is correlated to the amino acid sequence and composition of the RS signal peptide. Several extremely low abundant isoforms of RS post-translationally modified with amino acid charge change were also identified in intact retina. The biochemical significance of these isoforms, if any, is currently not known.

1.2 RS is a Peripheral Membrane Protein

The mature RS is a plasma membrane associated protein (Vijayasarathy et al., 2007). As is characteristic of peripheral membrane proteins, RS was dissociated from the membranes at high pH and segregated into the aqueous phase upon Triton X-114 solubilization and phase separation. Protease protection assays confirmed the presence of a great majority of RS (about 80%) on the outer leaflet of the plasma membrane and the rest around the plasma membrane in the cytoplasmic side. Immunoelectron microscopy observations show dense localization of RS on the plasma membrane of the photoreceptor inner segment (Fig. 1A and 1B). Little or no immunoreactivity was present on connecting cilia, outer segments, or in the extracellular space (Fig. 1A and 1B). Profound alterations were observed in photoreceptor ultrastructure following the loss of RS expression. In comparison to closely arranged photoreceptor inner and outer segments in wild type retina (Fig. 1C), the electron micrograph of the retina from $RS1^{-/y}$ mice shows disorganization of the inner and outer segment structure with associated changes in volume densities of the cytoplasm and size and shape of the mitochondria (Fig. 1D).

1.3 RS Interaction with Membrane Phospholipids

The finding that RS is present in the membrane fraction and can be extracted together with the glycerophospholipids after NP-40 treatment suggested that RS might be bound to membrane phospholipids (Vijayasarathy et al., 2007). The

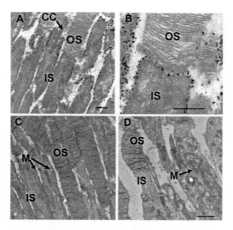

Fig. 1 Electron microscopy and localization of RS on the photoreceptor inner segment plasma membrane. In C57BL/6J mice retina, RS immunogold was distributed on the outer surfaces of inner segments (A and B). Transmission electron micrographs of retinas revealed normal photoreceptor architecture in wild type retina (C). $RS1^{-/y}$ mice retinas show disorganization of photoreceptor inner and outer segments (D). Scale Bars - A, B, and C: 500 nm; D: 100 nm. CC, connecting cilium; OS, outer segment; IS, inner segment; M, mitochondria

molecular basis of RS interactions has been extrapolated from knowledge about the conserved discoidin domain sequence, which comprises about 75% of the mature RS protein. Similar to the discoidin domains of blood coagulation factors V and VIII (Gilbert and Drinkwater, 1993), the fusion protein of RS discoidin domain (RS-DD) and glutathione-s-transferase displayed moderate to high affinity binding to negatively charged phospholipids in an in vitro protein-lipid overlay assay. RS-DD did not bind phosphatidylethanolamine (PE), phosphatidylcholine (PC), and other lysophospholipids (Vijayasarathy et al., 2007). The 3D structure model of RS predicted that three aromatic amino acid residues Tyr-89, Trp-92, and Phe-108 form the membrane lipid anchoring sites (Fraternali et al., 2003). These three aromatic residues are consistently mutated into cysteines in some families with XLRS disease (http://www.dmd.nl/rs/). Site-directed mutagenesis of these three aromatic residues either reduced or abolished the affinity of the mutant RS-DD binding to PS, while retaining varying affinities for binding to other phosphoinositides. These data suggest that the interactions with negatively charged glycerophospholipids are critical for RS binding to membranes and that RS exhibits a preference for binding to certain lipid moieties, such as phosphatidylserine.

1.4 Influence of Ionic Milieu on RS-membrane Association

The affinity of RS for membrane surface was also influenced by divalent cations (Vijayasarathy et al., 2007). Inclusion of either Ca^{2+} or Mg^{2+}(5 mM) in the buffer prevented the release of RS from the membranes, while similar concentrations of

EGTA or EDTA resulted in the highest release of RS. The lipid binding properties of RS as well its sensitivity to divalent cations is consistent with charge interactions, which are important structural and functional features of proteins. Divalent cations mediate interactions between proteins and their ligands and also influence the binding of proteins to phospholipids and carbohydrates. Ca^{2+} has also been shown to induce the restructuring and sugar binding affinity of discoidin 1, an adhesive protein from Dictyostelium discoideum (Valencia et al., 1989).

1.5 RS Interactions with Extracellular Matrix (ECM)

It is believed that RS may mediate the association of the extracellular matrix with the surface of photoreceptor and other retinal cells to promote cell adhesion and thereby stabilize the cellular architecture of the highly structured retinal tissue. In the homo-octameric form (Molday, 2007), RS bound to the cell membrane through phospholipids would have sites open to interact with other extracellular proteins such as collagens and with carbohydrates. Collagens have been shown to act as ligands for the discoidin domains (Vogel et al., 2006). In an enzyme-linked immunosorbent in vitro assay, the recombinant RS (amino acid 24–224) with the N-terminal 6XHis tag (His-RS) bound to Type I collagen more avidly than to Types II, III, and IV (Fig. 2A). Retinal membrane fractions enriched in RS also showed specific binding to Type I Collagen (Fig. 2B). However, there is no current evidence of Type I collagen in the retina, and collagen Types II, III, and XVII that are known to be

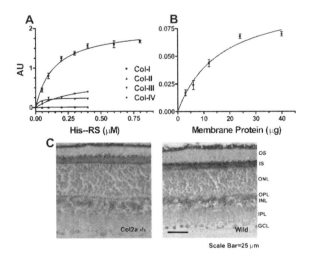

Fig. 2 Purified recombinant RS binds more avidly to Type I collagen than to collagen Types II, III, and IV. Increasing amounts of purified His-RS (A) or mice retinal membrane fractions (B) were incubated with collagen coated plates and the amount of bound RS was measured by ELISA using anti-RS antibody. (C) Immunohistochemical labeling of RS (brown staining) in 2 month old Col2a1 mutant and wild type mice retina using anti-RS antibody and goat anti-rabbit conjugated HRP (horseradish peroxidase) (Please see the color plate for a color version of this figure.)

present in the retina displayed no evidence of interaction with RS (Vijayasarathy et al., 2007). Furthermore, the Col2a1 mutant mouse in which retinoschisis was reported (Donahue et al., 2003) revealed normal retinal localization and distribution of RS (Fig. 2C). In summary these results do not suggest an interaction between RS and retinal cell collagens that have been tested in this study.

Blue native gels, resolve multi-protein complexes in accordance to their molecular masses (Schagger and von Jagow, 1991). On a blue native gel, RS from retinal cell lysates migrated with electrophoretic mobilties that corresponded to 200 kDa octamer and a >700 kDa diffuse complex (Fig. 3). Subfractionation of the gel slice corresponding to 700 kDa region, followed by in gel tryptic digestion and MS/MS peptide sequence analysis, identified RS in two of the three fractions. In both cases, the coverage was 15% by amino acid count in the discoidin domain region of RS. The RS sequence information did not indicate post-translational modification of amino acid residues. None of the extracellular matrix (ECM) protein sequences were found in this diffuse RS band to indicate RS interaction with ECM. The proteins identified in this diffuse band included NCAM (neural cell adhesion molecule), $Na^+ K^+$ ATPase, crystallins and other cytoskeletal and mitochondrial membrane proteins. Although a recent study (Steiner-Champliaud et al., 2006) suggested RS-crystallin interaction, further investigation is needed to determine the significance of intracellular protein–RS interactions as well as the authenticity of the multi-protein complex in terms of RS interacting proteins.

RS is a peripheral membrane protein bound by ionic forces to the outer leaflet of the photoreceptor inner segment plasma membrane. Most importantly, the high affinity of RS for membrane surfaces would restrict its diffusion into the extracellular matrix. The results suggest that RS may act locally to maintain photoreceptor inner segment stability and architecture, and it is not secreted only for export to the inner retina as previously proposed (Reid and Farber, 2005). We propose that

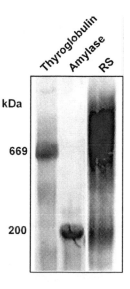

Fig. 3 RS-multiprotein complex. Whole cell lysates (40 μg protein) from mouse retina solubilized in Triton X-100 were adjusted to 0.5 M Bis-Tris pH 7.0. The smples were electrophoressed on 4–13% acrylamide gels under native conditions at 4°C as described by Schagger and von Jagow (1991). RS was localized by immunoblotting. The Serva-Blue G dye stained molecular weight markers: thyroglobulin (669 kDa) and amylase(200 kDa)

disruption of the inner segment architecture due to the loss of RS on inner segments might be the basic mechanism that underlies the displacement and disorganization of photoreceptors that we have seen in RS deficient mice retinas. RS bound by ionic forces or phospholipids on the membrane surface can participate in cell-matrix and cell-cell interactions which will influence cytoskeletal organization. Future studies will be needed to address the molecular mechanisms and the role of RS in such events.

Acknowledgments This study was supported by the NIH Intramural Research Program through National Institute on Deafness and Other Communication Disorders and National Eye Institute, Bethesda, MD 20892, USA.

References

Apushkin, M. A., and Fishman, G. A. (2006). Use of dorzolamide for patients with X-linked retinoschisis. Retina26, 741–745.

Donahue, L. R., Chang, B., Mohan, S., Miyakoshi, N., Wergedal, J. E., Baylink, D. J., Hawes, N. L., Rosen, C. J., Ward-Bailey, P., Zheng, Q. Y., et al. (2003). A missense mutation in the mouse Col2a1 gene causes spondyloepiphyseal dysplasia congenita, hearing loss, and retinoschisis. J Bone Miner Res18, 1612–1621.

Fraternali, F., Cavallo, L., and Musco, G. (2003). Effects of pathological mutations on the stability of a conserved amino acid triad in retinoschisin. FEBS Lett544, 21–26.

Gilbert, G. E., and Drinkwater, D. (1993). Specific membrane binding of factor VIII is mediated by O-phospho-L-serine, a moiety of phosphatidylserine. Biochemistry32, 9577–9585.

Molday, R. S. (2007). Focus on molecules: Retinoschisin (RS1). Exp Eye Res84, 227–228.

Reid, S. N., Akhmedov, N. B., Piriev, N. I., Kozak, C. A., Danciger, M., and Farber, D. B. (1999). The mouse X-linked juvenile retinoschisis cDNA: expression in photoreceptors. Gene227, 257–266.

Reid, S. N., and Farber, D. B. (2005). Glial transcytosis of a photoreceptor-secreted signaling protein, retinoschisin. Glia49, 397–406.

Sauer, C. G., Gehrig, A., Warneke-Wittstock, R., Marquardt, A., Ewing, C. C., Gibson, A., Lorenz, B., Jurklies, B., and Weber, B. H. (1997). Positional cloning of the gene associated with X-linked juvenile retinoschisis. Nat Genet17, 164–170.

Schagger, H., and von Jagow, G. (1991). Blue native electrophoresis for isolation of membrane protein complexes in enzymatically active form. Anal Biochem199, 223–231.

Sikkink, S. K., Biswas, S., Parry, N. R., Stanga, P. E., and Trump, D. (2006). X-Linked Retinoschisis: An Update. J Med Genet44, 225–232.

Steiner-Champliaud, M. F., Sahel, J., and Hicks, D. (2006). Retinoschisin forms a multi-molecular complex with extracellular matrix and cytoplasmic proteins: interactions with beta2 laminin and alphaB-crystallin. Mol Vis12, 892–901.

Takada, Y., Fariss, R. N., Møller, M., Bush, R. A., Rushing, E. J., Sieving, P. A., and Bush, R. A. (2006). Retinoschisin expression and localization in rodent and human pineal and consequences of mouse RS1 gene knockout. Mol Vis12, 1108–1116.

Takada, Y., Fariss, R. N., Tanikawa, A., Zeng, Y., Carper, D., Bush, R., and Sieving, P. A. (2004). A retinal neuronal developmental wave of retinoschisin expression begins in ganglion cells during layer formation. Invest Ophthalmol Vis Sci45, 3302–3312.

Valencia, A., Pestana, A., and Cano, A. (1989). Spectroscopical studies on the structural organization of the lectin discoidin I: analysis of sugar- and calcium-binding activities. Biochim Biophys Acta990, 93–97.

Vijayasarathy, C., Gawinowicz, M. A., Zeng, Y., Takada, Y., Bush, R. A., and Sieving, P. A. (2006). Identification and characterization of two mature isoforms of retinoschisin in murine retina. Biochem Biophys Res Commun349, 99–105.

Vijayasarathy, C., Takada, Y., Zeng, Y., Bush, R. A., and Sieving, P. A. (2007). Retinoschisin is a peripheral membrane protein with affinity for anionic phospholipids and affected by divalent cations. Invest Ophthalmol Vis Sci48, 991–1000.

Vogel, W. F., Abdulhussein, R., and Ford, C. E. (2006). Sensing extracellular matrix: An update on discoidin domain receptor function. Cell Signal18, 1108–1116.

Wang, T., Zhou, A., Waters, C. T., O'Connor, E., Read, R. J., and Trump, D. (2006). Molecular pathology of X linked retinoschisis: mutations interfere with retinoschisin secretion and oligomerisation. Br J Ophthalmol90, 81–86.

Weber, B. H., Schrewe, H., Molday, L. L., Gehrig, A., White, K. L., Seeliger, M. W., Jaissle, G. B., Friedburg, C., Tamm, E., and Molday, R. S. (2002). Inactivation of the murine X-linked juvenile retinoschisis gene, Rs1h, suggests a role of retinoschisin in retinal cell layer organization and synaptic structure. Proc Natl Acad Sci U S A99, 6222–6227.

Zeng, Y., Takada, Y., Kjellstrom, S., Hiriyanna, K., Tanikawa, A., Wawrousek, E., Smaoui, N., Caruso, R., Bush, R. A., and Sieving, P. A. (2004). RS-1 Gene delivery to an adult Rs1h knockout mouse model restores ERG b-wave with reversal of the electronegative waveform of X-linked retinoschisis. Invest Ophthalmol Vis Sci45, 3279–3285.

Part VII
Basic Science Underlying Retinal Degeneration

Proteomics Profiling of the Cone Photoreceptor Cell Line, 661W

Muayyad R. Al-Ubaidi, Hiroyuki Matsumoto, Sadamu Kurono, and Anil Singh

1 Introduction

Cultured retinal cells are convenient experimental systems offering great advantages in the assessment of numerous retinal processes. The two most important advantages are the ease of evaluation of an isolated cellular function without the effects of other retinal cell types and an avoidance of use of the more costly animal research. The Two obvious disadvantages are the loss of the architecture of the native tissue, and lack of functional influence of other retinal cell types. However, for most of the research applications, the advantages of use of in vitro systems offset the potential limitations.

Retinal cell culture can be used to determine effectiveness of promoter fragments from retina-specific genes, the functional role of domains on a retinal protein and how mutations would effect that function and to express retinal proteins for biochemical analyses. Last but not least, retinal cell culture can be used to determine the toxicity of pharmacologic agents, and for studies of cell death and differentiation.

Except for Müller cells, all other retinal cells are terminally differentiated, specialized neuronal cells with a limited, if any, capacity for cell division. However, immortalized cell lines currently exist for several retinal cell types including Müller cells (Roque et al., 1997). A cell line expressing retina-specific genes, including the photoreceptor proteins IRBP and cone transducin, has also been isolated from a mouse ocular tumor (Bernstin, Kutty, Wiggert, Albert, & Nickerson, 1994). Furthermore, Y-79 (Reid et al., 1974) and WERI-Rb (McFall, Sery, & Makadon, 1977) are immortalized cell lines derived from human retinoblastoma tumors. It was initially believed that the Y-79 cells had originated from a cone cell lineage (Bogenmann, Lochrie, & Simon, 1988), but later these cells were shown to express rod opsin, rod transducin, rod phosphodiesterase, and recoverin (Di Polo & Farber, 1995;

M.R. Al-Ubaidi
Department of Cell Biology, University of Oklahoma Health Sciences Center, 940 Stanton L. Young Blvd. (BMSB781), Oklahoma City, OK 73104, USA; IBERICA Holdings Co., Ltd, Kurume University Translational Research Center, Kurume, Fukuoka 830-0011, Japan, Tel: 405-271-2382, Fax: 405-271-3548
e-mail: muayyad-Al-ubaidi@ouhsc.edu

Wiechmann, 1996). Finally, primary retinal cultures, created from several mammalian donor retinas (Kelley, Turner, & Reh, 1995; Gaudin, Forster, Sahel, Dreyfus, & Hicks, 1996), were employed in vision research. These types of cell lines, besides being monotonous in preparation, are not sufficient for some types of experimentation due to their heterogeneity, and special conditions for their growth. Thus, there is a need for additional retinal cell models, which are homogeneous, passage able, and easily grown as a monolayer using standard tissue culture techniques. Rods are easier to study in primary cultures since they make about 60% of the total population of retinal cell. However, studying cones is most difficult, especially in primary cultures from murine retinas, since cones constitute no more than 1.8–3% of the total population of retinal cells. A cone photoreceptor cell line (661 W) has been immortalized by the expression of SV40-T antigen under control of the human IRBP promoter (Al-Ubaidi et al., 1992). Cellular, and molecular analyses have demonstrated that 661 W cells express cone but not rod photoreceptors markers (Tan et al., 2004) and respond to light stimulation and undergo cell death when stressed by bright light (Kanan, Moiseyev, Agarwal, Ma, & Al Ubaidi, 2007).

2 Materials and Methods

2.1 Immortalization of the Mouse Photoreceptor Cells

The 661 W cell line was established from retinal tumors arising in transgenic mice expressing the viral oncoprotein simian virus 40 (SV40) large tumor antigen (Tag) under control of a 1.3 kb fragment of the human IRBP promoter (Al-Ubaidi et al., 1992). Expression of T-antigen under the IRBP promoter resulted in bilateral retinal tumors. Multiple sub-cell lines were generated from one of the transgenic founders ($F_0 661$) with each receiving an alphabetical designation.

2.2 Culture Conditions and Morphology of 661 W Cells

The 661 W cell line was maintained in Dulbecco's modified Eagle's medium containing 10% fetal bovine serum, 300 mg/L glutamine, 32 mg/L Putrescine, 40 μL of β-mercaptoethanol, and 40 μg of each of cytidine-5'-diphosphoethanolamine, cytidine-5'-diphosphocholine, hydrocortisone 21-hemisuccinate and progesterone. The media also contained penicillin (90 units/ml) and streptomycin (0.09 mg/ml). Cells were grown at 37 °C in a humidified atmosphere of 5% CO_2 and 95% air.

2.3 Two-dimensional (2-DE) Gel Electrophoresis

The cell pellets or C57/BL6 mouse retinas were homogenized with an isoelectric focusing lysis solution and processed according to Matsumoto and Komori

(Matsumoto & Komori, 2000). In this homogenization the lysis buffer was diluted approximately two-thirds. The total proteins of ca 500 micrograms were loaded on each gel. The 2-DE gels were stained by Coomassie blue.

2.4 Peptide Mass Fingerprinting (PMF)

In-gel digestion of 2-DE gel spots were performed as described before (Matsumoto & Komori, 2000). The tryptic peptides dissolved in 0.2% TFA were mixed with a matrix solution (CHCA 10 mg/mL in 50% $CH_3CN/0.1\%$ TFA). Mass spectra were obtained using an MALDI-TOF Mass Spectrometer (Voyager Elite, Applied BioSystems, Foster City, CA). The spectra were analyzed in the positive-ion mode, and the mass peaks were assigned by PerSeptive GRAMS/386 v3.02. PMF search was performed by MASCOT (http://www.matrixscience.com) using NCBInr database 20061125. The search parameters for PMF were: animal species, *Rodentia* (Rodents); enzyme specificity, trypsin (maximum missed cleavage = 1); modification, propionamide (cysteine), N-acetyl (protein), oxidation (methionine), and pyro-glutamate (N-terminal glutamate and glutamine); mass tolerance, 0.5 Da. Protein identification was based on the probability-based MOWSE score to exceed 65 ($p<0.05$). In this scoring system the "protein score" is defined by $-10^*Log(P)$ where P is the probability that the observed match is a random event. Protein scores greater than 65, i.e., $p<0.05$, are considered significant. Such PMF criteria on protein spots isolated on 2-DE gels fulfills the requirement suggested by the Draft Guidelines for Proteomic Data Publication (Matsumoto, Kahn, & Komori, 1999; Carr et al., 2004).

3 Results

Comparison of the two 2DE gels presented in Fig. 1 to each other revealed the presence of at least 37 prominent protein spots that were either only observed in extracts of 661W cells or were highly enriched. The identities of these proteins are presented in Table 1.

3.1 Proteins that Have Not been Described in the Retina Before

Seventeen of the identified spots represent proteins that have not been studied in the retina before. Some of these proteins are quite interesting either due to their cellular localization, functional significance or role in differentiation and disease. Lamin B1, which is a nuclear structural protein that has been previously shown to be involved in apoptosis, upon gene duplication leads to autosomal dominant leukodystrophy (Padiath et al., 2006). The heat shock cognate protein is expressed on the surface of human embryonic stem cells and is involved in differentiation (Son et al., 2005).

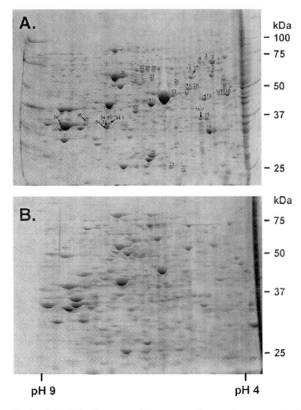

Fig. 1 2-D gel analysis of 661W cell extracts (A) compared to total mouse retinal extracts (B) 2-D gels were stained with Commassie Blue and scanned. The pH of the first dimension is shown at the bottom of (B) and the approximate molecular weights are shown on the right of each 2-D gel

Three heterogeneous nuclear ribonucleoproteins (hnRNP) were detected. Those are hnRNP-F, -H1 and -L. Significance of the rat hnRNP-F comes from it association with TATA-binding protein (Yoshida, Makino, & Tamura, 1999) and the hnRNP-H1, a protein involved in mRNA processing was induced by hypoxia, an event most likely mediated by hypoxia-inducible factor 1 (HIF-1) (Greijer et al., 2005). hnRNP-L was found to interact with the 3' border of the internal ribosomal entry site of hepatitis C virus (Hahm, Kim, Y. K., Kim, J. H., Kim, T. Y., & Jang, 1998) and its interaction with the 3'untranslated region of the murine inducible nitric-oxide synthase mRNA was found to be modulated with inflammation (Soderberg, Raffalli-Mathieu, & Lang, 2002). The Non-neuronal alpha enolase has been described only once in the retina but well studied in the brain whereby its levels were found increased in rats treated with methylazoxymethanol, the antimitotic agent (Nagayoshi et al., 1986).

Another protein that has not been studied in the retina is T-complex protein 1-alpha, which among other proteins, was altered in mesial temporal lobe epilepsy (Yang, Czech, Felizardo, Baumgartner, & Lubec, 2006). Yet another protein that is significant but has not been studied in the retina is dihydropyrimidinase-related

Table 1 List of identified protein spots from gels presented in Fig. 1. MW, theoretical molecular weight; pI, theoretical isoelectric point; MS, probability based MASCOT MOWSE score in PMF; Cov., the coverage of tryptic fragments in PMF; Matched, the matched number of tryptic fragments over the observed number of peaks; gi. #, gene identification number. Retina, denotes whether or not the identified protein has been described in the retina before.

Spot #	Protein Name/Description	MW	pI	MS(Score)	Cov.	Matched	gi. #	Retina
1	Lamin B 1	67029	5.11	219	41%	28/30	17865719	N
2	Heat shock cognate 71kDa protein (Heat Shock 70 kDa protein 8)	71045	5.24	255	52%	30/40	123647	N
3	Heat shock protein 9A	73838	5.91	161	31%	18/22	6754256	N
4	Serum albumin precursor	67518	5.75	222	35%	20/22	5915682	Y
5	Heterogeneous nuclear ribonucleoprotein K	48764	5.39	84	31%	14/35	13384620	Y
6	Heterogeneous nuclear ribonucleoprotein K	48764	5.39	110	38%	17/36	13384620	
7	**Mixture**							
	Heat shock protein 1 (chaperonin)	61131	5.67	124	60%	29/79	31981679	Y
	Alpha-internexin	55922	5.23	77	43%	19/79	94730353	Y
8	Vimentin	51604	4.96	277	63%	33/42	2078001	Y
9	ATP synthase, H+ transporting mitochondrial F1 complex, beta subunit	56265	5.19	132	43%	24/44	31980648	Y
10	Enolase 2, gamma neuronal	47693	4.99	193	51%	22/28	7305027	Y
11	Heterogeneous nuclear ribonucleoprotein F	46127	5.31	119	36%	15/31	19527048	N
12	Heterogeneous nuclear ribonucleoprotein F	46127	5.31	167	49%	23/41	19527048	N
13	Creatine kinase, brain	43041	5.4	129	47%	17/35	10946574	Y
14	Creatine kinase, brain	43041	5.4	148	55%	21/51	10946574	Y
15-1	Enolase 1, alpha non-neuron	47521	6.37	130	40%	18/33	12963491	N
15-2	Enolase 1, alpha non-neuron	47521	6.37	90	35%	16/36	12963491	N
16	Guanine nuleotide-binding protein, beta-1 subunit	38348	5.6	103	46%	18/56	6680045	Y
17	Chaperonin subunit 5 (epsilon)	60154	5.72	196	43%	29/39	6671702	N
18	Inosine-5'-monophosphate dehydrogenase 1	55686	6.29	80	27%	14/34	1708472	Y
19	Heterogeneous nuclear ribonucleoprotein H2	49603	5.89	79	28%	14/35	9845253	N
20	Heterogeneous nuclear ribonucleoprotein H1	49524	5.89	80	29%	16/45	10946928	N
21	Enolase 1, alpha non-neuron	47521	6.37	141	47%	23/60	12963491	Y
22	Guanylate Kinase 1	22046	6.12	92	46%	12--36	6680137	Y
23	Peroxiredoxin 6	24953	5.98	184	78%	20/41	6671549	Y
24	T-complex protein 1 subunit beta (TCP-1-beta)	57867	5.97	114	43%	19/50	22654291	N
25	Heterogeneous nuclear ribonucleoprotein L	60867	6.65	86	36%	24/71	33667042	N
26	Heterogeneous nuclear ribonucleoprotein L	60867	6.65	152	43%	21/40	33667042	N
27	**Mixture**							
	Dihydropyrimidinase-related protein 4	62633	6.51	148	50%	22/44	34328211	N
	Heterogeneous nuclear ribonucleoprotein L	60867	6.85	65	29%	13/44	33667042	N
28	Dihydrolipoamide dehydrogenase	54878	7.99	89	28%	13/29	31982856	N
29	Pyruvate Kinase 3	58518	7.18	266	62%	33/43	31981562	Y
30	Enolase 1, alpha non-neuron	47521	6.37	173	43%	23/32	12963491	Y
31	Glutamate-ammonia ligase	43014	6.64	122	41%	16/29	483918	Y
32	Aldolase 3, C isoform	39867	6.67	146	63%	17/34	60687506	N
33	Carbonic anhydrase	29216	6.52	145	67%	17/37	31981657	Y
34-1	glyceraldehyde-3-phosphate dehydrogenase	36142	8.44	84	40%	14/44	6679937	Y
34-2	Heterogeneous nuclear ribonucleoprotein A2/B1	32511	8.74	139	59%	24/57	32880197	Y
34-3	Heterogeneous nuclear ribonucleoprotein A2/B1	32511	8.74	174	59%	24/47	32880197	Y
35	Crystallin, Zeta	35602	8.18	141	50%	17/34	33859530	Y
36	Similar to glyceraldehyde-3-phosphate dehydrogenase	36142	8.44	140	50%	20/43	6679937	Y
37	Voltage - dependent anion channel 1	30879	8.62	147	67%	15/36	6755963	Y

protein-4 (DRP-4). A proteomic approach was used to link motor function to cerebellar protein expression in $129 \times 1/\text{SvJ}$, C57BL/6J and nNOS WT mice. Poor performance on the Rota rod, the standard test for motor coordination, was detected in $129 \times 1/\text{SvJ}$ mice. Identification and quantification of 48 proteins revealed increased expression of dihydropyrimidinase-related protein-4 (DRP-4) (Pollak et al., 2005). Furthermore, evaluation of DRP-4 in Downs syndrome brains revealed its significantly increased levels (Weitzdoerfer, Fountoulakis, & Lubec, 2001). Association of identified proteins spots with brain dysfunction is not limited to DRP-4. A novel mutation in the dihydrolipoamide dehydrogenase E3 subunit gene (DLD) resulted in an atypical form of alpha-ketoglutarate dehydrogenase deficiency

(Odievre et al., 2005) and DLD's deficiency has been associated with Alzheimer's disease in an Ashkenazi Jewish population (Brown et al., 2004).

3.2 Proteins that have been Studied in the Retina Before

Of the 37 spots of proteins selected for analysis, 20 have been shown to be present in the retina before. However, it is not clear at present whether that reflects their presence in cones only or in cones and any other retinal cell type.

Of the proteins that have been described in the retina, hnRNP-K, an RNA/DNA-binding protein that acts in several cellular compartments. It has been shown that insulin activates the import of hnRNP-K protein into the mitochondria and its over-expression modulates insulin-activated mitochondrial gene expression suggesting that hnRNP-K protein may be a mediator of mitochondrial response to insulin (Dzwonek, Mikula, & Ostrowski, 2006). Although yet to be shown, this may have implications in diabetic retinopathy.

Of the structural proteins that have been identified in the retina and were among the enriched spots in 661W extracts are neuronal intermediate filament, alpha-internexin and vimentin. Alpha-internexin is transiently expressed in amacrine cells in the developing mouse retina (Chien & Liem, 1995), but not in cones, while vimentin has been found to coexist with neuronfilaments in the axonless horizontal cell of the mouse retina (Drager, 1983). Developmentally, vimentin is present in all retinal cells between embryonic days 4 and 8 and by E10 it was restricted to Müller cells (Lemmon & Rieser, 1983).

A protein that was observed in multiple spots on the 2DE gel is neuron specific enolase (NSE). NSE immunoreactivity has been described in retinas of many species and was found in the large ganglion, amacrine cells and horizontal cells of the retina. Furthermore, photoreceptors were found to be labeled in the rat and human retina and only one cone type in the rabbit (Wilhelm, Straznicky, & Gabriel, 1992).

The ubiquitous mitochondrial creatine kinase (CK) is expressed in cells and tissues with high energy demands such as the brain and the retina. However, in mouse knockout studies, no phenotype was associated with absence of CK (Steeghs, Oerlemans, & Wieringa, 1995). This may be the result of high degree of redundancy either on the protein or the pathway levels. Pyruvate kinase and glyceraldehyde-3-phosphate dehydrogenase (G3PD) are two of the glycolytic enzymes that are present in the outer segments of rod and cone photoreceptor cells (Hsu & Molday, 1991). Interestingly, studies performed on retinas of early onset macular degeneration in cynomolgus monkeys detected increased albumin and decreased G3PD concentrations (Nicolas et al., 1996). Immunofluorescence microscopy and biochemical activity assays of bovine and chicken retina sections demonstrated the presence of G3PD enzyme in rod and cone outer segments (Hsu & Molday, 1991). However, no specific role for G3PD in retinal diseases has been described.

A guanine nucleotide-binding protein, beta-1 subunit has been cloned from human and bovine retinas which shows that a family of beta-subunit polypeptides exists in the retina (Levine, Smallwood, Moen, Helman, & Ahn, 1990). Guanylate kinase was found at high levels in all photoreceptor cellular compartments except the outer segments (Berger et al., 1980). However, for either protein, there are no descriptions of mutations in these genes.

Inosine 5'-monophosphate dehydrogenase type I (IMPDH1) catalyses the rate-limiting step in guanine nucleotide biosynthesis and also binds single-stranded nucleic acids. Two mutations, R224P and D226N, in IMPDH1 that disrupt nucleic acid binding have been found to cause autosomal dominant retinitis pigmentosa (Mortimer & Hedstrom, 2005).

Peroxiredoxin 6, a member of glutathione antioxidant cycle, is developmentally regulated in the retina whereby its levels are transiently elevated around time of eye opening in the neonatal rat and gradually decline to adult levels shortly thereafter (Fujii, Ikeda, Yamashita, & Fujii, 2003).

Glutamate-ammonia ligase (glutamine synthetase) is involved in glutamate metabolism, hence it is not surprising that it was demonstrated in the embryonic neural retina in Müller fibers and its expression is dependent on cell-cell interactions (Linser & Moscona, 1979).

An interesting enzyme that has received special attention in the treatment of retinitis pigmentosa is carbonic anhydrase (CA). CA activity has been observed in pigment epithelial cells in the optic cup of early mouse embryos. Later in the prenatal period the enzyme appears in Müller cells perikarya. During postnatal development, CA activity appears in the radial processes of the Muller cells, followed by increased activity in the plexiform layers. CA localization in pigment epithelial and Müller cells attains the adult pattern at about 16 postnatally (Bhattacharjee, 1976).

Current dogma suggests that oxidative stress can directly affect critical cellular components leading to lipid peroxidation which in turn and through the formation of 4-hydroxynonenal (4-HNE) can lead to the oxidation of other cellular targets. It was found that heterogeneous nuclear ribonucleoprotein A2/B1, albumin, glutamine synthetase and voltage-dependent anion channel are among those oxidized targets (Tanito et al., 2006). The observation made by the authors is that 4-HNE modifications of retinal proteins are specific to a particular set of proteins rather than random events on abundant proteins (Tanito et al., 2006).

A comprehensive analysis of the expression of crystallins in mouse retina demonstrated for the first time that mouse retinal cells express transcripts for 20 different members of the crystallin gene family. Among those is zeta-crystallin (Tanito et al., 2006). The significance of expression of these different crystallins in any retinal cell is yet to be realized.

4 Discussion

We have partially mapped the proteomic trajectory of the cone photoreceptor cell line 661W by establishing the identity of 37 proteins. These proteins were selected either due to their apparent absence on total retinal extract 2DE gels or because they were present on 661 W 2DE gels at much higher amounts. We have divided those proteins into two groups depending upon whether or not these proteins have been observed before in the retina. However, we do recognized that due to extraction protocols, some membrane and organelle proteins may have not be extracted and consequently are not presented in the selected protein spots.

One observation that is clearly obvious is some proteins identified were previously observed in retinal cells other than cone photoreceptors. This can be due to either epitope masking in cone cells due to association with other proteins or due to the presence of these proteins at much smaller amounts. Alternatively, one can argue that the 661 W cells represent a mixture of cells including amacrine and Müller cells. However, data previously published argue against the assumption of a heterogeneous cell line (Tanito et al., 2006).

Among the 37 proteins with determined trajectories, 7 protein groups showed heterogeneity by being displayed at more than one location on the 2-DE gels. Most of these heterogeneities are due to a difference in pI with a small or no difference in molecular weight (MW). This could be due to some differences in the post-translational modifications such as glycosylation or phosphorylation. One exception is the non-neuronal enolase 1, alpha which was displayed on 2-DE gels as four different spots (see spots 15-1, 15-2, 21 and 30, Fig. 1), with differences in both pI and MW. However, we identified the parent protein as one of two spots exhibiting MW of ~48 kDa and pI around 6 consistent with theoretical prediction (Haniu et al., 2006). In contrast, the proteins identified in this work have substantially smaller MWs, likely due to truncation of the parent protein.

Some of the proteins we identified have been shown to be specific targets for oxidation during light stress. The fact that these proteins are cone-specific makes the study of these proteins in age related macular degeneration (AMD) important, especially in light of the fact that light has been established as a factor in AMD (Seddon & Chen, 2004).

Acknowledgments This research was partially supported by grants from the NEI/NIH (EY14052 and EY13877), a COBRE grant (RR017703) from the NCRR/NIH, a NEI/NIH Vision Core Grant (EY012190) to the Department of Ophthalmology, Knights Templar Eye Foundation, Inc. We would like to thank Drs. Naoka Komori and Nobuaki Takemori for their contribution to the discussion.

References

Al-Ubaidi, M. R., Font, R. L., Quiambao, A. B., Keener, M. J., Liou, G. I., Overbeek, P. A., & Baehr, W. (1992). Bilateral retinal and brain tumors in transgenic mice expressing simian virus 40 large T antigen under control of the human interphotoreceptor retinoid-binding protein promoter. *J. Cell Biol., 119,* 1681–1687.

Berger, S. J., DeVries, G. W., Carter, J. G., Schulz, D. W., Passonneau, P. N., Lowry, O. H. et al., (1980). The distribution of the components of the cyclic GMP cycle in retina. *J Biol Chem, 255,* 3128–3133.

Bernstin, S. L., Kutty, G., Wiggert, B., Albert, D. M., & Nickerson, J. M. (1994). Expression of retina-specific genes by mouse retinoblastoma cells. *Invest. Ophthalmol. Vis. Sci., 35,* 3931–3937.

Bhattacharjee, J. (1976). Developmental changes of carbonic anhydrase in the retina of the mouse: a histochemical study. *Histochem. J., 8,* 63–70.

Bogenmann, E., Lochrie, M. A., & Simon, M. I. (1988). Cone cell-specific genes expressed in retinoblastoma. *Science, 240,* 76–78.

Brown, A. M., Gordon, D., Lee, H., Caudy, M., Hardy, J., Haroutunian, V. et al., (2004). Association of the dihydrolipoamide dehydrogenase gene with Alzheimer's disease in an Ashkenazi Jewish population. *Am. J. Med. Genet. B Neuropsychiatr. Genet., 131,* 60–66.

Carr, S., Aebersold, R., Baldwin, M., Burlingame, A., Clauser, K., & Nesvizhskii, A. (2004). The need for guidelines in publication of peptide and protein identification data: working group on publication guidelines for peptide and protein identification data. *Mol. Cell Proteomics., 3,* 531–533.

Chien, C. L. & Liem, R. K. (1995). The neuronal intermediate filament, alpha-internexin is transiently expressed in amacrine cells in the developing mouse retina. *Exp. Eye Res., 61,* 749–756.

Di Polo, A. & Farber, D. B. (1995). Rod photoreceptor-specific gene expression in human retinoblastoma cells. *Proc. Natl. Acad. Sci. U.S.A, 92,* 4016–4020.

Drager, U. C. (1983). Coexistence of neurofilaments and vimentin in a neurone of adult mouse retina. *Nature, 303,* 169–172.

Dzwonek, A., Mikula, M., & Ostrowski, J. (2006). The diverse involvement of heterogeneous nuclear ribonucleoprotein K in mitochondrial response to insulin. *FEBS Letters, 580,* 1839–1845.

Fujii, T., Ikeda, Y., Yamashita, H., & Fujii, J. (2003). Transient elevation of glutathione peroxidase 1 around the time of eyelid opening in the neonatal rat. *J. Ocul. Pharmacol. Ther., 19,* 361–369.

Gaudin, C., Forster, V., Sahel, J., Dreyfus, H., & Hicks, D. (1996). Survival and regeneration of adult human and other mammalian photoreceptors in culture. *Invest Ophthalmol. Vis. Sci., 37,* 2258–2268.

Greijer, A. E., van der, G. P., Kemming, D., Shvarts, A., Semenza, G. L., Meijer, G. A. et.al., (2005). Up-regulation of gene expression by hypoxia is mediated predominantly by hypoxia-inducible factor 1 (HIF-1). *J. Pathol., 206,* 291–304.

Hahm, B., Kim, Y. K., Kim, J. H., Kim, T. Y., & Jang, S. K. (1998). Heterogeneous nuclear ribonucleoprotein L interacts with the 3' border of the internal ribosomal entry site of hepatitis C virus. *J Virology, 72,* 8782–8788.

Haniu, H., Komori, N., Takemori, N., Singh, A., Ash, J. D., & Matsumoto, H. (2006). Proteomic trajectory mapping of biological transformation: Application to developmental mouse retina. *Proteomics., 6,* 3251–3261.

Hsu, S. C. & Molday, R. S. (1991). Glycolytic enzymes and a GLUT-1 glucose transporter in the outer segments of rod and cone photoreceptor cells. *J. Bio. Chem., 266,* 21745–21752.

Kanan, Y., Moiseyev, G., Agarwal, N., Ma, J. X., & Al Ubaidi, M. R. (2007). Light induces programmed cell death by activating multiple independent proteases in a cone photoreceptor cell line. *Invest Ophthalmol. Vis. Sci., 48,* 40–51.

Kelley, M. W., Turner, J. K., & Reh, T. A. (1995). Regulation of proliferation and photoreceptor differentiation in fetal human retinal cell cultures. *Invest Ophthalmol. Vis. Sci., 36,* 1280–1289.

Lemmon, V. & Rieser, G. (1983). The development distribution of vimentin in the chick retina. *Brain Res., 313,* 191–197.

Levine, M. A., Smallwood, P. M., Moen, P. T., Jr., Helman, L. J., & Ahn, T. G. (1990). Molecular cloning of beta 3 subunit, a third form of the G protein beta-subunit polypeptide. *Proc. Natl. Acad. Sci. U.S.A, 87,* 2329–2333.

Linser, P. & Moscona, A. A. (1979). Induction of glutamine synthetase in embryonic neural retina: localization in Muller fibers and dependence on cell interactions. *Proc. Natl. Acad. Sci. U.S.A,* 76, 6476–6480.

Matsumoto, H., Kahn, E. S., & Komori, N. (1999). The emerging role of mass spectrometry in molecular biosciences: studies of protein phosphorylation in fly eyes as an example. *Novartis. Found. Symp., 224,* 225–244.

Matsumoto, H. & Komori, N. (2000). Ocular proteomics: cataloging photoreceptor proteins by two-dimensional gel electrophoresis and mass spectrometry. *Methods Enzymol., 316,* 492–511.

McFall, R. C., Sery, T. W., & Makadon, M. (1977). Characterization of a new continuous cell line derived from a human retinoblastoma. *Cancer Res., 37,* 1003–1010.

Mortimer, S. E. & Hedstrom, L. (2005). Autosomal dominant retinitis pigmentosa mutations in inosine 5'-monophosphate dehydrogenase type I disrupt nucleic acid binding. *Biochem. J., 390,* 41–47.

Nagayoshi, M., Hirata, Y., Tamaru, M., Sugimoto, S., Shimizu, J., Hirabayashi, K. et al., (1986). A neurochemical study of rat brain maldevelopment induced by MAM treatment at different stages of gestation. *Nippon Seirigaku Zasshi, 48,* 14–25.

Nicolas, M. G., Fujiki, K., Murayama, K., Suzuki, M. T., Mineki, R., Hayakawa, M. et al., (1996). Studies on the mechanism of early onset macular degeneration in cynomolgus (Macaca fascicularis) monkeys. I. Abnormal concentrations of two proteins in the retina. *Exp. Eye Res., 62,* 211–219.

Odievre, M. H., Chretien, D., Munnich, A., Robinson, B. H., Dumoulin, R., Masmoudi, S. et al., (2005). A novel mutation in the dihydrolipoamide dehydrogenase E3 subunit gene (DLD) resulting in an atypical form of alpha-ketoglutarate dehydrogenase deficiency. *Hum. Mutat., 25,* 323–324.

Padiath, Q. S., Saigoh, K., Schiffmann, R., Asahara, H., Yamada, T., Koeppen, A. et al., (2006). Lamin B1 duplications cause autosomal dominant leukodystrophy. *Nat. Genet., 38,* 1114–1123.

Pollak, D., Weitzdoerfer, R., Yang, Y. W., Prast, H., Hoeger, H., & Lubec, G. (2005). Cerebellar protein expression in three different mouse strains and their relevance for motor performance. *Neurochem. Int., 46,* 19–29.

Reid, T. W., Albert, D. M., Rabson, A. S., Russell, P., Craft, J., Chu, E. W. et al., (1974). Characteristics of an established cell line of retinoblastoma. *J. Natl. Cancer Inst., 53,* 347–360.

Roque, R. S., Agarwal, N., Wordinger, R. J., Brun, A. M., Xue, Y., Huang, L. C. et al., (1997). Human papillomavirus-16 E6/E7 transfected retinal cell line expresses the Muller cell phenotype. *Expe. Eye Res., 64,* 519–527.

Seddon, J. M. & Chen, C. A. (2004). The epidemiology of age-related macular degeneration. *Int. Ophthalmol. Clin., 44,* 17–39.

Soderberg, M., Raffalli-Mathieu, F., & Lang, M. A. (2002). Inflammation modulates the interaction of heterogeneous nuclear ribonucleoprotein (hnRNP) I/polypyrimidine tract binding protein and hnRNP L with the 3'untranslated region of the murine inducible nitric-oxide synthase mRNA. *Mol. Pharmacol., 62,* 423–431.

Son, Y. S., Park, J. H., Kang, Y. K., Park, J. S., Choi, H. S., Lim, J. Y. et al., (2005). Heat shock 70-kDa protein 8 isoform 1 is expressed on the surface of human embryonic stem cells and downregulated upon differentiation. *Stem Cells, 23,* 1502–1513.

Steeghs, K., Oerlemans, F., & Wieringa, B. (1995). Mice deficient in ubiquitous mitochondrial creatine kinase are viable and fertile. *Biochimica et Biophysica Acta, 1230,* 130–138.

Tan, E., Ding, X. Q., Saadi, A., Agarwal, N., Naash, M. I., & Al-Ubaidi, M. R. (2004). Expression of cone-photoreceptor-specific antigens in a cell line derived from retinal tumors in transgenic mice. *Invest Ophthalmol. Vis. Sci., 45,* 764–768.

Tanito, M., Haniu, H., Elliott, M. H., Singh, A. K., Matsumoto, H., & Anderson, R. E. (2006). Identification of 4-hydroxynonenal-modified retinal proteins induced by photooxidative stress prior to retinal degeneration. *Free Radic. Biol. Med., 41,* 1847–1859.

Weitzdoerfer, R., Fountoulakis, M., & Lubec, G. (2001). Aberrant expression of dihydropyrimidinase related proteins-2,-3 and -4 in fetal Down syndrome brain. *J. Neural Transm. Suppl., 61,* 95–107.

Wiechmann, A. F. (1996). Recoverin in cultured human retinoblastoma cells: enhanced expression during morphological differentiation. *J. Neurochem., 67,* 105–110.

Wilhelm, M., Straznicky, C., & Gabriel, R. (1992). Neuron-specific enolase-like immunoreactivity in the vertebrate retina: selective labelling of Muller cells in Anura. *Histochemistry, 98,* 243–252.

Yang, J. W., Czech, T., Felizardo, M., Baumgartner, C., & Lubec, G. (2006). Aberrant expression of cytoskeleton proteins in hippocampus from patients with mesial temporal lobe epilepsy. *Amino. Acids, 30,* 477–493.

Yoshida, T., Makino, Y., & Tamura, T. (1999). Association of the rat heterogeneous nuclear RNA-ribonucleoprotein F with TATA-binding protein. *FEBS Lett., 457,* 251–254.

γ-Secretase Regulates VEGFR-1 Signalling in Vascular Endothelium and RPE

Michael E. Boulton, Jun Cai, Maria B. Grant, and Yadan Zhang

1 Introduction

Neovascular diseases of the eye include retinopathy of prematurity (ROP), proliferative diabetic retinopathy (PDR), and the exudative or "wet" form of age-related macular degeneration (AMD). Together these diseases affect all age groups and are the
leading causes of vision impairment in developed nations (Lee et al., 1998). The col-
lective evidence suggests that the vascular endothelial growth factor (VEGF) family
is critical for ocular angiogensis (Cai and Boulton, 2002; Grant et al., 2004). First,
increasing VEGF in animal models promotes ocular neovascularization and this can
be reversed by neutralizing VEGF or its receptors(vanWijngaarden et al., 2005;
Witmer et al., 2003). Second, VEGF is hypoxia-inducible and thus dramatically
upregulated by the hypoxic environment in ROP and PDR (Grant et al., 2004;
Witmer et al., 2003). Third, treatment of AMD patients with CNV with VEGF
inhibitors such as Macugen or Lucentis significantly reduces choroidal neovascularization (vanWijngaarden et al., 2005).

2 VEGF Ligands and Receptors

The VEGF family consists of VEGF-A, -B, -C, -D, -E and placental growth factor
(PlGF) which can exist in a number of different isoforms with varying potency and
specificity dependent on the local environmental cues and the vascular cell type
involved (Ferrara, 2005). VEGF receptors, VEGFR-1 (Flt-1), VEGFR-2 (KDR,
Flk1), and VEGFR-3, only bind certain isoforms of VEGF. The ligand-binding
region in the extracellular domain is localized within the second and third Ig
domains in both VEGFR1 and VEGFR-2 (Shibuya and Claesson-Welsh, 2006).
Ligands for VEGFR-1 include VEGF-A, -B, and PlGF; ligands for VEGFR-2

M. E. Boulton
Ophthalmology and Visual Sciences, University of Texas Medical Branch, Galveston, Texas
77550, Tel: 409-747-5410, Fax: 409-747-5402
e-mail: boultonm@utmb.edu

R.E. Anderson et al. (eds.), *Recent Advances in Retinal Degeneration*,
© Springer 2008

include VEGF-A, -C, -D, and -E, while ligands for VEGFR-3 are VEGF-C and -D (Shibuya and Claesson-Welsh, 2006). Thus, PlGF uniquely binds VEGFR-1, and VEGF-E uniquely binds VEGFR-2. Overall, there is greater than 40% sequence homology between VEGFR-1 and VEGFR-2. An interesting difference between VEGFR-1 and VEGFR-2 is that VEGF-A binds to VEGFR-1 with very high affinity ($K_d \approx 10^{-12}$), about an order of magnitude higher than its affinity to VEGFR-2 (Rahimi, 2006). Signalling through VEGFRs may also be further modified through receptor heterodimerization and their association with the co-receptors neuropilin-1 and –2. VEGFR-2 signalling plays a critical role in promoting neovascularization and vasculogenesis during development and in neovascularization under physiological and pathological conditions(Ferrara, 2005; Witmer et al., 2003). VEGFR2 signals via a strong tyrosine kinase signal which is able to regulate endothelial function and survival via a number of different signalling pathways including Ras/mitogen activated protein kinase (MAPK), Src, PI3K and NOS (Rahimi, 2006). We and others have shown that PlGF (a VEGFR-1 specific ligand) is able to promote and sustain pathological angiogenesis both in vitro (Cai and Boulton, 2002) and in vivo using several models including the OIR model (Luttun et al., 2002) and that ocular angiogenesis can be blocked by VEGFR-1 siRNA(Shen et al., 2006). Although the role of VEGFR-1 signalling has yet to be fully elucidated there is increasing evidence that VEGFR-1 is a potent negative regulator of VEGFR-2(Witmer et al., 2003).

VEGFR-1 is shown to have a regulatory role in vascular development since VEGFR-1 null mutant mice die at embryonic day 8.5 to 9.0 (E8.5 to E9.0) due to an overgrowth of endothelial cells and disorganization of blood vessels. However, mice lacking the tyrosine kinase domain of VEGFR-1 (VEGFR-1 TK(−) mice) develop an essentially normal vasculature(Hiratsuka et al., 1998) which suggests that the VEGFR-1 tyrosine kinase domain is not essential and that VEGFR-1 may signal via alternative pathways. Further support that VEGFR-1 may act through multiple signalling pathways is provided by the observation that VEGF-A and PlGF generate different patterns of VEGFR-1 autophosphorylation. VEGFR-1 signalling may also be regulated by extracellular matrix components since Nozaki and colleagues observed that the antiangiogenic capacity of VEGFR-1 can be silenced by secreted protein, acidic and rich in cysteine (SPARC) (Nozaki et al., 2006).

It is now becoming evident that "cross-talk" between VEGFR-1 and VEGFR-2 plays a critical role in regulating VEGFR-2-mediated signalling. Bussolati and colleagues showed that NO release from activated VEGFR-1 negatively regulates VEGFR-2-induced proliferation of HUVECs(Bussolati et al., 2001). Chimeric substitution of the intracellular domains of VEGFR-1 and VEGFR-2 with colony stimulating factor-1 confirmed that activation of VEGFR-1 suppresses VEGFR-2-mediated MAPK activation and endothelial cell proliferation (Rahimi et al., 2000). PI3 kinase-dependent pathways appear to play a role in the inhibitory effect of VEGFR-1 on VEGFR-2-mediated cell proliferation (Zeng et al., 2001). Increased VEGFR-2 phosphorylation is observed in embryonic stem cell cultures from VEGFR-1 knockout animals compared to wild type and the VEGFR-1 phenotype can be partially rescued by the selective VEGFR-2 inhibitor SU5416 (Roberts et al., 2004). Autiero and colleagues elegantly demonstrated PlGF activation of VEGFR-1 results in intermolecular transphosphorylation of VEGFR-2 thereby amplifying VEGF driven angiogenesis through VEGFR2 (Autiero et al., 2003). These observations substantiate the importance of the intermolecular communication between VEGFR-1 and VEGFR-2. To further support this we have recently identified an alternative signalling pathway for the regulation of VEGFR-2 that requires the intracellular translocation of both cleaved and full length VEGFR-1 within cells (Cai et al., 2006).

3 Regulated Intramembrane Proteolysis of VEGFR-1

Regulated intramembrane proteolysis (RIP) has recently emerged as a novel, but highly conserved mechanism in cell signalling (Landman and Kim, (2004)). γ-Secretase-dependent RIP has been extensively studied since it is central to Notch signalling. Processing of transmembrane proteins by γ-secretase-dependent RIP leads to the generation of biologically active peptides that function in both, nuclear and non-nuclear signalling (Landman and Kim, (2004)). RIP of membrane receptors usually requires two sequential proteolytic cleavages, carried out by distinct proteases. The first cleavage occurs at the cell surface, and usually leads to the shedding of the protein's extracellular domain in response to ligand binding (Rawson, 2002) allowing for the second intramembrane-dependent γ-secretase cleavage that releases the active cytoplasmic domain. The cytoplasmic domain subsequently translocates into the cells where it can either (1) locate to the nucleus where it serves to regulate gene expression through an association with DNA bound cofactors, as reported for Notch and erbB-4 (Ni et al., 2001; Selkoe and Kopan, (2003)) or (2) bind to cytsolic proteins and regulate their action (e.g. p75[NTR](Kanning et al., 2003) and E-cadherin (Marambaud et al., 2002)).

γ-secretase is a complex composed of four different integral membrane proteins: presenilin, nicastrin, Aph-1, and Pen-2 (Wolfe, 2006). The most studied component of the γ-secretase complex is presenilin that is an integral enzyme in the cleavage of amyloid precursor protein and cleavage of Notch. Although γ-secretase is ubiquitously expressed in a wide range of cell types which themselves express multiple substrates ranging from signalling receptors to junctional complexes there is clear evidence of substrate specificity. However, exactly how this specificity is achieved remains unclear(Mastrangelo et al., 2005).

We and others have identified a potential role for γ-secretase in vasculogenesis and angiogenesis(Cai et al., 2006; Murakami et al., 2006; Nakajima et al., 2006; Nakajima et al., 2003). Abnormal blood vessel development occurs in mice lacking presenilin-1 (Nakajima et al., 2003). Presenilin-1 controls the growth and differentiation of endothelial progenitor cells (Nakajima et al., 2006). An Ets domain is located on the presenilin promoter and Ets is known to be a key regulator of vasculogenesis and angiogenesis(Murakami et al., 2006). Furthermore, the transcriptional elements Ets and CREB are known to regulate expression of presenilin and these elements are themselves regulated by a variety of growth factors including VEGF. Little is known about the mechanism by which γ-secretase regulates angiogenesis but to date emphasis has largely been placed on the Notch signalling system and has shown that (1) upregulation of Notch ligand Delta-like 4 inhibits VEGF-induced endothelial cell function and this can be blocked by inhibiting γ-secretase(Hellstrom et al., 2007) and (2) γ-secretase is critical for cell-autonomous notch signalling and regulates endothelial cell branching and proliferation during vascular tubulogenesis (Sainson et al., 2005). However, we have recently shown that γ-secretase is able to regulate VEGFR-2-induced vascular permeability and angiogenesis in retinal microvascular endothelial cells via VEGFR-1 cleavage and translocation of the C-terminal domain and full length VEGFR-1 (Cai et al., 2006).

4 The Role of γ-Secretase in VEGFR-1 Signalling in Retinal Microvascular Endothelial Cells

We have been able to demonstrate that γ-secretase activity is present in retinal microvascular endothelial cells and that PEDF induces a greater than 8-fold increase in γ-secretase activity (Cai et al., 2006). γ-secretase induction by PEDF in the presence of VEGF resulted in the appearance of an intracellular cleaved 80kDa C-terminal domain of VEGFR-1 within 1 hour post-induction and a reduction in the localization of full length VEGFR-1 to the nucleus (Cai et al., 2006). A blocking antibody against VEGFR-1 added prior to γ-secretase induction abolished cleavage and translocation of the C-terminal domain of VEGFR-1. Interestingly, even though we were able to induce the formation of an active γ-secretase complex in the plasma membrane, VEGF binding to VEGFR-1 is essential before cleavage occurs (Cai et al., 2006) leading us to hypothesize that a change in VEGFR-1 conformation occurs which in turn exposes a cleavage site. Furthermore, unlike most other receptors cleaved by regulated intramembrane proteolysis cleavage of VEGFR-1 does not appear to require prior shedding of its extracellular domain.

The trafficking of Aph-1, nicastrin, presenilin and PEN-2 (the four molecules which constitute γ-secretase) to the plasma membrane is believed to be critical for constituting the enzymatically active γ-secretase complex (Wolfe, 2006). We have used both confocal microscopy and Western blotting to show that following γ-secretase induction both presenilin-1 and nicastrin can be mobilized to the plasma membrane of retinal endothelial cells within 30 minutes.

Tyrosine kinase phosphorylation of VEGFR-1 is reported to be relatively weak compared to VEGFR-2 (Rahimi, 2006). To assess the effect of γ-secretase induction on the phosphorylation state of VEGFR-1 receptor and its translocated domains, we immunoprecipitated phosphorylated proteins and, following western blotting, immunolocalized with antibodies against VEGFR-1 (Cai et al., 2006). VEGF induced an increase in autophosphorylation of VEGFR-1 compared to control with bands at 250 and 180 kDa in whole cell lysates. γ-secretase induction greatly reduced VEGFR-1 phosphorylation in both the 250 and 180 kDa bands and dephosphorylation was greatest when γ-secretase was induced by PEDF in combination with VEGF. Analysis of the subcellular fractions demonstrated that VEGF induced an increase in auto-phosphorylation of full length VEGFR-1 in membrane, cytoskeleton and nuclear fractions. Interestingly, γ-secretase induction almost completely blocked the tyrosine phosphorylation of full length VEGFR-1 in all fractions regardless of whether the endothelial cells were cultured in the presence or absence of VEGF and phosphorylation of the cleaved 80 kDa VEGFR-1 C-terminal domain was not observed. γ-secretase inhibition prevented dephosphorylation confirming a critical role for γ-secretase induction in VEGFR-1 cell signalling.

5 γ-Secretase Regulates Vascular Permeability and Angiogenesis VIA VEGFR-1

We have already confirmed that VE-cadherin plays a critical role in regulating vascular permeability via VEGFR-1 and shown that PlGF, a ligand specific for VEGF-1 is able to reduce VEGF-induced vascular permeability. Upon addition of VEGF to confluent vascular endothelial cell cultures there is a significant decrease in VE-cadherin expression within 1 hour. By contrast, PlGF causes an upregulation in VE-cadherin expression. γ-secretase induction by PEDF inhibits VEGF-induced vascular permeability in cultured vascular endothelial cells and this can be blocked by γ-secretase inhibition.

γ–secretase induction is also able to reduce endothelial cell proliferation and abolish migration and tubule formation in vitro and this could be blocked by the addition of γ-secretase inhibitor L685458(Cai et al., 2006). VEGFR-1 was confirmed to be a requirement for γ-secretase-induced inhibition of VEGF-induced angiogenesis since VEGFR-1 antisense abolishes the inhibitory effect of γ-secretase on VEGF-induced tubule formation, cell proliferation and cell migration (Cai et al., 2006).

6 The Role of γ-Secretase in VEGFR-1 Signalling In RPE Cells

The components of γ-secretase are expressed in RPE cells and both nicastrin and presenilin-1 are translocated to the plasma membrane following exposure to PEDF. Quiescent RPE cells demonstrated a number of different intracellular molecular weight C-terminal VEGFR-1 fragments as well as full length VEGFR-1. These were decreased following induction of γ-secretase by PEDF in the presence of VEGF.

7 Summary

In conclusion, γ-secretase is expressed in both retinal microvascular endothelial cells and RPE cells and is able to elicit regulated intramembrane proteolysis of VEGFR-1. Furthermore, γ-secretase regulates the translocation of the intracellular domain of

VEGFR1 as well as full length VEGFR1 in both cell types. γ-secretase is clearly able to act as a potent negative regulators of VEGFR2 induced in vitro angiogenesis but its role in the RPE has yet to be elucidated. We conclude that γ-secretase may offer a therapeutic target for the treatment of both retinal and choroidal neovascularization.

References

Autiero, M., et al., 2003. Role of PlGF in the intra- and intermolecular cross talk between the VEGF receptors Flt1 and Flk1. Nat Med. 9, 936–43.

Bussolati, B., et al., 2001. Vascular endothelial growth factor receptor-1 modulates vascular endothelial growth factor-mediated angiogenesis via nitric oxide. Am J Pathol. 159, 993–1008.

Cai, J., Boulton, M., 2002. The pathogenesis of diabetic retinopathy: old concepts and new questions. Eye. 16, 242–60.

Cai, J., et al., 2006. Pigment epithelium-derived factor inhibits angiogenesis via regulated intracellular proteolysis of vascular endothelial growth factor receptor 1. J Biol Chem. 281, 3604–13.

Ferrara, N., 2005. The role of VEGF in the regulation of physiological and pathological angiogenesis. Exs. 209–31.

Grant, M. B., et al., 2004. The role of growth factors in the pathogenesis of diabetic retinopathy. Expert Opin Investig Drugs. 13, 1275–93.

Hellstrom, M., et al., 2007. Dll4 signalling through Notch1 regulates formation of tip cells during angiogenesis. Nature. 445, 776–80.

Hiratsuka, S., et al., 1998. Flt-1 lacking the tyrosine kinase domain is sufficient for normal development and angiogenesis in mice. Proc Natl Acad Sci U S A. 95, 9349–54.

Kanning, K. C., et al., 2003. Proteolytic processing of the p75 neurotrophin receptor and two homologs generates C-terminal fragments with signaling capability. J Neurosci. 23, 5425–36.

Landman, N., Kim, T. W., 2004. Got RIP? Presenilin-dependent intramembrane proteolysis in growth factor receptor signaling. Cytokine Growth Factor Rev. 15, 337–51.

Lee, P., et al., 1998. Ocular neovascularization: an epidemiologic review. Surv Ophthalmol. 43, 245–69.

Luttun, A., et al., 2002. Revascularization of ischemic tissues by PlGF treatment, and inhibition of tumor angiogenesis, arthritis and atherosclerosis by anti-Flt1. Nat Med. 8, 831–40.

Marambaud, P., et al., 2002. A presenilin-1/gamma-secretase cleavage releases the E-cadherin intracellular domain and regulates disassembly of adherens junctions. Embo J. 21, 1948–56.

Mastrangelo, P., et al., 2005. Dissociated phenotypes in presenilin transgenic mice define functionally distinct gamma-secretases. Proc Natl Acad Sci U S A. 102, 8972–7.

Murakami, Y., et al., 2006. Ets-1-dependent Expression of vascular endothelial growth factor receptors is activated by latency-associated nuclear antigen of Kaposi's Sarcoma-associated herpesvirus through interaction with daxx. J Biol Chem. 281, 28113–21.

Nakajima, M., et al., 2006. Presenilin-1 controls the growth and differentiation of endothelial progenitor cells through its beta-catenin-binding region. Cell Biol Int. 30, 239–43.

Nakajima, M., et al., 2003. Abnormal blood vessel development in mice lacking presenilin-1. Mech Dev. 120, 657–67.

Ni, C. Y., et al., 2001. gamma -Secretase cleavage and nuclear localization of ErbB-4 receptor tyrosine kinase. Science. 294, 2179–81.

Nozaki, M., et al., 2006. Loss of SPARC-mediated VEGFR-1 suppression after injury reveals a novel antiangiogenic activity of VEGF-A. J Clin Invest. 116, 422–9.

Rahimi, N., 2006. VEGFR-1 and VEGFR-2: two non-identical twins with a unique physiognomy. Front. Biosci. 11, 818–829.

Rahimi, N., et al., 2000. Receptor chimeras indicate that the vascular endothelial growth factor receptor-1 (VEGFR-1) modulates mitogenic activity of VEGFR-2 in endothelial cells. J Biol Chem. 275, 16986-92.

Rawson, R. B., 2002. Regulated intramembrane proteolysis: from the endoplasmic reticulum to the nucleus. Essays Biochem. 38, 155–68.

Roberts, D. M., et al., 2004. The vascular endothelial growth factor (VEGF) receptor Flt-1 (VEGFR-1) modulates Flk-1 (VEGFR-2) signaling during blood vessel formation. Am J Pathol. 164, 1531–5.

Sainson, R. C., et al., 2005. Cell-autonomous notch signaling regulates endothelial cell branching and proliferation during vascular tubulogenesis. Faseb J. 19, 1027–29.

Selkoe, D., Kopan, R., 2003. Notch and Presenilin: regulated intramembrane proteolysis links development and degeneration. Annu Rev Neurosci. 26, 565–97.

Shen, J., et al., 2006. Suppression of ocular neovascularization with siRNA targeting VEGF receptor 1. Gene Ther. 13, 225–34.

Shibuya, M., Claesson-Welsh, L., 2006. Signal transduction by VEGF receptors in regulation of angiogenesis and lymphangiogenesis. Exp Cell Res. 312, 549–60.

vanWijngaarden, P., et al., 2005. Inhibitors of ocular neovascularization: promises and potential problems. Jama. 293, 1509–13.

Witmer, A. N., et al., 2003. Vascular endothelial growth factors and angiogenesis in eye disease. Prog Retin Eye Res. 22, 1–29.

Wolfe, M. S., 2006. The gamma-secretase complex: membrane-embedded proteolytic ensemble. Biochemistry. 45, 7931–39.

Zeng, H., et al., 2001. Vascular permeability factor (VPF)/vascular endothelial growth factor (VEGF) peceptor-1 down-modulates VPF/VEGF receptor-2-mediated endothelial cell proliferation, but not migration, through phosphatidylinositol 3-kinase-dependent pathways. J Biol Chem. 276, 26969–79.

Analysis of the Rate of Disk Membrane Digestion by Cultured RPE Cells

Tanja Diemer, Daniel Gibbs, and David S. Williams

1 Introduction

The retinal pigment epithelium (RPE) is a monolayer of polarized cells localized between the photoreceptor cell layer and Bruch's membrane. As part of an essential photoreceptor outer segment (ROS) renewal process, the RPE cells phagocytose and degrade the distal ROS disk membranes on a daily basis. It is hypothesized that even a minor delay in uptake or clearance of the daily outer segment load by the RPE can result in the accumulation of undigested material and ensuing retinal damage.

We are interested in the role of the RPE in retinal degeneration, and, in particular, factors that might affect the rate of disk membrane digestion and thus the health of the RPE. We are using genetic mouse models in combination with cultures of RPE cells. Here, we describe an assay of disk membrane digestion by primary mouse RPE cells and ARPE19 cells for these analyses.

2 Phagocytosis and Degradation by the RPE

In the mouse (and primates) the total outer segment renewal time is about 10 days, so that, each day, 10% of each ROS must be ingested and digested (Young, 1967; Young, 1971). The phagocytic step is receptor mediated, involving the integrin receptor alphaVbeta5 (Finnemann et al., 1997), the scavenger receptor CD36 (Ryeom et al., 1996) and Mer tyrosine kinase (Gal et al., 2000; Vollrath et al., 2001; Feng et al., 2002), all of which are located on the apical plasma membrane. Following ingestion, the ROS disks are transported from the apical RPE towards the basal side of RPE, where they fuse with lysosomes in order to be degraded (Bosch et al., 1993; Herman and Steinberg, 1982a,b).

T. Diemer

Departments of Pharmacology and Neurosciences, UCSD School of Medicine, La Jolla, California, 92093-0983, USA, Tel: 858-534-9550, Fax: 858-822-6950

e-mail: tdiemer@ucsd.edu

R.E. Anderson et al. (eds.), *Recent Advances in Retinal Degeneration*,
© Springer 2008

Defects in phagocytic uptake of ROS disks can promote photoreceptor degeneration, as reported for the RCS rat, which lacks functional Mer tyrosine kinase (Bok and Hall, 1971; D'Cruz et al., 2000). Deficiencies in the digestion of ROS disks lead to accumulation of undigested material in the RPE, basal deposits and photoreceptor cell death in transgenic mice, overexpressing mutant cathepsin D (Rakoczy et al., 2002). Digestion of ingested disk membranes can also be affected by defects in the transport of phagosomes or lysosomes, so that there is a delay in the fusion of the two. Lack of myosin VIIa was shown to retard the delivery of phagosomes to the basal RPE, and delay phagosome digestion (Gibbs et al., 2003).

Our particular method for measuring ROS digestion has been developed from phagocytosis assays described by other groups (Colley and Hall 1986; Chaitin and Hall, 1983; Finnemann et al., 1997; Finnemann et al., 2002), and optimized for our purposes with respect to ROS concentration, exposure time and intervals for sampling. Thus, we are able to measure defects in the digestion of ROS disks by primary mouse RPE cells, as well as the earlier events of binding and ingestion. The degradation of ROSs by the RPE is assessed by exposing the cells to ROSs for a short period, followed by complete removal of unbound ROSs and subsequent incubation in medium without ROSs. This exposure provides an initial "pulse" of ROSs to the cells, which is then followed by a "chase" period, the beginning of which is defined as the time when ROSs are removed. The rates of ingestion and digestion can then be measured by quantifying the number of bound and ingested ROSs over time.

This digestion assay also permits the identification of separate photoreceptor and RPE defects by feeding ROSs from mutant mice to RPE cells from normal mice, and vice versa (Gibbs et al., 2003).

3 Phagocytosis Assay

Fluorescent assays have been reported to study the interaction of ROSs with RPE cells. ROSs labeled with fluorescein isothiocyanate (FITC) have been used to measure total phagocytosis. Surface bound and ingested ROS can be distinguished by quenching external FITC fluorescence (Finnemann et al., 1997). In the indirect assay used by us, RPE cells are first treated with unlabeled ROSs and subsequently probed with opsin antibodies. The number of surface bound ROSs is distinguished from the ingested ROS by labeling of non-permeabilized and permeabilized cells (Colley and Hall 1986; Chaitin and Hall, 1983).

3.1 Mouse Primary RPE Cell and ARPE19 Cell Culture

The mouse RPE cells were isolated and cultured essentially as described earlier (Gibbs et al., 2003). Intact eyes were removed from 12 day old mice. The eyes were washed twice in 10 ml Dulbecco's modified eagle's medium (DMEM) containing high glucose. After incubation in Dispase solution (0.2% (w/v) Dispase dissolved in DMEM and sterile filtered) for 45 min at 37 °C in a 15 ml conical tube, the eyes were washed twice in growth medium (GM), which consisted of DMEM (high glucose), 10% FCS, 1% penicillin/streptomycin, 2.5 mM L-glutamine and 1 × MEM nonessential amino acids. Media and additives were purchased from Invitrogen. An incision was made around the ora serrata of each eye. Anterior cornea, lens capsule and associated iris pigmented epithelium were removed. After incubating the resulting eyecups in GM for 20 min at 37 °C, the neural retina was separated from the RPE. Intact sheets of RPE were peeled off the basement membrane and transferred into a tube containing 10 ml GM. The sheets were sedimented at 200 × g for 5 min and washed twice with GM. After the last wash the RPE cells were resuspended in GM (RPE cells from one eye per 0.3 ml GM). 0.3 ml cell suspension was transferred into transwell inserts or on glass. The cells were cultured 4–5 days at 37 °C, 5% CO_2 in a humidified incubator before being used for ROS phagocytosis assays. ARPE19 cells (ATCC), a spontaneously immortalized cell line that forms a monolayer and differentiates under specific conditions (Dunn et al., 1996), were grown at 37 °C with 5% CO_2 in DMEM-F12 with 10% FBS, 1% penicillin/streptomycin and glutamine. They were used in an undifferentiated state.

3.2 Phagocytosis of ROSs by Cultured Mouse RPE and ARPE19 Cells

ROSs were isolated and purified from adult mouse retinas as described previously (Tsang et al., 1998; Gibbs et al., 2003). A ROS suspension, containing 1×10^6–5×10^6 ROSs in 0.15 ml, was applied to cells grown on transwell filters or glass coverslips in 24-well plates. For the pulse-chase experiment, the cells were incubated at 37 °C, 5% CO_2 in a humidified incubator for 5 min for mouse RPE or 4 h for ARPE19 cells. After this interval, the unbound ROSs were removed by extensive washing with PBS (1 mM KH_2PO_4, 155 mM NaCl, 3 mM Na_2HPO_4 x $7H_2O$, pH 7.4), followed by an incubation in GM at 37 °C, 5% CO_2 for different lengths of time. The cells were washed 3 times for 5 min in PBS and fixed in 4% paraformaldehyde. Double immunofluorescence labeling of bound and total ROSs was performed using a bovine opsin polyclonal antibody, pAb01 (Liu et al., 1999), and the method described for rat RPE (Colley and Hall, 1986). After fixation, the ROSs bound to but not ingested by the cells are labeled with pAb01 followed by an Alexa 488 nm conjugated goat anti rabbit monoclonal secondary antibody (Molecular Probes). The cells were washed in PBS and permeabilized with 50% ethanol for 5 min at room temperature. Both bound and ingested ROSs were then labeled with pAb01 followed by an Alexa 594 nm conjugated goat anti rabbit monoclonal antibody (Molecular Probes). The nuclei were stained with 300 nM DAPI (4, 6 diamidino-2-phenylindole chloride) in PBS. RPE cells grown on glass were mounted with mowiol. For those grown on transwell filters, the filters were excised and mounted under a coverglass, also using mowiol mounting medium. Ingested

ROSs were determined by subtracting the bound from the total ROSs. ROSs (at least 0.5 μm in diameter) were counted at × 400 magnification in all cells within 10–15 fields of view, selected randomly. Images were collected with a Zeiss Axiophot microscope, equipped with an ORCA C4742-95 charge coupled device (CCD) camera. Image acquisition was performed using the OPENLAB V.2.2.5 software package, for image analysis ImageJ was used.

3.3 Pulse-chase Experiment for Primary Mouse RPE and ARPE19 Cells

We have used both mouse primary RPE cells and a stable RPE cell line, ARPE19, that has retained the ability of the native epithelium to phagocytose ROSs. Although a cell line has the advantage of unlimited availability of cells, the primary mouse RPE cells allow us to use tissue from mutant mice.

The ingestion of mouse ROSs by primary mouse RPE cells is initiated within 5 min. After adding a pulse of 1×10^6 ROSs in 0.15 ml GM to the RPE cells for 5 min, fewer than half the ROSs remained after a 30-min chase period in GM, and after a 60 min chase, the ROSs are almost completely digested (Fig. 1). Bound ROSs also declined during the 30- and 60-min chase period in GM. The small volume of medium in which the ROSs are provided to the cells allows a short exposure time without a lag time due to sedimentation of ROSs. The 5-min pulse of ROSs differs from other published studies (Finnemann et al., 2002; Colley and Hall, 1986), where longer times (2 hours) were used for other RPE cell cultures. Its brevity permits sharper resolution of the rate of digestion, but primary RPE cell cultures must be used with such a short pulse, since only they will ingest ROSs within a few minutes.

Gibbs et al., 2003 showed that, in RPE cells from myosin VIIa-deficient mice, the number of ingested ROSs remaining was double that in control RPE at 30-min and 60-min time points after the addition of ROSs, whereas the ingestion rate was unaffected. In vivo, MYO7A-null RPE cells have a larger proportion of phagosomes in the apical processes during a 2-h period around the time of peak shedding. Lack

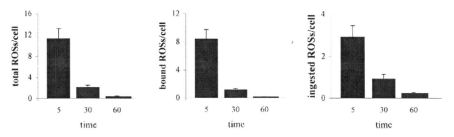

Fig. 1 Phagocytosis by primary mouse RPE cells. The number of total, bound and ingested ROSs per cell were quantified after a 5-min pulse of ROSs, followed by a chase of either 30 min or 60 min after the ROSs were removed. Double immunolabeling allows bound and ingested ROSs to be distinguished from each other

Fig. 2 Phagocytosis by
ARPE19 cell line. Confluent
ARPE19 cells were
challenged with ROSs for 4h
followed by a chase in growth
medium for 3h or over night.
Total ROSs per field of view
were counted

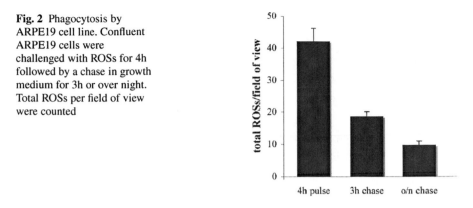

of myosin VIIa is thought to delay degradation of phagosomes by inhibiting their transport to basal RPE, where digestion occurs.

ARPE19 cells ingest (Finnemann et al., 1997) and digest ROSs more slowly than primary mouse RPE cells do. After a 4h pulse with ROSs, they show reduction in total opsin labeling after 3h and over night incubation in GM (Fig. 2).

4 Conclusions

This assay can be a valuable tool to analyze ingestion and digestion of ROS disk membranes by the RPE. By using primary RPE cultures, one can take advantage of mutant mouse models to study RPE-dependent retinal degeneration. We are using this system to dissect out roles for motor proteins in the transport of phagosomes and lysosomes in the RPE (e.g. Gibbs et al., 2003). We are also using it to help understand mechanisms underlying RPE pathologies; for example, in mouse models for macular dystrophy, such as Stargardt's macular degeneration type 3 (Karan et al., 2005).

Acknowledgments This research was supported by NIH grant EY07042.

References

Bok, D., and Hall, M. O., 1971, The role of the pigment epithelium in the etiology of inherited retinal dystrophy in the rat, *J. Cell Biol.* **49**:664–682.

Bosch, E., Horwitz, J., and Bok, D., 1993, Phagocytosis of outer segments by retinal pigment epithelium: phagosome- lysosome interaction, *J. Histochem. Cytochem.* **41**:253–263.

Chaitin, M. H., and Hall, M. O., 1983, Defective ingestion of rod outer segments by cultured dystrophic rat pigment epithelial cells, *Invest. Ophthalmol. Vis. Sci.* **24**(7):812–20.

Colley, N. J., and Hall, M. O., 1986, Phagocytosis of light- and dark-adapted rod outer segments by cultured RPE cells: a reassessment, *Exp. Eye Res.* **42**:323–329.

D'Cruz, P. M., Yasumura, D., Weir, J., Matthes, M. T., Abderrahim, H., LaVail, M. M., and Vollrath, D., 2000, Mutation of the receptor tyrosine kinase gene Mertk in the retinal dystrophic RCS rat, *Hum. Mol. Genet.* **9**(4):645–51.

Dunn, K. C., Aotaki-Keen, A. E., Putkey, F. R., and Hjelmeland, L. M., 1996, ARPE-19, a human retinal pigment epithelial cell line with differentiated properties, *Exp. Eye Res.* **62**:155–169.

Feng, W., Yasumura, D., Matthes, M. T., LaVail, M. M., and Vollrath, D., 2002, Mertk triggers uptake of photoreceptor outer segments during phagocytosis by cultured retinal pigment epithelial cells, *J. Biol. Chem.* **277**(19):17016–22.

Finnemann, S. C., Leung, L. W., and Rodriguez-Boulan, E., 2002, The lipofuscin component A2E selectively inhibits phagolysosomal degradation of photoreceptor phospholipid by the retinal pigment epithelium, *Proc. Natl. Acad. Sci. USA* **99**(6):3842–47.

Finnemann, S. C., Bonilha, V. L., Marmorstein, A. D., and Rodriguez-Boulan, E., 1997, Phagocytosis of rod outer segments by retinal pigment epithelial cells requires alpha(v)beta5 integrin for binding but not for internalization, *Proc. Natl. Acad. Sci. USA* **25**(24):12932–37.

Gal, A., Li, Y., Thompson, D. A., Weir, J., Orth, U., Jacobson, S. G., Apfelstedt-Sylla, E., and Vollrath, D., 2000, Mutations in MERTK, the human orthologue of the RCS rat retinal dystrophy gene, cause retinitis pigmentosa. *Nat. Genet.* **26**(3):270–71.

Gibbs, D., Kitamoto, J., and Williams, D. S., 2003, Myosin VIIa in RPE phagocytosis and a potential cause of blindness in Usher syndrome 1B, *Proc. Natl. Acad. Sci. USA* **100**(11):6481–86.

Herman, K. G., and Steinberg, R. H., 1982a, Phagosome degradation in the tapetal retinal pigment epithelium of the opossum, *Invest. Ophthalmol. Vis. Sci.* **23**:291–304.

Herman, K. G., and Steinberg, R. H., 1982b, Phagosome movement and the diurnal pattern of phagocytosis in the tapetal retinal pigment epithelium of the opossum, *Invest. Ophthalmol. Vis. Sci.* **23**:277–290.

Karan, G. , Lillo, C., Yang, Z., Cameron, D. J., Locke, K. G., Zhao, Y., Thirumalaichary, S., Li, C., Birch, D. G., Vollmer-Snarr, H. R., Williams, D. S., and Zhang, K., 2005, Lipofuscin accumulation, abnormal electrophysiology, and photoreceptor degeneration in mutant ELOVL4 transgenic mice: a model for macular degeneration, *Proc. Natl. Acad. Sci.* **102**, 4164–69

Liu X., Udovichenko I. P., Brown, S. D., Steel, K. P., and Williams, D. S., 1999, Myosin VIIa participates in opsin transport through the photoreceptor cilium, *J. Neurosci.* **19**:6267–74.

Rakoczy, P. E., Zhang, D., Robertson, T., Barnett, N. L., Papdimitriou, J., Constable, I. J., and Lai, C. M., 2002, Progressive age-related changes similar to age-related macular degeneration in a transgenic mouse model, *Am. J. Pathol.* **161**:1515–24.

Ryeom, S. W., Sparrow, J. R, and Silverstein, R. L., 1996, CD36 participates in the phagocytosis of rod outer segments by retinal pigment epithelium, *J. Cell Sci.* **109**:387–95.

Tsang, S. H., Burns, M. E., Calvert, P. D., Gouras, P., Baylor, D. A., Goff, S. P., and Arshavsky, V. Y., 1998, Role for the target enzyme in deactivation of photoreceptor G protein in vivo, *Science* **282**:117–21.

Vollrath, D., Feng, W., Duncan, J. L., Yasumura, D., D'Cruz, P. M., Chappelow, A., Matthes, M. T., Kay, M. A., and LaVail, M. M., 2001, Correction of the retinal dystrophy phenotype of the RCS rat by viral gene transfer of Mertk, *Proc. Natl. Acad. Sci. USA* **98**(22):12584–89.

Young, R. W., 1967, The renewal of photoreceptor cell outer segments, *J. Cell Biol.* **33**:61–72.

Young, R. W., 1971, Shedding of discs from rod outer segments in the rhesus monkey, *J. Ultrastruct. Res.* **34**(1):190–203.

Functional Expression of Cone Cyclic Nucleotide-Gated Channel in Cone Photoreceptor-Derived 661W Cells

J. Browning Fitzgerald, Anna P. Malykhina, Muayyad R. Al-Ubaidi, and Xi-Qin Ding

1 Introduction

Cone phototransduction mediated by cone cyclic nucleotide-gated (CNG) channel activation is essential for central and color vision. Rod or cone CNG channels are composed of two structurally related subunit types: the A and the B subunits. The stoichiometry of the rod CNG channel complex has been established by biochemical, biophysical and molecular biological means, showing a heterotetrameric complex composed of three A and one B subunits (Shammat and Gordon, 1999; Zheng et al., 2002). Naturally occurring mutations in the cone channel have been shown to affect cone function and to associate with varieties of cone diseases (Kaupp and Seifert, 2002). Unlike the rod channel, the biochemical properties and functional regulation of the cone CNG channel are much less understood; only recently has the molecular identity of the channel B subunit been revealed (Gerstner et al., 2000). This is primarily due to the difficulty of investigating the cone system in a mammalian retina and lack of an appropriate cone-specific cell line. The recently characterized cone-derived 661W cell line has been shown to be a useful model to study cone-specific proteins and cone function. The 661W cell line was originally cloned from retinal tumors of a transgenic mouse line expressing SV-40 T antigen under control of the human interphotoreceptor retinoid binding protein (hIRBP) promoter (Tan et al., 2004). These cells demonstrate cellular and biochemical characteristics of cone photoreceptors and resemble neuronal cells in morphology. They grow as a monolayer, exhibit processes characteristic of neuronal cells and express several markers of cone photoreceptors, including blue and green opsins, transducin and cone arrestin (Tan et al., 2004). However, they do not express rod opsin or arrestin, or rod and cone-specific proteins, such as phosducin, peripherin/*rds* and rom-1, or the retinal pigment epithelial cell specific protein, RPE65 (Tan et al., 2004). Moreover, these cells have been shown to respond to light stress, oxidative stress and other

X.-Q. Ding
Departments of Cell Biology, University of Oklahoma Health Sciences Center, 940 Stanton L. Young Blvd., Oklahoma City, OK 73104, USA, Tel: 405-271-8001 x47959, Fax: 405-271-3548
e-mail: xi-qin-ding@ouhsc.edu

R.E. Anderson et al. (eds.), *Recent Advances in Retinal Degeneration*,
© Springer 2008

types of toxic stimulation with apoptotic cell death, similar to observations recorded in normal retinal photoreceptor cells (Crawford et al., 2001; Tuohy et al., 2002; Tan et al., 2004). In a number of studies, 661 W cells have been used as a photoreceptor cellular model to study the apoptotic pathway and mechanism involved in photoreceptor degeneration (Castagnet et al., 2003; Sanvicens et al., 2004; Srinivasan et al., 2004). A recent study has described a mechanism involving multiple independent proteases in light induced programmed cell death using 661 W cells (Kanan et al., 2007). Convincingly, 661 W cell line has been shown to serve as a useful cellular model to study cone specific protein, cone biology and the associated diseases. This work was designed to functionally express cone CNG channel in 661 W cells to determine the feasibility of use of this cell line in studies of cone specific proteins and to explore the regulation of cone CNG channel and biochemical properties in a cone-derived cellular environment.

2 Materials and Methods

2.1 Antibodies Against Cone CNG Channel Subunits

Polyclonal antibodies against peptides corresponding to the sequences between residues 77 and 97 (SNAQPNPGEQKPPDGGEGRKE) of the mouse CNGA3 and between residues 278 and 293 (DSNELKRNYRSSTKFR) of the mouse CNGB3 were generated and affinity purified for Western blotting and immunocytochemistry (ICC). Antibody against human red/green opsin was generously provided by Dr. Jeremy Nathans at Johns Hopkins University.

2.2 Reverse Transcription-polymerase Chain Reaction (RT-PCR)

RT was carried out on total retinal RNA using an oligo-dT primer and superscript III reverse transcriptase. RT-PCR was performed using forward primer 5'-CGCGGATCCGCGTGAATGTGACCTGTGCAGAGATGG-3' and the reverse primer 5'-CCGCTCGAGCGGGGGCAGAGCCACCTGCATTTTCAGTCAG-3' for CNGA3 and forward primer 5'-CGCGGATCCGCGTTTCAGACCTGCCTCAGAG AA-3' and the reverse primer 5'-TGCTCTAGAGCACTTCCTTTGGAACTTTCAC CTTTATTTCTG-3' for CNGB3. The neuronal housekeeping gene hypoxanthine phosphoribosyltransferase (HPRT) was included as an internal control.

2.3 Heterologous Expression of the Cone CNG Channel Subunits in 661 W Cells

Construct encoding the full-length mouse CNGA3 was generated by ligating the cDNA into the BamH I and Xho I sites of the expression vector pcDNA3.1. The

CNGA3-HA was produced by inserting the coding sequence in-frame into the carboxyl terminus of CNGA3 using the quick-change site-directed mutagenesis strategy. The mouse CNGB3 construct was generously provided by Dr. Martin Biel (Ludwig-Maximilians-Universitat Munchen, Germany).

Cells were routinely cultured in Dubelcco's modified Eagle's medium supplemented with 10% fetal bovine serum and 1% penicillin/streptomycin at 37°C in a humidified atmosphere with 5% CO_2. Transfection was performed using nucleofector technology which is a highly efficient gene transfer method for hard-to-transfect cell lines and for most primary cells (Iversen et al., 2005; Leclere et al., 2005).

2.4 Western Blotting and ICC

Western blotting and ICC were carried out as previously described (Ding et al., 2004; Tan et al., 2004).

2.5 Electrophysiological Recordings

Standard whole-cell patch clamp recordings were performed as previously described (Malykhina et al., 2006) on transfected cells grown on 35 mm culture dishes. For voltage clamp experiments the external solution contained (in mM): NaCl 135, KCl 5.4, NaH_2PO_4 0.33, $MgCl_2$ 1, $CaCl_2$ 2, HEPES 5, D-glucose 5.5, adjusted with NaOH to pH 7.4. Pipette solution consisted of (in mM): K^+aspartate 100, KCl 30, NaCl 5, $MgCl_2$ 2, Na-ATP 2, EGTA 1, HEPES 5 with pH 7.2 adjusted with KOH. Patch electrodes had resistances of 3-5 $M\Omega$ when filled with internal solution. Whole cell currents were recorded by using voltage clamp, ramp, and gap-free protocols. For voltage clamp protocol cells were held at –70 mV and series of voltage steps from –70 mV up to +60 mV were applied with 10 mV increments. For ramp protocol cells were held at –50 mV and voltage changes were used in a ramp manner from –80 mV to +80 mV. For gap-free protocol the holding potential was also – 50 mV. All experiments were performed at room temperature (23°C) and recorded using an Axopatch 200B amplifier (Axon Instrument, Foster City, CA). pCLAMP software (Axon Instruments) was used for data acquisition and analysis.

3 Results

3.1 Expression of CNGA3 and CNGB3 in 661 W cells

RT-PCR was performed to determine whether there are endogenously expressed cone CNG channel subunits in 661 W cells. With primers amplifying the full-length mouse CNGA3, a single band was detected from the wild type and cone-dominant $Nrl^{-/-}$ retinas (generously provided by Dr. Anand Swaroop at the University of

Fig. 1 Expression of
CNGA3, CNGB3 and
red/green opsin in 661 W
cells and mouse retinas
(A–B). RT-PCR detection of
CNGA3 (A) and CNGB3 (B).
HPRT was used as internal
control (C–D). Western blot
detection of CNGB3 (C) and
green opsin (D) in 661 W
cells

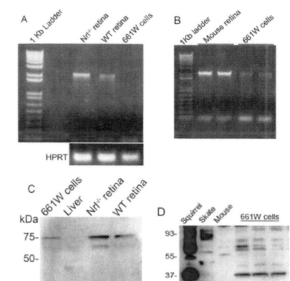

Michigan) but no signal was seen in 661 W cells (Fig. 1A). RT-PCR with primers amplifying the full-length mouse CNGB3 showed a weak band in 661 W cells, compared with the ample signal in the mouse retina (Fig. 1B). Consistent with the RT-PCR results, a weak expression of CNGB3 protein in 661 W cells was detected by Western blotting using the anti-CNGB3 antibody (Fig. 1C). With this antibody a single band that migrated at position of 75 kDa was detected in 661 W cells and in mouse retinas. The signal was more abundant in $Nrl^{-/-}$ retina than that in the WT. No CNGA3 was detected with the respective antibody (data not shown) which is consistent with the RT-PCR finding. Expression of green opsin in 661 W cells was detected by Western blotting (Fig. 1D). Thus, these results suggest that there is no detectable, endogenously expressed CNGA3 but a weak expression of CNGB3 in 661 W cells.

3.2 Heterologous Expression of Cone CNG Channel Subunits in 661 W Cells

To express CNGA3 in 661 W cells several transfection strategies were tested and only the nucleofector method showed to be effective in introducing the cDNA and expression. Figure 2 shows heterologous expression of CNGA3 and CNGA3-HA in 661 W cells 48 hours post-transfection detected by Western blotting (Fig. 2A) and ICC (Fig. 2B). Expression of the CNGA3 constructs was detected by both antibodies against CNGA3 or HA epitope. A single band migrated at ~70 kD was detected in the protein extracts from transfected cells. The aggregates on top of the lanes may reflect an incomplete solubilization or reduction. In ICC examination, the channel

Fig. 2 Heterologous expression of CNGA3 in 661 W cells detected by Western blotting (A) and immunocytochemistry (B). Antibodies against both CNGA3 and against HA epitope were used in both immunoblotting and ICC

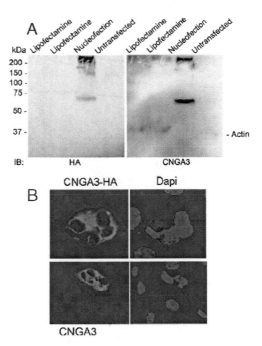

subunit was observed throughout the cell, predominantly localized at the plasma membrane (Fig. 2B).

3.3 Functional Activity of Cone CNG Channel Heterologously Expressed in 661 W Cells

Standard whole cell patch clamp recordings were performed on 661 W cells transfected with CNGA3 or co-transfected with CNGA3 and CNGB3 to examine the channel functional activity. Voltage clamp protocol was first applied on cells transfected with CNGA3 or CNGA3-HA in the absence of cGMP. As shown in Fig. 3, a steady increase of whole cell outward current was detected upon depolarization

Fig. 3 Patch clamp recordings from 661 W cells transfected with CNGA3 and CNGA3-HA. A steady increase of current amplitude was detected upon depolarization

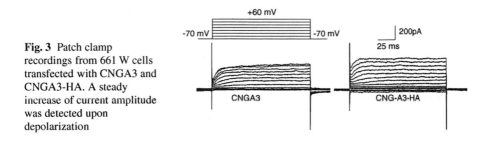

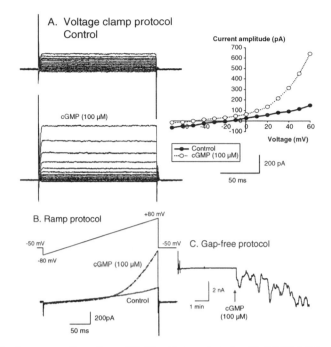

Fig. 4 Patch clamp recordings from 661 W cells transfected with CNGA3-HA + CNGB3 in response to cGMP (100 μM). A. Effect of cGMP application on current amplitude in 661 W cell and the corresponding current-voltage curve. B. Increase in current after cGMP application is more prominent at positive potentials. C. cGMP evoked oscillations in inward current recorded via gap-free mode (cell was held at −50 mV during recording)

steps in 661 W cells expressing CNGA3. Patch-clamp recording was also performed on the cells transfected with both CNGA3 and CNGB3 subunits in the presence of 100 μM cGMP. Whole cell voltage clamp, ramp, and gap-free protocols showed steady increase of total outward currents in response to cGMP stimulation (Fig. 4). A current-voltage relationship was generated from the voltage clamp recording at concentration of 100 μM cGMP in the presence of 2 mM extracellular Ca^{2+} (Fig. 4A, right panel). Thus, functional activity of the heterologously expressed cone CNG channel was established in the cone-derived 661 W cells.

4 Discussion

Rod and cone CNG channels localized at the plasma membrane of photoreceptor outer segment play a pivotal role in phototransduction. Proper subunit association, complex assembly, and accurate regulation are vital for the channel function. Compared to the more advanced understanding on the rod CNG channel our knowledge of the cone channel regarding biochemical features and functional regulation is quite limited. This is primarily due to the difficulty of investigating the cone system in a mammalian retina. There have been some studies using Xenopus oocytes or HEK293 cells as cellular models to investigate cone CNG channel but many of the results developed from these studies appeared controversial. Studies from Zhong et al using HEK293 cells proposed a 3A:1B stoichiometry of the cone channel complex (Zhong et al., 2002) while a 2A:2B stoichiometry was proposed by Peng et al from studies using Xenopus oocytes (Peng et al., 2004). Similarly, functional importance of calmodulin binding to the cone CNG channel was documented in studies using Xenopus oocytes (Peng et al., 2003) while the irrelevance of calmodulin to the cone CNG channel regulation was proposed by Muller et al from studies using HEK293 cells (Muller et al., 2001). CNG channel is an important component in the phototransduction cascade. The nature that 661 W cells possess includes exhibiting characteristic of neuronal cells and expressing cone specific proteins that are involved in photoactivation and phototransduction (cone opsins, transducin and arrestin, etc) (Tan et al., 2004) provides an ideal internal environment to study the functional regulation and biochemical properties of cone CNG channel. This work was designed to establish the potential use of the cone-derived photoreceptor cell line, the 661 W cell line, as a valuable cellular model to study cone CNG channel. The channel A and B subunits were successfully expressed in these cells and their response to cGMP stimulation was demonstrated by electrophysiological recording. Although this cell line is known to be difficult for transfection, the novel DNA nucleofector technology has proven to be effective in this matter. 661 W cell line stably expressing Bcl2 has been generated and used in a number of studies investigating apoptosis in photoreceptors (Crawford et al., 2001; Kanan et al., 2007). The availability of an in vitro model of cone photoreceptor that closely resembles the native setting will facilitate studies of the cone channel and help understand its physiology and any mutation-related pathology.

Acknowledgments This work was supported by the National Institutes of Health (NIH) COBRE grant P20 RR017703, National Eye Institute (NEI) grant EY14052 and a research grant from American Health Assistance Foundation (AHAF). We thank Dr. Muna Naash's support in providing experimental facilities.

References

Castagnet P, Mavlyutov T, Cai Y, Zhong F, Ferreira P (2003) RPGRIP1s with distinct neuronal localization and biochemical properties associate selectively with RanBP2 in amacrine neurons. *Hum Mol Genet* **12**:1847–1863.

Crawford MJ, Krishnamoorthy RR, Rudick VL, Collier RJ, Kapin M, Aggarwal BB, Al-Ubaidi MR, Agarwal N (2001) Bcl-2 overexpression protects photooxidative stress-induced apoptosis of photoreceptor cells via NF-kappaB preservation. *Biochem Biophys Res Commun* **281**: 1304–1312.

Ding XQ, Nour M, Ritter LM, Goldberg AF, Fliesler SJ, Naash MI (2004) The R172W mutation in peripherin/rds causes a cone-rod dystrophy in transgenic mice. *Hum Mol Genet* **13**:2075–2087.

Gerstner A, Zong X, Hofmann F, Biel M (2000) Molecular cloning and functional characterization of a new modulatory cyclic nucleotide-gated channel subunit from mouse retina. *J Neurosci* **20**:1324–1332.

Iversen N, Birkenes B, Torsdalen K, Djurovic S (2005) Electroporation by nucleofector is the best nonviral transfection technique in human endothelial and smooth muscle cells. *Genet Vaccines Ther* **3**:2.

Kanan Y, Moiseyev G, Agarwal N, Ma JX, Al-Ubaidi MR (2007) Light induces programmed cell death by activating multiple independent proteases in a cone photoreceptor cell line. *Invest Ophthalmol Vis Sci* **48**:40–51.

Kaupp UB, Seifert R (2002) Cyclic nucleotide-gated ion channels. *Physiol Rev* **82**:769–824.

Leclere PG, Panjwani A, Docherty R, Berry M, Pizzey J, Tonge DA (2005) Effective gene delivery to adult neurons by a modified form of electroporation. *J Neurosci Methods* **142**:137–143.

Malykhina AP, Qin C, Greenwood-van Meerveld B, Foreman RD, Lupu F, Akbarali HI (2006) Hyperexcitability of convergent colon and bladder dorsal root ganglion neurons after colonic inflammation: mechanism for pelvic organ cross-talk. *Neurogastroenterol Motil* **18**:936–948.

Muller F, Vantler M, Weitz D, Eismann E, Zoche M, Koch KW, Kaupp UB (2001) Ligand sensitivity of the 2 subunit from the bovine cone cGMP-gated channel is modulated by protein kinase C but not by calmodulin. *J Physiol* **532**:399–409.

Peng C, Rich ED, Varnum MD (2004) Subunit configuration of heteromeric cone cyclic nucleotide-gated channels. *Neuron* **42**:401–410.

Peng C, Rich ED, Thor CA, Varnum MD (2003) Functionally important calmodulin-binding sites in both NH2- and COOH-terminal regions of the cone photoreceptor cyclic nucleotide-gated channel CNGB3 subunit. *J Biol Chem* **278**:24617–24623.

Sanvicens N, Gomez-Vicente V, Masip I, Messeguer A, Cotter TG (2004) Oxidative stress-induced apoptosis in retinal photoreceptor cells is mediated by calpains and caspases and blocked by the oxygen radical scavenger CR-6. *J Biol Chem* **279**:39268–39278.

Shammat IM, Gordon SE (1999) Stoichiometry and arrangement of subunits in rod cyclic nucleotide-gated channels. *Neuron* **23**:809–819.

Srinivasan B, Roque CH, Hempstead BL, Al-Ubaidi MR, Roque RS (2004) Microglia-derived pronerve growth factor promotes photoreceptor cell death via p75 neurotrophin receptor. *J Biol Chem* **279**:41839–41845.

Tan E, Ding XQ, Saadi A, Agarwal N, Naash MI, Al-Ubaidi MR (2004) Expression of cone-photoreceptor-specific antigens in a cell line derived from retinal tumors in transgenic mice. *Invest Ophthalmol Vis Sci* **45**:764-768.

Tuohy G, Millington-Ward S, Kenna PF, Humphries P, Farrar GJ (2002) Sensitivity of photoreceptor-derived cell line (661 W) to baculoviral p35, Z-VAD.FMK, and Fas-associated death domain. *Invest Ophthalmol Vis Sci* **43**:3583–3589.

Zheng J, Trudeau MC, Zagotta WN (2002) Rod cyclic nucleotide-gated channels have a stoichiometry of three CNGA1 subunits and one CNGB1 subunit. *Neuron* **36**:891–896.

Zhong H, Molday LL, Molday RS, Yau KW (2002) The heteromeric cyclic nucleotide-gated channel adopts a 3A:1B stoichiometry. *Nature* **420**:193–198.

Phosphorylation of Caveolin-1 in Bovine Rod Outer Segments in vitro by an Endogenous Tyrosine Kinase

Michael H. Elliott and Abboud J. Ghalayini

1 Introduction

Caveolin-1 (Cav-1), the principal protein component of caveolar membrane domains (Glenney, Jr. and Soppet, 1992; Kurzchalia et al., 1992; Rothberg et al., 1992), was originally identified as a major tyrosine phosphoprotein in Rous sarcoma virus (v-Src) transformed cells (Glenney, Jr. and Zokas, 1989). Although Cav-1 can be phosphorylated on several tyrosine residues (Nomura and Fujimoto, 1999; Schlegel et al., 2001), the most well-characterized phosphorylation site on Cav-1 is tyrosine-14, a site specifically recognized by monoclonal antibodies developed to detect this phosphorylated residue (Lee et al., 2000; Nomura and Fujimoto, 1999). Cav-1 was identified as a phosphoprotein over fifteen years ago, yet surprisingly, little is known about the functional significance of Cav-1 tyrosine phosphorylation. Cav-1 is reportedly phosphorylated by several Src family non-receptor tyrosine kinases (Labrecque et al., 2004; Li et al., 1996; Sanguinetti et al., 2003; Sanguinetti and Mastick, 2003) and is phosphorylated following growth factor, insulin, and estrogen stimulation (Kim et al., 2000; Kiss et al., 2005; Lee et al., 2000; Maggi et al., 2002; Mastick et al., 1995; Orlichenko et al., 2006). Importantly, Cav-1 phosphorylation occurs in response to a variety of cellular stresses (Cao et al., 2004; Chen et al., 2005; Sahasrabuddhe et al., 2006; Sanguinetti et al., 2003; Sanguinetti and Mastick, 2003; Volonte et al., 2001) and has been implicated in the regulation of apoptosis (Shajahan et al., 2006).

Cav-1 is expressed in several retinal cell-types including photoreceptors (Boesze-Battaglia et al., 2002; Elliott et al., 2003; Kachi et al., 2001; Nair et al., 2002; Senin et al., 2004), retinal pigment epithelium (Bridges et al., 2001; Mora et al., 2006), and retinal vascular endothelial cells (Feng et al., 1999; Stitt et al., 2000). The protein is specifically enriched in detergent-resistant membranes derived from rod outer segment (ROS) membranes (Elliott et al., 2003; Martin et al., 2005; Nair et al., 2002;

M.H. Elliott
Department of Ophthalmology, University of Oklahoma Health Sciences Center; Dean A. McGee Eye Institute, Oklahoma City, OK 73104, USA, Tel: 405-271-8316, Fax: 405-271-8128
e-mail: michael-elliott@ouhsc.edu

R.E. Anderson et al. (eds.), *Recent Advances in Retinal Degeneration*,
© Springer 2008

Senin et al., 2004) and disk preparations (Boesze-Battaglia et al., 2002). Immuno-cytochemistry suggests that it is more abundant in photoreceptor inner segments (Elliott et al., 2003) and that it is also present in synaptic termini (Kachi et al., 2001; Kim et al., 2006). To date, there is little information regarding Cav-1 phosphorylation in retinal cells and its potential functional significance. In the current study, we investigated the phosphorylation of Cav-1 by an endogenous tyrosine kinase(s) in rod outer segment preparations in vitro.

2 Methods

2.1 Preparation of Bovine ROS, in Vitro Phosphorylation and Inhibition by PP2

Bovine ROS were prepared from retinas on continuous sucrose gradients (25–50%) as previously described (Zimmerman and Godchaux III, 1982) with slight modification (Elliott et al., 2003). Tyrosine-phosphorylated ROS were prepared by incubation in phosphorylation buffer [50mM Tris-HCl (pH 7.4), 100 mM NaCl, 2 mM $MgCl_2$, 1 mM ATP, 1 mM Na_3VO_4] for 30 minutes at 37°C as previously described (Bell et al., 1999; Bell et al., 2000). Control ROS were incubated in the same buffer without ATP. In some experiments, ROS (1 mg/ml) were incubated (30 min; 37°C) with or without PP2 (10 μM), a specific Src kinase family inhibitor prior to addition of ATP.

2.2 Preparation of Detergent-resistant Membranes (DRM) from ROS

Detergent-resistant membranes (DRM) were prepared from bovine ROS using ice-cold 1% Triton X-100 according to a previously described modification (Elliott et al., 2003; Martin et al., 2005) of the method of Seno et al., (2001). The detergent:phospholipid molar ratio under these conditions is ~3:1 (Martin et al., 2005).

2.3 Immunoprecipitation

Immunoprecipitations from solubilized ROS membranes (100–200 μg) were carried out as previously described (Ghalayini et al., 2002) except that the buffer was supplemented with 60 mM octylglucoside to efficiently solubilize Cav-1 (Elliott et al., 2003). Antibodies (1–2 μg) used for immunoprecipitations were: monoclonal anti phosphotyrosine (PY99); polyclonal anti-Cav-1 (N-20); polyclonal anti-c-Src (SRC2) and normal rabbit or mouse IgG to control for non-specific binding. All antibodies were from Santa Cruz Biotechnology, Inc. (Santa Cruz, CA). Immune complexes were recovered by binding to protein A/G-coupled agarose and were washed four times with solubilization buffer prior to elution with reducing SDS-PAGE sample buffer.

2.4 SDS-PAGE and Western Blot Analysis

Proteins were resolved by reducing SDS-PAGE, transferred to PVDF membranes (0.45 μm) and blots were incubated with anti-PY99 (1:500), anti-Cav-1 (1:200), anti-PY14-Cav-1 (1:2500; BD Biosciences, San Jose, CA), or anti-c-Src (1:200) followed by incubation with appropriate HRP-coupled secondary antibody. In some experiments, parallel gels were stained with GelCode Blue staining reagent (Pierce, Rockford, IL) according to the manufacturer's instructions.

3 Results

To determine whether Cav-1 can be phosphorylated by endogenous kinases in ROS, purified ROS membranes were incubated with ATP, followed by immunoprecipitation with several antibodies. As shown in Fig. 1A, Cav-1 phosphorylated on tyrosine-14, was recovered in immunoprecipitates only from ROS membranes incubated with ATP. Phosphorylated Cav-1 migrated as a cluster of distinct bands that may represent different phosphospecies. In other experiments, Cav-1 was also recovered when total tyrosine phosphoproteins were immunoprecipitated with anti-phosphotyrosine (Fig. 1B). Finally, Cav-1 was recovered in anti-c-Src immunoprecipitates in an ATP-independent manner and was found to be phosphorylated on tyrosine-14 only in immune complexes recovered from ROS incubated with ATP (Fig. 1C).

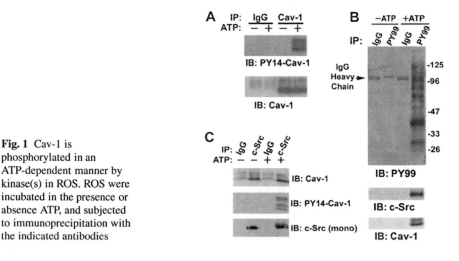

Fig. 1 Cav-1 is phosphorylated in an ATP-dependent manner by kinase(s) in ROS. ROS were incubated in the presence or absence ATP, and subjected to immunoprecipitation with the indicated antibodies

Fig. 2 Cav-1
phosphorylation does not
alter its localization to DRM
fractions. ROS were
incubated in the presence
(right column) or absence
(left column) of 1 mM ATP,
DRM fractions were isolated,
and subjected to immunoblot
analysis with the indicated
antibodies

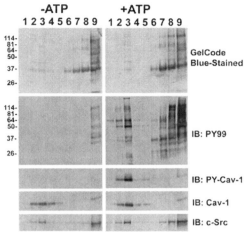

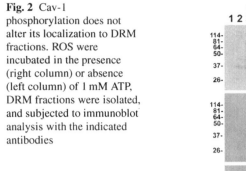

To determine whether Cav-1 phosphorylation affects its partitioning into raft domains, we isolated DRM fractions from ROS incubated with or without ATP. DRM are low buoyant density, membrane fractions resistant to solubilization with some non-ionic detergents and are suggested to represent biochemically-isolated raft domains (Pike, 2004). As indicated in Fig. 2, although DRMs represent a small fraction of the total ROS protein (upper panels), Cav-1 is dramatically-enriched in these fractions (4th panels). Several tyrosine phosphoproteins (including Cav-1, 3rd panel, right column) are detectable in DRM fractions only after ATP incubation. As is apparent, phosphorylation of Cav-1 does not affect its partitioning into DRM fractions (4th panel).

Cav-1 is reportedly phosphorylated by several Src family tyrosine kinases (Labrecque et al., 2004; Li et al., 1996; Sanguinetti et al., 2003; Sanguinetti and Mastick, 2003). In order to investigate a putative role for Src family kinases in the in vitro phosphorylation of Cav-1 in ROS, purified ROS membranes were incubated with the Src selective inhibitor, PP2 (10 μM) prior to their incubation with ATP. As shown, in Fig. 3, PP2 dramatically reduced the tyrosine phosphorylation of

Fig. 3 Cav-1
phosphorylation is reduced
by the Src family kinase
inhibitor PP2. ROS
membranes were incubated
with 10 μM PP2 prior to
addition of 1 mM ATP. Blots
were probed with the
indicated antibodies as
described in the methods
section. Cav-1
phosphorylation is
dramatically reduced in
PP2-treated ROS

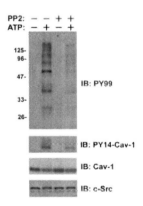

Cav-1 (as well as several other tyrosine phosphoproteins) suggesting that the kinase responsible for Cav-1 phosphorylation in ROS, in vitro, is likely to be a Src family kinase.

4 Discussion

The results presented herein indicate that Cav-1 can be phosphorylated on tyrosine -14 in vitro by an endogenously-expressed Src family kinase in isolated ROS membranes. The conditions that trigger Cav-1 phosphorylation in vivo and the functional consequences resulting from this phosphorylation remain unknown. Light exposure stimulates tyrosine phosphorylation of several protein targets in ROS in vivo (Ghalayini et al., 1998) including the insulin receptor β-subunit (Rajala et al., 2002) and triggers the binding of c-Src to ROS membranes, in vivo (Ghalayini et al., 2002). Our preliminary studies suggest that Cav-1 is not a target of light-dependent phosphorylation (Elliott and Ghalayini, *unpublished results*), but it remains unclear if damaging light or another form of stress could result in Cav-1 phosphorylation in vivo. In other cell-types, Cav-1 is phosphorylated in response to both oxidative and osmotic stresses (Cao et al., 2004; Chen et al., 2005; Sahasrabuddhe et al., 2006; Sanguinetti et al., 2003; Sanguinetti and Mastick, 2003; Volonte et al., 2001) and may regulate the apoptotic response (Shajahan et al., 2006). A possible role of Cav-1 phosphorylation in photoreceptor stress response remains to be elucidated.

Acknowledgments This work was supported by grants from the National Institutes of Health (EY012190, EY005235, EY11504, and RR017703), Research to Prevent Blindness, Inc., and the Foundation Fighting Blindness.

References

Bell, M. W., Alvarez, K., and Ghalayini, A. J., 1999, Association of the tyrosine phosphatase SHP-2 with transducin-alpha and a 97-kDa tyrosine-phosphorylated protein in photoreceptor rod outer segments, *J. Neurochem.* 73:2331.

Bell, M. W., Desai, N., Guo, X. X., and Ghalayini, A. J., 2000, Tyrosine phosphorylation of the alpha subunit of transducin and its association with Src in photoreceptor rod outer segments, *J. Neurochem.* 75:2006.

Boesze-Battaglia, K., Dispoto, J., and Kahoe, M. A., 2002, Association of a photoreceptor-specific tetraspanin protein, ROM-1, with triton X-100-resistant membrane rafts from rod outer segment disk membranes, *J. Biol. Chem.* 277:41843.

Bridges, C. C., El Sherbeny, A., Roon, P., Ola, M. S., Kekuda, R., Ganapathy, V., Camero, R. S., Cameron, P. L., and Smith, S. B., 2001, A comparison of caveolae and caveolin-1 to folate receptor alpha in retina and retinal pigment epithelium, *Histochem. J.* 33:149.

Cao, H., Sanguinetti, A. R., and Mastick, C. C., 2004, Oxidative stress activates both Src-kinases and their negative regulator Csk and induces phosphorylation of two targeting proteins for Csk: caveolin-1 and paxillin, *Exp. Cell Res.* 294:159.

Chen, D. B., Li, S. M., Qian, X. X., Moon, C., and Zheng, J., 2005, Tyrosine phosphorylation of caveolin 1 by oxidative stress is reversible and dependent on the c-src tyrosine kinase but not mitogen-activated protein kinase pathways in placental artery endothelial cells, *Biol. Reprod.* **73**:761.

Elliott, M. H., Fliesler, S. J., and Ghalayini, A. J., 2003, Cholesterol-dependent association of caveolin-1 with the transducin alpha subunit in bovine photoreceptor rod outer segments: disruption by cyclodextrin and guanosine 5'-O-(3-thiotriphosphate), *Biochemistry.* **42**:7892.

Feng, Y., Venema, V. J., Venema, R. C., Tsai, N., Behzadian, M. A., and Caldwell, R. B., 1999, VEGF-induced permeability increase is mediated by caveolae, *Invest Ophthalmol. Vis. Sci.* **40**:157.

Ghalayini, A. J., Desai, N., Smith, K. R., Holbrook, R. M., Elliott, M. H., and Kawakatsu, H., 2002, Light-dependent association of Src with photoreceptor rod outer segment membrane proteins in vivo, *J. Biol. Chem.* **277**:1469.

Ghalayini, A. J., Guo, X. X., Koutz, C. A., and Anderson, R. E., 1998, Light stimulates tyrosine phosphorylation of rat rod outer segments In vivo, *Exp. Eye Res.* **66**:817.

Glenney, J. R., Jr. and Soppet, D., 1992, Sequence and expression of caveolin, a protein component of caveolae plasma membrane domains phosphorylated on tyrosine in Rous sarcoma virus-transformed fibroblasts, *Proc. Natl. Acad. Sci. U. S. A.* **89**:10517.

Glenney, J. R., Jr. and Zokas, L., 1989, Novel tyrosine kinase substrates from Rous sarcoma virus-transformed cells are present in the membrane skeleton, *J. Cell Biol.* **108**:2401.

Kachi, S., Yamazaki, A., and Usukura, J., 2001, Localization of caveolin-1 in photoreceptor synaptic ribbons, *Invest Ophthalmol. Vis. Sci.* **42**:850.

Kim, H., Lee, T., Lee, J., Ahn, M., Moon, C., Wie, M. B., and Shin, T., 2006, Immunohistochemical study of caveolin-1 and -2 in the rat retina, *J. Vet. Sci.* **7**:101.

Kim, Y. N., Wiepz, G. J., Guadarrama, A. G., and Bertics, P. J., 2000, Epidermal growth factor-stimulated tyrosine phosphorylation of caveolin-1. Enhanced caveolin-1 tyrosine phosphorylation following aberrant epidermal growth factor receptor status, *J. Biol. Chem.* **275**:7481.

Kiss, A. L., Turi, A., Mullner, N., Kovacs, E., Botos, E., and Greger, A., 2005, Oestrogen-mediated tyrosine phosphorylation of caveolin-1 and its effect on the oestrogen receptor localisation: an in vivo study, *Mol. Cell Endocrinol.* **245**:128.

Kurzchalia, T. V., Dupree, P., Parton, R. G., Kellner, R., Virta, H., Lehnert, M., and Simons, K., 1992, VIP21, a 21-kD membrane protein is an integral component of trans-Golgi-network-derived transport vesicles, *J. Cell Biol.* **118**:1003.

Labrecque, L., Nyalendo, C., Langlois, S., Durocher, Y., Roghi, C., Murphy, G., Gingras, D., and Beliveau, R., 2004, Src-mediated tyrosine phosphorylation of caveolin-1 induces its association with membrane type 1 matrix metalloproteinase, *J. Biol. Chem.* **279**:52132.

Lee, H., Volonte, D., Galbiati, F., Iyengar, P., Lublin, D. M., Bregman, D. B., Wilson, M. T., Campos-Gonzalez, R., Bouzahzah, B., Pestell, R. G., Scherer, P. E., and Lisanti, M. P., 2000, Constitutive and growth factor-regulated phosphorylation of caveolin-1 occurs at the same site (Tyr-14) in vivo: identification of a c-Src/Cav-1/Grb7 signaling cassette, *Mol. Endocrinol.* **14**:1750.

Li, S., Seitz, R., and Lisanti, M. P., 1996, Phosphorylation of caveolin by src tyrosine kinases. The alpha-isoform of caveolin is selectively phosphorylated by v-Src in vivo, *J. Biol. Chem.* **271**:3863.

Maggi, D., Biedi, C., Segat, D., Barbero, D., Panetta, D., and Cordera, R., 2002, IGF-I induces caveolin 1 tyrosine phosphorylation and translocation in the lipid rafts, *Biochem. Biophys. Res. Commun.* **295**:1085.

Martin, R. E., Elliott, M. H., Brush, R. S., and Anderson, R. E., 2005, Detailed characterization of the lipid composition of detergent-resistant membranes from photoreceptor rod outer segment membranes, *Invest Ophthalmol. Vis. Sci.* **46**:1147.

Mastick, C. C., Brady, M. J., and Saltiel, A. R., 1995, Insulin stimulates the tyrosine phosphorylation of caveolin, *J. Cell Biol.* **129**:1523.

Mora, R. C., Bonilha, V. L., Shin, B. C., Hu, J., Cohen-Gould, L., Bok, D., and Rodriguez-Boulan, E., 2006, Bipolar assembly of caveolae in retinal pigment epithelium, *Am. J. Physiol Cell Physiol.* **290**:C832.

Nair, K. S., Balasubramanian, N., and Slepak, V. Z., 2002, Signal-dependent translocation of transducin, RGS9-1-Gbeta5L complex, and arrestin to detergent-resistant membrane rafts in photoreceptors, *Curr. Biol.* **12**:421.

Nomura, R. and Fujimoto, T., 1999, Tyrosine-phosphorylated caveolin-1: immunolocalization and molecular characterization, *Mol. Biol. Cell.* **10**:975.

Orlichenko, L., Huang, B., Krueger, E., and McNiven, M. A., 2006, Epithelial growth factor-induced phosphorylation of caveolin 1 at tyrosine 14 stimulates caveolae formation in epithelial cells, *J. Biol. Chem.* **281**:4570.

Pike, L. J., 2004, Lipid rafts: heterogeneity on the high seas, *Biochem. J.* **378**:281.

Rajala, R. V., McClellan, M. E., Ash, J. D., and Anderson, R. E., 2002, In vivo regulation of phosphoinositide 3-kinase in retina through light-induced tyrosine phosphorylation of the insulin receptor beta-subunit, *J. Biol. Chem.* **277**:43319.

Rothberg, K. G., Heuser, J. E., Donzell, W. C., Ying, Y. S., Glenney, J. R., and Anderson, R. G., 1992, Caveolin, a protein component of caveolae membrane coats, *Cell.* **68**:673.

Sahasrabuddhe, A. A., Ahmed, N., and Krishnasastry, M. V., 2006, Stress-induced phosphorylation of caveolin-1 and p38, and down-regulation of EGFr and ERK by the dietary lectin jacalin in two human carcinoma cell lines, *Cell Stress. Chaperones.* **11**:135.

Sanguinetti, A. R., Cao, H., and Corley, M. C., 2003, Fyn is required for oxidative- and hyperosmotic-stress-induced tyrosine phosphorylation of caveolin-1, *Biochem. J.* **376**:159.

Sanguinetti, A. R. and Mastick, C. C., 2003, c-Abl is required for oxidative stress-induced phosphorylation of caveolin 1 on tyrosine 14, *Cell Signal.* **15**:289.

Schlegel, A., Arvan, P., and Lisanti, M. P., 2001, Caveolin-1 binding to endoplasmic reticulum membranes and entry into the regulated secretory pathway are regulated by serine phosphorylation. Protein sorting at the level of the endoplasmic reticulum, *J. Biol. Chem.* **276**:4398.

Senin, I. I., Hoppner-Heitmann, D., Polkovnikova, O. O., Churumova, V. A., Tikhomirova, N. K., Philippov, P. P., and Koch, K. W., 2004, Recoverin and rhodopsin kinase activity in detergent-resistant membrane rafts from rod outer segments, *J. Biol. Chem.* **279**:48647.

Seno, K., Kishimoto, M., Abe, M., Higuchi, Y., Mieda, M., Owada, Y., Yoshiyama, W., Liu, H., and Hayashi, F., 2001, Light- and guanosine 5'-3-O-(thio)triphosphate-sensitive localization of a G protein and its effector on detergent-resistant membrane rafts in rod photoreceptor outer segments, *J. Biol. Chem.* **276**:20813.

Shajahan, A. N., Wang, A., Decker, M., Minshall, R. D., Liu, M. C., and Clarke, R., 2006, Caveolin-1 tyrosine phosphorylation enhances paclitaxel-mediated cytotoxicity, *J. Biol. Chem.* **282**:5934.

Stitt, A. W., Burke, G. A., Chen, F., McMullen, C. B., and Vlassara, H., 2000, Advanced glycation end-product receptor interactions on microvascular cells occur within caveolin-rich membrane domains, *FASEB J.* **14**:2390.

Volonte, D., Galbiati, F., Pestell, R. G., and Lisanti, M. P., 2001, Cellular stress induces the tyrosine phosphorylation of caveolin-1 (Tyr(14)) via activation of p38 mitogen-activated protein kinase and c-Src kinase. Evidence for caveolae, the actin cytoskeleton, and focal adhesions as mechanical sensors of osmotic stress, *J. Biol. Chem.* **276**:8094.

Zimmerman, W. F. and Godchaux, W., III, 1982, Preparation and characterization of sealed bovine rod cell outer segments, *Methods Enzymol.* **81**:52.

Regulation of Neurotrophin Expression and Activity in the Retina

Abigail S. Hackam

1 Introduction

Growth factors and their receptors are upregulated during retinal degeneration as an intrinsic tissue response that may protect remaining photoreceptors (Harada et al., 2002; Wen et al., 1995; Yu et al., 2004). Growth factor delivery to animal models of retinal degeneration leads to various degrees of preservation of photoreceptor morphology and function (Chaum, 2003). A major class of neuroprotective growth factors in the retina are the neurotrophins NGF, BDNF, NT3 and NT4/5. Therapeutic use of these molecules is complicated by their ability to activate pro-death as well as pro-survival pathways. Understanding mechanisms that induce neurotrophin upregulation during injury and controlling the cellular response to exogenous growth factors will be essential for taking full advantage of their neuroprotective activity while minimizing deleterious side-effects. This review summarizes the complex regulation of neurotrophin ligands and receptors that together promote neuronal survival.

2 TRK Receptor Activation: The Retinal Expression Paradox

Neurotrophins bind to two types of receptors, the high affinity Trk receptor tyrosine kinases (TrkA, B and C) and the low affinity $p75^{NTR}$ receptor. The neurotrophins have selective binding to the Trk receptors but bind equally well to $p75^{NTR}$. Trk receptors contain a tyrosine kinase intracellular domain, a single-pass transmembrane domain and a large extracellular domain containing three leucine-rich motifs, two cysteine-rich regions and two immunoglobulin-like C2 type domains that bind neurotrophins.

A.S. Hackam
Bascom Palmer Eye Institute, University of Miami Miller School of Medicine, 1638 NW10th Ave., Miami, FL 33136, Tel: 305-547-3723, Fax: 305-547-3658
e-mail: ahackam@med.miami.edu

R.E. Anderson et al. (eds.), *Recent Advances in Retinal Degeneration*,
© Springer 2008

Fig. 1 Major signaling pathways that lead to cell survival or apoptosis upon activation of Trk or p75^{NTR} receptors, respectively. Both receptors induce mitochondrial and nuclear processes. p75^{NTR} can also promote cell survival by regulating NFκB and Akt, and Trk receptors can promote cell death via MAPK and PI3K

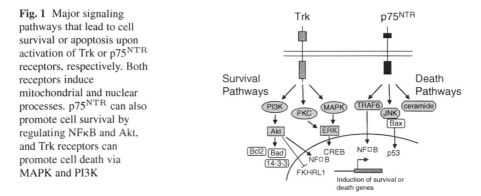

Neurotrophin binding to Trk receptors induces a multitude of signaling cascades that are initiated by phosphorylation-dependent recruitment of adaptor proteins, enzymes and small GTP binding proteins to the receptor complex (Fig. 1). Neurotrophin-dependent survival pathways are primarily mediated by engagement of MAP kinases, PI3 kinase and protein kinase C (PKC) (Kalb, 2005). MAPK and PKC lead to activation of the ERK survival pathway and PI3K activates the pro-survival protein kinase Akt that phosphorylates and inhibits the pro-apoptotic protein Bad. Bad phosphorylation induces association with 14-3-3 proteins and leads to activation of the anti-apoptotic proteins Bcl2 and Bcl$_{XL}$. Trk receptor activation also regulates transcriptional pathways. Akt activates NF-kB pro-survival transcriptional pathways by phosphorylating and promoting the degradation of the inhibitor IkB. Akt-dependent inhibition of the Forkhead transcription factor FKHRL1 blocks transcription of the pro-apoptotic gene FasL, and MAPK activates CREB and induces expression of pro-survival genes. Additionally, Trk activation inhibits the JNK-Bax-p53 pathway and increases expression of inhibitor of apoptosis (IAP) protein.

The ERK and Akt pathways promote cell survival by acting intracellularly in target cells expressing Trk receptors. Paradoxically, retinal injection of BDNF in mice induced transient p-ERK and c-fos expression not in photoreceptors but in Muller glia, RGC and amacrine cells (Wahlin et al., 2000). Further, TrkB receptors are absent from rodent photoreceptors. These findings contributed to the "Muller glia hypothesis" of neuroprotection, in which the protection of photoreceptors proceeds through an intermediate cell type (Harada et al., 2002). TrkB and TrkC are present in adult human photoreceptors (Nag and Wadhwa, 1999), suggesting that direct photoreceptor protection by neurotrophins may play a role in the human retina.

3 Variable Outcomes of Neurotrophin Receptor Activation

The p75^{NTR} receptor is a member of the TNF superfamily and contains extracellular cysteine-rich domains and an intracellular death domain. Engagement of p75^{NTR} by NGF and other neurotrophins induces apoptosis by several routes, including activation of the JNK-p53-Bax pro-death pathway and by increasing levels of the pro-apoptotic molecule ceramide from sphingomyelin hydrolysis (Fig. 1). In some neurons, Trk receptors compete for binding with adaptor proteins to $p75^{NTR}$ and block the apoptotic signal.

$p75^{NTR}$ is expressed primarily in Muller glia and at low levels in RGC. During photoreceptor degeneration in *rd1* mice, $p75^{NTR}$ protein is upregulated in Muller glia and in the ONL (Nakamura et al., 2005). Reducing $p75^{NTR}$ levels by crossing $p75^{NTR}$-/- and $p75^{NTR}$+/- mice with retinal degeneration *rd1* mice did not alter the rate of photoreceptor death (Nakamura et al., 2005). Similarly, Rohrer et al showed that lack of $p75^{NTR}$-/- did not reduce apoptosis from light toxicity (Rohrer et al., 2003). These studies demonstrate that neurotrophin-independent death pathways primarily mediate photoreceptor death in $p75^{NTR}$-/- mice. However, these experiments are complicated by data showing that the $p75^{NTR}$-/- mice express a fragment of $p75^{NTR}$ that could potentially retain death-inducing activity (von Schack et al., 2001). Further, $p75^{NTR}$+/- retinas had reduced light damage (Rohrer et al., 2003) and a $p75^{NTR}$ blocking antibody had a small neuroprotective effect for light damage (Harada et al., 2000), indicating that $p75^{NTR}$ – dependent apoptosis may play a role in the retina.

The pro-death outcome of $p75^{NTR}$ binding depends on the specific interacting adapter proteins and their downstream pathways. $p75^{NTR}$ also promotes neuronal survival in response to neurotrophins by regulating NF-kB, which induces survival or death signals (Kalb, 2005). $p75^{NTR}$ also activates the Akt pro-survival pathway through PI3K signaling (Roux et al., 2001). Unexpectedly, Trk receptors can induce death signals in some situations. For example, cortical neuronal cultures undergo necrosis with BDNF and TrkB activation (Kim et al., 2003), BDNF increases susceptibility to excitotoxicity in spinal cord neurons (Fryer et al., 2000) and medulloblastoma cell lines undergo apoptosis from TrkA receptor activation by NGF (Muragaki et al., 1997). The mechanism of death-promoting Trk signaling may be through activation of MAPK and PI3K pathways. That these pathways also promote survival in some situations illustrates the complexity of the death and survival choices induced by neurotrophins. It will be intriguing to determine whether these non-traditional activities for neurotrophin receptors play a role in the retina.

4 Regulation of Neurotrophin Expression

Neurotrophins are expressed locally in the retina, by Muller glia, microglia and other cells, or are transported retrogradely by RGCs. Retrograde transport of neurotrophins, which is regulated by $p75^{NTR}$, has not been explored during photoreceptor degeneration. At the transcriptional level, the regulation of BDNF is the best described of the neurotrophins and has proven to be very complex. The BDNF gene has four 5' non-coding exons and each exon has its own promoter elements and cell-specific expression patterns. Promoter III has been investigated in detail and contains numerous transcription factor binding elements, including sites for USF1/2, CREB and Brn3c (Timmusk et al., 1993). Since CREB is activated by Trk binding, the regulation of BDNF transcription by CREB suggests positive feedback mechanisms that may sustain the activity of BDNF.

Several signaling networks leading to transcription factor binding to the BDNF promoter have been characterized. For example, neuronal calcium signaling induces BDNF through binding of upstream stimulatory factors (USF) 1 and 2 to Ca^{2+}-responsive E-box elements (Chen et al., 2003), and dopamine-induced transcription involves cAMP/CREB binding. Understanding the regulation of the BDNF promoter in the retina would provide insight into its activity during retinal degeneration.

Neurotrophin release from astrocytes is regulated differentially by signals from adjacent neurons. For example, in basal forebrain astrocyte cultures BDNF transcripts but not NGF are increased by KCl, Ca^{2+} and the muscarinic agonist carbachol, both BDNF and NGF are increased by glutamate, and NT3 is not regulated by any of these stimuli (Wu et al., 2004). In rat Muller glia cultures, glutamate upregulated expression and secretion of all four neurotrophins (Taylor et al., 2003).

In the retina, neurotrophins increase expression of other growth factors, which may influence the efficacy of therapeutic delivery strategies. In rat Muller glia cultures, microglia-derived GDNF and CNTF increased BDNF and bFGF, and BDNF increased CNTF and bFGF levels (Harada et al., 2002). Injection of NGF in retinal degeneration RCS rats induced BDNF, bFGF, TGFβ, VEGF and neuropeptide Y (Lenzi et al., 2005). In contrast, exogenous NGF decreased bFGF expression by activating p75^{NTR} (Harada et al., 2000). Withdrawal of bFGF-mediated survival signals from Muller glia was proposed to contribute to photoreceptor death (Harada et al., 2002). Therefore, protection by neurotrophins may be indirect by inducing the release of additional secreted factors or by stimulating other protective trophic pathways. This effect could amplify the protective response, possibly by recruiting other glia that are not proximal to the injury site.

In our laboratory, we investigate cellular pathways that regulate neurotrophin expression during degeneration. One example is the Wnt pathway, an essential signaling cascade that mediates retinal development and stem cell proliferation and is a critical regulator of cell survival in degenerative conditions of the brain such as Alzheimers disease. Wnt signaling regulates growth factor expression in several tissues, including NT3 in the limb bud (Patapoutian et al., 1999), GDNF during kidney development and TGFβ during adult chondrogenesis (Tuli et al., 2003). The Wnt pathway is active during photoreceptor death in the *rd1* mouse (Yi et al., submitted), suggesting that Wnt signaling may regulate neurotrophin expression and activity during retinal degeneration.

5 Regulation of Receptor Activity

The signaling response to neurotrophin injections in the retina is transient (Wahlin et al., 2001). Cellular mechanisms down-regulate the signal in order to precisely control neurotrophin signaling for the proper time period and in the correct location. One regulatory mechanism is the degradation of Trk receptors through ligand-dependent ubiquitination (Arevalo et al., 2006). p75^{NTR} may regulate the ubiquitination of Trk receptors. Additionally, stimulation of the target cell by cAMP, Ca^{2+} or electrical activity induces exocytosis of intracellular vesicles containing Trk receptors into the plasma membrane (Meyer-Franke et al., 1998). Other sources of regulation include tyrosine phosphatases to terminate the signaling, differential expression of the adaptor proteins and enzymes, membrane sorting of Trk receptors and association with Trk splice variants. How these regulatory mechanisms contribute to the regulation of Trk receptors during retinal degeneration is an important topic that requires further exploration.

6 Conclusions

Over-expression of neurotrophins and other growth factors could elevate the threshold for apoptosis and halt or delay degeneration. Delaying blindness by even a few years would have a meaningful impact on quality of life. Furthermore, delivering a combination of growth factors, or using a factor that upregulates multiple endogenous growth factors, may be a more effective photoreceptor protector than growth factor delivery alone. This improved rescue would be similar to combining BDNF with its TrkB receptor which protected more ganglion cells than BDNF alone (Cheng et al., 2002). Growth factor mediated rescue will be applicable to all photoreceptor degenerations, regardless of the primary cause or genetic mutation. Much effort has focused on the downstream signaling cascades induced by neurotrophins. However, a key question is the identity of the upstream signaling pathways that regulate growth factor expression in Muller glia and other cells. Elucidating the molecular mechanisms and signaling pathways that regulate neurotrophin expression and activity will be important for taking advantage of the therapeutic potential of these important molecules and may lead to the identification of novel treatments.

Acknowledgments Funding was provided by a Research for the Prevention of Blindness Career Development Award, the Karl Kirchgessner Foundation, a Fight for Sight Grant-in-Aid and the International Retina Research Foundation. Institutional support was provided by an unrestricted grant to Bascom Palmer Eye Institute from the Research to Prevent Blindness and an NEI core grant (P30 EY014801).

References

Arevalo J. C., Waite J., Rajagopal R., Beyna M., Chen Z. Y., Lee F. S. and Chao M. V., 2006, Cell survival through Trk neurotrophin receptors is differentially regulated by ubiquitination. *Neuron* **50**, 549–59.
Chaum E., 2003, Retinal neuroprotection by growth factors: a mechanistic perspective. *J Cell Biochem* **88**, 57–75.

Chen W. G., West A. E., Tao X., Corfas G., Szentirmay M. N., Sawadogo M., Vinson C. and Greenberg M. E., 2003, Upstream stimulatory factors are mediators of Ca2+-responsive transcription in neurons. *J Neurosci* **23**, 2572–81.

Cheng L., Sapieha P., Kittlerova P., Hauswirth W. W. and Di Polo A., 2002, TrkB gene transfer protects retinal ganglion cells from axotomy-induced death in vivo. *J Neurosci* **22**, 3977–86.

Fryer H. J., Wolf D. H., Knox R. J., Strittmatter S. M., Pennica D., O'Leary R. M., Russell D. S. and Kalb R. G., 2000, Brain-derived neurotrophic factor induces excitotoxic sensitivity in cultured embryonic rat spinal motor neurons through activation of the phosphatidylinositol 3-kinase pathway. *J Neurochem* **74**, 582–95.

Harada T., Harada C., Kohsaka S., Wada E., Yoshida K., Ohno S., Mamada H., Tanaka K., Parada L. F. and Wada K., 2002, Microglia-Muller glia cell interactions control neurotrophic factor production during light-induced retinal degeneration. *J Neurosci* **22**, 9228–36.

Harada T., Harada C., Nakayama N., Okuyama S., Yoshida K., Kohsaka S., Matsuda H. and Wada K., 2000, Modification of glial-neuronal cell interactions prevents photoreceptor apoptosis during light-induced retinal degeneration. *Neuron* **26**, 533–41.

Kalb R., 2005, The protean actions of neurotrophins and their receptors on the life and death of neurons. *Trends Neurosci* **28**, 5–11.

Kim H. J., Hwang J. J., Behrens M. M., Snider B. J., Choi D. W. and Koh J. Y., 2003, TrkB mediates BDNF-induced potentiation of neuronal necrosis in cortical culture. *Neurobiol Dis* **14**, 110–9.

Lenzi L., Coassin M., Lambiase A., Bonini S., Amendola T. and Aloe L., 2005, Effect of exogenous administration of nerve growth factor in the retina of rats with inherited retinitis pigmentosa. *Vision Res* **45**, 1491–500.

Meyer-Franke A., Wilkinson G. A., Kruttgen A., Hu M., Munro E., Hanson M. G., Jr., Reichardt L. F. and Barres B. A., 1998, Depolarization and cAMP elevation rapidly recruit TrkB to the plasma membrane of CNS neurons. *Neuron* **21**, 681–93.

Muragaki Y., Chou T. T., Kaplan D. R., Trojanowski J. Q. and Lee V. M., 1997, Nerve growth factor induces apoptosis in human medulloblastoma cell lines that express TrkA receptors. *J Neurosci* **17**, 530–42.

Nag T. C. and Wadhwa S., 1999, Neurotrophin receptors (Trk A, Trk B, and Trk C) in the developing and adult human retina. *Brain Res Dev Brain Res* **117**, 179–89.

Nakamura K., Harada C., Okumura A., Namekata K., Mitamura Y., Yoshida K., Ohno S., Yoshida H. and Harada T., 2005, Effect of p75NTR on the regulation of photoreceptor apoptosis in the rd mouse. *Mol Vis* **11**, 1229–35.

Patapoutian A., Backus C., Kispert A. and Reichardt L. F., 1999, Regulation of neurotrophin-3 expression by epithelial-mesenchymal interactions: the role of Wnt factors. *Science* **283**, 1180–83.

Rohrer B., Matthes M. T., LaVail M. M. and Reichardt L. F., 2003, Lack of p75 receptor does not protect photoreceptors from light-induced cell death. *Exp Eye Res* **76**, 125–9.

Roux P. P., Bhakar A. L., Kennedy T. E. and Barker P. A., 2001, The p75 neurotrophin receptor activates Akt (protein kinase B) through a phosphatidylinositol 3-kinase-dependent pathway. *J Biol Chem* **276**, 23097–104.

Taylor S., Srinivasan B., Wordinger R. J. and Roque R. S., 2003, Glutamate stimulates neurotrophin expression in cultured Muller cells. *Brain Res Mol Brain Res* **111**, 189–97.

Timmusk T., Palm K., Metsis M., Reintam T., Paalme V., Saarma M. and Persson H., 1993, Multiple promoters direct tissue-specific expression of the rat BDNF gene. *Neuron* **10**, 475–89.

Tuli R., Tuli S., Nandi S., Huang X., Manner P. A., Hozack W. J., Danielson K. G., Hall D. J. and Tuan R. S., 2003, Transforming growth factor-beta-mediated chondrogenesis of human mesenchymal progenitor cells involves N-cadherin and mitogen-activated protein kinase and Wnt signaling cross-talk. *J Biol Chem* **278**, 41227–36.

von Schack D., Casademunt E., Schweigreiter R., Meyer M., Bibel M. and Dechant G., 2001, Complete ablation of the neurotrophin receptor p75NTR causes defects both in the nervous and the vascular system. *Nat Neurosci* **4**, 977–8.

Wahlin K. J., Adler R., Zack D. J. and Campochiaro P. A., 2001, Neurotrophic signaling in normal and degenerating rodent retinas. *Exp Eye Res* **73**, 693–701.

Wahlin K. J., Campochiaro P. A., Zack D. J. and Adler R., 2000, Neurotrophic factors cause activation of intracellular signaling pathways in Muller cells and other cells of the inner retina, but not photoreceptors. *Invest Ophthalmol Vis Sci* **41**, 927–36.

Wen R., Song Y., Cheng T., Matthes M. T., Yasumura D., LaVail M. M. and Steinberg R. H., 1995, Injury-induced upregulation of bFGF and CNTF mRNAS in the rat retina. *J Neurosci* **15**, 7377–85.

Wu H., Friedman W. J. and Dreyfus C. F., 2004, Differential regulation of neurotrophin expression in basal forebrain astrocytes by neuronal signals. *J Neurosci Res* **76**, 76–85.

Yu D. Y., Cringle S., Valter K., Walsh N., Lee D. and Stone J., 2004, Photoreceptor death, trophic factor expression, retinal oxygen status, and photoreceptor function in the P23H rat. *Invest Ophthalmol Vis Sci* **45**, 2013–19.

Involvement of Guanylate Cyclases in Transport of Photoreceptor Peripheral Membrane Proteins

Sukanya Karan, Jeanne M. Frederick and Wolfgang Baehr

Guanylate cyclase 1 (GC1) is present in mouse rod and cone outer segments while guanylate cyclase 2 (GC2) is present only in rods. Accordingly, deletion of GC1 (gene symbol *Gucy2e*) affects predominantly cones while knockout of GC2 (gene symbol *Gucy2f*) has no major effect on rod and cone physiology since GC1 can substitute for the loss of GC2. Simultaneous inactivation of GC1 and GC2 abolishes rod and cone phototransduction, generating a phenotype affecting viability of both rods and cones, and resembling human Leber Congenital Amaurosis. While studying the GC single and double knockout mice, we observed that GCAP1, GRK1, cone PDE and cone transducin subunits were either severely reduced or absent in GC1-/- cone outer segments, while GCAP1, GCAP2 and rod PDE6 subunits were downregulated and/or absent in GCdko rods. Based on the absence of several peripheral membrane-associated proteins in GC1-/- and GCdko outer segments, we have developed a model in which GCs serve a role in transport of peripheral membrane proteins from the inner segment, where biosynthesis occurs, to the outer segment.

1 Introduction

In photoreceptors, guanylate cyclases are essential components responsible for the production of cGMP, the internal transmitter of phototransduction. In darkness, the cytoplasm of the rod contains high levels of cGMP ($1-10$ μM) maintaining a number of cGMP-gated (CNG) cation channels in an open state. Within milliseconds after a light flash, CNG channels close and photoreceptor cells hyperpolarize. CNG channel closure terminates the influx of cations (mostly Na^+ and Ca^{2+}), while the Na^{2+}, Ca^{2+}/K^+ exchanger (NCKX) continues to extrude Ca^{2+}. The consequence of channel closure and continued NCKX activity is a rapid drop in internal free Ca^{2+}, and formation of Ca^{2+}-free guanylate cyclase-activating proteins (GCAPs)

S. Karan

John A. Moran Eye Center, University of Utah, Salt Lake City, UT 84132, Tel: 801-585-7621, Fax: 801-585-7686

e-mail: sukanyat15@yahoo.com

R.E. Anderson et al. (eds.), *Recent Advances in Retinal Degeneration*,
© Springer 2008

351

which stimulate membrane-bound guanylate cyclases (GC) to accelerate production of cGMP from GTP. This is an important step in the recovery of photoreceptors to the dark state, which requires the re-opening of CNG channels (for a recent review, see Lamb and Pugh, 2006).

2 Guanylate Cyclases and Their Activators, GCAPS

There are two known retina-specific guanylate cyclases in mammals termed GC-E and GC-F in mice (here GC1 and GC2, respectively). GC1 and GC2 cDNA clones were isolated from human retinal cDNA libraries in 1992 and 1995, respectively (Shyjan et al., 1992; Lowe et al., 1995) and recognized to be members of a large guanylate cyclase multigene family. The polypeptides have a size of about 120–124 kDa. The GCs have all features characteristic of a membrane GC – a signal sequence, a large amino-terminal extracellular domain (ECD), a single membrane-spanning region (TM), a kinase-like homology domain (KHD) and a carboxy-terminal catalytic domain (CD). In situ hybridization of each cyclase shows expression in the photoreceptor cell bodies and inner segments (Imanishi et al., 2002). Immunocytochemistry showed GCs to be associated with the rod and cone outer segment disk membranes. GC1 was also detected in the pineal gland, an organ developmentally related to the retina, the olfactory bulb (Duda and Koch, 2002) as well as the cochlear nerve and the organ of Corti (Seebacher et al., 1999). The cyclase catalytic domains are the most conserved regions followed by the kinase-like domains. The extracellular domains have no known function and are the most divergent. The purified membrane cyclases are Ca^{2+} insensitive. Ca^{2+}-sensitivity is mediated by GCAPs.

GCAPs are Ca^{2+}-binding proteins of the calmodulin (CaM) gene superfamily (Palczewski et al., 2004). In the mammalian retina, two GCAPs (GCAP1 and GCAP2) have been identified as part of a complex regulatory system responsive to fluctuating levels of free Ca^{2+}. A third GCAP, GCAP3 is expressed in human and zebrafish retinas, but not in mouse (Imanishi et al., 2002). Immunocytochemistry in bovine and mouse retinas has shown that GCAP1 is present in rods and cones, while GCAP2 is seen nearly exclusively in rods (Baehr et al., 2007). In vitro, Ca^{2+}-free GCAP1 stimulates GC1 while GCAP2 stimulates both GC1 and GC2; both GCAPs are inactive when Ca^{2+} is high (>1 μM). The GCAP polypeptides are typically 175 to 205 amino acids in length, are acidic and contain four EF-hand motifs for Ca^{2+}-binding, three of which are functional (EF2–4). EF-hand motifs consist of a 12 amino acid loop flanked by helical regions (helix-loop-helix configuration).

3 Knockout of GC1

In humans, null mutations in the GC1 gene cause Leber Congenital Amaurosis-type 1 (LCA1), an autosomal recessive, early-onset dystrophy affecting rods and cones (Tucker et al., 2004; Hanein et al., 2004). A naturally occurring retinal degeneration in chicken (*rd* chicken), caused also by a null mutation in the GC1 gene (Semple-Rowland et al., 1998), mimics the human LCA phenotype. GC1-/- mice were generated by the laboratory of David Garbers several years ago by replacing a portion of exon 1 with a *neo* cassette (Yang et al., 1999). Surprisingly, the null mutation in the mouse GC1 gene produced a slowly progressing cone dystrophy, but not a rod/cone dystrophy as observed in LCA. In contrast to cones, the GC1-/- rods remain viable and responsive to light, most likely due to the presence in GC2. The number of cones in 4- and 5-week-old GC1-/- mice gradually decreased by 6 months, forming a from the inferior retinal region with relatively few survivors to the superior region where more cones survived (Coleman et al., 2004).

4 Knockout of GC2

In human, no retina disease has been linked to a mutation in the GC2 gene on the X-chromosome. Since a GC1 null allele in human causes a severe rod/cone dystrophy and GC2 cannot substitute for the loss of GC1, a recessive disease based on a GC2 null allele seems rather unlikely. To elucidate the role of GC2 in the mouse retina, we deleted the GC2 gene by targeted recombination (Baehr et al., 2007). We replaced a portion of exon 2, which contains the translation start codon ATG, by the *neo* cassette, thereby eliminating the peptide leader sequence which is important for translocation of GC2 into the ER, and also a part of the mature N-terminus of GC2. This construct is unable to initiate translation of a GC2 polypeptide. GC2-/- photoreceptors function nearly as well as WT in electroretinography and single rod cell recordings, and retina histology is normal (Baehr et al., 2007).

5 GC Double Knockout Retinas

GC double knockouts (GCdko) mice were generated by crossbreeding GC1-/- and GC2-/- mice (Baehr et al., 2007). The GCdko mice were fertile and developed normally, thereby excluding a vital role for GC1 or GC2 in embryonic development. An immunoblot of GC1-/-, GC2-/- and GCdko retinal lysates using polyclonal antibodies raised against the hinge domain present in both GC1 and GC2 (Tucker et al., 1999) revealed that GC2 is less abundant than GC1 and that both GCs are absent in the GCdko retina (not shown). Further, immunoblots with anti-GC1 and anti-GC2 antibodies showed that the GC1 expression level is maintained in GC2-/- retina, and that the GC2 expression level is also maintained in GC1-/- retina (Baehr et al., 2007). At 2 months of age, outer segment lengths are approximately 50–70% of normal suggesting that degeneration progresses relatively slowly in GCdko mice (Fig. 1). At six months of age, the GCdko ONL contains only four-to-six rows of nuclei, and rod outer segment lengths are severely reduced in superior/inferior and nasal/temporal quadrants.

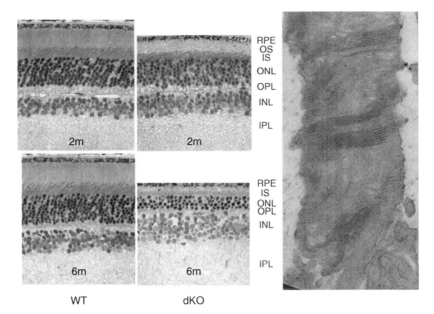

Fig. 1 Left panels, bright-field micrographs showing plastic sections of two-month and six-month old WT and GCdko retinas. Note that OS, IS and ONL layers are severely reduced in the double knockout at 6 months. Right panel, ultrastructure of a pre-degenerate ROS from a one-month old GCdko retina fixed conventionally for electron microscopy. Note the atypical striated appearance which is attributed to regions of electron-dense membrane stacks alternating with regions containing tubular profiles

6 Downregulation of Peripheral Membrane-associated Proteins in GC Double Knockout Photoreceptors

We observed downregulation of GCAP1, GCAP2, and rod PDE subunits in GCdko rods (Fig. 2) while rhodopsin, rod Tα, PrBP/δ (PDEδ), and CNGA1 levels were

Fig. 2 Immunoblots of WT, GC1-/-, GC2-/- and GCdko retina lysates probed with (left panel) anti-rhodopsin, anti-rod Tα, anti-rod PDE, anti-GCAP1, anti-GCAP2 antibodies; (right panel) anti-cone Tα, anti-cone arrestin, and anti-GRK1 antibodies. Internal controls with β-actin demonstrate approximately equal loading levels (Please see the color plate for a color version of this figure.)

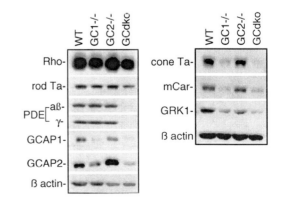

unaffected. Interestingly, rod arrestin protein levels were elevated relative to WT. The downregulations of GCAPs and PDE in double knockout retinas are likely post-translational since *Guca1a* (encoding GCAP1), *Guca1b* (encoding GCAP2), *and Pde6a* (encoding PDE6-α subunit) RNA concentrations in WT and GCdko are identical, as evidenced by semiquantitative real-time RT/PCR (Baehr et al., 2007). Independent microarray analysis confirmed that RNA levels of these and other photo-transduction genes are unchanged (results not shown). In GC1-/- and GCdko cones, myristoylated cone Tα, farnesylated cone Tγ, geranylgeranylated cone PDEα', and farnesylated GRK1 were undetectable by immunocytochemical analysis (not shown).

The posttranslational downregulation of these proteins could result from several mechanisms, including proteolytic degradation, protein instability, cGMP dependence, and/or lack of vesicular transport. Concerning proteolytic degradation, GCAPs have been shown to be susceptible to proteolysis in low free Ca^{2+} in vitro (Rudnicka-Nawrot et al., 1998), conditions presumed to be predominant in the GCdko and GC1-/- photoreceptor cells where cation channels are closed. In the Ca^{2+}-bound form, GCAPs assume a compact conformation which is resistant to proteolysis, whereas in the Ca^{2+}-free form, GCAPs open up and become accessible to proteases. Thus, proteolytic degradation of GCAPs in low [Ca^{2+}] could provide a mechanism for GCAP downregulation. However, transducin and PDE subunits are Ca^{2+} insensitive and do not change their conformation depending on Ca^{2+}. PDE subunits can be expressed stably (although inactive) in tissue culture in the absence of GC, Ca^{2+}, or cGMP (Qin and Baehr, 1994). It seems unlikely that low occupation of non-catalytic cGMP binding sites (GAF domains) (Mou and Cote, 2001) present on catalytic subunits influences PDE stability. However, we cannot exclude a functional deficit of an unidentified cGMP-dependent pathway essential for protein stabilization.

7 GCS and Rhodopsin as Key Molecules in Vesicular Transport

Common to all "destabilized" proteins (GCAPs, rod PDE) or proteins absent from cone outer segments (cone Tα, cone Tγ, GRK1, cone PDEα') is their membrane association, either directly via prenyl or acyl anchors (PDE subunits, GRK1) or indirectly by interaction with integral membrane proteins (GCAPs and GCs). Since membrane-associated proteins are firmly bound to the membrane surface and do not diffuse, they must be transported to the ROS post-synthesis. To explain down-regulation, we therefore favor a model in which vesicular transport of peripher-ally membrane-associated PDE subunits and GC-associated GCAPs is impaired in GC1-/- and GCdko photoreceptors. Failure of transport of essential outer seg-ment proteins disrupts phototransduction, renders outer segments non-functional and labile. Presumably, ER-associated proteins that are not competent for vesicular transport are eventually degraded by the ER quality control machinery, a mecha-nism similar to that degrading mutant or misfolded integral membrane proteins that cannot exit the ER (Frederick et al., 2001).

8 Transport of Rhodopsin and GCS in Rods

In mouse retina, photoreceptors are postmitotic after PN7 and renew their entire outer segments roughly every ten days. This high turnover requires very active biosynthesis and transport of transmembrane and membrane-associated proteins from the ribosomes and endoplasmic reticulum to the outer segment. Transport of the GPCR, rhodopsin (R), consists of several steps – including budding of vesicular R transport carriers (RTCs) from the trans-Golgi network (TGN), vectorial translocation of RTCs through the inner segment, fusion of the RTCs with the plasma membrane near the cilium and transport of R through the cilium to the outer segment. Mechanistic details of these steps are complex and not fully elucidated. However, it is obvious that R is essential for ROS morphogenesis, since R-/- mice (Lem et al., 1999; Humphries et al., 1997) and mice expressing misfolded mutant rhodopsin on a R-/- background (Frederick et al., 2001) do not form ROS. Expression of R (McNally et al., 1999), but not of C-terminally truncated R (Concepcion et al., 2002), restores ROS formation. The truncation removes a C-terminal sorting motif of rhodopsin (VXPX) which regulates budding of rhodopsin transport carriers (RTCs) from the TGN (Deretic, 1998; Deretic et al., 2005). The VXPX motif is recognized by Arf4, a small GTPase which regulates incorporation of R into RTCs (Deretic et al., 2005). Once fused with the plasma membrane, R transport is mediated by heterotrimeric kinesin II, a motor powering intraflagellar transport (IFT). A *Cre-loxP* knockout of the KIF3A subunit of kinesin II resulted in accumulation of opsin, arrestin, and membranes within the photoreceptor inner segment, and prevented transport of R through the cilium (Marszalek et al., 2000).

In polarized epithelial Madin-Darby canine kidney (MDCK) cells, the R C-terminal was shown to interact with TcTex-1, a component of the 1.2 MDa dynein motor complex, which transports cargo towards the minus end of microtubules (Tai et al., 1999). Tctex-1 elimination failed to transport R to the apical surface of MDCK cells (Tai et al., 2001). However, the delivery of R to the ROS is unchanged in the presence of microtubule (MT) depolymerizing agents in explanted *Xenopus* eyecups (Vaughan et al., 1989), and therefore the significance of MT-dependent transport of R in vivo is somewhat controversial.

Our results suggest a role for GC1 and GC2 in protein trafficking pathways, analogous to the role played by rhodopsin, but with important differences. Knockout of GCs does not affect the rhodopsin transport pathway since rhodopsin is found at near normal levels in GCdko ROS. Therefore, GC transport and rhodopsin transport in rods must occur independently. Knockout of rhodopsin, on the other hand, prevents ROS formation and affects all other rod transport pathways, assigning a key regulatory role for intracellular transport to rhodopsin. Deletion of one GC does not affect transport of PDE subunits in rods, but deletion of both GCs prevents transport entirely and leads to PDE degradation as evidenced by an absence of PDE signal on immunoblots (Fig. 2). A similar downregulation of PDE subunits was reported in transgenic mouse retinas expressing cone $T\alpha$(Q204L) and rod $T\alpha$(Q200L), mutants deficient in GTPase activity (Raport et al., 1994; Kerov et al., 2005). One probable interpretation is that these mutants do not associate effectively with transport carriers and/or impede transport of PDE subunits.

9 Model of Protein Transport in Cones

Cones, a small minority (3–5%) among mouse photoreceptors, express distinct sets of genes encoding cone-specific pigments, cone $T\alpha$, cone PDE (PDEα') and distinct channel subunits (CNGA3, CNGB3). Little is known regarding the transport of newly synthesized cone phototransduction proteins. Our results suggest that separate pathways have evolved in rods and cones for transport of membrane proteins to the outer segment due to the following: First, knockout of GC1, the only GC present in cone outer segments, affects S-cone and M/L-cone pigments, but not rhodopsin. Cone pigments are either missing from the GC1-/- COS or are mislocalized in vesicles that appear detached from the cone inner segments while the distribution of rhodopsin in GC1-/- and GCdko rod outer segments is normal. Second, cone $T\alpha$ and cone $T\gamma$ were undetected in GC1-/- cone outer segments while rod $T\alpha$ and rod $T\gamma$ distributed normally in GC1-/- and GCdko rods. Thus, rod transducin localizes to ROS independently of GC transport, while the appearance of cone transducin in cone outer segments depends on presence of GC, perhaps reflecting tighter membrane association of cone $T\alpha$. Tight membrane association of cone $T\alpha$ provides a possible explanation for lack of light-induced translocation in WT mice (Coleman and Semple-Rowland, 2005; Elias et al., 2004).

We conclude that, following biosynthesis, distinct pathways have evolved for transport of membrane proteins from the inner to the outer segment. GC1 deletions have the most profound effect on structure and function of cone outer segments. Transmembrane proteins such as GC1 are synthesized on ER-associated ribosomes, exported to the Golgi and assembled into transport carriers which are moved along microtubules with molecular motors (e.g., dynein-1) (Rosenbaum and Witman, 2002). We envision that GCAP1 is biosynthesized as a cytosolic protein and associates with GC1 soon after emerging from the TGN, embedded in vesicles. Most likely GC1 has a C-terminal sorting signal similar to that observed for rhodopsin. GRK1 and PDE catalytic subunits are prenylated proteins, and are ER-associated during C-terminal processing (cleavage of C-aaX and carboxymethylation). Prenylated proteins may be delivered to the transport carrier by prenyl binding proteins like PrBP/δ (PDEδ) where they are anchored in the membrane. Such a delivery pathway is supported by the phenotype of a PrBP(PDEδ) knockout, in which GC1 and GCAP1 are present in mutant cone outer segments, but prenylated GRK1 and PDEα' are at very low levels (Zhang et al., 2007). The transport carrier delivers its cargo to the distal end of the inner segment for intraflagellar transport through the connecting cilium. A transport defect arises when the integral membrane protein is not produced (e.g., GC1 null mutations), but not when a peripheral protein is absent.

In summary, the particulate GCs have roles in transport of peripherally membrane-associated proteins to the rod and cone outer segments in addition to their enzymatic activities. In the absence of GC1, associated proteins (GCAP1, cone transducin, cone PDE and GRK1) fail to transport to cone outer segments and are subsequently downregulated.

References

Baehr, W., Karan, S., Maeda, T., Luo, D. G., Li, S., Bronson, J. D., Watt, C. B., Yau, K.-W., Frederick J. M., and Palczewski, K., 2007, The function of Guanylate Cyclase 1 (GC1) and Guanylate Cyclase 2 (GC2) in rod and cone photoreceptors, *J. Biol. Chem.* **282**:8837–8847.

Coleman, J. E., Zhang, Y., Brown, G. A., and Semple-Rowland, S. L., 2004, Cone cell survival and downregulation of GCAP1 protein in the retinas of GC1 knockout mice, *Invest Ophthalmol. Vis. Sci.* **45**:3397–3403.

Coleman, J. E., and Semple-Rowland, S. L., 2005, GC1 deletion prevents light-dependent arrestin translocation in mouse cone photoreceptor cells, *Invest Ophthalmol. Vis. Sci.* **46**:12–16.

Concepcion, F., Mendez, A., and Chen, J., 2002, The carboxyl-terminal domain is essential for rhodopsin transport in rod photoreceptors, *Vision Res.* **42**:417–426.

Deretic, D., 1998, Post-Golgi trafficking of rhodopsin in retinal photoreceptors *Eye* **12 (Pt 3b):** 526–530.

Deretic, D., Williams, A. H., Ransom, N., Morel, V., Hargrave, P. A., and Arendt, A., 2005, Rhodopsin C terminus, the site of mutations causing retinal disease, regulates trafficking by binding to ADP-ribosylation factor 4 (ARF4), *Proc. Natl. Acad. Sci U.S.A.* **102**:3301–3306.

Duda, T., and Koch, K. W., 2002, Calcium-modulated membrane guanylate cyclase in synaptic transmission? *Mol. Cell Biochem.* **230**:107–116.

Elias, R. V., Sezate, S. S., Cao, W., and McGinnis, J. F., 2004, Temporal kinetics of the light/dark translocation and compartmentation of arrestin and alpha-transducin in mouse photoreceptor cells, *Mol. Vis.* **10**:672–681.

Frederick, J. M., Krasnoperova, N. V., Hoffmann, K., Church-Kopish, J., Ruether, K., Howes, K. A., Lem, J., and Baehr, W., 2001, A P23H-containing mutant rhodopsin transgene expressed on a null background forms a non-functional, cytotoxic product and accelerates retinal degeneration, *Invest Ophthalmol. Vis. Sci.* **42**:826–833.

Hanein, S., Perrault, I., Gerber, S., Tanguy, G., Barbet, F., Ducroq, D., Calvas, P., Dollfus, H., Hamel, C., Lopponen, T., Munier, F., Santos, L., Shalev, S., Zafeiriou, D., Dufier, J. L., Munnich, A., Rozet, J. M., and Kaplan, J., 2004, Leber congenital amaurosis: comprehensive survey of the genetic heterogeneity, refinement of the clinical definition, and genotype-phenotype correlations as a strategy for molecular diagnosis, *Hum. Mutat.* **23**:306–317.

Humphries, M. M., Rancourt, D., Farrar, G. J., Kenna, P., Hazel, M., Bush, R. A., Sieving, P. A., Sheils, D. M., McNally, N., Creighton, P., Erven, A., Boros, A., Gulya, K., Capecchi, M. R., and Humphries, P., 1997, Retinopathy induced in mice by targeted disruption of the rhodopsin gene. *Nature Genet.* **15**:216–219.

Imanishi, Y., Li, N., Sowa, M. E., Lichtarge, O., Wensel, T. G., Saperstein, D. A., Baehr, W., and Palczewski, K., 2002, Characterization of retinal guanylate cyclase-activating protein 3 (GCAP3) from zebrafish to man, *Eur. J. Neurosci.* **15**:63–78.

Kerov, V., Chen, D., Moussaif, M., Chen, Y. J., Chen, C. K., and Artemyev, N. O., 2005, Transducin activation state controls its light-dependent translocation in rod photoreceptors, *J. Biol. Chem.* **280**:41069–41076.

Lamb, T. D., and Pugh, E. N. Jr., 2006, Phototransduction, dark adaptation, and rhodopsin regeneration the proctor lecture, *Invest Ophthalmol. Vis. Sci.* **47**:5138–5152.

Lem, J., Krasnoperova, N. V., Calvert, P. D., Kosaras, B., Cameron, D. A., Nicol. O, M., Makino, C. L., and Sidman, R. L., 1999, Morphological, physiological, and biochemical changes in rhodopsin knockout mice, *Proc. Natl. Acad. Sci. U.S.A.* **96**:736–741.

Lowe, D. G., Dizhoor, A. M., Liu, K., Gu, Q., Spencer, M., Laura, R., Lu, L., and. Hurley, J. B., 1995, Cloning and expression of a second photoreceptor-specific membrane retina guanylyl cyclase (RetGC), RetGC-2, *Proc. Natl. Acad. Sci. U.S.A.* **92:**5535–5539.

Marszalek, J. R., Liu, X., Roberts, E. A., Chui, D., Marth, J. D., Williams, D. S., and Goldstein, L. S., 2000, Genetic evidence for selective transport of opsin and arrestin by kinesin-II in mammalian photoreceptors, *Cell.* **102:**175–187.

McNally, N., Kenna, P., Humphries, M. M., Hobson, A. H., Khan, N. W., Bush, R. A., Sieving, P. A., Humphries, P., and Farrar, G. J., 1999, Structural and functional rescue of murine rod photoreceptors by human rhodopsin transgene, *Hum. Mol. Genet.* **8:** 1309–1312.

Mou, H., and Cote, R. H., 2001, The catalytic and GAF domains of the rod cGMP phosphodiesterase (PDE6) heterodimer are regulated by distinct regions of its inhibitory gamma subunit, *J Biol. Chem.* **276:**27527–27534.

Palczewski, K., Sokal, I., and Baehr, W., 2004, Guanylate cyclase-activating proteins: structure, function, and diversity, *Biochem. Biophys. Res. Commun.* **322:**1123–1130.

Qin, N., and Baehr, W., 1994, Expression and mutagenesis of mouse rod photoreceptor cGMP phosphodiesterase, *J. Biol. Chem.* **269:**3265–3271.

Raport, C. J., Lem, J., Makino, C., Chen, C.-K., Fitch, C. L., Hobson, A., Baylor, D., Simon, M. I., and Hurley, J. B., 1994, Downregulation of cGMP phosphodiesterase induced by expression of GTPase-deficient cone transducin in mouse rod photoreceptors, *Invest. Ophthalmol. Vis. Sci.* **35:** 2932–2947.

Rosenbaum, J. L., and Witman, G. B., 2002, Intraflagellar transport, *Nat. Rev. Mol. Cell Biol.* **3:**813–825.

Rudnicka-Nawrot, M., Surgucheva, I., Hulmes, J. D., Haeseleer, F., Sokal, I., Crabb, J. W., Baehr, W., and Palczewski, K., 1998, Changes in biological activity and folding of guanylate cyclase-activating protein 1 as a function of calcium, *Biochemistry* **37:**248–257.

Seebacher, T., Beitz, E., Kumagami, H., Wild, K., Ruppersberg, J. P., and Schultz, J. E., 1999, Expression of membrane-bound and cytosolic guanylyl cyclases in the rat inner ear, *Hear. Res.* **127:**95–102.

Semple-Rowland, S. L., Lee, N. R., Van Hooser, J. P., Palczewski, K., and Baehr, W., 1998, A null mutation in the photoreceptor guanylate cyclase gene causes the retinal degeneration chicken phenotype, *Proc. Natl. Acad. Sci. U.S.A.* **95:**1271–1276.

Shyjan, A. W., de Sauvage, F. J., Gillett, N. A., Goeddel, D. V., and Lowe, D. G., 1992, Molecular cloning of a retina-specific membrane guanylyl cyclase, *Neuron.* **9:**727–737.

Tucker, C. L., Ramamurthy, V., Pina, A. L., Loyer, M., Dharmaraj, S., Li, Y., Maumenee, I. H., Hurley, J. B., and Koenekoop, R. K., 2004, Functional analyses of mutant recessive GUCY2D alleles identified in Leber congenital amaurosis patients: protein domain comparisons and dominant negative effects, *Mol. Vis.* **10:**297–303.

Tai, A. W., Chuang, J. Z., Bode, C., Wolfrum, U., and Sung, C. H., 1999, Rhodopsin's carboxy-terminal cytoplasmic tail acts as a membrane receptor for cytoplasmic dynein by binding to the dynein light chain Tctex-1, *Cell.* **97:**877–887.

Tai, A. W., Chuang, J. Z., Sung, C. H., 2001, Cytoplasmic dynein regulation by subunit heterogeneity and its role in apical transport, *J. Cell Biol.* **153:**1499–1509.

Tucker, C. L., Woodcock, S. C., Kelsell, R. E., Ramamurthy, V., Hunt, D. M., and Hurley, J. B., 1999, Biochemical analysis of a dimerization domain mutation in RetGC-1 associated with dominant cone-rod dystrophy, *Proc. Natl. Acad. Sci. U.S.A.* **96:**9039–9044 .

Vaughan, D. K., Fisher, S. K., Bernstein, S. A., Hale, I. L., Linberg, K. A., Matsumoto, B., 1989, Evidence that microtubules do not mediate opsin vesicle transport in photoreceptors, *J. Cell Biol.* **109:**3053–3062.

Yang, R. B., Robinson, S. W., Xiong, W. H., Yau, K. W., Birch, D. G., and Garbers, D. L., 1999, Disruption of a retinal guanylyl cyclase gene leads to cone-specific dystrophy and paradoxical rod behavior, *J. Neurosci.* **19:**5889–5897.

Zhang, H., Li, S., Doan, T., Rieke, F., Detwiler, P. B., Frederick, J. M., and Baehr, W., 2007, Deletion of PrBP/{delta} impedes transport of GRK1 and PDE6 catalytic subunits to photoreceptor outer segments, *Proc. Natl. Acad. Sci U.S.A.* **104:** 8857–8862.

Rod Progenitor Cells in the Mature Zebrafish Retina

Ann C. Morris, Tamera Scholz, and James M. Fadool

1 Introduction

In mammals, neuronal cell death during retinal degenerative diseases or following acute retinal injury often leads to irreversible visual impairment because, as is true for most regions of the adult central nervous system, the mammalian retina harbors little capacity for regeneration. In contrast, the neural retinas of urodele amphibians and teleost fishes show remarkable regenerative ability in response to many types of experimental damage. In teleost fishes, retinal regeneration is mediated in part by the proliferation of a specialized population of cells called the rod progenitor cells. These cells possess some of the properties characteristic of transit amplifying cells, such as steady-state proliferation and a commitment to the rod photoreceptor cell fate. However, these cells are also able to respond to rod photoreceptor damage by increasing their rate of proliferation. Therefore, an understanding of the signals that induce rod progenitor cells to proliferate and differentiate following retinal damage may help us to understand the barriers to photoreceptor regeneration in higher vertebrate organisms.

Although it has been many years since the discovery that rod progenitor cells are a source for new neurons in the regenerating fish retina, the in vivo factors that regulate rod progenitor proliferation and differentiation, as well as the source of the proliferative cues, remain poorly defined. This chapter will review the phenomena of persistent and injury-induced neurogenesis in the zebrafish retina, with particular emphasis on the role of rod progenitor cells, and will describe a new genetic model that should further our understanding of the regulation of rod progenitor proliferation.

A.C. Morris
Department of Biological Science, Florida State University, Tallahassee, Florida, 32306,
Tel: 850-644-5420, Fax: 850-644-0989
e-mail:amorris@bio.fsu.edu

R.E. Anderson et al. (eds.), *Recent Advances in Retinal Degeneration,*
© Springer 2008

2 Barriers to Retinal Regeneration in Mammals

Neuronal degeneration associated with ocular diseases such as retinitis pigmentosa, macular degeneration, and retinal detachment is a significant cause of visual impairment and blindness. In recent years, there has been tremendous interest in the potential of neural stem/progenitor cells to repopulate the damaged retina and/or to rescue degenerating retinal neurons. This interest has been sparked both by the discovery of putative neural stem/progenitor cells in the adult mammalian eye (Ahmad et al., 2000; Haruta et al., 2001; Tropepe et al., 2000), and by the demonstration that neural stem/progenitor cells isolated from adult ocular tissues could be incorporated into the retina upon transplantation and could express proteins consistent with their laminar position (Ahmad et al., 2000; Tropepe et al., 2000; Chacko et al., 2003). Recent work indicates that newly post-mitotic rod progenitor cells isolated from the post-natal mouse retina are able to integrate more effectively than stem cells upon transplantation, suggesting that the ontogenetic state of transplanted cells is critical for their successful incorporation into the degenerating retina (MacLaren et al., 2006). While these results are very exciting, several basic developmental questions remain: What are the intrinsic and extrinsic properties of neural progenitor cells in the eye? How do environmental signals direct migration and differentiation of these cells? Can the intrinsic and extrinsic properties be manipulated to direct neural replacement? The retinas of teleost fish have long been known to possess the capacity to regenerate following injury, owing to the presence of two distinct populations of stem/progenitor cells in the adult visual system. Therefore, the teleost retina represents a valuable model system in which to study the mechanisms of neural stem/progenitor proliferation, differentiation, and neuronal regeneration.

3 The Anatomy of the Zebrafish Retina

Like most classes of extant vertebrates, the zebrafish retina is composed of seven major cell types (six classes of neurons and one glial cell type) organized into three nuclear layers (the ganglion cell, inner, and outer nuclear layers) and two synaptic layers (the inner and outer plexiform layers). However, this simplified view grossly understates that true diversity of neuronal types that contribute to the complex circuitry of the vertebrate retina. Unlike rodents, the zebrafish is diurnal and its retina contains a large number of diverse cone subtypes in addition to rod photoreceptors [reviewed in Morris and Fadool (2005)]. The cones are subdivided into four classes based upon spectral sensitivity and morphology (Raymond et al., 1993; Robinson et al., 1993.) The four cone subtypes are stereotypically tiered within the outer nuclear layer. Just below the level of the cone nuclei, the rod cell bodies reside closest to the outer plexiform layer. In the tangential plane, the cone and rod photoreceptors form a highly ordered mosaic that serves to ensure an even sampling of the visual field (Robinson et al., 1993; Fadool, 2003.) One of our goals is to make use of this highly ordered spatial arrangement as a model to explore the importance of cell-cell interactions during normal retinal development and in retinal dystrophies.

4 Persistent Neurogenesis in the Teleost Retina

Zebrafish, similar to many teleost fish and amphibians, continue to grow throughout their life, and the increase in body size is matched by an increase in the size of the eye and the area of the retina [reviewed in Hitchcock et al. (2004), Fadool (2003)]. As the animal grows, enlargement of retinal area is accomplished by two mechanisms. First, new retinal neurons are added to the existing retina from a population of mitotic progenitor cells that reside in a specialized region termed the circumferential germinal zone (CGZ), at the junction between the neural retina and the iris epithelium (Fig. 1). The newly differentiated retinal neurons at the retinal periphery are integrated into the existing retina in an annular fashion (Fadool, 2003; Otteson and Hitchcock, 2003).

The second mechanism of retinal growth in teleost fish involves the gradual stretching of the existing retina within the expanding optic cup in a balloon-like manner (Fadool, 2003; Otteson and Hitchcock, 2003). This results in a corresponding reduction in the packing density of the retinal neurons. While visual acuity is

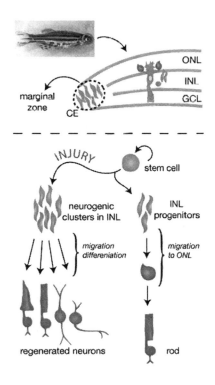

Fig. 1 Persistent neurogenesis in the teeost retina and injury-induced regeneration

preserved through an increase in the size of the retinal image (proportional to the increase in size of the eye), visual sensitivity must be maintained by the addition of new rod photoreceptors in the central retina. These rod photoreceptors are generated from another population of mitotically active neural progenitors, the rod progenitor cells.

Rod progenitor cells were first described over 20 years ago in the goldfish and cichlid retina (Johns and Fernald, 1981; Johns, 1982; Sandy and Blaxter, 1980), and have since been observed in numerous species of teleost fish (Otteson and Hitchcock, 2003). These germinal cells are interspersed throughout the outer nuclear layer, positioned at the level of the rod photoreceptor nuclei. Labeling experiments with various markers of mitotic activity have demonstrated that rod progenitors are actively dividing cells which also produce daughter cells that go on to differentiate into retinal neurons (Johns and Fernald, 1981; Johns, 1982). As their name implies, the differentiated progeny of the rod progenitors are normally only rod photorecep-tors. It was formerly thought that rod progenitors were also capable of producing multiple retinal cell types in response to retinal damage (see below). This view has been revised in light of more recent work suggesting that stem cells of the inner nuclear layer (INL) are the source for new neurons in the regenerating retina (Wu et al., 2001; Yurco and Cameron, 2005; Fausett and Goldman, 2006). The rod pro-genitors themselves appear to arise from a population of more slowly dividing cells in the INL (Julian et al., 1998; Otteson et al., 2001). These rounded, stationary cells give rise to radially arranged, fusiform-shaped cells that appear to migrate from the INL to the outer nuclear layer (ONL) where they develop into the rod progenitors (Fig. 1). Furthermore, the proliferative cells of the INL express Pax6, a marker of retinal progenitor cells, whereas the rod progenitor cells are Pax6-negative (Otteson et al., 2001; Hitchcock et al., 1996). Therefore, the slowly-dividing INL cells have been suggested to be the true neuronal stem cells of the retina that in the intact retina give rise to the cells of the rod lineage, whereas the rod progenitor may be thought of as a transit amplifying cell. However, as with the rod progenitor cells, the putative INL stem cells have not been purified or propagated in vitro, preventing a thorough examination of their developmental potential.

As mentioned above, the mechanisms that regulate the proliferative capacity of rod progenitor cells are poorly understood. Because the generation of new rods is associated with the continued growth of the animal, it is not surprising that stimu-lation of the growth hormone/IGF-I signaling pathway induces an increase in rod progenitor proliferation (Mack et al., 1995; Otteson et al., 2002; Zygar et al., 2005). However, IGF-I regulation of rod progenitor cells has not yet been demonstrated in vivo. Recently, expression of the bHLH transcription factor NeuroD was demon-strated in the rod progenitors and putative INL stem cells of the adult goldfish and larval zebrafish retina (Hitchcock et al., 2004; Hitchcock and Kakuk-Atkins, 2004; Ochocinska and Hitchcock, 2007). However, not all of the rod progenitor cells were positive for NeuroD expression, so it may not be a ubiquitous marker of rod pro-genitors, nor is it known whether NeuroD plays a role in regulating rod progenitor proliferation or differentiation.

5 Retinal Regeneration in Fish

The ability of the retina of teleost fish to regenerate following injury has been known for over 30 years [reviewed in Fadool (2003), Otteson and Hitchcock (2003)]. Numerous methods have been used to damage retinal neurons in fish, including surgical excision of a portion of the retina (Yurco and Cameron, 2005; Cameron, 2000; Cameron et al., 2005), cytotoxic destruction with chemicals such as ouabain, tunicamycin, or 6-hydroxydopamine (Raymond et al., 1988; Negishi et al., 1991; Braisted and Raymond, 1993; Braisted and Raymond, 1992), laser ablation (Wu et al., 2001; Braisted et al., 1994), phototoxicity (Vihtelic and Hyde, 2000; Vihtelic et al., 2005) and heat lesioning (Raymond et al., 2006). In each experimental paradigm, the damaged retina regenerates within several days to weeks. While these studies were able to demonstrate regeneration of retinal neurons, it should be recognized that the reintegration of these neurons into the existing retinal circuitry, as well as the functionality of the newly generated neurons, has not been fully examined. In fact, in many cases, regenerated photoreceptors fail to reform a correctly patterned mosaic (Braisted et al., 1994; Vihtelic and Hyde, 2000; Raymond et al., 2006) .

While some experimental methods for injuring retinal neurons cause more damage than others – for example, ouabain destroys all retinal neurons whereas photodamage kills only the rod and cone photoreceptors – generation of new retinal neurons appears in many cases to involve an increase in proliferation of the rod progenitor cells (Raymond et al., 1988; Negishi et al., 1991; Braisted and Raymond, 1993; Braisted and Raymond, 1992; Vihtelic and Hyde, 2000; Hitchcock et al., 1992). This originally led to the hypothesis that the rod progenitors are the primary source of regenerating retinal neurons. However, this view has recently been challenged by work indicating that Muller cells respond to retinal damage by proliferating and producing the INL stem cells (Wu et al., 2001; Yurco and Cameron, 2005; Fausett and Goldman, 2006). It is possible that both the INL stem cells and the rod progenitor cells can serve as sources of regenerating retinal neurons and the choice of cell population depends on the extent of damage (see below).

Just as we know little about the regulation of rod progenitor proliferation in the intact fish retina, our knowledge of the factors that regulate the increase in rod progenitor proliferation in the regenerating retina is correspondingly thin. It has been shown that some of the genes, such as the *Notch* and *Delta* genes, *N-cadherin*, *rx1*, and *vsx2*, that are expressed during embryonic development of the retina, are also expressed during regeneration of photoreceptors in the goldfish and zebrafish (Wu et al., 2001; Raymond et al., 2006), supporting the idea that retinal regeneration in the adult fish recapitulates the developmental program of the embryonic retina. However, the factors involved in inducing the regenerative program remain to be discovered. A comparison of the gene expression profiles of intact and regenerating zebrafish retinas was recently reported (Cameron et al., 2005). This study identified several genes whose expression is increased in the regenerating zebrafish retina. However, because the retina was damaged by surgical excision, many of the identified factors were involved in processes that are most likely unrelated to proliferation of rod progenitor cells, such as activation of the immune system, clearance of cellular debris, and wound healing.

6 XOPS-mCFP Transgenic Zebrafish

As mentioned above, studies of rod progenitor cell proliferation in response to retinal injury are complicated by the extent of damage caused by the acute injury methods typically employed. Furthermore, the behavior of the rod progenitors must be studied during a discrete window of time following injury. Clearly, these studies would benefit from the development of genetic models of photoreceptor degeneration in zebrafish. Our laboratory has characterized a transgenic line of zebrafish, the XOPS-mCFP line, which experiences selective degeneration of the rod photoreceptor cells (Morris et al., 2005) due to the toxic effect of a rod-targeted fluorescent reporter gene. This rod degeneration is accompanied by a significant increase in rod progenitor activity, leading to an ongoing cycle of rod photoreceptor birth and death, mediated by the continued proliferation of the rod progenitor cells. Therefore, this line offers a unique opportunity to study the rod progenitors in more detail.

Because the XOPS-mCFP line is a genetic model, we are able to examine rod progenitor responses to photoreceptor degeneration continually throughout the life of the animal as opposed to during a discrete window of time following acute injury. For example, we have found that rod progenitor activity is detectable in XOPS-mCFP animals as early as 7 days post fertilization, long before rod progenitor proliferation is observable in wild type animals (in preparation).

The XOPS-mCFP line is also currently the only transgenic zebrafish line that exhibits selective degeneration of the rod photoreceptors, without any other secondary cell loss. Therefore, we can compare the response to rod degeneration alone with that observed by others after loss of rods and cones and/or multiple retinal neurons. Interestingly, we have found that selective rod degeneration in XOPS-mCFP animals does not lead to an increase in proliferation of either Muller cells or the putative stem cells in the INL (in preparation). This suggests that the rod progenitors possess an intrinsic ability to respond to cues in the ONL, and to upregulate their own proliferation when needed. Further studies of the XOPS-mCFP line should yield important insights into the intrinsic and extrinsic factors that regulate proliferation of the rod progenitors in response to rod degeneration.

7 Summary

The zebrafish is an excellent model organism in which to study the retina's response to photoreceptor degeneration and/or acute injury. While much has been learned about the retinal stem and progenitor cells that mediate the damage response, several questions remain that cannot be addressed by acute models of injury. The development of genetic models, such as the XOPS-mCFP transgenic line, should further efforts to understand the nature of the signals that promote rod progenitor proliferation and differentiation following photoreceptor loss. This in turn may help to refine future approaches in higher vertebrates aimed at enhancing retinal progenitor cell activity for therapeutic purposes.

References

Ahmad, I., Tang, L., and Pham, H., 2000, Identification of neural progenitors in the adult mammalian eye, *Biochem. Biophys. Res. Commun.* **270**:517.

Braisted, J.E., Essman, T.F., and Raymond, P.A., 1994, Selective regeneration of photoreceptors in goldfish retina, *Development* **120**:2409.

Braisted, J.E., and Raymond, P.A., 1993, Continued search for the cellular signals that regulate regeneration of dopaminergic neurons in goldfish retina, *Brain Res. Dev. Brain Res.* **76**:221.

Braisted, J.E., and Raymond, P.A., 1992, Regeneration of dopaminergic neurons in goldfish retina. *Development* **114**:913.

Cameron, D.A., 2000, Cellular proliferation and neurogenesis in the injured retina of adult zebrafish, *Vis. Neurosci.* **17**:789.

Cameron, D.A., Gentile, K.L., Middleton, F.A., and Yurco, P., 2005, Gene expression profiles of intact and regenerating zebrafish retina, *Mol. Vis.* **20**:775.

Chacko, D.M., Das, A.V., Zhao, X., James, J., Bhattacharya, S., and Ahmad, I., 2003, Transplantation of ocular stem cells: the role of injury in incorporation and differentiation of grafted cells in the retina, *Vision Res.* **43**:937.

Fadool, J.M., 2003, Development of a rod photoreceptor mosaic revealed in transgenic zebrafish. *Dev. Biol.* **258**:277.

Fadool, J.M., 2003, Rod genesis in the teleost retina as a model of neural stem cells. *Exp. Neurol.* **184**:14.

Fausett, B.V., and Goldman, D., 2006, A role for alpha1 tubulin-expressing Muller glia in regeneration of the injured zebrafish retina, *J. Neurosci.* **26**:6303.

Haruta, M., Kosaka, M., Kanegae, Y., Saito, I., Inoue, T., Kageyama, R. et al., 2001, Induction of photoreceptor-specific phenotypes in adult mammalian iris tissue. *Nat. Neurosci.* **4**:1163.

Hitchcock, P., and Kakuk-Atkins, L., 2004, The basic helix-loop-helix transcription factor neuroD is expressed in the rod lineage of the teleost retina, *J. Comp. Neurol.*, **477**:108.

Hitchcock, P.F., Lindsey Myhr, K.J., Easter, S.S., Jr., Mangione-Smith, R., and Jones, D.D., 1992, Local regeneration in the retina of the goldfish, *J. Neurobiol.* **23**:187.

Hitchcock, P.F., Macdonald, R.E., VanDeRyt, J.T., and Wilson, S.W., 1996, Antibodies against Pax6 immunostain amacrine and ganglion cells and neuronal progenitors, but not rod precursors, in the normal and regenerating retina of the goldfish, *J. Neurobiol.* **29**:399.

Hitchcock, P., Ochocinska, M., Sieh, A., and Otteson, D., 2004, Persistent and injury-induced neurogenesis in the vertebrate retina, *Prog. Retin. Eye Res.* **23**:183.

Johns, P.R., 1982, Formation of photoreceptors in larval and adult goldfish. *J. Neurosci.* **2**:178.

Johns, P.R., and Fernald, R.D., 1981, Genesis of rods in teleost fish retina, *Nature* **293**:141.

Julian, D., Ennis, K., and Korenbrot, J.I., 1998, Birth and fate of proliferative cells in the inner nuclear layer of the mature fish retina, *J. Comp. Neurol.* **394**:271.

Mack, A.F., Balt, S.L., and Fernald, R.D., 1995, Localization and expression of insulin-like growth factor in the teleost retina, *Vis. Neurosci.* **12**:457.

MacLaren, R.E., Pearson, R.A., MacNeil, A., Douglas, R.H., Salt, T.E., Akimoto, M. et al., 2006, Retinal repair by transplantation of photoreceptor precursors, *Nature* **444**:203.

Morris, A.C., and Fadool, J.M., 2005, Studying rod photoreceptor development in zebrafish, *Physiol. Behav.* **86**:306.

Morris, A.C., Schroeter, E.H., Bilotta, J., Wong, R.O., and Fadool, J.M., 2005, Cone survival despite rod degeneration in XOPS-mCFP transgenic zebrafish, *Invest. Ophthalmol. Vis. Sci.* **46**:4762.

Negishi, K., Stell, W.K., Teranishi, T., Karkhanis, A., Owusu-Yaw, V., and Takasaki, Y., 1991, Induction of proliferating cell nuclear antigen (PCNA)-immunoreactive cells in goldfish retina following intravitreal injection with 6-hydroxydopamine, *Cell. Mol. Neurobiol.* **11**: 639.

Ochocinska, M.J., and Hitchcock, P.F., 2007, Dynamic expression of the basic helix-loop-helix transcription factor neuroD in the rod and cone photoreceptor lineages in the retina of the embryonic and larval zebrafish, *J. Comp. Neurol.* **501**:1.

Otteson, D.C., Cirenza, P.F., and Hitchcock, P.F., 2002, Persistent neurogenesis in the teleost retina: evidence for regulation by the growth-hormone/insulin-like growth factor-I axis, *Mech. Dev.* **117**:137.

Otteson, D.C., D'Costa, A.R., and Hitchcock, P.F., 2001, Putative stem cells and the lineage of rod photoreceptors in the mature retina of the goldfish, *Dev. Biol.* **232**:62.

Otteson, D.C., and Hitchcock, P.F., 2003, Stem cells in the teleost retina: persistent neurogenesis and injury-induced regeneration, *Vision Res.* **43**:927.

Raymond, P.A., Barthel, L.K., Bernardos, R.L., and Perkowski, J.J., 2006, Molecular characterization of retinal stem cells and their niches in adult zebrafish, *BMC Dev. Biol.* **6**:36.

Raymond, P.A., Barthel, L.K., Rounsifer, M.E., Sullivan, S.A., and Knight, J.K., 1993, Expression of rod and cone visual pigments in goldfish and zebrafish: a rhodopsin-like gene is expressed in cones, *Neuron* **10**:1161.

Raymond, P.A., Reifler, M.J., and Rivlin, P.K., 1988, Regeneration of goldfish retina: rod precursors are a likely source of regenerated cells, *J. Neurobiol.* **19**:431.

Robinson, J., Schmitt, E.A., Harosi, F.I., Reece, R.J., and Dowling, J.E., 1993, Zebrafish ultraviolet visual pigment: absorption spectrum, sequence, and localization, *Proc. Natl. Acad. Sci. U. S. A.* **90**:6009.

Sandy, J.M., and Blaxter, J.H.S., 1980, A study of retinal development in larval herring and sole, *J Marine Biol Assoc (UK).* **60**:59.

Tropepe, V., Coles, B.L., Chiasson, B.J., Horsford, D.J., Elia, A.J., McInnes, R.R. et al., 2000, Retinal stem cells in the adult mammalian eye, *Science* **287**:2032.

Vihtelic, T.S., and Hyde, D.R., 2000, Light-induced rod and cone cell death and regeneration in the adult albino zebrafish (Danio rerio) retina, *J. Neurobiol.* **44**:289.

Vihtelic, T.S., Soverly, J.E., Kassen, S.C., and Hyde, D.R., 2005, Retinal regional differences in photoreceptor cell death and regeneration in light-lesioned albino zebrafish, *Exp. Eye. Res.* **82**:558.

Wu, D.M., Schneiderman, T., Burgett, J., Gokhale, P., Barthel, L., and Raymond, P.A., 2001, Cones regenerate from retinal stem cells sequestered in the inner nuclear layer of adult goldfish retina, *Invest. Ophthalmol. Vis. Sci.* **42**:2115.

Yurco, P., and Cameron, D.A., 2005, Responses of Muller glia to retinal injury in adult zebrafish, *Vision Res.* **45**:991.

Zygar, C.A., Colbert, S., Yang, D., and Fernald, R.D., 2005, IGF-1 produced by cone photoreceptors regulates rod progenitor proliferation in the teleost retina, *Brain Res. Dev. Brain Res.* **154**:91.

αvβ5 Integrin Receptors at the Apical Surface of the RPE: One Receptor, Two Functions

Emeline F. Nandrot, Yongen Chang, and Silvia C. Finnemann

1 Introduction

Photoreceptors and retinal pigment epithelial (RPE) cells, two adjacent cells types of the outer retina, interact with each other functionally in numerous ways. Maintenance of permanent retinal adhesion and cyclic phagocytosis of shed photoreceptor outer segment fragments (POS) by RPE cells are two forms of these interactions that are crucial for vision. RPE cells form a polarized monolayer and extend apical microvilli that ensheath photoreceptor outer segments. Outer segments consist of stacked membranous disks containing the phototransduction machinery and are permanently renewed. To maintain constant outer segment length photoreceptors eliminate their most aged tips by daily shedding (Young, 1967), which precedes a burst of phagocytosis by the RPE that efficiently clears POS from the subretinal space and recycles many of their components (Young and Bok, 1969). POS shedding and subsequent phagocytosis by RPE cells are critical for photoreceptor cell function and long term survival. Indeed, complete failure to ingest POS by RPE cells from the Royal College of Surgeons (RCS) rat strain causes debris accumulation and rapid photoreceptor degeneration (Mullen and LaVail, 1976; Edwards and Szamier, 1977). Clearing their daily load of POS renders post-mitotic RPE cells the most active phagocytes in the body.

Synchronized POS clearance is tightly regulated and any delay in completing the shedding or digestion process can cause accumulation of autofluorescent lipofuscin inclusion bodies containing a complex mix of proteins and lipids that likely result from incomplete turnover of POS material (Feeney, 1978). In vitro studies have recently shown that lipofuscin components may directly impair RPE function and viability (Finnemann et al., 2002; Schutt et al., 2006). These data suggest that defective digestion of POS by RPE cells may contribute to development or progression of age-related retinal diseases such as age-related macular degeneration.

E.F. Nandrot
Margaret M. Dyson Vision Research Institute, Department of Ophthalmology, Weill Medical College of Cornell University, Box 233, 1300 York Avenue, New York, NY 10021, USA,
Tel: 212-746-2327, Fax: 212-746-8101
e-mail: efn2001@med.cornell.edu

R.E. Anderson et al. (eds.), *Recent Advances in Retinal Degeneration*,
© Springer 2008

Outer segment renewal in higher vertebrates is synchronized by circadian rhythms influenced by the daily dark-light cycle (Goldman et al., 1980). Animal studies in rod- or cone-dominant species revealed that rods mainly shed their POS within 2 hours after onset of light and cones shed within 2 hours after dusk (LaVail, 1976; Young, 1977). The increase in the number of phagosomes present in RPE cells at these two time points suggests a peak in phagocytic activity every 12 or 24 hours for RPE cells depending on whether they serve rods, cones or both. No untimely phagocytosis has been observed so far, suggesting that RPE cells may downregulate their phagocytic activity if not "on duty".

Retinal adhesion is equally essential for vision as daily POS phagocytosis but must be maintained permanently. Different factors such as intraocular pressure and a net fluid transport from retina to RPE contribute to retinal adhesion. Additionally, receptors expressed at the RPE apical surface are thought to adhere to ligands in the interphotoreceptor matrix (IPM), a complex mix of proteins and proteoglycans filling the subretinal space and ensheathing cone and rod POS (Hageman et al., 1995; Hollyfield et al., 1989; Hollyfield, 1999). IPM proteoglycan rearrangement and RPE microvilli collapse are early responses to retinal detachment that, if persistent, result in RPE dedifferentiation and proliferation, POS degeneration and photoreceptor cell death by apoptosis (Cook et al., 1995).

Despite their obvious importance for vision, we still know little about mechanisms that regulate the rhythm of RPE phagocytosis and RPE surface receptors or IPM ligands that mediate retinal adhesion.

2 Studying POS Phagocytosis by RPE Cells In vitro and In vivo

Studies seeking to identify the molecular machinery used by photoreceptors and RPE cells for photoreceptor outer segment renewal greatly benefit from the fact that RPE cells in tissue culture retain their phagocytic activity towards POS. Recording the binding and internalization kinetics of POS by RPE in culture ideally complements the classical microscopic characterization of OS uptake by RPE in vivo. First, OS recognition cannot be studied separately from OS internalization in vivo because shed OS in the subretinal space are juxtaposed to the RPE surface whether or not they are recognized or bound by RPE receptors. Second, far greater numbers of RPE cells can be evaluated in each sample in in vitro assays than in tissue sections. Therefore, small but significant alterations in RPE phagocytic activity may be detected in in vitro assays that may be missed in the light and electron microscopy studies of post-mortem tissues. Third, RPE cells in vitro can be studied following specific manipulation of their phagocytic mechanism by pharmacological compounds, recombinant proteins, protein overexpression or down-regulation, just to name a few. Gain- and loss-of-function approaches are well suited to unequivocally identify critical components of the RPE phagocytic machinery. Fourth, in vitro phagocytic challenge of RPE cells allows one to test directly the phagocytic activity of RPE cells towards POS, while altered photoreceptor shedding or IPM may indirectly

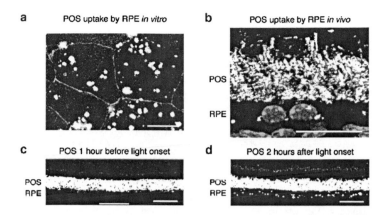

Fig. 1 Fluorescence microscopy quantification of POS phagocytosis by RPE cells in vitro and in vivo. (**a**) Maximal projection of confocal microscopy sections of primary wild-type mouse RPE cells in culture. RPE cells show vigorous uptake of FITC-labeled POS (white) after 1 hour of phagocytic challenge. RPE cell junctions stained with ZO-1 (gray outlines). (**b–d**) Cryosections of 2-month-old wild-type mice eyecups labeled with rhodopsin antibody. (**b**) RPE-photoreceptor outer segment interface close-up showing intact rod outer segments and opsin-positive phagosomes (bright white dots) adjacent to RPE nuclei (gray). (**c–d**) Low magnification view of similar stainings without nuclei illustrates that these images can be used to count phagosome numbers in the RPE. (**c**) One hour before light onset, the RPE cell layer shows few opsin-labeled phagosomes. (**d**) Two hours after light onset, the RPE cell layer shows numerous opsin-labeled phagosomes confirming the daily burst of rod POS phagocytosis by the RPE. Scale bars: 20 μm. Modified from Finnemann and Chang with permission from Humana Press Inc

alter the phagocytic activity by RPE cells in vivo. Importantly, however, RPE cells in vitro only provide a phagocytic assay system with relevance to RPE phagocytosis in vivo if cells are studied as differentiated, polarized epithelial monolayers that assemble their phagocytic machinery at their apical surface. Finally, while all evidence suggests that the phagocytic activity of polarized RPE cells in vitro retains the primary characteristics of the phagocytic activity of RPE cells in vivo, this is not the case for the nature of particle contact. In experimental phagocytosis assays, RPE cells must establish firm binding of isolated POS that is stable enough to withstand shear forces during sample processing, including vigorous washing steps. This is in sharp contrast to the contact of apical RPE receptors with shedding/shed POS in the subretinal space, where mechanical stress is absent and a stable binding event per se may not occur. Thus, comparison of in vivo and in vitro RPE phagocytosis counting fluorescence- or opsin antibody-labeled POS as illustrated in Fig. 1 are both required to fully elucidate the phagocytic machinery of the RPE.

3 RPE Phagocytosis In vitro and In vivo Uses αvβ5 Integrin

αvβ5 integrin expression at the apical surface of rodent RPE in vivo coincides with postnatal establishment of mature interactions between photoreceptors and RPE including the onset of POS renewal (Finnemann et al., 1997). Stable binding of POS to the cell surface of RPE cells in culture is largely dependent on $\alpha v \beta 5$ integrin receptors (Finnemann et al., 1997). In addition to POS recognition or tethering RPE cells also use $\alpha v \beta 5$ integrin receptors to activate signaling pathways through focal adhesion kinase that are necessary to activate MerTK (Finnemann, 2003; Nandrot et al., 2004). As $\beta 5$ integrin only dimerizes with αv integrin subunits, $\beta 5$ integrin knockout mice provide the opportunity to study RPE cells that permanently and exclusively lack $\alpha v \beta 5$ receptors (Huang et al., 2000).

To determine whether $\alpha v \beta 5$ integrin plays a role in RPE phagocytosis, we used the technology outlined above to quantify phagocytosis of photoreceptor outer segment fragments (POS) by $\beta 5$-deficient RPE in vivo and in vitro (Nandrot et al., 2004). Indeed, RPE cells in $\beta 5$ integrin knockout mice in vivo retain basal levels of phagocytic activity but lack the characteristic burst of phagocytosis upon early morning rod shedding. Moreover, $\alpha v \beta 5$ integrin is essential for POS binding in vitro, as RPE cells derived from $\beta 5$ integrin knockout mice in primary culture largely fail to bind isolated POS. These data demonstrate that $\alpha v \beta 5$ integrin has a key function in RPE phagocytosis.

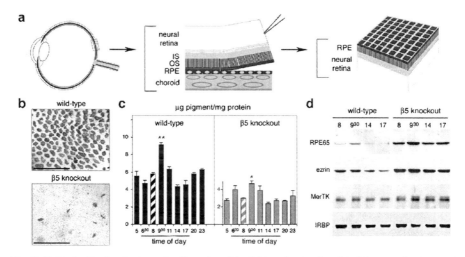

Fig. 2 Retinal adhesion is dramatically reduced in $\beta 5$ knockout mice. (**a**) After enucleation and lens/cornea removal, retinas are swiftly peeled off opened eyecups creating shearing forces to assess retinal adhesion. In retinas with normal retinal adhesion, apical cellular domains of RPE largely remain attached to the outer surface of the neural retina. (**b**) Whole-mount of peeled retina, shown outer retina up, demonstrating that $\beta 5$ knockout retina retains significantly less RPE pigment than wild-type retina. (**c**) Quantification of RPE pigment in retina peeled at different times of day. $\beta 5$ knockout retina shows reduced pigment contents and attenuated adhesiveness peak compared to wild-type retina. (**d**) Representative immunoblots of individual peeled retina confirming the melanin pigment results. Modified from Finnemann and Chang and from Nandrot et al. (2006) with permission from Humana Press Inc. and the American Physiological Society

4 Studying the Strength of Retinal Adhesion

Integrins can directly mediate adhesive interactions of cells with their extracellular substrate or with neighboring cells. Because of the fragility of isolated neural retinas, in vitro assays that study let alone quantify adhesive interactions between photoreceptor outer segments and RPE cells of mammalian origin do not exist. Furthermore, retinal adhesion of intact tissue is known to rapidly decline postmortem in rodent retina. To measure strength of retinal adhesion in retinal tissue immediately post-mortem, we adapted a published protocol to directly compare strength of retinal adhesion from wild-type and knockout mice of different ages as depicted in Fig. 2a (Endo et al., 1988; Nandrot et al., 2006).

During peeling, the apical domain of RPE cells separates from the basal domain and fractions with the isolated neural retina from wild-type mice if adhesion between the photoreceptors and RPE microvilli is sufficiently strong (Fig. 2b). After peeling, both proteins and melanin pigment derived from RPE cells can be analyzed and quantified. Control experiments established that neural retina content of the RPE specific protein RPE65 and of melanin directly correlated with each other and very well represented the number of RPE apical patches attached to the neural retina. Interestingly, both melanin pigment quantification (Fig. 2c) and analysis of proteins on western blots (Fig. 2d) indicated that retinal adhesion, like retinal phagocytosis, followed a diurnal rhythm with maximum strength of adhesion at ~9.30 AM (3.5 hours after light onset).

5 A Role for αvβ5 Integrin in Retinal Adhesion

To determine whether αvβ5 integrin receptors at the surface of RPE cells participated in retinal adhesion, we used the neural retina separation technique to quantify strength of retinal adhesion in age- and background-matched β5 knockout and wild-type mice (Nandrot et al., 2006). RPE pigment was transferred onto peeled retina from β5 knockout mice to a much lower extent, showing a decreased adhesion due to the absence of αvβ5 integrin receptors (Fig. 2b).

Furthermore, melanin and RPE protein quantification revealed that retinal adhesion was significantly reduced at all times in β5 knockout mice (Fig 2 c,d). Interestingly the daily cyclic rhythm of retinal adhesion was attenuated, as the peak was less prominent compared to other time points in these mice. These data demonstrate that αvβ5 integrin receptors at the surface of RPE cells contribute significantly to retinal adhesion.

6 Perspectives

Our results show that lack of αvβ5 integrin receptors eliminates the rhythm of POS phagocytosis in the retina and weakens retinal adhesion. The two functions may be largely independent of each other since both are defective immediately following the establishment of mature RPE-photoreceptor interactions in β5 knockout mouse retina. We also found that retinal adhesion and POS phagocytosis, each a crucial function for vision, follow independent diurnal rhythms that peak at different times of day.

αvβ5 integrin can recognize a number of extracellular ligands such as thrombospondin, vitronectin and MFG-E8. It is therefore an intriguing possibility that apical αvβ5 receptors of the RPE may respond to two different ligands in the subretinal space to either promote POS phagocytic signaling or to mediate retinal adhesion. We are currently exploring candidates to identify the ligand for each of αvβ5 integrin's function in the retina in vivo.

Acknowledgments This work was supported by NIH grant EY13295 and the Dyson Foundation. S.C.F. is the recipient of a William and Mary Greeve Scholarship by Research To Prevent Blindness, Inc., and of an Irma T. Hirschl Career Scientist Award.

References

Cook, B., Lewis, G. P., Fisher S. K., and Adler, R., 1995, Apoptotic photoreceptor degeneration in experimental retinal detachment, *Invest. Ophthalmol. Vis. Sci.* **36**:990–996.

Edwards, R. B., and Szamier, R. B., 1977, Defective phagocytosis of isolated rod outer segments by RCS rat retinal pigment epithelium in culture, *Science.* **197**:1001–1003.

Endo, E. G., Yao, X. Y., and Marmor, M. F., 1988, Pigment adherence as a measure of retinal adhesion: dependence on temperature, *Invest. Ophthalmol. Vis. Sci.* **29**:1390–1396.

Feeney, L., 1978, Lipofuscin and melanin of human retinal pigment epithelium. Fluorescence, enzyme cytochemical, and ultrastructural studies, *Invest. Ophthalmol. Vis. Sci.* **17**:583–600.

Finnemann, S. C., Bonilha, V. L., Marmorstein, A. D., and Rodriguez-Boulan, E., 1997, Phagocytosis of rod outer segments by retinal pigment epithelial cells requires αvβ5 integrin for binding but not for internalization, *Proc. Natl. Acad. Sci. U. S. A.* **94**:12932–12937.

Finnemann, S. C., Leung, L. W., and Rodriguez-Boulan, E., 2002, The lipofuscin component A2E selectively inhibits phagolysosomal degradation of photoreceptor phospholipid by the retinal pigment epithelium, *Proc. Natl. Acad. Sci. U. S. A.* **99**:3842–3847.

Finnemann, S. C., 2003, Focal adhesion kinase signaling promotes phagocytosis of integrin-bound photoreceptors, *EMBO J.* **22**:4143–4154.

Finnemann, S. C., and Chang, Y., Photoreceptor-RPE interactions: physiology and molecular mechanisms. (In press) In: *Visual Transduction and Non Visual Light Perception*, J. Tombran-Tink and C.J. Barnstable, ed., Humana Press, Totowa, New Jersey.

Goldman, A. I., Teirstein, P. S., and O'Brien, P. J., 1980, The role of ambient lighting in circadian disc shedding in the rod outer segment of the rat retina, *Invest. Ophthalmol. Vis. Sci.* **19**: 1257–1267.

Hageman, G. S., Marmor, M. F., Yao, X. Y., and Johnson, L. V., 1995, The interphotoreceptor matrix mediates primate retinal adhesion, *Arch. Ophthalmol.* **113**:655–660.

Hollyfield, J. G., Varner, H. H., Rayborn, M. E., and Osterfeld, A. M., 1989, Retinal attachment to the pigment epithelium, *Retina.* **9**:59–68.

Hollyfield, J. G., 1999, Hyaluronan and the functional organization of the interphotoreceptor matrix, *Invest. Ophthalmol. Vis. Sci.* **40**:2767–2769.

Huang, X., Griffiths, M., Wu, J., Farese, R. V., Jr., and Sheppard, D., 2000, Normal development, wound healing, and adenovirus susceptibility in β5-deficient mice, *Mol. Cell. Biol.* **20**: 755–759.

LaVail, M. M., 1976, Rod outer segment disk shedding in rat retina: relationship to cyclic lighting, *Science.* **194**:1071–1074.

Mullen, R. J., and LaVail, M. M., 1976, Inherited retinal dystrophy: primary defect in pigment epithelium determined with experimental rat chimeras, *Science.* **192**:799–801.

Nandrot, E. F., Kim, Y., Brodie, S. E., Huang, X., Sheppard, D., and Finnemann, S. C., 2004, Loss of synchronized retinal phagocytosis and age-related blindness in mice lacking αvβ5 integrin, *J. Exp. Med.* **200**:1539–1545.

Nandrot, E. F., Anand, M., Sircar, M., and Finnemann, S. C., 2006, Novel role for αvβ5-integrin in retinal adhesion and its diurnal peak, *Am. J. Physiol. Cell. Physiol.* **290**:C1256-C1262.

Schutt, F., Bergmann, M., Holz, F. G., Dithmar, S., Volcker, H. E., and Kopitz, J., 2006, Accumulation of A2-E in mitochondrial membranes of cultured RPE cells, *Graefes. Arch. Clin. Exp. Ophthalmol.* [epub ahead of print].

Young, R.W., 1967, The renewal of photoreceptor cell outer segments, *J. Cell Biol.* **33**:61–72.

Young, R. W., 1977, The daily rhythm of shedding and degradation of cone outer segment membranes in the lizard retina, *J. Ultrastruct. Res.* **61**:172–185.

Young, R. W., and Bok, D., 1969, Participation of the retinal pigment epithelium in the rod outer segment renewal process, *J. Cell Biol.* **42**:392–403.

Implantation of Mouse Eyes with a Subretinal Microphotodiode Array

Machelle T. Pardue, Tiffany A. Walker, Amanda E. Faulkner, Moon K. Kim, Christopher M. Bonner, and George Y. McLean

1 Introduction

Retinal prosthetics are designed to restore vision in patients with photoreceptor degenerative diseases, such as retinitis pigmentosa (RP) and macular degeneration. Subretinal microphotodiode arrays (MPAs), which response to incident light in a gradient fashion, have been designed to replace degenerating photoreceptors. Such devices have been implanted into rats (Ball et al., 2001), cats (Chow et al., 2001) and humans (Chow et al., 2004). These studies have revealed that implantation of a MPA device is capable of restoring some visual function in patients (Chow et al., 2004) and eliciting a superior colliculus response in normal and degenerating rats (DeMarco et al., 2007). Furthermore, the low level electrical stimulation produced by the MPA device has been shown to have neuroprotective properties (Pardue et al., 2005).

When RCS rats are implanted with an MPA device at the beginning of the degenerative process, photoreceptor function and morphology are preserved (Pardue et al., 2005). Subretinal electrical stimulation may provide protection to the photoreceptors by stimulating the selective expression of FGF-2 in the RCS rat (Ciavatta et al., 2006). While these studies show promise for subretinal electrical stimulation as a treatment of RP, implantation of MPA devices in S334ter rats does not preserve photoreceptors (Walker et al., 2005). We hypothesize that this may be due to the underlying mutations between RCS and S334ter rats. RCS rats have a recessive mutation in a tyrosine kinase gene, *Mertk*, which results in failed phagocytosis of shed outer segments by the retinal pigment epithelium (Mullen and LaVail, 1976; D'Cruz et al., 2000) while S334ter rats have a rhodopsin mutation which leads to photoreceptor death (Lee et al., 2003).

Rat models with photoreceptor degeneration are few while there are numerous mouse models of RP that have been described (Chang et al., 2002; Dalke and

M.T. Pardue
Rehab R&D, Atlanta VA Medical Center, Decatur, GA 30033, USA; Department of Ophthalmology, Emory University, Atlanta GA 30322, USA, Tel: 404-321-6111 x 7342, Fax: 404-728-4847
e-mail: mpardue@emory.edu

Graw, 2005). Thus, to further elucidate whether the neuroprotective effect of sub-retinal electrical stimulation is generalized to all types of photoreceptor degeneration, implantation of mouse models of RP would be advantageous. This study describes the development of surgical techniques and the success of implanting a small mouse eye with a subretinal MPA device.

2 Methods

2.1 Experimental and Implant Design

Adult wild-type C57Bl/6J mice (n = 6) were obtained from an in-house breeding colony originating from mice purchased from Jackson Laboratories (Bar Harbor, ME). Mice were implanted at 21–28 days of age and retinal function was measured every two weeks until 8 weeks post-implantation. After the final measurement, mice were euthanized and the eyes enucleated for histological assessment. All procedures were approved by the local Institutional Animal Care and Use Committee and carried out in accordance with the Association for Research in Vision and Ophthalmology statement concerning the use of animals in ophthalmic and vision research.

The MPA device was identical in electrical properties to devices described previously (Chow et al., 2001). Briefly, each device consisted of a silicon disk covered on the top side with a microphotodiode array. However, the devices were manufactured in a smaller size to accommodate the small mouse eye, measuring 23 μm thick and 0.5 mm in diameter.

2.2 Surgical Procedures

Surgical procedures were similar to that described for the rat eye (Ball et al., 2001). After dilation of the pupils (1% mydriacyl, 2.5% phenylephrine) and anaesthetization of the cornea (0.5% tetracine HCl), the anaesthetized (ketamine 80 mg/kg; xylazine 16 mg/kg) mouse was placed on a heating pad. A traction suture (8-0) placed in the superior lid was used to retract the upper lid while a second traction suture placed in the superior limbus was used to rotate the eye inferiorly (Fig. 1). The conjunctiva and underlying tenon capsule were opened using iris spring scissors to reveal the superior limbus. The tip of a 16 gauge stiletto blade was used to make a 0.6 mm long incision through the sclera, choroids, RPE, and retina, about 1 mm posterior to the limbus (Fig. 1). The eye was wet with saline (0.9% NaCl) and the retina was allowed to detach naturally along the incision over a period of 10 minutes, after which the implant was gently manipulated into the subretinal space using the tips of two IOL manipulators. The eye was then rotated back to primary position and the fundus was examined to confirm subretinal placement of the device. A drop of antibiotic solution was applied to the eye (Neosporin Ophthalmic Solution) and

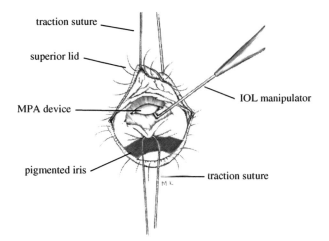

Fig. 1 Sketch of the mouse eye during surgery of the subretinal MPA device. The eye is rotated inferiorly and the superior sclera is exposed. See text for details of surgery

the mouse was given yohimbine (2.1 mg/kg) to reverse the effects of the xylazine and speed recovery from anesthesia (Turner and Albassam, 2005).

2.3 Electroretinography (ERG)

Retinal function was monitored by recording electroretinograms (ERGs) with an automated system (LKC system; Gaithersburg, MD). After overnight dark-adaptation, mice were anesthetized (ketamine 80 mg/kg; xylazine 16 mg/kg) and their pupils dilated (1% mydriacyl, 2.5% phenylephrine) under dim red light. Mice were placed on a homeothermic heating pad inside a Faraday cage. ERGs were recorded from both eyes simultaneously with a nylon fiber electrode contacting the center of the cornea through a layer of 1% methylcellulose. Platinum needle electrodes placed in the cheek and tail served as reference and ground, respectively.

Dark-adapted responses to stimuli from a Ganzfeld xenon flash lamp were recorded in a series presented in order of increasing strength, ranging from 0.001 to 137 cd s/m^2. The interstimulus intervals were increased from 15 to 60 seconds with increasing flash strenth. To record cone-mediated responses, mice were light-adapted for 10 minutes (30 cd/m^2) and then presented with a series of flashes at 2.1 Hz, ranging from 0.15 to 75 cd s/m^2.

2.4 Histology

After eight weeks of implantation, mice were euthanized and their eyes enucleated. Each eye was marked on the corneal surface to indicate its orientation and was

immersion fixed overnight by immersion in 2% paraformaldehyde/2.5% glutaraldehyde. Eyes were rinsed in phosphate buffer, dehydrated through a graded ethanol
series and embedded in plastic resin (Embed 812/Der736; Electron Microscopy
Science, Hatfield, PA). Retinal sections were cut on an ultramicrotome (Reichert;
0.5 μm) and stained with toluidine blue. Morphological analysis was made by exam-
ining retinal layers adjacent and overlying the MPA device.

3 Results

3.1 Retinal Function

Implantation of a subretinal MPA device produced no significant differences in
retinal function between the implanted and opposite (unoperated) eye. Figure 2A
shows the dark-adapted ERG waves recorded from a mouse in which one eye was
implanted with the MPA device while the other eye served as an unoperated control.
Amplitude and implicit time of both the a- and b-waves are similar between the
two eyes. Note that the electrical activity of the implant is seen as a fast negative
spike in the ERG trace. As expected, the microphotodiodes respond in a gradient
fashion to the incident light, producing an implant spike that becomes larger with
increasing intensities. At the brightest flash intensities, the implant spike amplitude
was 180 μV (4.1 cd sec/m^2) and 1300 μV (137 cd sec/m^2).

Figure 2B shows the maximal dark-adapted b-wave amplitude across time. At
two weeks after implantation, retinal function of the implanted eyes is reduced. Similar reductions in ERG amplitudes 1–2 weeks after subretinal surgery were reported
previously for rats (Pardue et al., 2005) and cats (Chow et al., 2002). However, by

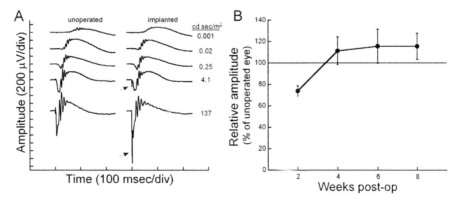

Fig. 2 (A) Dark-adapted ERG waves to a series of flash intensities, as indicated on the right. The
electrical activity of the implant (arrow) can be seen in the two brightest flash intensities as a fast
(0.5 msec) spike. (B) Plot of the dark-adapted ERG b-wave response to a bright stimulus (137 cd
sec/m^2) across the follow-up period. The average amplitude of the implanted eye is plotted in
proportion to the opposite control eye. Error bars represent standard error of the mean

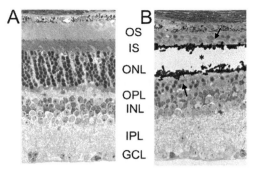

Fig. 3 Photomicrographs of mouse retina (A) from an unoperated eye and (B) directly overlying the implant. The black material in (B) is the remnants of the MPA device that shattered during sectioning. The asterisk indicates the position of the MPA device. The arrows indicate the remnants of photoreceptor nuclei around the implant

4 weeks after surgery, retinal function is equal to or greater than the opposite, unimplanted eye. Cone-mediated response also showed no differences between implanted and unoperated eyes.

3.2 Retinal Morphology

Figure. 3 shows the histological appearance of an unoperated mouse retina (A) compared to retina directly overlying the MPA device (B). Areas adjacent to the implant had the same appearance as unoperated eyes, with all retinal layers intact. However, directly overlying the implant device, there is a localized loss of photoreceptors segments and decreased number of photoreceptor nuclei (Fig. 3B). This same reaction has also been found in normal rats (Ball et al., 2001) and cats (Chow et al., 2001; Pardue et al., 2001) implanted with a subretinal MPA device. At 8 weeks post-op, photoreceptors are still present immediately adjacent to the implant. The inner retina has normal morphology and thickness in areas adjacent to and directly over the implant.

4 Discussion

These data demonstrate the feasibility of implanting a 0.5 mm subretinal MPA device into normal mouse eyes. The normal mouse retina reacts to a solid foreign object in the subretinal space in the same way as other mammalian species with dual retinal circulation: the photoreceptors nourished by the choroid degenerate. The loss of photoreceptors and subsequent inner retinal changes that have been documented in cats parallel the changes found in retinal detachment models (Pardue et al., 2001). Thus, we hypothesize that the solid nature of the MPA implant causes a localized retinal detachment. However, the presence of the MPA device and its electrical activity appear to be well tolerated by the retina as a whole, with no other indications of rejection, inflammation, or toxicity. With the demonstration of successful subretinal implantation of the normal mouse eye, various mouse models of retinal degeneration can now be tested to determine the generalized effect of subretinal electrical stimulation on photoreceptor preservation.

References

Ball, S.L., Pardue, M.T., Chow, A.Y., Chow, V.Y., and Peachey, N.S., 2001, Subretinal implantation of photodiodes in rodent models of photoreceptor degeneration, In: *New Insights into Retinal Degenerative Diseases*, R.E. Anderson, M.M. LaVail, and J.G. Hollyfield, eds., Kluwer/Plenum, New York, pp.175–182.

Chang, B., Hawes, N.L., Hurd, R.E., Davisson, M.T., Nusinowitz, S., and Heckenlively, J.R., 2002, Retinal degeneration mutants in the mouse. *Vision Res.* **42**:517–25.

Chow, A.Y., Pardue, M.T., Chow, V.Y., Peyman, G.A., Liang, C., Perlman, J.I., and Peachey, N.S., 2001, Implantation of silicon chip microphotodiode arrays into the cat subretinal space. *IEEE Trans. Neural Syst. Rehabil. Eng.* **9**:86–95.

Chow, A.Y., Pardue, M.T., Perlman, J.I., Ball, S.L., Chow, V.Y., Hetling, J.R., Peyman G.A., Liang, C., Stubbs, E.B., Jr., and Peachey, N.S., 2002, Subretinal implantation of semiconductor-based photodiodes: durability of novel implant designs. *J. Rehabil. Res. Dev.* **39**:313–321.

Chow, A.Y., Chow, V.Y., Peyman, G.A., Packo, K.H., Pollack, J.S., and Schuchard, R., 2004, The artificial silicon retina^{TM} (ASR^{TM}) chip for the treatment of vision loss from retinitis pigmentosa. *Arch. Ophthalmol.* **122**:460–469.

Ciavatta, V.T., Chrenek, M., Wong, P., Nickerson, J.M., and Pardue, M.T., 2006, Growth factor expression following implantation of microphotodiode arrays in RCS rats. ARVO E-abstract 3177.

Dalke, C., and Graw, J., 2005, Mouse mutants as models for congenital retinal disorders. *Exp. Eye Res.* **81**:503–512.

D'Cruz, P.M., Yasumura, D., Weir, J., Matthes, M.T., Abderrahim, H., LaVail, M.M., and Vollrath, D., 2000, Mutation of the receptor tyrosine kinase gene MertK in the retina dystrophic RCS rat. *Hum. Mol. Genet.* **9**:645–51.

DeMarco, P.J., Jr., Yarbrough, G.L., Yee, C.W., McLean, G.Y., Sagdullaev, B.T., Ball, S.L., and McCall, M.A., 2007, Stimulation via a subretinally placed prosthetic elicits central activity and induces a trophic effect on visual responses. *Invest. Ophthalmol. Vis. Sci.* **48**:916–26.

Lee, D., Geller, S., Walsh, N., Valter, K., Yasumura, D., Matthes, M., LaVail, M., and Stone, J., 2003, Photoreceptor degeneration in Pro23His and S334ter transgenic rats. *Adv. Exp. Med. Biol.* **533**:297–302.

Mullen, R.J., and LaVail, M.M., 1976, Inherited retinal dystrophy: primary defect in pigment epithelium determined with experiment rat chimeras. *Science* **192**:799–801.

Pardue, M.T., Phillips, M.J., Yin, H., Sippy, B.D., Webb-wood, S., Chow, A.Y., and Ball, S.L., 2005, Neuroprotective effect of subretinal implants in the RCS rat. *Invest. Ophthalmol. Vis. Sci.* **46**:674–682.

Pardue, M.T., Stubbs, E.B., Jr., Perlman, J.I., Narfstrom, K., Chow, A.Y., and Peachey, N.S., 2001, Immunohistochemical studies of the retina following long-term implantation with subretinal microphotodiode arrays. *Exp. Eye Res.* **73**:333–343.

Turner, P.V., and Albassam, M.A., 2005, Susceptiblity of rats to corneal lesions after injectable anesthesia. *Comp. Med.* **55**:175–182.

Walker, T.A., Faulkner, A.E., Cheng, Y., Yin, H., Fernandes, A., Phillips, M.J., Ball, S.L., Chow, A.Y., and Pardue, M.T., 2005, Subretinal implantation induces photoreceptor preservation in RCS rat not seen in wild-type long evans or S334ter rats. ARVO E-Abstract 5267.

Variation in the Electroretinogram of C57BL/6 Substrains of Mouse

Alison L. Reynolds, G. Jane Farrar, Pete Humphries, and Paul F. Kenna

1 Introduction

The electroretinogram (ERG) is one of the most commonly used clinical techniques to measure visual function. The ERG records the impulse generated by retinal cells in response to a single flash of light (Fishman et al., 2001). By altering the light or dark adapted status of the subject and recording at different light intensities and/or flicker frequencies, rod and cone function can be recorded and analysed in isolation, as can the function of second order neurons (Marmor et al., 2004). The ERG is a complex waveform and alterations can be used to diagnose and follow the progress of a variety of retinal disorders. Since this system is non-invasive, it can also be adapted to record from anaesthetised mice, specifically those with either spontaneous or targeted mutations in retinal genes (Nusinowitz and Ridder , 2002; Peachey and Ball, 2003).

Many external variables can influence the ERG, such as the anaesthetic used, dilation of the pupil, dark or light adaptation, location of the electrode on the cornea or repeated flashing in the rod (dark adapted) series (Smith et al., 2002). In order to filter out such variables, ERG recordings must be undertaken in a standard manner in every animal, in any given laboratory or series of investigations. It is important to limit biological variation while recording the ERG in genetically manipulated mice, paying particular attention to genetic background.

Strain-specific variation in both retinal and ocular phenotypes of genetically manipulated mice has been reported in a number of studies. p53-deficient mice have been shown, for example, to develop ocular abnormalities including optic nerve hypoplasia, retinal folds and abnormal inner retinal vessels when on a C57BL/6J genetic background, but such mice have a normal-appearing fundus on a 129Sv genetic background (Ikeda et al., 1999). In studies of light-induced apoptosis, some strains of mouse, including C57BL/6J are resistant to light damage, whereas others,

A.L. Reynolds

Ocular Genetics Unit, Smurfit Institute of Genetics, Trinity College Dublin, Ireland,

Tel: 353 1 608 2482, Fax: 353 1 608 3848

e-mail: alison.reynolds@tcd.ie

R.E. Anderson et al. (eds.), *Recent Advances in Retinal Degeneration*,

© Springer 2008

such as 129/Ola, are very much more susceptible (Wenzel et al., 2001). Mice carrying the recessive mutation of the Tubby gene develop, among other symptoms, a retinal degeneration, variation in the thickness of the retina outer nuclear layer (ONL) in these animals having been observed when the primary mutation is expressed on different genetic backgrounds (Ikeda et al., 2002). Mice with a targeted disruption of the rhodopsin gene develop a severe retinopathy which has been shown to be less severe on a C57BL/6J than on a 129Sv genetic background (Humphries et al., 2001). Such variation is attributable to differences in genetic background and such studies highlight just how important an isogenic background is for studies of vision. Strain-specific variation in ERG has also been reported between different wild type inbred strains, for example, between pigmented and albino mice (Green et al., 1994; Gresh et al., 2003) and in differences in eye size, lens weight and retinal area between C57BL/6J and DBA/2J strains (Zhou and Williams, 1999). Ganglion cell number is known to differ between the recombinant inbred strains BXD and BXH (Williams et al., 1998). Age-related variation in the thickness of the outer nuclear layer has also been reported between two albino mouse strains, C57BL/6J-c(2J) and BALB/cByJ (Danciger et al., 2003).

In this study, an electroretinographic comparison of three substrains of the commonly used C57BL/6 inbred mouse was performed to see whether any phenotypic variability could be observed. One of these substrains, C57BL/6JOlaHsd, is known to contain a 365Kb deletion on chromosome 6, making this substrain a functional knockout for both the synuclein alpha (Snca) and multimerin 1 (Mmrn1) genes (Specht and Schoepfer, 2004). The protein product of Snca plays a role in the molecular pathologies of degenerative neuropathies, such as Alzheimer's disease and Parkinson's disease (Farrer et al., 2001). Variation in the murine ERG can be used to search for genetic causes of such variation, with a view to isolating the genes involved.

2 Materials and Methods

2.1 Animals

All procedures involving animals were performed in accordance with the ARVO statement for the Use of Animals in Ophthalmic and Vision Research, with approval from the institutional ethics committee and under licence. Electroretinograms were recorded in mice at 4–6 months of age. Three substrains of C57BL/6 mouse were used: C57BL/6 (Bantin & Kingman Universal Ltd, Hull, UK), C57BL/6J (The Jackson Laboratory, Bar Harbor, Maine) and C57BL/6JOlaHsd (Harlan, UK).

2.2 Electroretinography

Animals were dark-adapted overnight and prepared for electroretinography under dim red light. The subjects were anaesthetised by means of ketamine (110 mg/kg) and xylazine (11 mg/kg) injected intraperitoneally. Pupil dilation was achieved by administering drops of tropicamide 1% and phenylephrine HCl 2.5% to each eye. The core temperature of each mouse was measured digitally using a rectal temperature probe attached to a heating pad (TH-2kmr Thermistor Probe, Cell Microcontrols, Norfolk, VA) so that the temperature of the animal could be maintained at 37°C +/–0.5°C. Standardized flashes of light were presented to the mouse in a Ganzfeld bowl (full field stimulator Q400; Roland Consult, Germany) to ensure uniform retinal illumination. The ERG responses were recorded simultaneously from both eyes by means of contact lens electrodes (Medical Workshop, Groningen, Netherlands) using Vidisic® (Dr Mann Pharma, Germany) as a conducting agent and to maintain corneal hydration. A reference electrode was positioned subcutaneously approximately 1mm from the temporal canthus and the ground electrode placed subcutaneously anterior to the tail. The responses were analysed using RetiScan RetiPort electrophysiology equipment (Roland Consult, Germany). The protocol used was based on that approved by the International Society for Clinical Electrophysiology of Vision (ISCEV). A series of six responses to flash stimuli varying in intensity from 1 to 3500 mcds/m^2 were used to record rod-dominated responses, each one averaged over four flashes. Flashes were presented from –25 dB to 0 dB in steps of 5 dB (1 dB = 1/10 of a log unit, i.e. the –25 dB flash is 2.5 log units less intense than the 0 dB flash, the maximal flash output of 3500 mcds/m^2). An inter-stimulus interval of 15 s was used at the three lowest flash intensities, followed by 30 s at 350 mcds/m^2 (–10 dB), 45 s at 1000 mcds/m^2 (–5 dB) and 60 s at 3500 mcds/m^2 (0 dB), the maximal combined rod – cone response. Following light adaptation for 10 min at a background illumination of 30 cd/m^2, the cone-isolated responses were recorded at the maximal intensity flash (3.5 cds/m^2) presented as a single flash and as a 10 Hz flicker. Oscillatory potentials were recorded at the maximum intensity flash, altering the bandpass filters to 100–200 Hz to isolate them. Timings and amplitudes were averaged over the two eyes to give a per animal value. a-waves were measured from the baseline to the trough and b-waves from the a-wave trough to the peak of the b-wave.

2.3 Statistical Analysis

For each animal the a- and b-wave timings and amplitudes at all flash intensities were used for statistical analysis. An unpaired 2-sample t-test was used to evaluate significance ($p \leq 0.05$) between substrains. Results were graphed by averaging by strain, using the standard error of the mean as y-error bars.

2.4 Genotyping

Genomic DNA was extracted from tail snips of all C57BL/6 substrains, using a standard phenol/chloroform protocol. PCR was performed in to confirm the presence or absence of a deletion on chromosome 6, a known sequence variant in C57BL/6JOlaHsd mice (Specht and Schoepfer, 2004). In addition, C57BL/6JOlaHsd DNA was commercially genotyped in 112 SNPs, spaced across the entire mouse genome (Kbioscience, UK; identity of the SNPs available on request). Experimental SNP genotypes were compared to published SNP genotypes for the C57BL/6J strain (Petkov et al., 2004).

3 Results

ERG analysis of retinal responses was carried out in three substrains of C57BL/6 mouse. There were no significant differences in the light adapted ERG between any of the three substrains (single flash or 10Hz flash) or in the oscillatory potentials. An initial comparison of the dark-adapted ERG of the C57BL/6JOlaHsd and C57BL/6 strains showed no strain-specific variation in the timing of the a- or b-waves (Fig. 1, Tables 1a and 1b). However, amplitude did show strain-specific variation in the a- and b-waves at higher flash intensities (Fig. 2, Tables 2a and 2b).

Given that the C57BL/6JOlaHsd strain is a naturally occurring functional knockout for the Snca gene, it was hypothesized that the absence of expression of this gene could result in the 10–16% depression in a- and b-wave amplitudes observed in this strain; without Snca, dopamine levels may increase and thus the amplitude decrease. In support of this theory, intravitreal administration of dopamine in rabbit is known

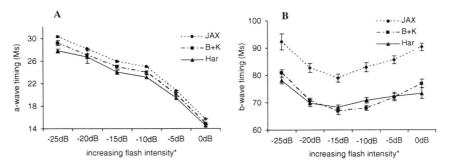

Fig. 1 Graphs showing the average timing values (in milliseconds) for the dark-adapted ERG a-wave (A) and b-wave (B) in three C57BL/6 substrains: JAX= C57BL/6J, B+K= C57BL/6, HAR = C57BL/6JOlaHsd. Y-error bars are S.E.M. *increasing flash intensities are given in dB (1dB = 1/10 log unit of max flash: 3500 mcds/m²)

Table 1a Summary of dark-adapted ERG a-wave timing (milliseconds): strain average ± standard deviation

Substrain	−25dB	−20dB	−15dB	**−10dB**	−5dB	0dB
JAX*	30.3 ± 2.1	28.1 ± 1.8	25.9 ± 1.2	24.9 ± 1.1	20.7 ± 1.2	15.6 ± 0.9
B+K^	29.2 ± 2.1	26.9 ± 1.5	24.9 ± 1.4	23.9 ± 1.4	20.1 ± 1	14.8 ±0.6
HAR+	27.8 ± 7.4	26.7 ± 6.8	24 ± 6.2	23.2 ± 6	19.4 ± 4.9	14.5 ± 3.8

JAX*= C57BL/6J, B+K^= C57BL/6, HAR+ = C57BL/6JOlaHsd.

Table 1b Summary of dark-adapted ERG b-wave timing (milliseconds): strain average ± standard deviation

Substrain	−25dB	−20dB	−15dB	−10dB	−5dB	0dB
JAX*	92.3 ± 12.5	82.7 ± 6.9	78.9 ± 6.2	82.9 ± 7.2	85.6 ± 6.6	90.4 ± 5.7
B+K^	80.8 ± 6	70.7 ± 4.5	66.8 ± 4.9	68.0 ± 4.3	72 ± 5.5	76.9 ± 6.5
HAR+	78.2 ± 5.9	69.8 ± 5.6	68.3 ± 4.5	70.8 ± 5	72.3 ± 6.7	73.4 ± 9.5

JAX*= C57BL/6J, B+K^ = C57BL/6, HAR+ = C57BL/6JOlaHsd.

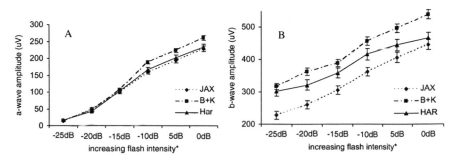

Fig. 2 Graphs showing the average amplitude values (μV) for the dark-adapted ERG a-wave (A) and b-wave (B) in three C57BL/6 substrains: JAX= C57BL/6J, B+K= C57BL/6, HAR = C57BL/6JOlaHsd. Y-error bars are S.E.M. *increasing flash intensities are given in dB (1dB = 1/10 log unit of max flash: 3500mcds/m²)

to decrease b-wave amplitude (Jagadeesh and Sanchez, 1981). A third substrain, C57BL/6J was also included in the study. The latter did not display any significant differences in the light-adapted ERG or oscillatory potentials when compared to the other two strains, however, the dark-adapted ERG of the C57BL/6J mouse was different to that in both of the other substrains. Timings of the dark-adapted a- and b-waves were significantly slower in the C57BL/6J substrain ($p \leq 0.05$) and amplitudes were lower ($p \leq 0.0001$), when compared to the other substrains.

Table 2a Summary of dark adapted ERG a-wave amplitude (μV): strain average ± standard deviation

Substrain	−25dB	−20dB	−15dB	−10dB	−5dB	0dB
JAX*	14.1 ± 7.5	49.6 ± 16.2	99.7 ± 20.4	158.2 ± 26.2	192.8 ± 29.5	228.7 ± 34.6
B+K^	15.4 ± 7.5	45.2 ± 10.3	106.4 ± 13.9	188.1 ± 19.1	222.9 ± 26.1	260.5 ± 28.9
HAR+	17.5 ± 5.6	42.5 ± 12.4	103.9 ± 19.6	165.8 ± 34.6	202 ± 35.4	233.9 ± 43

JAX*= C57BL/6J, B+K^= C57BL/6, HAR+ = C57BL/6JOlaHsd.

Table 2b Summary of dark-adapted ERG b-wave amplitude (μV): strain average ± standard deviation

Substrain	−25dB	−20dB	−15dB	−10dB	−5dB	0dB
JAX*	228.1 ± 53.1	260.5 ± 53.1	306 ± 54.5	363.2 ± 57.3	406.6 ± 67.6	446.5 ± 69.8
B+K^	317.5 ± 40.1	362.8 ± 48.7	388.8 ± 47.7	457.9 ± 56.8	497.4 ± 59	539.2 ± 59.6
HAR+	302 ± 69.5	321.8 ± 76.1	358.3 ± 73.7	416.8 ± 86.1	445.8 ± 85.8	466.2 ± 85.6

JAX*= C57BL/6J, B+K^ = C57BL/6, HAR+ = C57BL/6JOlaHsd.

Table 3 Differences observed between published C57BL/6J SNP data (Petkov et al., 2004) when compared with C57BL/6JOlaHsd SNP data

Marker (Rs #)	Chr	C57BL/6J	C57BL/6JOlaHsd	Problem
3664528	1	C:C	T:C	Heterozygous
3674936	2	T:T	C:T	Heterozygous
3707236	18	A:A	G:A	Heterozygous

The genotyping results of 112 SNPs across the entire C57BL/6JOlaHsd genome revealed that three SNPs (2.7%) were heterozygous i.e. they were of a different genotype to the published C57BL/6J SNPs (Table 3). This suggests that C57BL/6JOlaHsd mice may be more separate from the C57BL/6J on the genomic level than previously thought. SNP genotyping was not performed in the C57BL/6 substrain.

4 Discussion

An electroretinographic analysis of three C57BL/6 substrains was performed in order to determine primarily whether a deletion on chromosome 6 in the C57BL/6JOlaHsd (Harlan) substrain may influence the ERG. This deletion has been well characterised and is known to contain two genes, those encoding synuclein alpha (Snca) and multimerin 1 (Mmrn1) (Specht and Schoepfer, 2001; Specht and Schoepfer, 2004). The absence of Snca was confirmed in all C57BL/6JOlaHsd mice used in these experiments (data not shown).

An initial comparison of the C57BL/6JOlaHsd (Harlan) and C57BL/6 (B&K) substrains indicated no observable differences between the light adapted ERG and oscillatory potentials. In the dark-adapted series, an increase of 10–16% was observed in the amplitude of both a- and b-waves of the C57BL/6 (B&K) mouse when compared to C57BL/6JOlaHsd (Harlan). This difference was significant at higher, but not at lower flash intensities ($p \leq 0.05$). There were no significant differences observed between these two substrains (Harlan and B&K) when the dark-adapted timing was analysed. It was hypothesised that the absence of Snca, a putative regulator of dopamine transmission, may depress the C57BL/6JOlsHsd dark-adapted ERG, as observed in this comparison.

In order to explore this hypothesis further, ERG recordings were made on a third C57BL/6 substrain, C57BL/6J (obtained from The Jackson Laboratory) known to contain the Snca locus. If this substrain had a similar dark-adapted ERG then it would add weight to the hypothesis that the comparatively low amplitudes in the C57BL/6JOlaHsd mouse were due to the lack of Snca. The dark-adapted ERG of the C57BL/6J mouse was different to both C57BL/6JOlaHsd and C57BL/6 substrains. Unlike the other substrains, C57BL/6J mice exhibited significantly slower a- and b-wave timings. In the a-wave, the timings were 7-10% slower ($p \leq 0.05$) and in the b-wave timings were 15–23% slower ($p \leq 0.0001$) at all flash intensities (Fig. 1; Tables 1a and 1b). When the dark-adapted amplitudes were analysed,

C57BL/6J mice had similar a-wave amplitudes to C57BL/6JOlaHsd mice, both of which had decreased amplitudes in comparison to C57BL/6 ($p \leq 0.005$ at higher flash intensities comparing C57BL/6 and C57BL/6J; Fig. 2(A); Table 2a). Thus, absence of Snca is unlikely to be responsible for differences observed in a-wave amplitude between C57BL/6JOlaHsd and C57BL/6 substrains. Analysis of b-wave amplitudes showed that all three substrains were different, C57BL/6 having the highest amplitudes, followed by C57BL/6JOlaHsd, with C57BL/6J having the lowest (Fig. 2(B); Table 45.2b). The difference between C57BL/6 and C57BL/6J amplitudes was highly significant ($p \leq 0.0001$) at all flash intensities. Since both C57BL/6 and C57BL/6J substrains contain the Snca locus, it is extremely unlikely that any differences in amplitude are being mediated through this locus.

Given that so many differences have been observed during the analysis of dark-adapted retinal function in these three substrains, it possible that unknown genomic differences could account for such differences. To date the only reported sequence variation between C57BL/6 substrains has been the Snca locus deletion (MGI Database, 2007), which may have arisen as far back as the 1970s (Specht and Schoepfer, 2004). In a study presented here, 112 SNPs were genotyped in C57BL/6JOlaHsd mice, of which three were found to be heterozygous (commercial genotyping performed by Kbiosciences, UK). While this comprises only 2.7% of the 112 SNPs, it highlights variation between the published SNPs in the C57BL/6J mouse (Petkov et al., 2004) and substrains. A rapid comparison of the ERG variation (standard deviation; Tables 1a, 1b, 2a and 45.2b) shows more variation in C57BL/6JOlaHsd mice when compared to the other substrains. The C57BL/6J mouse, which has the least variation in the dark-adapted ERG is regularly genotyped for genetic purity (Taft et al., 2006; The Jackson Laboratory, 2006). Other mouse strains, such as the 129 strain, have been shown to be heterozygous (Simpson et al., 1997). Genotypes of inbred strains of mice raised in private colonies at different locations can be influenced by genetic drift, neutral mutation occurring randomly within a population. Variation in the dark-adapted ERG among substrains highlights the need to be vigilant about the use of an exact substrain for all experiments, particularly those involving the ERG.

In summary, characteristics associated with Ganzfeld ERG have been studied in three substrains of C57BL/6 mouse. We have observed that whereas there are no differences in oscillatory potentials or in the light-adapted ERG within these substrains, there are significant differences in the dark-adapted ERG responses. Such differences are unlikely to be mediated by synuclein alpha, since the ERG of two substrains containing the Snca locus was different. Studying variation in retinal function, especially in closely related inbred mouse strains, offers a unique opportunity to search for genes controlling such properties. Knowledge of the functions of such genes will lead to a more comprehensive understanding of retinal function and dysfunction.

Acknowledgments This work was supported by grants from the Higher Education Authority of Ireland, Health Research Board of Ireland and Science Foundation Ireland. We thank Sylvia Mehigan and Caroline Woods for technical assistance.

References

Danciger M, Lyon J, Worrill D, LaVail MM, Yang H (2003) A strong and highly significant QTL on chromosome 6 that protects the mouse from age-related retinal degeneration. Invest Ophthalmol Vis Sci 44: 2442–49

Farrer M, Maraganore D, Lockhart P, Singleton A, Lesnick T, de Andrade M, West A, de Silva R, Hardy J, Hernandez D (2001) alpha-Synuclein gene haplotypes are associated with Parkinson's disease. Hum Mol Genet. 10: 1847–51

Fishman GA, Birch DG, Holder GE, Birgell MG (2001) Electrophysiologic testing in disorders of the retina, optic nerve, and visual pathway (2nd Ed) American Academy of Ophthalmology Monograph Series, No. 2.

Green D, Herreros de Tejada P, Glover M (1994) Electrophysiological estimates of visual sensitivity in albino and pigmented mice. Vis Neurosci 11: 919–25

Gresh J, Goletz P, Crouch R, Rohrer B (2003) Structure-function analysis of rods and cones in juvenile, adult, and aged C57bl/6 and Balb/c mice. Vis Neurosci 20: 211–20

Humphries MM, Kiang S, McNally N, Donovan MA, Sieving PA, Bush RA, Machida S, Cotter T, Hobson A, Farrar J, Humphries P, Kenna P (2001) Comparative structural and functional analysis of photoreceptor neurons of Rho-/- mice reveal increased survival on C57BL/6J in comparison to 129Sv genetic background. Vis Neurosci 18: 437–43

Ikeda A, Naggert JK, Nishina PM (2002) Genetic modification of retinal degeneration in tubby mice. Exp Eye Res. 74: 455–61

Ikeda S, Hawes NL, Chang B, Avery CS, Smith RS, Nishina PM (1999) Severe ocular abnormalities in C57BL/6 but not in 129/Sv p53-deficient mice. Invest. Ophthalmol. Vis Sci 40: 1874–78

Jagadeesh J, Sanchez R (1981) Effects of apomorphine on the rabbit electroretinogram. Invest Ophthalmol Vis Sci 21: 620–24

Marmor M, Holder GE, Seeliger MW, S. Y (2004) Standard for clinical electroretinography (update). Doc Ophthalmol 108: 107–114

MGI Database (2007) The Jackson Laboratory. http://www.informatics.jax.org/menus/strain_menu.shtml

Nusinowitz S, Ridder W. H. III, JR. H (2002) Electrophysiological testing of the mouse visual system. In: Sundberg J (ed) Systematic evaluation of the mouse eye: anatomy, pathology and biomethods., vol 1. CRC Press, Boca Raton, pp 320–344

Peachey N, Ball S (2003) Electrophysiological analysis of visual function in mutant mice. Doc Ophthalmol. 107: 13–36

Petkov P, Ding Y, Cassell M, Zhang W, Wagner G, Sargent E, Asquith S, Crew V, Johnson K, Robinson P, Scott V, Wiles M (2004) An efficient SNP system for mouse genome scanning and elucidating strain relationships. Genome Res 14: 1806–11

Simpson E, Linder CC, Sargent EE, Davisson MT, Mobraaten LE, Sharp, JJ (1997) Genetic variation among 129 substrains and its importance for targeted mutagenesis in mice. Nature Genetics 16: 19–27

Smith R, John S, Nishina P, Sundberg J (2002) Systematic evaluation of the mouse eye: anatomy, pathology and biomethods. CRC Press LLC, Boca Raton, FL

Specht C, Schoepfer R (2001) Deletion of the alpha-synuclein locus in a subpopulation of C57BL/6J inbred mice. BMC Neurosci 2: 11

Specht CG, Schoepfer R (2004) Deletion of multimerin-1 in [alpha]-synuclein-deficient mice. Genomics 83: 1176–78

Taft R, Davisson M, Wiles M (2006) Know thy mouse. Trends Genet 22: 649–53

The Jackson Laboratory (2006) Genetic background: understanding its importance in mouse-based biomedical research. http://jaxmice.jax.org/literature/manuals/mouse_ genetics_resource_manual.pdf

Wenzel A, Reme CE, Williams TP, Hafezi F, Grimm C (2001) The Rpe65 Leu450Met variation increases retinal resistance against light-induced degeneration by slowing rhodopsin regeneration. J Neurosci 21: 53–58

Williams RW, Strom RC, Goldowitz D (1998) Natural variation in neuron number in mice is linked to a major quantitative trait Locus on Chr 11. J Neurosci 18: 138–46

Zhou G, Williams R (1999) Eye1 and Eye2: gene loci that modulate eye size, lens weight, and retinal area in the mouse. Invest Ophthalmol Vis Sci 40: 817–25

A2E, A Pigment of RPE Lipofuscin, is Generated from the Precursor, A2PE by a Lysosomal Enzyme Activity

Janet R. Sparrow, So Ra Kim, Ana M. Cuervo and Urmi Bandhyopadhyayand

1 Introduction

The lipofuscin that accumulates in retinal pigment epithelial cells with age and that is abundant in some retinal disorders, is sequestered within the interior of membrane bound organelles of the lysosomal compartment of the cell. RPE lipofuscin pigments form in large part due to reactions of vitamin A aldehyde. Evidence to support the contention that RPE lipofuscin derives primarily as a byproduct of the visual cycle, comes from work demonstrating that when the 11-*cis*-retinal (11-cisRAL) and all-*trans*-retinal (atRAL) chromophores are absent, as in $Rpe65^{-/-}$ mice, the lipofuscin-specific autofluorescence eminating from RPE whole-mounts is reduced by more than 90% (Katz and Redmond, 2001). RPE lipofuscin is also lacking in patients with early – onset retinal dystrophy associated with mutations in RPE65, a visual cycle protein shown to be the isomerohydrolase essential to the production of 11-*cis*-retinal (Lorenz et al., 2004). For some time it was thought that these lipofuscin fluorophores might form within the acidic environment of the lysosome. However, the detection of RPE lipofuscin precursors in photoreceptor outer segments, together with studies in the Royal College of Surgeon (RCS) rat showing that when outer segment phagocytosis fails, RPE lipofuscin is substantially diminished (katz et al., 1986), demonstrates an origin from photoreceptor cells. Nevertheless, questions still remain regarding the extent to which processing of the lipofuscin precursors occurs in lysosomes. For instance, the di-retinal conjugate A2E, a prominent pigment of RPE lipofuscin, is generated in photoreceptor outer segments by a multi-step pathway involving the formation of A2PE, the phosphatidyl-pyridinium bisretinoid that is the immediate precursor of A2E. Our finding that A2E is generated from A2PE by phosphate hydrolysis and that this cleavage can be mediated by phospholipase-D indicates that enzyme-mediated mechanisms may be important in releasing A2E from its precursor; acid hydrolysis of A2PE occurs at a slow rate

J.R. Sparrow
Departments of Ophthalmology; Pathology and Cell Biology,
Columbia University, New York, NY 10032, Tel: 212-305-9944, Fax: 212-305-9638
e-mail: jrs88@columbia.edu

R.E. Anderson et al. (eds.), *Recent Advances in Retinal Degeneration,*
© Springer 2008

(Liu et al., 2000; Ben-Shabat et al., 2002). The significance of enzyme-mediated hydrolysis as the mechanism responsible for generating at RAL-derived lipofuscin chromophores from their precursors, is dependent in part on demonstrating an activity in RPE cell lysosomes that can serve this function. Here we probe for such an activity.

2 Methods

2.1 Synthesis of A2E and A2PE

A2E was synthesized from at RAL and ethanolamine as described previously (Parish et al., 1998). A2PE was synthesized using atRAL and phosphatidylethanolamine from egg yolk or dipalmitoyl-phosphatidylethanolamine (DP-A2PE) as described previously (Liu et al., 2000).

2.2 Preparation of a Lysosomal Fraction of ARPE-19 Cells

Lysosomes from ARPE-19 cells were isolated by modification of a previously described method (Storrie and Madden, 1990). Briefly, ARPE-19 cells, grown to confluence (11 flasks) and serum-deprived for 24 hours, were scraped from flasks and centrifuged at 500 g for 5 min at 4°C. Pellets were resuspended in 1–2 ml of 0.25 M sucrose and the cells were disrupted in a nitrogen cavitation chamber at 35 psi pressure, on ice for 7 min. The resulting suspension of fragmented cells was centrifuged at 2500 x g for 15 min 4°C to sediment nuclei, unbroken cells and heavy mitochondria and the post-nuclear supernatant (~3 ml) was fractionated on a discontinuous metrizamide/percoll density gradient (35% metrizamide, 17% metrizamide and 6 % Percoll in 0.25% sucrose) with centrifugation (20,000 rpm, 35 min, 4°C; SW40.1 rotor). The fraction containing lysosomes and light mito-chondria (band 2) was collected, adjusted to 40% metrizamide and separated in a second discontinuous metrizamide density gradient (17% metrizamide, 5% metriza-mide and 0% metrizamide in 0.25% sucrose) by centrifugation (20,000 rpm, 35 min, 4°C). In addition, from male Wistar rats (200–250 g) fasted for 24 hours, liver lyso-somes were isolated from a light mitochondrial-lysosomal fraction in a discontin-uous metrizamide density gradient as described (Cuervo et al., 1997). Lysosomal matrices and membranes were isolated after hypotonic shock and centrifugation (200,000 g, 20 min, 4°C) (Ohsumi et al., 1983).

2.3 Incubation with Phospholipase-D and the Lysosomal Fraction

Fifteen microliters of 2 mM DP-A2PE in DMSO was added to 285 μl of 40 mM morpholinepropanesulfonic acid buffer (pH 6.5) containing 300 units/ml phospholipase-D from S. chromofuscus (Sigma-Aldrich, St. Louis, MO) and 15 mM

CaCl$_2$ or 100 μg protein of the lysosomal fraction of ARPE-19 cells or rat liver. The mixtures were incubated for 3 h at 37°C and were then extracted with 2:1 v/v chloroform/methanol containing 0.1 % TFA, dried under argon and re-dissolved in 300 μl of 50% methanolic chloroform. In some experiments, calphostin C (5 μM; Sigma-Aldrich, St. Louis, MO), and 100 μL of a protease inhibitor mixture (Sigma-Aldrich, St. Louis, MO) were added to inhibit the activity of phospholipase-D (Ben-Shabat et al., 2002). A2PE and A2E were detected by HPLC using a reverse phase C4 column, monitoring at 430 nm and injection of authentic standards of A2PE or A2E.

2.4 HPLC Analysis

For quantification of A2E and A2PE an Alliance system (Waters, Corp, Milford, MA) equipped with 2695 Separation Module, and 2996 Photodiode Array Detector and operating with Empower® software was used with a C4 column

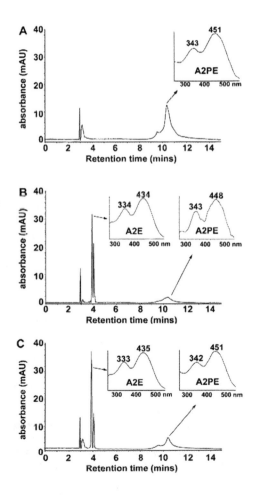

Fig. 1 An activity present in lysosomes isolated from ARPE-19 cells cleaves A2PE to generate A2E. A2PE was incubated in the absence (A) and presence (B) of the lysosomal fraction or with phospholipase-D (C). Samples were analyzed by reverse phase HPLC with 430 nm detection. A peak with UV-visible absorbance and retention time indicative of A2E appears in B and C

(4 × 250 mm, 5 μm). A2PE and A2E were eluted with the following gradients of acetonitrile in water (containing 0.1% trifluoroacetic acid): 75% (5 min; flow rate, 1 ml/min), 75–100% (5 min; flow rate, 1.5 ml/min), and 100% (10 min; flow rate, 1.5 ml/min), and were monitored at 430 nm. Injection volumes were 10 μL; each sample was injected three times for reliability.

3 Results

To assay for an enzyme activity that can release A2E from its precursor A2PE, lyso-somes were isolated from ARPE-19 cells and rat liver by differential centrifugation followed by centrifugation through a discontinuous metrizamide gradient. Incubation of an HPLC purified sample of DP-A2PE (Fig. 1A) with the RPE lysosomal fraction followed by HPLC analysis revealed the appearance of a chromatographic peak that on the basis of UV-visible absorbance and retention time could be identified as A2E. The peak attributable to A2PE was concomitantly decreased in height (Fig. 1B). Incubation of A2PE in the presence of phospholipase-D also resulted in the appearance of A2E in the chromatographic profile (Fig. 1C). A hydrolytic activity that could mediate phosphate cleavage of A2PE was also present in the liver lysosomal fraction (Fig. 2A, B). Additionally, the activity in liver lysosomes that released A2E from A2PE was efficiently suppressed by the phospholipase-D inhibitor calphostin C (Fig. 2C) and by a protease inhibitor cocktail (Fig. 2D).

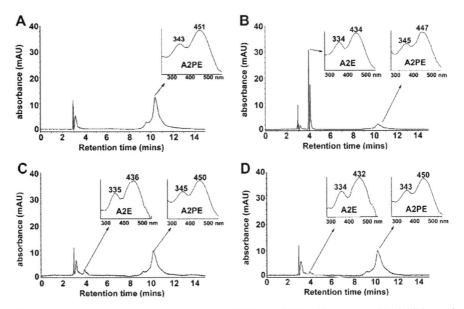

Fig. 2 An activity in liver lysosomes generates A2E from A2PE and is suppressed by inhibitors of phospholipase-D. A2PE was incubated in the absence (A) and presence (B, C, D) of a liver lyso-somal fraction. The phospholipase-D inhibitor calphostin C (C) and a protease inhibitor mixture with phospholipase-D inhibitory activity (D) were added to some reaction mixtures. Reverse phase HPLC chromatograms with 430 nm detection

4 Conclusions

Understanding the steps involved in the biosynthesis of A2E is vital to the development of therapies that would reduce the deposition of A2E in RPE cells. In the current work we have shown that an enzyme activity is present in RPE cell lysosomes that can generate A2E by phosphate hydrolysis of the precursor A2PE. The ability of phospholipase-D inhibitors to suppress the cleavage activity in the lysosomal fractions, indicates that phospholipase-D may be the enzyme in RPE cell lysosomes. The detection of small amounts of A2E in extracts of photoreceptor cell outer segments (Ben-Shabat et al., 2002), together with reports of a phospholipase-D activity in outer segments isolated from bovine eyes suggests that some A2PE may also undergo hydrolysis before internalization by RPE cells (Salvador and Giusto, 1998).

A2PE, the precursor of the lipofuscin pigment A2E, forms in outer segments (Liu et al., 2000; Ben-Shabat et al., 2002). Because shedding of outer segment membrane with deposition in RPE cells leads to the complete replacement of the outer segment every 10–14 days (Young, 1971), A2PE is not continually amassed in outer segments; rather it is transferred to RPE cells along with the phagocytosed outer segment material. Nonetheless, A2PE is not detectable in RPE cells, because as we have shown here, A2PE is efficiently processed to generate A2E. However, although other macromolecules phagocytosed by the RPE are degraded by lysosomal enzymes to small molecules that can diffuse out of the lysosome (Feeney-Burns and Eldred, 1983), after phosphate cleavage of A2PE no further degradation of the molecule occurs. This is likely because the structure of A2E is unprecedented and as such is not recognized by the lysosomal enzymes of the RPE cell. Being undigestible it accumulates. The presence of an enzyme activity in RPE lysosomes that can release di-retinal RPE lipofuscin pigments and phosphatidic acid from precursors is also significant to more recently characterized lipofuscin pigments. Specifically, we have shown that the RPE pigment atRAL dimer-E can be generated by phosphate cleavage of atRAL dimer-PE, a compound that is generated when two molecules of atRAL condense to form an aldehyde-bearing dimer that then reacts with PE to form a protonated Schiff base. The pigments atRAL dimer-PE and atRAL dimer-E have absorbances in the visible spectrum at ~ 510 nm and structures and biosynthetic pathways that are distinct from A2E/isoA2E. We have identified these compounds in RPE isolated from human eyes and in the lipofuscin-filled RPE of mice homozygous for a null mutation in the *Abca4/Abcr* gene (Fishkin et al., 2004).

Acknowledgments The work was supported by National Institutes of Health Grant EY12951 and Research to Prevent Blindness. JRS is the recipient of an Alcon Research Institute Award.

References

Ben-Shabat S, Parish CA, Vollmer HR, Itagaki Y, Fishkin N, Nakanishi K, Sparrow JR. 2002, Biosynthetic studies of A2E, a major fluorophore of RPE lipofuscin. *J Biol Chem* 277: 7183–7190.

Cuervo AM, Dice JF, Knecht E. 1997, A population of rat liver lysosomes responsible for the selective uptake and degradation of cytosolic proteins. *J Biol Chem* 272:5606–5615.

Feeney-Burns L, Eldred GE. 1983, The fate of the phagosome: conversion to 'age pigment' and impact in human retinal pigment epithelium. *Trans Ophthalmol Soc U K* 103:416–421.

Fishkin N, Pescitelli G, Sparrow JR, Nakanishi K, Berova N. 2004, Absolute configurational determination of an all-*trans*-retinal dimer isolated from photoreceptor outer segments. *Chirality* 16:637–641.

Fishkin NE, Pescitelli G, Itagaki Y, Berova N, Allikmets R, Nakanishi K, Sparrow JR. 2004, Isolation and characterization of a novel RPE cell fluorophore: all-trans-retinal dimer conjugate. *Invest Ophthalmol Vis Sci* 45:E-abstract 1803.

katz ML, Drea CM, Eldred GE, Hess HH, Robison WG, Jr. 1986, Influence of early photoreceptor degeneration on lipofuscin in the retinal pigment epithelium. *Exp Eye Res* 43:561–573.

Katz ML, Redmond TM. 2001, Effect of Rpe65 knockout on accumulation of lipofuscin fluorophores in the retinal pigment epithelium. *Invest Ophthalmol Vis Sci* 42:3023–3030.

Liu J, Itagaki Y, Ben-Shabat S, Nakanishi K, Sparrow JR. 2000, The biosynthesis of A2E, a fluorophore of aging retina, involves the formation of the precursor, A2PE, in the photoreceptor outer segment membrane. *J Biol Chem* 275:29354–29360.

Lorenz B, Wabbels B, Wegscheider E, Hamel CP, Drexler W, Presing MN. 2004, Lack of fundus autofluorescence to 488 nanometers from childhood on in patients with early-onset severe retinal dystrophy associated with mutations in RPE65. *Ophthalmol* 111:1585–1594.

Ohsumi Y, Ishikawa T, Kato K. 1983, A rapid and simplified method for the preparation of lysosomal membranes from rat liver. *J Biochem* 93:547–556.

Parish CA, Hashimoto M, Nakanishi K, Dillon J, Sparrow JR. 1998, Isolation and one-step preparation of A2E and iso-A2E, fluorophores from human retinal pigment epithelium. *Proc Natl Acad Sci U S A* 95:14609–14613.

Salvador GA, Giusto NM. 1998, Characterization of phospholipase-D activity in bovine photoreceptor membranes. *Lipids* 33:853–860.

Storrie B, Madden E. 1990, Isolation of subcellular organelles. *Methods Enzymol* 182:203–225.

Young RW. 1971, The renewal of rod and cone outer segments in the rhesus monkey. *J Cell Biol* 49:303–318.

Endothelin Receptors: Do They Have a Role in Retinal Degeneration?

Vanesa Torbidoni, María Iribarne, and Angela M. Suburo

1 Introduction

Although endothelins (ETs) were originally discovered as potent vasoconstrictors secreted by the endothelium (Yanagisawa et al., 1988), it has become evident that they also fulfill important roles in the nervous system (Schinelli, 2006). ETs are a family of 21-amino-acid peptides with three isoforms, ET-1, ET-2 and ET-3. ET-1 and ET-3 are present in most ocular structures. They are present in most regions of the anterior segment and in blood vessels of the choroid and the sclera (Chakrabarti and Sima, 1997). Precursor mRNAs of the three endothelins have been detected in the retina (Chakrabarti et al., 1998; Rattner and Nathans, 2005). ET-1 and ET-3 precursor mRNA appear in several retinal cell phenotypes (Ripodas et al., 2001), but the largest protein concentration appears in astrocytes (Torbidoni et al., 2005).

ETs mediate their action through binding to two G-protein-linked receptors, ET-A and ET-B, which have been isolated and cloned from mammalian tissues (Davenport and Maguire, 2006). ET-A is characterized by the rank affinity order ET-1=ET-2>ET-3 whereas ET-B accepts all ET isopeptides with similar affinity (Kis et al., 2006). Activation of ET receptors triggers various short- and long-term changes at cellular level but their effects on brain and retinal physiology and pathophysiology are still poorly understood, since the ET system can behave completely differently in each cell type. Complex interactions occur between both endothelinergic receptors at different levels of the signaling pathways (Blomstrand et al., 2004), and it can sometimes be difficult to recognize receptor-specific responses. ET-B, however, is unique in its ability to internalize bound ligand, reducing extracellular levels of ETs (D'Orleans-Juste et al., 2002).

Brain astrocytes are major endothelinergic effectors. ET-1 has been implicated in astrocytic regulation of the blood-brain barrier (Abbott et al., 2006), gap junctional coupling, proliferation, and pathological responses (Ostrow and

V. Torbidoni
Facultad de Ciencias Biomédicas, Universidad Austral, Pilar B1629AHJ, Buenos Aires, Argentina,
Tel: 54-2322-482959, Fax: 54-2322-482205
e-mail: atorbidoni@cas.austral.edu.ar

R.E. Anderson et al. (eds.), *Recent Advances in Retinal Degeneration*,
© Springer 2008

Sachs, 2005), Endothelinergic stimulation of astrocytes induces phosphorylation of cAMP response element-binding protein (CREB) and transcription of immediate early genes (Schinelli et al., 2001). At the neuronal level, ET-1 can modulate activity-dependent synaptic plasticity (Drew et al., 1998), and anterograde fast axonal transport (Stokely et al., 2002).

If we consider that ET-A and ET-B receptors can be expressed by neurons, glial cells and endothelia, several endothelinergic intercellular signaling circuits could be operating simultaneously in the retina. Therefore, we have characterized the retinal localization of ET-A and ET-B since this is of paramount importance to know where endothelinergic signaling is occurring. Moreover, since each of these pathways could have a specific role in retinal disease, we have focused on their participation in light-induced retinal degeneration.

2 Endothelin Receptors in the Inner Retina and Optic nerve

In the inner retina we have found that both receptors are present in blood vessels. Cells of the ganglion cell layer (GCL) exhibit a large concentration of ET-A receptor, whereas lighter immunostaining is also detected in a subpopulation of still unidentified amacrine cells. We have not detected ET-A in retinal astrocytes or Müller cells. However, a distinctive group of ET-A immunoreactive cells cover the surface of the optic nerve head (ONH) and central retina vessels. ET-B receptors were specifically found in astrocytes, both in the retina and optic nerve (Fig. 1, A–D). The large concentration of ET-1 in astrocytes could not only reflect local synthesis of this peptide, but also the capacity of ET-B receptors to internalize bound ligand. Astrocytes produce their own ET-1, but they could also obtain it from the vascular endothelium. In addition, ET-1 can be synthesized by cells of the GCL since they contain the protein precursor Pre-pro-ET-1. However the lack of ET-B receptor would preclude accumulation of the mature peptide in these cells. Astrocytes might function as reservoirs for ET-1. By regulating levels of this peptide in the extracellular space they could control permeability of the blood-retinal barrier and neuronal functions such as axonal transport and survival (Siren et al., 2002; Yagami et al., 2005). Saturation of the astrocytic ET-1 load capacity could be one of the factors involved in the loss of ganglion cells and their axons in glaucoma, where there is a high increase of intraocular ET-1 (Prasanna et al., 2005), or after chronic administration of ET-1 (Chauhan et al., 2004). On the other hand, the close association of ET-A immunoreactive glia with central vessels of the retina suggests a specific function for these cells in the control of optic nerve blood flow.

3 Endothelin Receptors in the Outer Retina

The outer plexiform layer (OPL) contains the first synapses of the visual pathway. These are complex contacts – triads – formed by photoreceptor axonic ends, bipolar dendrites and horizontal processes (Wassle, 2004). Both ET-A and ET-B receptors

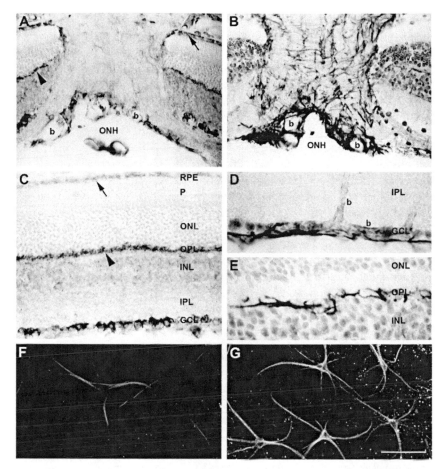

Fig. 1 A–E are sections from normal retinas stained with an immunoenzymatic procedure. (A) In the optic nerve, ET-A only labels a subpopulation of glial cells covering the ONH and central retinal vessels (b). The RPE (arrow) and OPL (arrowhead) are also labeled. (B) A similar section shows ET-B labeling of astrocytes in the optic nerve and very strong staining of ONH and perivascular glial cells. (C) This retina section demonstrates ET-A immunoreactivity in the RPE (arrow), OPL (arrowhead), and GCL cells. (D) ET-B immunoreactivity appears in a blood vessel coursing along the vitreal surface that is surrounded by strongly stained astrocytic processes. (E) In the OPL, ET-B immunoreactivity appears in branched cell processes occupying the innermost aspect of this layer. Their structure and localization identify them as horizontal cells

Figures F–G are confocal images of retinal wholemounts showing ET-B immunofluorescence in astrocytes. (F) In a control retina, immunolabeled astrocytes are sparsely distributed and show few processes. (G) After exposure to 1,500 lux during 6 days there is a higher density of astrocyte cell bodies showing a larger number of processes and stronger immunofluorescence. Calibration Bar, A to C, F and G, 50 μm; D and E, 25 μm

Illustrations reprinted from Exp. Eye Res. 81, V. Torbidoni et al., Endothelin-1 and its receptors in light-induced retinal degeneration, 265–275 (2005), with permission from Elsevier

are present in the OPL (Fig. 1A, C and E). ET-A appears in a layer of regularly distributed varicosities that partially co-localize with SV2, a marker of photoreceptor synaptic vesicles, and PSD95, a molecular scaffold protein also found in photoreceptor terminals. ET-B labels elongate processes with irregular branches located at the inner boundary of the OPL, suggesting its presence in horizontal cells. This was confirmed by co-localization of ET-B with a phosphorylated 200 Kd neurofilament (identified by monoclonal antibody RT-97) that is selectively found in horizontal cells. Horizontal networks supply continuous information regarding average light intensity over an area of the retina and maintain bipolar cell threshold constant when illumination varies (Sjostrand, 2003). Therefore, the presence of a specific endothelinergic receptors on complementary members of the triad synapse could perhaps contribute to control neurotransmitter release and/or synaptic thresholds. ET-A is also present in the retinal pigment epithelium (RPE).

Thus, differently from previous studies (MacCumber et al., 1989; Iandiev et al., 2005), we have demonstrated that retinal vascular endothelium expresses both endothelinergic receptors, whereas ET-A receptors are characteristically present in retinal neuronal structures and ET-B receptors seem to be restricted to astrocytes and horizontal cells (Torbidoni et al., 2005).

4 Endothelinergic Receptors After Light Exposure

Our experiments are carried out on male BALB/c mice, bred under a light (60 lux)/darkness cycle. Light damage is induced by constant exposure to 1,500 lux. Under these conditions, lesions begin in the temporal hemisphere, near the equator, where disappearance of photoreceptor outer and inner segments can be detected after 2–3 days, and about half of the nuclear rows in the outer nuclear layer (ONL) are missing after 6 days. At 18 days the ONL becomes reduced to one or two nuclear rows (Torbidoni et al., 2005).

A slight increase of ET-B immunofluorescence in astrocytes and its appearance in Müller radial glia follows short (1–2 days) light exposures (Torbidoni et al., 2006). Quantitative image analysis demonstrated that ET-B increase was statistically significant after 6 days of exposure (Fig. 1F and G). This increase parallels a rise of astrocytic ET-1 levels and glial fibrillary acidic protein (GFAP) labeling of astrocytes and Müller cells. At the same time, ET-A labeling of amacrine cells becomes stronger. Thus, endothelinergic changes in the inner retina resemble those described in a rat model of glaucoma (Prasanna et al., 2005). We have not detected changes in the intensity or distribution of endothelinergic receptors in the OPL after short light exposures. ET-A- and ET-B-immunoreactive structures gradually disappear after longer exposures, with significant reductions occurring in the temporal hemisphere after 4 days of exposure. Similar phenomena occur in every region of the retina, but at a slower rate. At the same time there is a large increase of ET-A in the RPE.

Increases of ET-1 and ET-B in the inner retina are compatible with the gliosis accompanying retinal degeneration (de Raad et al., 1996; Wu et al., 2003). On the other hand, the presence of ET-A and ET-B in degenerating structures of the OPL, coupled with the increase of ET-A in the RPE, suggests that endothelinergic circuits could be involved in the response to photo-injury.

5 Blocking Endothelinergic Receptors Can Reduce Light-induced Retinal Injury

A decrease in apoptotic photoreceptors and gliosis is observed when experimental animals are treated with tezosentan (10 mg/kg/day, sc, Actelion Pharmaceuticals, Switzerland) (Clozel et al., 1999) during light exposure (4 days) (Torbidoni et al., 2006). Cleaved caspase-3 (CC-3) immunostaining is a good marker of apoptosis. Retinal wholemounts from control animals treated with saline injections show 27.3 ± 3.0 CC-3+ cells/field, almost duplicating the scores in tezosentan-treated animals (17.0 ± 2.7 CC-3+ cells/field) (Torbidoni et al., 2006).

Tezosentan also reduces GFAP-immunoreactivity as measured by image analysis in retinal wholemounts. Western blots show that the highest GFAP levels correspond to animals submitted to 1,500 lux and receiving saline injections. They also show that GFAP levels in light-exposed retinas from mice receiving tezosentan are not significantly different from retinas under basal illumination conditions (Torbidoni et al., 2006).

6 Conclusions

Our findings indicate a selective distribution of ET-1 and its receptors in different layers of the neural and pigmented retina. Localization of receptors ET-A and ET-B supports the existence of physiologically important endothelinergic circuits. One would be related to astrocytes and is probably similar to that described in the blood-brain barrier (Abbott et al., 2006). In the retina, however, it seems to be coupled to endothelinergic activity of GCL cells and might be related with their survival and other physiological activities. Dysfunction of this circuit could play a role in glaucoma. Another circuit, related to photoreceptors, might regulate efficiency of synaptic transmission in the triad complex. Sources of ligand are still unclear, since prepro-ET-1 mRNA has not been found in this region of the retina but is present in the RPE (Ripodas et al., 2001). Prepro-ET-1 protein, however, seems to be present in OPL structures (Torbidoni et al., 2005). On the other hand, light injury can induce expression of ET-2 (Rattner and Nathans, 2005). The importance of this circuit is demonstrated by the reduction of light-induced photoreceptor apoptosis after blockade of endothelinergic receptors. Endothelinergic blockade also decreases the gliosis associated with photoreceptor degeneration. This downregulation would reflect both a direct inhibition of the glial hypertrophic response and the improvement of neuronal survival. Thus, the endothelinergic system appears as a crucial mediator in the crosstalk between neurons and glial cells in healthy and diseased retinas.

Acknowledgments Research has been supported by Universidad Austral, Consejo Nacional de Investigaciones Científicas y Técnicas, and Secretaría de Estado de Ciencia y Tecnología, Argentina.

References

Abbott, N. J., Ronnback, L., Hansson, E., 2006, Astrocyte-endothelial interactions at the blood-brain barrier, *Nat. Rev. Neurosci.* **7**:41.

Blomstrand, F., Venance, L., Siren, A. L., Ezan, P., Hanse, E., Glowinski, J., Ehrenreich, H., Giaume, C., 2004, Endothelins regulate astrocyte gap junctions in rat hippocampal slices, *Eur. J. Neurosci.* **19**:1005.

Chakrabarti, S., Gan, X. T., Merry, A., Karmazyn, M., Sima, A. A., 1998, Augmented retinal endothelin-1, endothelin-3, endothelinA and endothelinB gene expression in chronic diabetes, *Curr. Eye Res.* **17**:301.

Chakrabarti, S., Sima, A. A., 1997, Endothelin-1 and endothelin-3-like immunoreactivity in the eyes of diabetic and non-diabetic BB/W rats, *Diabetes Res. Clin. Pract.* **37**:109.

Chauhan, B. C., LeVatte, T. L., Jollimore, C. A., Yu, P. K., Reitsamer, H. A., Kelly, M. E., Yu, D. Y., Tremblay, F., Archibald, M. L., 2004, Model of endothelin-1-induced chronic optic neuropathy in rat, *Invest. Ophthalmol. Vis. Sci.* **45**:144.

Clozel, M., Ramuz, H., Clozel, J. P., Breu, V., Hess, P., Loffler, B. M., Coassolo, P., Roux, S., 1999, Pharmacology of tezosentan, new endothelin receptor antagonist designed for parenteral use, *J. Pharmacol. Exp. Ther.* **290**:840.

Davenport, A. P., Maguire, J. J., 2006, Endothelin, *Handb. Exp. Pharmacol.* **176** Pt 1:295.

de Raad, S., Szczesny, P. J., Munz, K., Reme, C. E., 1996, Light damage in the rat retina: glial fibrillary acidic protein accumulates in Muller cells in correlation with photoreceptor damage, *Ophthalmic. Res.* **28**:99.

D'Orleans-Juste, P., Labonte, J., Bkaily, G., Choufani, S., Plante, M., Honore, J. C., 2002, Function of the endothelin(B) receptor in cardiovascular physiology and pathophysiology, *Pharmacol. Ther.* **95**:221.

Drew, G. M., Coussens, C. M., Abraham, W. C., 1998, Effects of endothelin-1 on hippocampal synaptic plasticity, *Neuroreport* **9**:1827.

Iandiev, I., Uhlmann, S., Pietsch, U. C., Biedermann, B., Reichenbach, A., Wiedemann, P., Bringmann, A., 2005, Endothelin receptors in the detached retina of the pig, *Neurosci. Lett.* **384**:72.

Kis, B., Chen, L., Ueta, Y., Busija, D. W., 2006, Autocrine peptide mediators of cerebral endothelial cells and their role in the regulation of blood-brain barrier, *Peptides* **27**:211.

MacCumber, M. W., Ross, C. A., Glaser, B. M., Snyder, S. H., 1989, Endothelin: visualization of mRNAs by in situ hybridization provides evidence for local action, *Proc. Natl. Acad. Sci. U S A* **86**:7285.

Ostrow, L. W., Sachs, F., 2005, Mechanosensation and endothelin in astrocytes – hypothetical roles in CNS pathophysiology, *Brain Res. Brain Res. Rev.* **48**:488.

Prasanna, G., Hulet, C., Desai, D., Krishnamoorthy, R. R., Narayan, S., Brun, A.-M., Suburo, A. M., Yorio, T., 2005, Effect of elevated intraocular pressure on endothelin-1 in a rat model of glaucoma, *Pharmacol. Res.* **51**:41.

Rattner, A., Nathans, J., 2005, The genomic response to retinal disease and injury: evidence for endothelin signaling from photoreceptors to glia, *J. Neurosci.* **25**:4540.

Ripodas, A., de Juan, J. A., Roldan-Pallares, M., Bernal, R., Moya, J., Chao, M., Lopez, A., Fernandez-Cruz, A., Fernandez-Durango, R., 2001, Localisation of endothelin-1 mRNA expression and immunoreactivity in the retina and optic nerve from human and porcine eye. Evidence for endothelin-1 expression in astrocytes, *Brain Res.* **912**:137.

Schinelli, S., 2006, Pharmacology and physiopathology of the brain endothelin system: an overview, *Curr. Med. Chem.* **13**:627.

Schinelli, S., Zanassi, P., Paolillo, M., Wang, H., Feliciello, A., Gallo, V., 2001, Stimulation of endothelin B receptors in astrocytes induces cAMP response element-binding protein phosphorylation and c-fos expression via multiple mitogen-activated protein kinase signaling pathways, *J. Neurosci.* **21**:8842.

Siren, A. L., Lewczuk, P., Hasselblatt, M., Dembowski, C., Schilling, L., Ehrenreich, H., 2002, Endothelin B receptor deficiency augments neuronal damage upon exposure to hypoxia-ischemia in vivo, *Brain Res.* **945**:144.

Sjostrand, F. S., 2003, Color vision at low light intensity, dark adaptation, Purkinje shift, critical flicker frequency and the deterioration of vision at low illumination. Neurophysiology at the nanometer range of neural structure, *J. Submicrosc. Cytol. Pathol.* **35**:117.

Stokely, M. E., Brady, S. T., Yorio, T., 2002, Effects of endothelin-1 on components of anterograde axonal transport in optic nerve, *Invest. Ophthalmol. Vis. Sci.* **43**:3223.

Torbidoni, V., Iribarne, M., Ogawa, L., Prasanna, G., Suburo, A. M., 2005, Endothelin-1 and its receptors in light-induced retinal degeneration, *Exp. Eye Res.* **81**:265.

Torbidoni, V., Iribarne, M., Suburo, A. M., 2006, Endothelin receptors in light-induced retinal degeneration, *Exp. Biol. Med. (Maywood)* **231**:1095.

Wassle, H., 2004, Parallel processing in the mammalian retina, *Nat. Rev. Neurosci.* **5**:747.

Wu, K. H., Madigan, M. C., Billson, F. A., Penfold, P. L., 2003, Differential expression of GFAP in early v late AMD: a quantitative analysis, *Br. J. Ophthalmol.* **87**:1159.

Yagami, T., Ueda, K., Sakaeda, T., Okamura, N., Nakazato, H., Kuroda, T., Hata, S., Sakaguchi, G., Itoh, N., Hashimoto, Y., Fujimoto, M., 2005, Effects of an endothelin B receptor agonist on secretory phospholipase A2-IIA-induced apoptosis in cortical neurons, *Neuropharmacology* **48**:291.

Yanagisawa, M., Kurihara, H., Kimura, S., Tomobe, Y., Kobayashi, M., Mitsui, Y., Yazaki, Y., Goto, K., Masaki, T., 1988, A novel potent vasoconstrictor peptide produced by vascular endothelial cells, *Nature* **332**:411.

CNTF Negatively Regulates the Phototransduction Machinery in Rod Photoreceptors: Implication for Light-Induced Photostasis Plasticity

Rong Wen, Ying Song, Yun Liu, Yiwen Li, Lian Zhao, and Alan M. Laties

1 Introduction

CNTF is a member of the interleukin-6 (IL-6) family of neuropoietic cytokines, which includes IL-6, IL-11, LIF (leukemia inhibitory factor), OsM (oncostatin M), and CT-1 (cardiotropin 1).

LaVail and colleagues (LaVail et al., 1992) were the first to report that CNTF promotes photoreceptor survival. Since then, the protective effect of CNTF has been confirmed in many animal models cross several species. These findings have raised the hope that CNTF could be a potential treatment for retinal degenerations.

Experiments using adeno-associated viral vectors to deliver cDNA of CNTF to retinal cells in animal models confirm the long-term protection of photoreceptors by CNTF (Liang et al., 2001; Bok et al., 2002; Schlichtenbrede et al., 2003). However, the treated retinas showed no improvement in the amplitudes of ERG responses. In some cases, the ERG responses in treated retinas had even lower amplitudes than in controls, despite the fact that many more rod photoreceptors survived than would have without the treatment. These unexpected and seemingly contradictory results raised the question whether CNTF might be detrimental to the function of photoreceptors.

To understand CNTF-induced suppression of ERG waves in rodent retina, we investigated the effects of CNTF on rods using recombinant human CNTF protein. Our results indicate that CNTF negatively regulates the phototransduction machinery in rod photoreceptors, leading to a decrease in their photon-catching capability. As a result, the ERG amplitudes are lower in CNTF-treated retinas at a given intensity of light stimulus (Wen et al., 2006). The similarity between CNTF-induced changes and light-induced photoreceptor plasticity strongly suggests that the same underlying mechanism operates under both conditions.

R. Wen

Department of Ophthalmology, University of Pennsylvania, School of Medicine; Philadelphia, PA 19104, Tel: 215-746-0207, 215-746-0209
e-mail: rwen@mail.med.upenn.edu

R.E. Anderson et al. (eds.), *Recent Advances in Retinal Degeneration*,
© Springer 2008

2 CNTF-Induced Changes IN ERG

To investigate CNTF-induced changes in the ERG, adult Long-Evans rats were injected with CNTF into the left eyes (intravitreal injection, 10 μg in 5 μl of phosphate buffered saline, or PBS) and the right eyes with PBS (5 μl). The same treatment was used in all experiments described in this chapter.

ERGs were recorded from both eyes simultaneously in the same animals 6 and 21 days after injection. The a-waves were measured from baseline to trough and b-waves were measured from the baseline or from the trough of the a-wave when present. The Naka-Rushton function is used to evaluate changes in the scotopic b-wave amplitude and sensitivity ($1/k$) (Fulton and Rushton, 1978).

Substantial decreases in the a- and b-wave responses were observed in eyes 6 days after CNTF injection (Fig. 1). The log-log plots of the a-wave (Fig. 1A, B) show proportional amplitude reduction at every intensity 6 days after injection, which is completely reversed by 21 days. The log-linear plots of b-wave amplitude versus intensity (Fig. 1C, D) illustrate the substantial reduction in amplitude as well as the shift to the right in the half-maximal intensity value (k), indicating a decrease

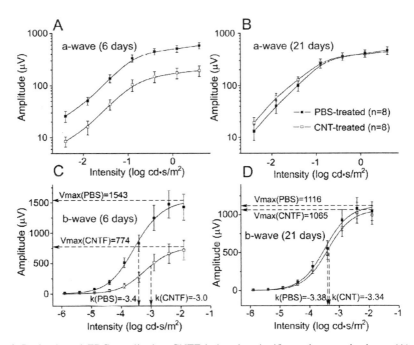

Fig. 1 Dark-adapted ERG amplitudes. CNTF induced a significant decrease in the a- (A) and b-wave (C) 6 days after injection. No significant difference between CNTF- and PBS-treated eyes in either a- (B) or b-wave (D) 21 days after injection. Solid lines in A and B are B-spline curves through the data points. Solid lines in C and D are the averaged Naka-Rushton function fits. Dashed lines indicate V_{max} and k values from these fits. Data are means ± SEM (n = 8). From Wen et al., 2006 (© 2006 by the Society for Neuroscience)

in sensitivity. These changes also recovered completely by 21 days along with the a-wave.

3 Changes in Phototransduction Related Proteins

The levels of several phototransduction related proteins, including rhodopsin, the transducin α, β subunits, and arrestin were measured by immunoblot analysis. Decreases in rhodopsin, transducin α and β were observed 6 days after CNTF treatment (Fig. 2A). The level of arrestin increased 3 and 6 days after CNTF treatment. All changes fully recovered 21 days after CNTF injection. In comparison, the level of Nrl was not significantly altered (Fig. 2A).

There was also a decrease in rhodopsin level in animals after exposure to 400 lx light, 10 hr daily, for 7 days (Fig. 2B). An increase in the arrestin level was also seen (Fig. 2B). All these changes fully recovered to pre-exposure levels after 7 days in the normal habitat cyclic light of 50 lx (Fig. 2B).

The transcriptional expression of rhodopsin and arrestin was examined by quantitative real-time PCR. A significant decrease in rhodopsin mRNA was seen 3 days and 6 days after CNTF injection (Fig. 2C). There was little change in arrestin mRNA after CNTF treatment (Fig. 2D), indicating that the increase in arrestin protein level was not due to an increase in transcription.

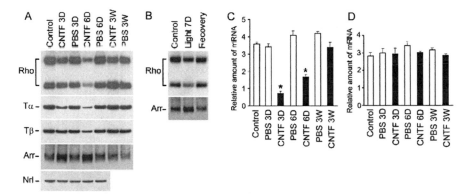

Fig. 2 CNTF- and light-induced changes phototransduction related proteins. Decrease in rhodopsin (Rho), transducin α and β subunit (Tα, Tβ) are observed after CNTF injection. An increase in arrestin (Arr) was also seen after treatment. No change was found in the Nrl level. All changes fully recovered by 21 days. A decrease in rhodopsin protein was seen after exposure to 10 hr 400 lx light for 7 days (B), along with an increase in arrestin. The light-induced changes fully recovered 7 days after exposure. CNTF induced a significant decrease in rhodopsin mRNA 3 and 6 days after treatment (C). Expression of arrestin was not altered (D). Asterisks indicate $p < 0.001$ (ANOVA). Modified from Wen et al., (2006) (© 2006 by the Society for Neuroscience)

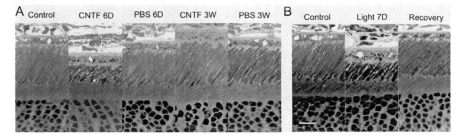

Fig. 3 Changes of ROS induced by CNTF and light exposure. CNTF induced a shortening of ROS with narrow regions along ROS length 6 days after treatment, which completely recovered 3 weeks after treatment (A). No alteration was seen in eyes treated with PBS (A). A shortening of ROS was seen after 7 days of light exposure (400 lx, 10 hr daily) (B). The ROS length recovered to normal after 7 days in cyclic 50 lx light (B). Scale bar: 10 μm. Modified from Wen et al., (2006) (© 2006 by the Society for Neuroscience)

4 CNTF- and Light-induced Changes in Rod Outer Segments

Six days after CNTF treatment, the length of rod outer segments (ROS) in CNTF-treated eyes was ($15.38 \pm 1.39\,\mu$m, mean $\pm$ SD, n = 13), shortened by about half (46% $p < 0.0001$, Student t test) compared to that ($28.31 \pm 2.72\,\mu$m, mean $\pm$ SD, n = 13) in the PBS-treated eye (Fig. 3A). The shape of the ROS in CNTF-treated eye became irregular with narrow regions along the length (Fig. 3A), which was not seen in the PBS-treated eye. Changes in ROS length and shape fully recovered 21 days after treatment (Fig. 3A).

A shortening of ROS comparable to that in CNTF-treated animals was observed in retinas that had received 10 hr daily light exposure (400 lx) for 7 days (Fig. 3B). The shape of the ROS also became somewhat irregular (Fig. 3B). These changes were fully recovered after 7 days in the normal cyclic habitat illuminance of 50 lx (Fig. 3B).

5 Discussion

We have demonstrated that CNTF treatment induces a series of biochemical and morphological changes in rod photoreceptors, which work in concert to down regulate the phototransduction machinery, leading to a lower photoresponsiveness. As a result, the amplitudes of the ERG a- and b-waves are lower in CNTF-treated retinas at a given intensity of stimulus. These biochemical and morphological changes in photoreceptors as well as changes in the ERG waves are fully reversible.

Photoreceptors are not directly responsive to CNTF. The effects of CTNF must be mediated through cells that are directly responsive to CNTF. In the retina, Müller cells directly respond to CNTF (Wen et al., 2006; Peterson et al., 2000). It is therefore likely that they are the mediators. In this scenario, CNTF activates Müller cells, which in turn send signals to rods (Fig. 4). The nature of the signals from Müller cells is not clear, but it is likely a diffusible factor (Fig. 4). Identification of the putative factor would shed light on Müller-photoreceptor interaction. It may also have potential medical applications.

CNTF-induced changes in rods are very similar to those found in animals exposed to higher habitat illuminance. Rhodopsin content in the retina is reduced in cyclic light-reared albino rats compared to dark-reared ones (Organisciak and Noell, 1977). Battelle and LaVail (Battelle and LaVail, 1978) demonstrated dynamic changes in rhodopsin content and ROS length under different light conditions. They found that dark adaptation for 10 days increased the rhodopsin content in light-reared animals to the level comparable to dark-reared animals. Returning animals to previous habitat illuminance reverse the change. Changes in ROS length follow a similar pattern (Battelle and LaVail, 1978). Moving animals from dark to cyclic light induces a decrease in rhodopsin expression, a decrease in transducin α expression, and an increase in arrestin expression (Organisciak et al., 1991; Farber et al., 1991). In addition, animals reared in high habitat illuminance have lower amplitude ERG a-waves than those reared in lower light levels (Reiser et al., 1996). The similarity between CNTF- and light-induced changes indicates that CNTF mimics light exposure in this regard, and suggests a common underlying mechanism (Fig. 4).

ROS undergo continual renewal (Young, 1967; Young and Droz, 1968). New disks are assembled at the base of ROS to displace the existing ones outward (Hall et al., 1969; Bargoot et al., 1969) and disks at the tip are shed and phagocytized by

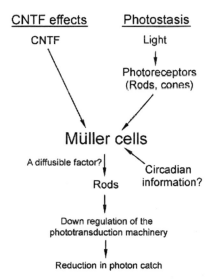

Fig. 4 Schematic illustration of hypothesized mechanism. CNTF activates Müller cells, which in turn send a signal to rods. In photostasis, Müller cells collect information of the number of photons captured by photoreceptors and circadian information from photosensitive ganglion cells. When the number of photons captured exceeds the daily quota for the retina, Müller cells inform rods to down regulate their phototransduction machinery. The CNTF and photostasis pathways converge in Müller cells

RPE cells (Young and Bok, 1969). Penn and Williams (Penn and Williams, 1986) offered the photostasis hypothesis to explain the light-induced adjustment in photoreceptors and the role ROS renewal plays. They proposed that the continual renewal of ROS allows rods to adjust the ROS length and rhodopsin content to a new light environment by regulating the rates of disk addition and removal. They further hypothesized that the adjustment is to allow the retina to catch a constant number of photons per day regardless of the light conditions the animal is chronically exposed to. In other words, there is a "set point" toward which rods adjust their photon-catching apparatus in changing light conditions. In albino rats, the daily quota of photons for a retina is about 10^{16} (Penn and Williams, 1986). Although numerous studies have provided evidence supporting this hypothesis, some fundamental questions remain. It is not clear how the number of photons captured by the entire retina is counted; where the photon counting mechanism is located; and how the information is fed back to individual photoreceptors so they can adjust their phototransduction machinery accordingly. Since intravitreal administration of CNTF regulates the phototransduction machinery, the regulatory mechanism should be inside the retina and input from outside the retina is not required. If the mechanism mediating the effects of CNTF is the same that mediates light-induced photoplasticity, then the mechanism of photostasis must be located inside the retina. We therefore hypothesize that Müller cells are the photon counters. They may integrate information from photoreceptors and circadian information from photosensitive ganglion cells (Berson et al., 2002), then signal rods to regulate their phototransduction machinery.

In summary, we have demonstrated that CNTF negatively regulates rod phototransduction machinery, resulting in lower amplitude ERG waves. The similarity between CNTF treatment and light exposure strongly suggests that regulation of the phototransduction machinery by CNTF and light is through a common mechanism, the mechanism mediating photostasis in which Müller cells play a central role. Our work highlights the glia-neuron interaction to control the behavior of neurons.

Acknowledgments Supported by NIH grants EY12727, EY015289, the Foundation Fighting Blindness, and the Karl Kirchgessner Foundation.

References

Bargoot, F. G., Williams, T. P. and Beidler, L. M., 1969, The localization of radioactive amino acid taken up into the outer segments of frog (Rana pipiens) rods. *Vision Res* **9**:385–391.

Battelle, B. A. and LaVail, M. M., 1978, Rhodopsin content and rod outer segment length in albino rat eyes: modification by dark adaptation. *Exp Eye Res* **26**:487–497.

Berson, D. M., Dunn, F. A. and Takao, M., 2002, Phototransduction by retinal ganglion cells that set the circadian clock. *Science* **295**:1070–1073.

Bok, D., Yasumura, D., Matthes, M. T., Ruiz, A., Duncan, J. L., Chappelow, A. V., Zolutukhin, S., Hauswirth, W. and LaVail, M. M., 2002, Effects of adeno-associated virus-vectored ciliary neurotrophic factor on retinal structure and function in mice with a P216L rds/peripherin mutation. *Exp Eye Res* **74**:719–735.

Farber, D. B., Danciger, J. S. and Organisciak, D. T., 1991, Levels of mRNA encoding proteins of the cGMP cascade as a function of light environment. *Exp Eye Res* **53**:781–786.

Fulton, A. B. and Rushton, W. A., 1978, The human rod ERG: correlation with psychophysical responses in light and dark adaptation. *Vision Res* **18**:793–800.

Hall, M. O., Bok, D. and Bacharach, A. D., 1969, Biosynthesis and assembly of the rod outer segment membrane system. Formation and fate of visual pigment in the frog retina. *J Mol Biol* **45**:397–406.

LaVail, M. M., Unoki, K., Yasumura, D., Matthes, M. T., Yancopoulos, G. D. and Steinberg, R. H., 1992, Multiple growth factors, cytokines, and neurotrophins rescue photoreceptors from the damaging effects of constant light. *Proc Natl Acad Sci U S A* **89**:11249–11253.

Liang, F. Q., Aleman, T. S., Dejneka, N. S., Dudus, L., Fisher, K. J., Maguire, A. M., Jacobson, S. G. and Bennett, J., 2001, Long-term protection of retinal structure but not function using RAAV.CNTF in animal models of retinitis pigmentosa. *Mol Ther* **4**:461–472.

Organisciak, D. T. and Noell, W. K., 1977, The rod outer segment phospholipid/opsin ratio of rats maintained in darkness or cyclic light. *Invest Ophthalmol Vis Sci* **16**:188–190.

Organisciak, D. T., Xie, A., Wang, H. M., Jiang, Y. L., Darrow, R. M. and Donoso, L. A., 1991, Adaptive changes in visual cell transduction protein levels: effect of light. *Exp Eye Res* **53**: 773–779.

Penn, J. S. and Williams, T. P., 1986, Photostasis: regulation of daily photon-catch by rat retinas in response to various cyclic illuminances. *Exp Eye Res* **43**:915–928.

Peterson, W. M., Wang, Q., Tzekova, R. and Wiegand, S. J., 2000, Ciliary neurotrophic factor and stress stimuli activate the Jak-STAT pathway in retinal neurons and glia. *J Neurosci* **20**: 4081–4090.

Reiser, M. A., Williams, T. P. and Pugh, E. N., Jr., 1996, The effect of light history on the aspartate-isolated fast-PIII responses of the albino rat retina. *Invest Ophthalmol Vis Sci* **37**:221–229.

Schlichtenbrede, F. C., MacNeil, A., Bainbridge, J. W., Tschernutter, M., Thrasher, A. J., Smith, A. J. and Ali, R. R., 2003, Intraocular gene delivery of ciliary neurotrophic factor results in significant loss of retinal function in normal mice and in the Prph2Rd2/Rd2 model of retinal degeneration. *Gene Ther* **10**:523–527.

Wen, R., Song, Y., Kjellstrom, S., Tanikawa, A., Liu, Y., Li, Y., Zhao, L., Bush, R. A., Laties, A. M. and Sieving, P. A., 2006, Regulation of rod phototransduction machinery by ciliary neurotrophic factor. *J Neurosci* **26**:13523–13530.

Young, R. W., 1967, The renewal of photoreceptor cell outer segments. *J Cell Biol* **33**:61–72.

Young, R. W. and Droz, B., 1968, The renewal of protein in retinal rods and cones. *J Cell Biol* **39**:169–184.

Young, R. W. and Bok, D., 1969, Participation of the retinal pigment epithelium in the rod outer segment renewal process. *J Cell Biol* **42**:392–403.

About the Editors

Robert E. Anderson, M.D., Ph.D., is George Lynn Cross Research Professor and Chair of Cell Biology, Dean A. McGee Professor of Ophthalmology, and Adjunct Professor of Biochemistry & Molecular Biology and Geriatric Medicine at The University of Oklahoma Health Sciences Center in Oklahoma City, Oklahoma. He is also Director of Research at the Dean A. McGee Eye Institute. He received his Ph.D. in Biochemistry (1968) from Texas A&M University and his M.D. from Baylor College of Medicine in 1975. In 1968, he was a postdoctoral fellow at Oak Ridge Associated Universities. At Baylor, he was appointed Assistant Professor in 1969, Associate Professor in 1976, and Professor in 1981. He joined the faculty of the University of Oklahoma in January of 1995. Dr. Anderson has published extensively in the areas of lipid metabolism in the retina and biochemistry of retinal degenerations. He has edited 13 books, 12 on retinal degenerations and one on the biochemistry of the eye. Dr. Anderson has received the Sam and Bertha Brochstein Award for Outstanding Achievement in Retina Research from the Retina Research Foundation (1980), and the Dolly Green Award (1982) and two Senior Scientific Investigator Awards (1990 and 1997) from Research to Prevent Blindness, Inc. He received an Award for Outstanding Contributions to Vision Research from the Alcon Research Institute (1985), and the Marjorie Margolin Prize (1994). He has served on the editorial boards of *Investigative Ophthalmology and Visual Science, Journal of Neuroscience Research, Neurochemistry International, Current Eye Research,* and *Experimental Eye Research.* Dr. Anderson has received grants from the National Institutes of Health, The Retina Research Foundation, the Foundation Fighting Blindness, and Research to Prevent Blindness, Inc. He has been an active participant in the program committees of the Association for Research in Vision and Ophthalmology (ARVO) and was a trustee representing the Biochemistry and Molecular Biology section. He has served on the Vision Research Program Committee and Board of Scientific Counselors of the National Eye Institute and the Board of the Basic and Clinical Science Series of The American Academy of Ophthalmology. Dr. Anderson is a past Councilor and Treasurer, and is current President-Elect, of the International Society for Eye Research.

Matthew M. LaVail, Ph.D., is Professor of Anatomy and Ophthalmology at the University of California, San Francisco School of Medicine. He received his Ph.D. degree in Anatomy (1969) from the University of Texas Medical Branch in

Galveston and was subsequently a postdoctoral fellow at Harvard Medical School. Dr. LaVail was appointed Assistant Professor of Neurology-Neuropathology at Harvard Medical School in 1973. In 1976, he moved to UCSF, where he was appointed Associate Professor of Anatomy. He was appointed to his current position in 1982, and in 1988, he also became director of the Retinitis Pigmentosa Research Center at UCSF, later named the Kearn Family Center for the Study of Retinal Degeneration. Dr. LaVail has published extensively in the research areas of photoreceptor-retinal pigment epithelial cell interactions, retinal development, circadian events in the retina, genetics of pigmentation and ocular abnormalities, inherited retinal degenerations, light-induced retinal degeneration, and pharmaceutical and gene therapy for retinal degenerative diseases. He has identified several naturally occurring murine models of human retinal degenerations and has developed transgenic mouse and rat models of others. He is the author of more than 150 research publications and has edited 12 books on inherited and environmentally induced retinal degenerations. Dr. LaVail has received the Fight for Sight Citation (1976); the Sundial Award from the Retina Foundation (1976); the Friedenwald Award from the Association for Research in Vision and Ophthalmology (ARVO, 1981); two Senior Scientific Investigators Awards from Research to Prevent Blindness (1988 and 1998); a MERIT Award from the National Eye Institute (1989); an Award for Outstanding Contributions to Vision Research from the Alcon Research Institute (1990); the Award of Merit from the Retina Research Foundation (1990); the first John A. Moran Prize for Vision Research from the University of Utah (1997); the first Trustee Award from The Foundation Fighting Blindness (1998); and the Llura Liggett Gund Award from the Foundation Fighting Blindness (2007). He has served on the editorial board of *Investigative Ophthalmology and Visual Science* and is currently an Executive Editor of *Experimental Eye Research*. Dr. LaVail has been an active participant in the program committee of ARVO and has served as a Trustee (Retinal Cell Biology Section) of ARVO. He has been a member of the program committee and a Vice President of the International Society for Eye research. He has also served on the Scientific Advisory Board of the Foundation Fighting Blindness since 1973.

Joe G. Hollyfield, Ph.D., is Director of Ophthalmic Research in the Cole Eye Institute at The Cleveland Clinic Foundation, Cleveland, Ohio. He received his Ph.D. from the University of Texas at Austin and did postdoctoral work at the Hubrecht Laboratory in Utrecht, The Netherlands. He has held faculty positions at Columbia University College of Physicians and Surgeons in New York City and at Baylor College of Medicine in Houston, TX. He was Director of the Retinitis Pigmentosa Research Center in The Cullen Eye Institute at Baylor from 1978 until his move to The Cleveland Clinic Foundation in 1995. He is currently Director of the Foundation Fighting Blindness Research Center at The Cleveland Clinic Foundation. Dr. Hollyfield has published over 170 papers in the area of cell and developmental biology of the retina and retinal pigment epithelium in both normal and retinal degenerative tissue. He has edited 13 books, 12 on retinal degenerations and one destructor of the eye. Dr. Hollyfield has received the Marjorie W. Margolin Prize (1981, 1994), the Sam and Bertha Brochstein Award (1985) and the Award of Merit in Retina Research (1998) from the Retina Research Foundation;

the Olga Keith Wiess Distinguished Scholars' Award (1981), two Senior Scientific Investigator Awards (1988, 1994) from Research to Prevent Blindness, Inc.; an award for Outstanding Contributions to Vision Research from the Alcon Research Institute (1987); the Distinguished Alumnus Award (1991) from Hendrix College, Conway, Arkansas; and the Endre A. Balazs Prize (1994) from the International Society for Eye Research (ISER). He is currently Editor-in-Chief of the journal, *Experimental Eye Research* published by Academic Press. Dr. Hollyfield has been active in the Association for Research in Vision and Ophthalmology (ARVO) serving on the Program Committee, as a Trustee and as President. He is also a past President and former Secretary of the International Society of Eye Research. He currently serves on the Scientific Advisory Boards of The Foundation Fighting Blindness, Research to Prevent Blindness, The Helen Keller Eye Research Foundation, The South Africa Retinitis Pigmentosa Foundation, and is Co-Chairman of the International Retinitis Pigmentosa Foundation Medical and Scientific Advisory Board.

Index

AAV-Opsin-rds, 136
ABI Prism GeneMapper Software v3.0, 231
ADRP associated rhodopsin mutation
  riboenzyme knockdown in vitro analysis,
    97–98
A2E from precursor A2PE generation,
  395–396
A2E-mediated RPE cell damage, 40
Affymetrix GeneChip® mouse Genome 430
  2.0 microarrays, 76
Age-related maculopathy
  degeneration, 45
  genetic association studies for
    chromosome 10q26 locus, 216–217
    RCA locus, 214–216
  and genetics risks of, 211
  Hardy-Weinberg equilibrium, 213
  macrophages role of, 186
  risk factors for, 185
  Utah population in, 253
Ala69Ser polymorphism, 217
Allele-independentADRP gene therapy, 107
AMD. see Age-related macular degeneration
AMD Bruch's membrane, 261–262
AMD higher fidelity model, 185
AMD-related pathways, 166
Anti-angiogenic factor like PEDF
  expression, 187
ARM. see Age-related maculopathy
ARPE19 cell line phagocytosis, 325
Aryl-hydrocarbon interacting protein-like 1
  (AIPL1), 231
Autosomal dominant form of RP (ADRP), 97
Autosomal dominant retinitis pigmentosa
  (adRP)
  causes of, 203
  genes and, 204
  genetic testing of probands and families
    with, 207

PRPF31 deletions in six adRP families,
  206–207
Autosomal Dominant Retinitis Pigmentosa
  (ADRP) mouse model and gene
  therapy, 107

Bassen- Kornzweig disease. see Hereditary
  abetalipoproteinemia
Bcl-x gene role in photoreceptor survival, 69
BCL-X$_L$ expression, 70
BDNF activity, 346
Best macular dystrophy, 22
Bonferroni post test and light induced
  apoptosis, 63
Bovine ROS, in vitro phosphorylation and
  inhibition by PP2, 336
Brain enriched genes, 182

Cu^{2+}/K$^+$ exchanger (NCKX), 351
Calcium-binding mitochondrial carriers
  (CaMCs), 239
Calmodulin (CaM) gene, 352
cAMP response element-binding protein
  (CREB), 400
Canine retina and brain gene profiles
  Principal Component Analysis (PCA)
    of, 183
  by retinal cDNA microarray, 179
Cathepsin D and Cathepsin Z, 187
Caveolin-1 (Cav-1), 335
Cav-1 phosphorylation, 338
C57BL/6 substrains, variation in
  electroretinogram, 386–388
CEP induced angiogenesis, 263
Cep induces neovascularization, 262–263
cGMP-gated (CNG), 351
Chick chorioallantoic membrane (CAM) assay,
  262–263
Choroidal neovascularization (CNV), 261

Ciliary neurotrophic factor (CNTF), 42, 45
    induced changes in rods, 405
    induced suppression of ERG waves in
        rodent retina, 401
    intraocular side-effects of, 45–49
    and light-induced changes in Rod Outer
        Segments, 404
    and light-induced changes photo-
        transduction related proteins,
        403
    photoreceptor cells and, 46
Clonning of stem cells, 4
CNGA3 and CNGB3 expression in 661W
    cells, 329–330
Complement factor H (CFH) on chromosome
    1q31, 211
Conditional Bcl-x Knockout mice analysis, 70
Cone/cone-rod dystrophies (CORDs), 229, 235
Cone cyclic nucleotide-gated (CNG) channel
    activation, 327
    antibodies and, 328
    electrophysiological recordings, 329
    heterologous expression of, 328–329
Cone-expressed cDNAs and microarray
    screening, 236
Cone function in RPE65-deficient animal
    models after AAV gene transfer, 89–90
Cone photoreceptors
    cell line 661W profiling, 301
        culture conditions and morphology of,
            302
        immortalization of mouse photoreceptor
            cells and, 302
        Peptide Mass Fingerprinting (PMF),
            303
    and molecular defects, 235
Cone phototransduction, 327
Cones and rods
    induced optomotor response, 90–91
    retinal degenerations, 23
Cone-specific Bcl-x Knockout mice
    characterization, 71
Congenital achromatopsia, 23
CORD5 haplotypes, 230
Cre-activatable lacZ reporter (R26R) mice, 71
C214S mutation in Rds, 132
    functional rescue of, 132–133
    histological rescue of, 133–135
Cytomegalovirus promoter (CBA-CMV), 188

Decosahexanoic acid (DHA), 61
Diabetic retinopathy (DR), 53
Dipalmitoyl-phosphatidylethanolamine
    (DP-A2PE), 394

3-(4,5-Dimethylthiazol-2-yl)-
    2,5-Diphenyltetrazolium bromide
    (MTT), 62
Docosahexaenoic acid, 39
Drusen-positive phenotype, 188
Dulbecco's modified eagle's medium
    (DMEM), 322

EFEMP1and diseased human retina, 279–280
Elovl4 5-bp deletion, 283
ELOVL4 role in fatty acid metabolism,
    283–285
Embryonic development and molecular
    recycling, 7–9
Embryonic stem cells, 4
Encapsulated cell therapy (ECT) device, 46
Endothelinergic receptors
        after light exposure, 396
        light-induced retinal injury, 397
Endothelin receptors in inner retina and optic
        nerve, 400–401
ERG. see Ganzfeld Electroretinography
ERGs. see Full-field electroretinograms
ERK and Akt pathways, 344

Fatty acid
    metabolism and ELOVL4 role, 283–285
    profiles of the eye balls of Elovl4 $^{del/del}$ and
        Elovl4 $^{+/del}$ pups, 286–287
F4/80$^+$CD11c$^+$ staining cells, 188
Flag-tagged RDH expression, 62
Full-field electroretinograms, 23

Ganglion Cell Layer (GCL), 400
Ganzfeld Electroretinography, 172
GC1 and GC2 knockout, 352–353
GC double knockouts (GCdko), 353
GCS and rhodopsin as key molecules in
    vesicular transport, 355
Glutamate-ammonia ligase (glutamine
    synthetase), 307
γ-Secretase-dependent RIP, 315
GTPase regulator (RPGR) gene, 24
Guanylate Cyclase-activating Proteins
    (GCAPs), 351
Guanylate Cyclase 1 (GC1) and Guanylate
    Cyclase 2 (GC2), 351
Guanylate Cyclases (GC), 352
GUCY2D gene, 229
Gyrate atrophy of choroid and retina, 22

Hereditary abetalipoproteinemia, 24
hnRNP-K protein, 306
HP2 hairpin ribozyme multiple turnover
    cleavage reaction, 104

Human 15A15 Clone characterization
  computer analysis of sequence, 240
Human congenital stationary night blindness
  (CSNB), 245
  causes of, 246
  electroretinogram for, 248
Human mitochondrial carrier protein
  family, 240
Human Red Green Pigment Promoter-
  controlled *cre* (HRGPPC) mice, 70
Human retina
  a- and b- waves amplitudes of ERG
    changes, 109
  adeno associated viral vectors and, 121
  changes recordings by electroretinogram
    (ERG), 167
  degenerations
    animal models studies, 29–32
    clinical findings of, 21–23
    murine model of age related, 165
    stem cell mediated therapy, 33
    treatment and, 24–25
  diseases and genes involved, 23–24
  EFEMP1and, 279–280
  enriched genes of, 182
  and Epo receptor expression, 76
  functions of, 161
  fundus examination of, 223–225
  GC double knockout, 353–354
  hypotoxic transcriptome of
    biological classification, 79–80
    hypoxic preconditioning and Affymetrix
      microarrays, 76
    light exposure and quantification of cell
      death, 77
    morphology, 77–78
    neuroprotective impact of p21, 80–81
    real-time PCR and, 77
    statistical analysis, 78–79
  light induced atopsis and, 61
  neuroprotection by hypoxic
    preconditioning, 81
  neurotrophin expression and activity, 343
  outer nuclear layer thinning, 109–110
  Principal Component Analysis (PCA)
    of, 183
  proteins study, 305–306
  response to hypoxia study, 75–76
  rods and cones distribution of, 23
  scotopic rearing and, 196
  targeting cell types with rAAV in, 125
Human retinal pigment epithelial (hRPE)
  cells

  cell cultures and cellular proliferation,
    269–270
  immunoprecipitation assay, 270–271
  statistical analysis, 271
4-Hydroxynonenal (4-HNE), 307
Hypoxia-inducible-factor 1a (HIF-1a), 71

Inner Nuclear Layer (INL), 364
Inosine 5'-monophosphate dehydrogenase
  type I (IMPDH1), 307
Insulin effect on 3H-thymidine incorporation
  of hRPE cells, 271
αvβ5Integrin receptors, 369–375
International Society for Clinical
  Electrophysiology of Vision
  (ISCEV), 385
Interphotoreceptor Matrix (IPM), 370
Intracellular ROI production measurement, 54
Intraflagellar Transport (IFT), 356–357

Kinase-like Homology Domain (KHD), 352

Leber Congenital Amaurosis (LCA), 121
Leber Congenital Amaurosis-type 1
  (LCA1), 352
Lentiviral vector expressing *Rpe65* mouse
  cDNA, 90
Light induced apoptosis
  experiments and cells growth
    chromophore role in 661W Cells and,
      63
    clone selection and viability assay, 62
    membrane fraction preparation and
      RDH, 63
  and human retina, macular degeneration, 61
  PEDF and DHA as drugs in, 64
  RDH expression in cure, 65
Light-induced photoreceptor degeneration
  and intravitreal injection,
    54–55
LINKAGE program package, 231
Lipofectamine 2000 reagent, 62
LOC387715 hypothetical gene, 216
Loess normalization curve, 181
Lucentis® for retinal degeneration, 24

Macugen® for retinal degeneration, 24
Madin-darby Canine Kidney (MDCK), 356
Malattia Leventinese cell
  compartmentalization, 277
Marfan syndrome, 278
MASCOT database, 303
Matrix remodeling like TIMP-2 inhibitors, 187
Mertk, tyrosine kinase gene, 372, 377

Mesopia-induced degradation of
    ERG, 196
Mice with rhodopsin, T17M mutation, 30
Microphotodiode Arrays (MPAs), 377
Mouse 21D1 characterization
    analysis of, 238–239
    molecular cloning, 238
Mouse Eyes Implantation, 380–381
Mouse primary RPE cell and ARPE19 cell
    culture, 322–323
    pulse-chase experiment for, 324–325
    ROSs phagocytosis, 323–324
Müller-photoreceptor interaction, 405
Multiplex ligation-dependent probe
    amplification (MLPA), 205
Murine model of age related retinal
    degeneration, 165

Nanoceria particles, 54
    and intracellular ROIs accumulation, 55
    and photoreceptor cells, 57–58
    radical-scavenging mechanism and, 58
    retina rescue by, 57
Neosporin Ophthalmic Solution, antibiotic
    solution, 378
Neuroprotectin D1 (NPD1), 39
    PEDF-induced NPD1 synthesis, 42
    synthesis and bioactivity, 41
Neurotrophin receptor
    activation, 344–345
    expression regulation, 345–346
NF-kB pro-survival transcriptional
    pathways, 344
Notch/Delta signalling pathway, 279
Nyctalopi 3D structure, 251

Optic Nerve Head (ONH), 400
Optomotor response in RPE65-/- mice,
    92–93
Ornithine amino transferase (OAT) gene, 24

Pax6 expression, 8–9
PD 98059 effect on insulin-stimulated
    3H-thydimine incorporation of hRPE
    cells, 272
PEDF-induced NPD1 synthesis, 42
Peripheral membrane-associated proteins
    downregulation, 354–355
Peroxiredoxin 6, 307
Phosphatidyl inosytol transfer protein (PITP)
    family, 231
Photoreceptor cells
    and CNTF, 46
    differentiation, 6–7

electroretinography and, 55
    synaptogenesis, 12
Photoreceptor outer segment fragments
    (POS), 369
P23H-3 rats
    dark-adapted flash-evoked electroretino-
        gram (ERG), 194–195
    light restriction and degeneration, 193–194
Pigment epithelial-derived factor-stimulated
    NPD1 synthesis, 39
Pigment epithelium derived factor
    (PEDF), 61
PITPNM3 gene genomic structure, 232
POS phagocytosis study by RPE cells,
    370–371
Preparation of detergent-resistant membranes
    (DRM) from ROS, 336
Progenitors. see Stem cells
Proliferative diabetic retinopathy (PDR), 313
Protein transport model in cones, 357–358
PRPF31 (RP11) gene, 205
PRSS11 serine protease gene, 216
Putative dilysine (KXKXX) endoplasmic
    reticulum retention
    signal, 283

Q626H mutation, 233

rAAV vector persistance, 124
rcd1 dog model (PDE6B mutation), 46
Rds-associated retinal diseases, 135
Rds expression levels in C214S transgenic
    retinas, 135
Recombinant adeno-associated viral (rAAV)
    vectors, 187
Refsum disease, 25
Re-growth of ERG, mechanisms of, 198
Regulation of complement activation (RCA)
    locus, 216
Remote Analysis Computation for gene
    Expression data (RACE) online tool, 76
Reproductive cloning, 5
Retina enriched genes, 182
Retinal adhesion, role for $\alpha v \beta 5$ integrin,
    372–373
Retinal cDNA microarray, 179
Retinal degeneration in chicken (rd
    chicken), 353
Retinal gene therapy, 121
Retinal neurons, primary culture, 54
Retinal pigment epithelium (RPE), 39, 261,
    369, 393
    phagocytosis and degradation by, 321–322
Retinal regeneration

in fish, 365–366
in mammals barriers, 362
Retina structure
in C214S transgenics, 134
in VPP transgenics, 101
Retinitis pigmentosa, 23
clinical trials for
red blood cell docosahexaenoic (RBC DHA) levels and, 27
vitamin A intake for, 26, 28
Retinitis Pigmentosa (RP), 377
Retinopathy of prematurity (ROP), 313
Retinoschisin (RS) in photoreceptor
interactions with Extracellular Matrix (ECM), 294–295
and interaction with membrane phospholipids, 292–293
ions and, 293–294
isoforms of, 292
multiprotein complex, 295
organization and molecular interaction, 291
Rhodopsin (R), 354–357, 365, 371, 378, 403, 405
and arrestin transcriptional expression by uantitative real-time PCR, 403
content in retina, 405
and GCs transport in rods, 354, 356–357
gene (RHO), 24, 107
mutant P23H-3 transgenic rat, 193
Ribozymes, 99–100
design for treatment of P23H associated ADRP, 101–102
and siRNA treatment, 108–109
in vitro catalytic efficiency of, 102–104
Rod and cone electroretinography (ERG), 131
Rod-/Cone-specific Bcl-x Knockout mice generation, 69–70
Rodents vision and optomotor response (OR), 90
ROD progenitor cells, 361–368
Rod-specific Bcl-x Knockout mice characterization, 70
Royal College of Surgeons (RCS), 369
RPE cells and A2E accumulation, 40
RPE phagocytosis, role of $\alpha v \beta 5$ integrin, 371–372
RPGRIP knock-out/KO mouse and gene replacement therapy, 31
R Transport Carriers (RTCs), 356
Rz397 and siRNA301 expression, 110

SAM algorithm and retina cDNA targets, 181
Scanning-laser Ophthalmoscopy (SLO), 172
Short Mouse Opsin Promoter-controlled cre (SMOPC1) mice, 69–70

Single membrane-spanning region (TM), 352
siRNA301 expression, 110
Stargardt disease, 22
Stargardt like macular dystrophy (STGD3), 283
animal maintenance and tissue collection, 284–285
Stem cells
clonning and, 4–5
as photoreceptors, 5–6
Synuclein alpha (Snca), 384

Teleost retina, neurogenesis in, 363–364
tg6-mouse
retinal function of, 174–175
retinal vasculature, 173
Therapeutic cloning, 4–5
Transcription factor expression and microenvironmental signals, 9
Transgenic mice generation, 130–131
Trans-golgi Network (TGN), 356
Treated eye
bilateral ERG recordings from, 141
morphometry of fundic regions of, 142
Trizol reagent (Invitrogen), 180
TRK receptor activation in retina, 343–344

USH2A gene, 24
Usher syndrome, 222

VEGFR 1
γ-Secretase-dependent RIP and, 317
regulated intramembrane proteolysis (RIP), 315–316
signalling in vascular endothelium and RPE, 313–314
Viral vectors, 148
with transgene expression for ocular gene therapy, 113
Virus mediated gene delivery and neuronal progenitors, 147
Visual and retinal function loss in light stressed mice, 157
VPP transgenic mouse models of ADRP, 100–101

a-Wave in rhodopsin-mutant degeneration, 197
Whole-cell patch clamp, 329

X-linked recessive RP (XLRP), 221
XOPS-mCFP transgenic zebrafish, 366

ZBED4
molecular cloning, 241
subcellular localization of, 241–242
Zebrafish retina anatomy, 362–363

Printed in the United States
112010LV00001BB/171/P